Advances in Esthetic Implant Dentistry

Advances in Esthetic Implant Dentistry

Dr. Abdelsalam Elaskary

The owner of the Elaksary & Associates Institute
and Clinic for Dental Implants and Oral Reconstruction,
Alexandria, Egypt
Visiting lecturer, University of New York NYU
The current President of the Arab Society of Oral Implantology, Cairo

WILEY Blackwell

This edition first published 2019

Edition History
John Wiley & Sons (1e, 2003); John Wiley & Sons (2e, 2007)

Registered Office(s)
John Wiley & Sons, Inc., 111 River Street, Hoboken, NJ 07030, USA
John Wiley & Sons Ltd, The Atrium, Southern Gate, Chichester, West Sussex, PO19 8SQ, UK

Editorial Office
9600 Garsington Road, Oxford, OX4 2DQ, UK

For details of our global editorial offices, customer services, and more information about Wiley products visit us at www.wiley.com.

Wiley also publishes its books in a variety of electronic formats and by print-on-demand. Some content that appears in standard print versions of this book may not be available in other formats.

Library of Congress Cataloging-in-Publication data has been applied for

Hardback ISBN: 9781119286677

Cover Design: Wiley
Cover image: © Abdelsalam Elaskary

Set in 10/12pt Warnock by SPi Global, Pondicherry, India
Printed and bound in Singapore by Markono Print Media Pte Ltd

10 9 8 7 6 5 4 3 2 1

About the Author

Dr. Abdelsalam Elaskary is the founder and owner of Elaskary & Associates clinic and educational institute located in Alexandria, Egypt. Dr. Elaskary is a former visiting professor at the University of Florida and currently an assistant visiting lecturer at the University of New York. He has authored two previously published text books in the field of dental Implantology; *Reconstructive Aesthetic Implant Surgery* (Wiley Blackwell, 2003) and *Fundamentals of Esthetic Implant Dentistry* (Wiley Blackwell, 2007), which have both been translated into five languages. In addition, Dr. Elaskary has made a rich contribution to the literature evidenced by numerous articles published in recognized reputable journals. He is a fellow and an ambassador for the International Congress of Oral Implantologists, where he was awarded the Ralph McKinney Annual Award in 1999. He is the current president of the Arab Society of Oral Implantology in Cairo and a former founding board member of the Arabian Academy of Aesthetic Dentistry.

Dedication

I dedicate this work to the one who teacheth by pen. Teacheth man that which he knew not. Exalted are you; we have no knowledge except what you have taught us.

Contents

Foreword

This text is a summary of the surgical and prosthetic treatment regimens that are encountered for implants placed in the esthetic region of the mouth together with their outcomes. Each chapter provides an insight to the reader on how to accomplish and preserve an anticipated esthetic result with osseointegration.

The chapters carve a pathway from the classical methods originally proposed to the contemporary contributions that are currently available. There is a clear understanding that the longevity of the results obtained using implants will be a combination of the implantologst's capabilities and the compliance of the patient. The outcome of treatment will be tempered by diagnostics and a realistic treatment plan. Considerations that will add to the results will be components of the smile, the shape of adjacent teeth, and the age and gender of the patient.

Immediate implants are easily accepted by the patient as this technique reduces the number of visits, the number of surgeries, and incur a smaller financial commitment; however, there are many factors that can make this technique less desirable. The periodontal health of the surrounding tissues can be an impediment as can the position in the dental arch of the tooth to be extracted. This text offers a step-by-step clinical protocol that enables the resolution of many problems. The state of the labial plate is recognized as a limitation; there are strong histologic and clinical chapters guiding the readership towards the redevelopment of damaged hard tissue. It is very important for the implantologist to discern the differences between the various osteogenic materials available so that the appropriate material for the procedure being used is selected. This text also focuses on possible gingival recession and indicates the soft tissue surgical procedures that may be helpful in preventing this problem, as well as strategies for correcting it when it occurs. Detailed attention is also paid to various surgical procedures and flap designs that will lead to the best possible outcomes.

The ultimate satisfaction of the patient to the collective procedures evidenced in this text will be found in cases of implant restoration. Esthetic satisfaction is mandated by the position of the implant. It is absolutely necessary for the non-surgical delivery of implants to use a navigation system that produces a guide to take the place of the visibility of bone. This is especially true in the treatment of periodontally compromised patients who have demonstrated their susceptibility to inflammation. We, therefore, must take care that the level of the collar of the implant and the adjoining bone result in a minimal probing depth of the gingiva for this population.

It is critical to prepare for potential biologic complications and to be realistic when treating advanced problems. This text presents a lucid, multidisciplinary approach for implant treatment throughout the mouth, but it is especially dedicated to implants placed in the esthetic position. There should be a place on the book shelf in every dental office for this textbook.

Myron Nevins, DDS

List of Contributors

Alessandro Acocella
Prato, Italy

Raquel Rezende Martins de Barros
Department of Oral and Maxillofacial Surgery and Traumatology and Periodontology
School of Dentistry of Ribeirão Preto
University of São Paulo
São Paulo, Brazil

Giampiero Ciabattoni
Faenza, Italy

Flavia Adelino Suaid Malheiros
Department of Oral and Maxillofacial Surgery and Traumatology and Periodontology
School of Dentistry of Ribeirão Preto
University of São Paulo
São Paulo, Brazil

Valdir Antonio Muglia
Department of Prosthodontics
School of Dentistry of Ribeirão Preto
University of São Paulo
São Paulo, Brazil

Arthur Belém Novaes, Jr.
Department of Oral and Maxillofacial Surgery and Traumatology and Periodontology
School of Dentistry of Ribeirão Preto
University of São Paulo
São Paulo, Brazil

Roberto Sacco
Barts and The London School of Medicine and Dentistry
and
Eastman Dental Institute
and
King's College Hospital
London, UK

Rawad Samarani
Department of Periodontology
Saint-Joseph University
Beirut, Lebanon

Preface

Modern implant dentistry has continued to evolve over the years. To provide optimal treatment results, new knowledge has offered advancements to digital dentistry, accurate and precise diagnostic aids that include three-dimensional imaging, accurate treatment planning – which is imperative to any clinical procedure, minimally invasive surgery, microsurgery, digital smile design, and novel materials and techniques to treat and restore osseous defects and compensate for missing soft tissue profiles.

In this book, there is a wide variety of choices for optimizing the esthetic and functional treatment outcomes with dental implants, especially in the esthetic zone. You will find many novel and customized ideas and methods for restoring and optimizing deficient bone in the alveolar ridge and the labial plate. The most peculiar and significant aspect of this book includes the true challenges a clinician faces while executing oral implant procedures on a day-to-day basis, and not just the mere cream of the cake scenarios. My prime focus as the author of the book is not to impress the reader with the outstanding and immediate fabulous clinical outcome, but to depict the complications and failures that could happen to any of us, and to show the clinical and radiographic outcomes of the cases completed over several years that epitomise my "philosophy of failure". This term relates mainly to the handling of implant-related complications: to plan not to fail, to plan how to deal with failures, and to transform a failed case to a success story, as well as dealing with patient psychology when treatment failure occurs.

This book includes nine chapters. *Chapter 1 Modern Trends in Esthetic Implant Therapy:* Progressive scientific breakthroughs have rapidly changed the face of modern implant therapy. There has been a paradigm shift in the success criteria; where survival and longevity were once considered the optimum standard, esthetics has now become the goal of the hour. This chapter takes a sojourn from where we, the implant surgeons, started off decades ago with a basic knowledge of implantology, and where we stand in the present era. Also, it emphasizes the patient's role in the success or failure of the treatment proposed, the influence of dental teamwork, co-ordination between the patient–clinician to balance the expectation and the meagre realities in a given clinical situation, the utmost need for referrals amongst clinicians, and exit plans for any untoward events.

Chapter 2 Extraoral Clinical Reflections: In this chapter, the value of integrating the facial components of the treatment plan has been emphasized, reinforcing the value of the smile as a reflection of an individual's social and personal well-being, and the impact a smile has on the individual and on society. Emphasis is laid on the components of the smile in terms of smile art, smile patterns, smile design, smile landmarks, smile arc, the vestibular reveal, the influence of the lips on the smile, the morphology of teeth, and patient-related factors such as age, gender, personality, and symmetry. The understanding of these parameters is paramount to the implant therapy and thus the success of the treatment outcome.

Chapter 3 Esthetic Outcome of Immediately Implanted and Loaded Implants in the Esthetic Region – A Discussion of Pre-Clinical and Clinical Evidence: In this chapter, the authors provide unique information about histological, histomorphometrical, and more recently, microtomografic features of peri-implant tissues. The authors detail the immediate implant placement from a physiological perspective to pronounce its effects and stability in the esthetic region. They overview their animal studies as well as pre-clinical studies on the effect of immediate implant placement to the labial plate of bone, and they provide valuable conclusions to this topic.

Chapter 4 Novel Concepts in Restoring Labial Plate of Bone in Immediate Implant Therapy: In this chapter, a step-by-step clinical protocol has been described that guides the reader in decision making as well as in the operating room. The author details non-traditional methods of restoring defective labial bone plate in the esthetic zone, that is fitted autogenous bone lumineers, the use of modified composite autograft for treating implant-related ridge deficiencies, and the use of PDLLA shields to restore missing contours. The socket template for restoring minor deficiencies of the labial plate of bone is also described. This chapter marks the incorporation of age-old knowledge and state-of-the-art technology to attain the best possible functional, stable, and esthetic results for the patient.

Chapter 5 Peri-implant Soft Tissue Stability – Prevalence, Etiology, Prevention and Treatment: Implant-related gingival recession is an ever present clinical dilemma for many clinicians. For the first time ever in the field of esthetic implant dentistry, the author has introduced a novel classification for implant-related gingival recession, detailed the etiology of implant-related recession, highlighted a novel guide scoring template to measure the degree of success of the treatment, and proposed and described a treatment protocol for each recession category that involves preventive measures, soft tissue solutions, the use of a novel combination of surgical techniques, three-dimensional bone grafting techniques, and the use of inter-positioned osteotomies (sandwich osteotomy).

Chapter 6 Revisiting Guided Bone Regeneration in the Esthetic Zone: In this chapter the author discusses the various surgical protocols and special considerations especially employed in the esthetic zone, which involve flap design, incisions on the edentulous site, vertical releasing incisions, flap advancements, and alternatives to achieve soft tissue bulk in any regenerative procedure. It also includes a guide to identify the type of bone graft to be used, along with choosing the membrane best suited to maximize the use of an autogenous graft. This chapter also includes information on what might go wrong and how that ultimately affects the treatment outcome and may jeopardize success.

Chapter 7 Perfecting Implant Related Esthetics via Using Optimum Surgical Guides: The authors emphasize the optimal protocol to apply CAD/CAM technology for implant placement. They have also implemented using computer-guided surgery to identify areas with better bone quality. The chapter concludes with a detailed discussion indicating the available software, the processing method, incorporating into the clinical scenario, and patient satisfaction, as well as the application of the immediate loading concept with a one-day teeth delivery.

Chapter 8 Restorative Space and Implant Position Optimization: This chapter defines the magnitude and means to optimize the restorative space, both in horizontal and vertical dimensions. With a thorough knowledge of the factors that influence the optimal positioning of the implant, the clinician will be better equipped to understand the rationale and predictability of the treatment. Although things go wrong when one least expects them, encountering improper implant positioning is not an uncommon complication, and the author clearly elaborates on the management of such complications.

Chapter 9 Treatment Complications and Failures with Dental Implants: In this chapter the author shows the long-term assessment and evaluation of the regenerative techniques available in implant dentistry. With assessments spanning eight years of follow-up, the author has determined the fate of using allografts, alloplasts, and xenografts over a long-term evaluation either when using them solely or when using them in particulate form. The author has evaluated the problems of using titanium mesh, sandwich osteotomies, and many other procedures. In this chapter, a conclusion has been drawn for the reader to help maximize the clinical outcome of any regenerative procedure based on the long-term follow-ups of the previous regenerative procedures.

Finally, I hope that this text will be an addition to your library as well as to your daily practice. I hope that it will enlighten you with new ideas and novel treatment strategies. Kindly visit the web pages of this book to find many educational videos for the surgeries listed within the text and many more interesting materials.

Acknowledgments

Foremost I pay my regards to Allah, "My dear Lord, enable me to be grateful for your favors which you have bestowed upon me and my parents, parents and to do righteousness of which You approve. And admit me by Your mercy into (the ranks of) Your righteous servants." *Solomon request in the Holy Quran – Anamel 27:19*

To Dad: your glorious heart, selfless attitude, unconditional endowing and incredible patience, are a few of your many qualities that have taught me to have the standing that I have today. I wish to imbibe your generosity in each and every sphere of my life. I thank you for making me what I aspire to be when I look at you. I wish Allah to have your soul in Heaven.

To Mom: thank you for being my constant driving force, for the unconditioned support, and your self-denial. To be around just to bless me for my undying aspirations. I wholeheartedly appreciate your positive impact in my life.

To my family: Mahy, Ibrahim, Ameen, and Princess Moushira – profound thanks for understanding the nature of my job, my long periods of absence, and bearing the stress of my workload so beautifully. I couldn't have done it without you.

To the legend Mohammad Ali: I really learnt a lot from you though now you have passed away. I learnt what versatility is, respect to the others no matter who they are, your tolerance, and I admire your patience, persistence, and inner zeal. May your soul rest in Heaven.

To Rolly Meffert: A true legend of your time, you have strongly impacted my career, your support for me during my early jump start was huge, you were a great humble scientist, your imprints are remarkable on teaching many scholars that are presently leaders in the field of implantology. May your soul rest in Heaven.

To Carl Misch: You were a scientific legend, we have all learnt from your vision in Oral Implantology. All of us have followed the earlier guidelines that you set through various publications. Your loss is greatly felt in this field; we will definitely miss you. May your soul rest in Heaven.

To Charles English: I personally did not meet you in person, but I have followed in the footsteps of your work on bone biomechanics; your work is a state of art in this field, and had a tremendous impact on the clinicians of today. May your soul rest in heaven.

To Ken Judy: The maestro and founder of the ICOI, you have supported many like myself along the road; you are now a real global icon that should be applauded for inspiring young minds.

To Ken Beacham: You are a real game changer! You have changed the way implant dental education has evolved over the years, your vision educated thousands of clinicians from all over the globe, your passionate work has also inspired high quality speakers in the field. I really admire your rare personal qualities and the work you provide. Your encouragement and support means a lot to me.

To Denis Tarnow: A real gem and icon in this field, an inspirer to many around the globe, a great mind and thinker, above all a humble human being. You have supported, taught, and inspired many clinicians across the globe including myself. Heartfelt thanks to you Denis for the opportunities that you have offered me along the road.

To Khaled Abdelghaffar: I really enjoyed your sincere friendship, your kind personal qualities and your highly professional skills. No wonder you became the minister of higher education in Egypt; being the top authority responsible for higher education is a hard task for sure, but you surely deserve it.

To Steve Boggan: Being the CEO of Biohorizons is surely a great professional achievement. I can see how you have uplifted your firm to the highest level. On a personal note, I truly thank you for just being who you are, the real friend, the one who is always supportive and responsive, which I have really appreciated.

To Terrence Griffin: Terry, I still recall those good old times watching you teaching and watching you doing surgeries with your magic hands definitely inspired me and many others, which is how I got my surgical skills. Thank you for your support at the outset of my carreer. No wonder you are now the president of the AAP.

To Elsaied Mahrous: Your teachings to me and many others 30 years ago, remains as a witness that you are a great person who has imparted all your knowledge to others without restriction; thank you dear Dr. Mahrous.

To my coworkers: I sincerely thank the co-authors of the chapters in this book for the great job they have done. Also, thank you dear Samia for your generous contribution to the artwork of this book, a fabulous job.

To the emerging young clinicians: All those that I meet locally and internationally, I wholeheartedly wish to thank you for your eagerness to learn and climb to the professional summit. I would like to share with you some tips for while you are climbing. **Set your vision**: It may sound hard, but try to develop your own vision; for example, where and what would you like to be in the coming 10 years? Usually visions don't work out as exactly as planned but having a defined path is critical to your life, and this vision will help you to set your goals later. **Widen the scope of your imagination:** Imagination is more important than the work itself! Fly in the field of your thoughts and remember that imagination has led the way to many useful inventions. Without imaginative minds, this world would not look the same as it does today, so don't be shy. Your dreams should be close to reality; the closer they are, the easier they will be to achieve; your dreams need to be in a delicate balance between what exists and what can be achieved in the future, tinged with a touch of optimism. **Creativity** is a feature of successful people. Try to acquire it. It is not inherited, so you can develop the potential of your brain throughout your path, to learn to reach a higher level of creativity. I know that creativity is the inseparable mate of sincerity. **Combine your hard work with faith**: Faith should be a constant companion to your hard work. You must have faith that your work will be recognized one day. Remember to develop your way with honor and dignity, not via intimidation or hypocrisy. **Let your work be ahead of your glory**, not the opposite. No matter how great your achievements are, stay close to Earth – always have your feet on the ground. Realize that success is not linked to any geographical location; you can achieve success from anywhere. Realize that the world has many people other than you who work silently and in the background, contribute to most of what we currently enjoy. **You might provoke others by your achievements**, but you will also please many others. Only your inner power will bear and endure the repetitive work that lies along your path. A few people might exceed your fast pace for no clear or valid reason, some of them bought their (fake) glory with (a price) either via their tribal profile or influential social profile, etc. At some point they might force you to rotate in their Galaxy or do their best to dull your radiance. Be sure this is temporary! Realize that stabs at your back only mean that you are at the forefront. All that is required is patience and biding your time. **Pay others back**, and consider while climbing your path, that many hands lifted you up along your journey; please don't forget those hands when you reach the top. Be supportive to others, including your competitors, engage with your immediate society because your active participation in your local environment is important; don't be like those who are always at the forefront when verbal participation is needed, but who shrink from their participation in a supporting financial role or in active reform. **On the social level**, the average person works six hours a day, while the successful person wants to work 24 hours every day! The successful person goes to work as if he/she is going to a date! However, life with a successful person is not always fun for those closest to them; it requires patience from the their life partner – the happiest life mate (in my opinion) is the one who provides unconditional support while witnessing both victories and defeats. The feeling of sharing the glory making is indeed pleasurable; it can be by encouragement, support, patience, and steadfastness. Or silence!

To the book readers: Thank you for your confidence and support, and thanks to those of you who have purchased my previous books in English or any other language versions; without your support this book would not have become reality, so my sincere thanks.

Thanks to one and all who have helped make me who I am today and who I aspire to be in future.

About the Companion Website

Don't forget to visit the companion website for this book:

www.wiley.com/go/elaskary/esthetic

There you will find valuable material designed to enhance your learning, including:

- Videos
- Case studies

The password to view the videos and case studies is the last word of the second paragraph in Chapter 9.

1

Modern Trends in Esthetic Implant Therapy

1.1 Predictability of Esthetic Implant Therapy

> The journey of the sun and moon is predictable.
> But yours is your own ultimate art.
>
> *Suzy Kassem (2011)*

This quote also applies to your future esthetic treatment plan. Scientific breakthroughs have rapidly changed the practice of implant prosthetics in dentistry today with fascinating inventions. Just as structural engineering principles must be combined with artistic skills to build an accurate building, so the same applies to implant dentistry, which should offer suitable (durable) prosthesis, using optimal designs and fabrication. Implant dentistry has come a long way from the era of the incidental discovery of osseointegration (Branemark et al. 1969). With high implant survival rates relished in the field, the focus has shifted toward creating an esthetic restoration that is indistinguishable from the adjacent natural teeth and that has stable long-lasting adjoining tissues over time. Yet the longevity of the esthetic outcome in implant therapy is now becoming the main focus for many clinicians because the current understanding is to provide not only an immediate fabulous esthetic result but also long-term success. The chauvinistic standard of having an immediate esthetic result that is promoted to conference audiences and in textbooks and publications is no longer sufficient without showing the actual outcome for patients in the long term. Therefore, more emphasis should be placed on the long-term follow-up for esthetic cases to offer clinicians predictable treatment protocols. The current shift in the understanding of esthetic implant therapy is the longevity of the treatment outcome that is documented year after year and which shows stable, healthy peri-implant tissue architecture and astonishingly durable esthetics.

In the early years of practicing oral implantology, the chief concerns were tissue health and implant survival. Over the past decade there has been a paradigm shift of increasing appreciation from long-lasting esthetics to the success of the final restoration. However, a modern affluent society often demonstrates an obsessive interest in achieving unrealistic forms of beauty, which may be detrimental to the final outcomes and perceptions of the patient. The role of the clinician is to smoothly direct the patient to her/his best interest and prescribe the best treatment protocol that can predictably work for longer while also giving the best possible esthetic result.

Market research has identified esthetics as one of the major reasons why clinicians advocate dental implants over conventional restoration methods for partial or complete edentulism. However, achieving an esthetic outcome with implant-supported restorations is significantly more challenging than with conventional restorations on natural teeth. Enhancement of the esthetic appearance supports effective and successful interactions among the soft and hard tissues (Palacci 2000). Indeed, the rationale for peri-implant plastic surgery should go well beyond pure esthetics to address issues concerning the quality of life and the psychological well-being of patients. Esthetic outcomes are based upon many variables. It is not just the implant design, surface characteristics, or type of abutment that will guarantee an esthetic result; it is rather the time spent on data collection in reaching a correct diagnosis that pays dividends in terms of function and esthetics (Jivraj and Chee 2006). This gives the patient a complete understanding of their desires by formulating the right treatment protocol. Thus, comprehending the patient's demands, and transforming them into a deliverable plan will be the best forward for the patient.

Though duplicating what nature has provided can be a formidable challenge, the placement of a dental implant in the esthetic zone is a technique-sensitive procedure with little room for error. A subtle mistake in the positioning of the implant or the mishandling of soft or hard tissue can lead to esthetic failure and patient dissatisfaction or a disastrous esthetic outcome. Since both dental and gingival esthetics act together to provide a smile with harmony and balance, the clinician must be aware of parameters

Advances in Esthetic Implant Dentistry, First Edition. Abdelsalam Elaskary.

Companion website: www.wiley.com/go/elaskary/esthetic

related to gingival morphology, form and dimension, characterization, surface texture, and color. Therefore, the ultimate aim should be for the implant restoration to fit harmonically with the frame of the natural smile.

A preoperative assessment of the patient's expectation is of paramount importance to depict the predictability of the esthetic vector. To achieve a successful esthetic result, implant placement in the esthetic zone demands a thorough preoperative diagnosis and treatment plan combined with excellent clinical skills. The predictability of the esthetic outcome of an implant restoration is dependent on many variables, including but not limited to the following: (1) patient selection, (2) tooth position, (3) root position of adjacent teeth, (4) phenotype of periodontium and tooth shape and the osseous crest height, (5) the available osseous anatomy of the implant site, (6) position of the implant, and (7) the related facial anatomy, which impacts the overall fate of the treatment plan (Elaskary 1999).

Garber (1995) and David, Garber and Salama (2000) described restoration-driven implant placement as a process where the final form of the restoration is decided upon first and then backwards, while the implant fixture is seen merely as an apical extension of the restoration. It emphasizes the importance of providing high-quality and esthetically demanding fixed prosthodontics. Since the ideal placement of dental implants should be determined by prosthetic parameters, the exact positioning of the implant with respect to location and angulation is often a delicate procedure (Misch 1997). In complete hybrid prosthetics supported with multiple fixtures, implant positioning might be more forgiving than in single or partial implant supported restorations with single tooth implant-supported restorations where a minimal error might be magnified and might lead to a serious esthetic outcome (Misch 1997).

With increasing demand toward patient-driven esthetics, numerous types of radiological and surgical innovationshavebeenproposed.Forexample,CAD/CAM-assisted (Computer Aided Design/Manufacture) implant placement provided a major leap in reducing implant alignment problems and ensures better esthetics, with many studies emphasizing the radiographic diagnostics (Engelman et al. 1988), computed tomography (CT)-based prosthetic treatment planning, or precise bone-mapping (Pesun 1997) and then guidance for the surgical implant placement (Minoretti, Merz, and Triaca 2000).

1.2 Where We Were

Esthetic implant therapy started many years ago, taking advantage of the ever flourishing nonstop human need for esthetics and adornment (Elaskary 2003). Although some of the procedures used were groundbreaking in their day, several have now become obsolete.

Over the years clinicians have thrived by reproducing only natural tooth shape, color, with gingival contours as close as possible to natural oral conditions. Surgical advancements started to evolve using esthetic surgical protocols that enabled esthetic implant-supported restorations to duplicate the original contours and profile characters of the natural teeth from all aspects. Elaskary (2008) consequently made several attempts to provide a protocol for 3D implant positing along with several soft tissue sculpturing procedures.

In esthetic sites, the goal of surgical therapy was to achieve successful implant–tissue integration and to sustain healthy esthetic peri-implant tissue contours that re-establish both function and esthetics. Therefore, a clear understanding of the specific needs of a patient in a given clinical situation and the need to master the necessary surgical techniques to achieve the treatment objectives were considered paramount. In non-esthetic sites, however, the primary goal of surgical therapy was to achieve a predictable hard and soft tissue integration of the implant to re-establish a long-lasting function with the implant-supported prosthesis.

Many factors were used to the optimize the implant fixture position in relation to its adjacent tissue contours (either when placed with guided assistance or non-guided), including the available soft tissue thickness, the overall original tissue volume prior to surgery, the degree of accuracy of the fabrication of the surgical template, the condition of the adjacent natural teeth and its relationship to the gingival architecture, the available occlusion, and the ability of the dental technician to develop natural-looking prosthetic contours (Elaskary 2003).

It has also been learned that the gingival tissues around dental implant fixture components should be enhanced and developed, at several phases to acquire the same dimensions and configurations of the original tissues around natural dentition. The original soft tissue configuration around natural teeth possess a flat profile at the point where they emerge from the free gingival margin after implant fixture placement. The subgingival area, and particularly the biological width, is the part that harbors the development of the emergence profile of the final prosthesis to match the dimensions of the tooth to be replicated. The clinician understood early on that an implant fixture design differed from a natural tooth in its morphological characteristics. This understanding facilitated the development of an ideal gingival scalloping and papillae simulation, thus creating a natural emergence profile that was supported by the final restoration at a later point in time. The optimal three-dimensional implant position of the implant head had to be within 2 mm apical to the gingival zenith of the natural teeth, preferably with a buccal bone wall at least 1–2 mm thick. This compelled the clinician to the accurately fabrice a provisional restoration that transferred the cylindrical shape of the implant to the cross-sectional shape of the root of the natural tooth at the gingival margin. The importance of developing a proper emergence profile was considered critical to achieving an esthetic final restoration that mimics the adjacent natural teeth. Thus, the ability of the clinician to duplicate the emergence of the natural teeth to the implant-supported restorations became a vital factor in achieving natural esthetics (Garber 1995).

A surgical guide (or a template as it used to be called) was sometimes made of an old partial denture with indented markings on the acrylic teeth indicating the site of the future implants (with palatal or lingual relief). The partial denture replicas lacked precise implant positioning because the template did not provide any control for buccolingual movement of the drill or apicocoronal movement; any deviation in the direction of the drilling angulation subsequently altered the future implant position. CAD/CAM surgical guides were then used to help ensure accurate implant positioning relative to the adjacent dentition or for future prosthetics; however, some guides lacked perfect precision. There have now been many outstanding developments in the field of CAD/CAM guides that offer many improvements on past techniques. Thus, the ability of the clinician to understand and control the relationship between the implant and its associated gingival and dental structures lead to the establishment of esthetic soft tissue contours and a harmoniously scalloped gingival line, which was important in achieving an esthetical final implant-supported restoration (Elaskary et al. 1999).

Regional soft tissue, bone morphology, and prosthetic contours affect the final shape and profile of the prosthesis and can be critical to its final appearance. For instance, implants placed in the interproximal areas may cause serious oral maintenance problems, while implants placed too far from the labial plate of bone can lead to esthetic disharmony and induce resorption of the labial plate of bone and possible related gingival recession. It might also lead to an undesired labial location of the opening for a screw hole on the facial surface of the prosthesis. Implants placed too far lingually relative usually result in a bulky prosthesis with unfavorable contours, which may also interfere with speech, impinge on the tongue space and surely lead to a poor esthetic result.

In attempts to optimize the esthetic outcome when using dental implants, various methods have been used to measure the height of the papilla with the aid of clinical photographs (Olson et al. 1992), while other clinicians (Jemt 1997; Nemcovsky et al. 2000) have developed an index for assessing the contour of the proximal papillae. Yet other researchers measured papilla-height using a bone sounding technique, thus relating papilla with the interdental bone. The latter studies (Grunder 2000; Tarnow et al. 2003) explained methods to measure the height of the interdental papilla, such as bone probing under local anesthesia. However, the relationship between the crestal bone and interdental papilla could not be evaluated accurately when using clinical photos or an index (Jemt 1997; Nemcovsky et al. 2000).

Some authors proposed the use of underexposing radiography X-ray dosage to reveal soft tissue changes around dental implants. Although the results obtained using this technique were found to have a high correlation with the actual soft tissue changes, it was not always easy to use in every clinical situation because underexposed radiography usually did not contain enough information on osseous structures for the clinician. A more useful method was to detect both soft tissue and hard tissue in a single radiographic image. This was made possible by applying contrast media on the soft tissue side (Rustemeyer and Martin 2013).

The clinician needed to evaluate the future crestal bone-to-implant interface closely using the available radiographic views to ensure the optimal implant housing. In any suspected or confirmed facial bone loss, the treatment of the osseous deficiency should be determined according to the type and severity of the bone defect, whether vertical or horizontal, or one wall, two walls, or a more osseous deficiency. An anatomical cast can be fabricated by transferring the subgingival contours of the provisional restoration to the working cast for gingival contouring. Gingival augmentation procedures can also be performed at any time to resolve discrepant gingival and mucosal contours, enhance existing thin facial tissues, and mask any metal show, creating a satisfactory treatment outcome; however, the clinical outcome was not always predictable.

The site, angulation, and depth of implants can be designed based on the presurgical imaging that provides important information for osseointegrated dental implant treatment procedure. The use of cross-sectional images in the buccolingual direction, which can be delivered by CT (Besimo and Kempf 1995; Israelson et al. 1992), or conventional X-ray tomography, allowed clinicians to plan a more accurate design of implant placement before surgery.

Obtaining study casts paved the clinician's way to exceptional clinical skills since it provides information about the edentulous site in three-dimensional (3D) views as well as information about existing occlusion, the relationship with the adjacent teeth, and the inter-arch relationship. Mapping of the alveolar bony topography or using ultrasound to view the underlying bone architecture of the future implant site on the study cast was used to detect the exact width of the alveolar ridge without outsourcing a CT scan. Using contrast media produced readings that were almost accurate reproducible measurements, enabling the resulting image to be analyzed with confidence. Measuring bone width at multiple sites improved the accuracy of recording and reduction of measurement errors (Mecall and Rosenfeld 1996).

In the past, the utilization of a panoramic radiograph and/or periodical radiographs was impressive to many clinicians. Quite often, the panoramic radiographs were combined with steel balls of 5 mm diameter to measure the magnification error factor of the radiograph. The use of conventional dental panoramic radiography and plain films radiography was usually performed with the patient wearing a radiographic template with integrated metal spheres or rods, sleeves, and guide posts at the position of the wax-up. Calculating the magnification factor, allowed the planning of the accurate location and dimensions of the implants were planned (Buser et al. 1990).

The surge of advancements in digital applications have provided clinicians with superior techniques that have replaced some of these older methods.

1.3 Where We Are Now

The past decade witnessed breakthrough inventions in almost every aspect in dentistry; they are inventions beyond anyone's imagination. Breath-taking surgical and prosthetic tools and fascinating diagnostic aids, all of which are currently in the hands of the modern up-to-date clinician. Truly vast numbers of immensely thrilling diagnostic aids have emerged using high-resolution, very accurate cone-beam CT scan machines to help process an implant case from A to Z using digital workflow. This became a routine clinical work at many dental clinics. The workflow could start from analyzing the available soft and hard tissue architecture accurately, developing a surgical guide that saves time, reduces pain, and allows an implant placement precision that is close to 98% (Deeb et al. 2017), as shown in Figure 1.1a–n. Using the available modern implant planning software has also become integrated into routine office practice, where the software allows clinicians not only to preplan the future fixture position and the implant-supported restoration design, but also to offer a new marvelous smile by having a final restoration that is ready milled even prior to the implant surgery. Unfortunately, the only constraint at the moment is the high cost of these inventions; however, our previous experiences has shown that the use of these expensive devices is more economical than traditional low-cost methods. An in-house CT scan machine has been developed that evaluates alveolar ridge anatomy in 3D, while the clinician is even able to design his/her own case for implant placement and order the CAD/CAM

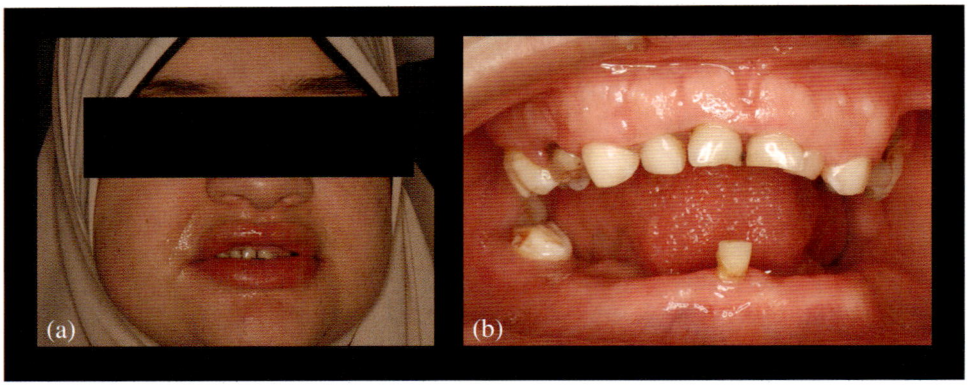

Figure 1.1 (a and b) Preoperative view of a female patient presented with Cleidocranial Dysostosis syndrome showing partial anodontia and many supernumerary teeth in an underdeveloped jaw.

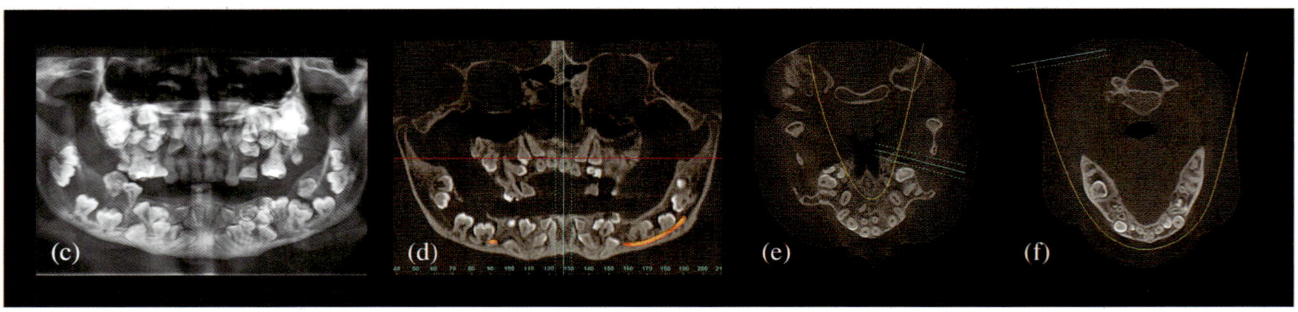

Figure 1.1 (c, d, e, and f) Cone-beam CT scan radiographic views showing multiple supernumerary unerupted teeth.

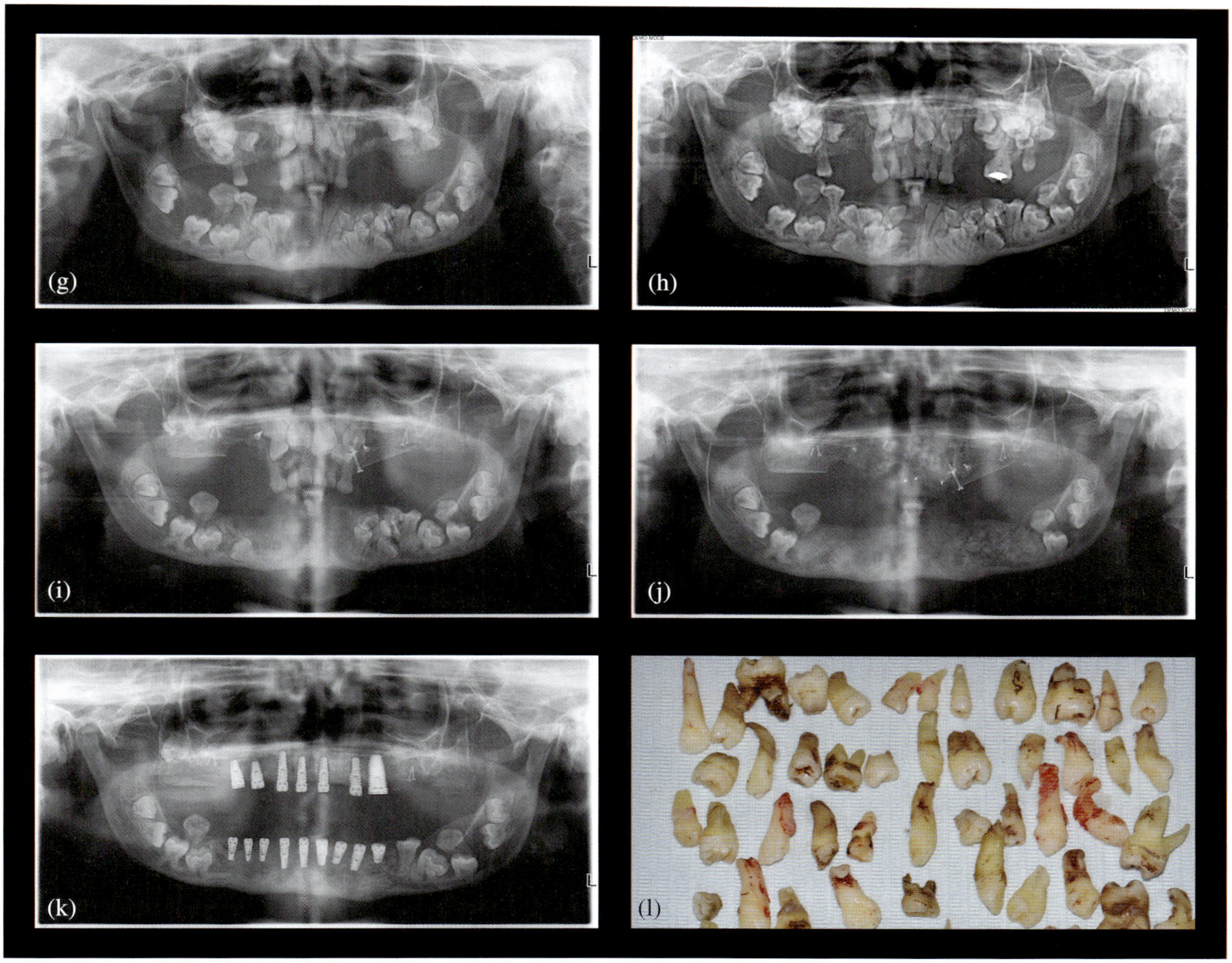

Figure 1.1 (g, h, i, and j) Serial panoramic chronological views showing the extraction of the supernumerary teeth with simultaneous jaw grafting. (k) The grafted jaw bones showing received dental implants; the remaining supernumerary teeth in the mandible are scheduled for removal later on before the construction of the final prosthesis. (l) Supernumerary teeth extracted over a 12 month period.

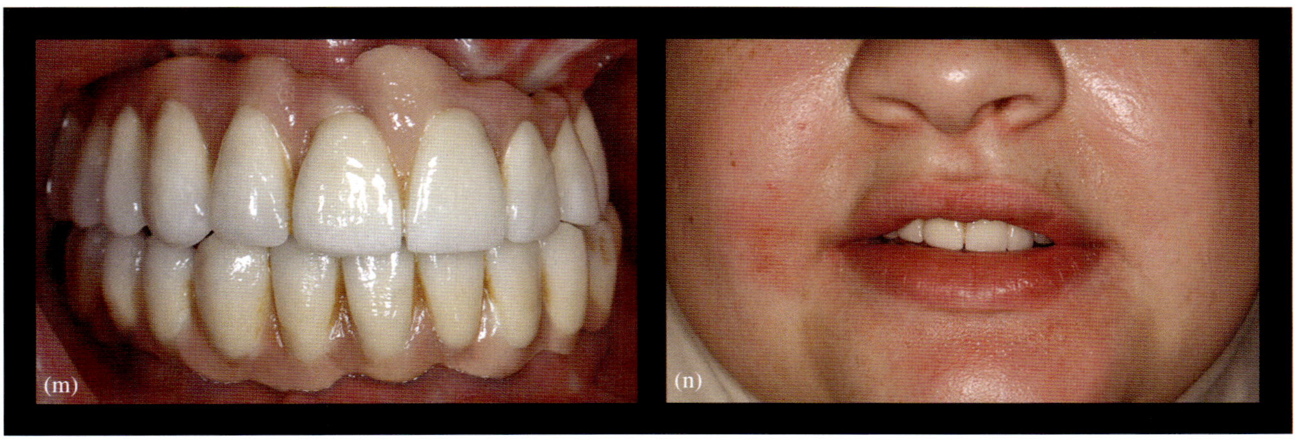

Figure 1.1 (m and n) Intra and extraoral views after implant-supported restoration showing a remarkable esthetic outcome.

surgical guide, has the outstanding ability to check the outcome of the surgical placement of dental implants in real time. In addition, a virtual design of the future implant-supported prostheses can be made ready prior to the start of implant placement surgery.

The investigators stated early on that 3D planning resulted in a far better implant position associated with bone quality and quantity than manual placement, improved biomechanics, and better esthetics (Basten 1995; Israelson et al. 1992; Verdi and Morgano 1993). The advancements minimized the likelihood of complications occurring, such as, for example, mandibular nerve damage, sinus perforations, fenestrations, or dehiscence. Thus, the 3D planning system is a reliable tool for the preoperative evaluation of implant placement. The surgeon and restorative dentist can now simulate an ideal implant placement procedure using the exact dimensions of the implant in its ideal depth and angulation on the CT images.

The rationale for the utilization of this CAD/CAM surgical guides depends on the following objectives:

1) In the CT evaluation, the radiopaque markers incorporated into the radiographic template should provide proper guidance in determining the location and the axis of the implant and the abutment. Relevant data should be transferred to the working cast through the markers, which dictate accurate reorientation of the surveying table for guiding channel preparation. An effective radiopaque marker should stay in place during modification procedures. Thus, if the design of the guide utilizes removal of the markers for channel preparation, the procedure must also include another guide for accurate transfer of the data from two to three dimensions.
2) Conversion of the radiographic template to a surgical aid should facilitate correct placement of the implants with the desired path of insertion, which is correlated with the data obtained from a two-dimensional scan image. The surgical guide should rest firmly on available structures and provide the surgeon with ease in site preparation and accurate visualization of the implant sites.

With the advent of computer-assisted surgery, the surgeon may now navigate through the entire implant procedure with extremely high accuracy. The emergence of cone-beam CT scanning 3D volumetric imaging systems now provides clinicians and specialists with complete views of all oral and maxillofacial structures, giving the dental profession the most thorough diagnostic information available to date for a variety of treatment areas (Sanderink et al. 1997). The combination of CT scanning, laboratory-based laser scanning technology, along with intraoral digital impression capture technology, in harmony with the design capabilities of state-of-the-art software, gave an accurate representation of a virtual patient. Clinicians can now preview and even test different treatment options to enhance patient care, combining data to develop a comprehensive treatment plan for patient analysis with treatment to create solutions that include all functional–esthetic aspects of oral rehabilitation.

Unique types of dental software were also found available for the clinician; a thrilling digital smile design software has enabled the restoration of many lost smiles virtually before proceeding to the actual treatment and also offers a guide to the fabrication of the final restoration. A close cooperation and working relationship among the dentist/technician team promises to enhance the utilization of new technology. 'Digital waxing' using a diagnostic wax-up and provisional restorations and their digital replicas to guide the creation of CAD/CAM restorations will become a clinician's 'standard operating procedure,' replacing hand waxing. Not to mention the availability of wide range of fascinating unique implant designs with outstanding endless prosthetic options that minimized the bone loss and maximized esthetics. On another level, and in order to allow a highly precise bone cutting, with minimal tissue trauma; Piezoelectric ultrasound units were devolved to enable highly efficient and precise bone cutting with minimal tissue trauma.

Newly devolved prosthetic materials that are available now, such as Prettau (Zirkonzahn, Tyrol, Italy), which was introduced as the future of highly esthetic Zirconia restorations, offer versatile clinical options for the clinician. Prettau® Zirconia is far more translucent than Zirconia cores of the past.

High-performance polymers reinforced with ceramic particles, such as Bio-HPP (Bredent GmbH & Co·KG Senden, Germany), have also found their way into the vast array of restorative materials. Bio-HPP offers elasticity (E-modulus of around 4000 MPa) that is very similar to human bone, offers no exchange of ions in the mouth, no discoloration, is biocompatible, and demonstrates chemical stability. It also exhibits high esthetics and customization and is plaque resistant (Han, Lee, and Shin 2016). It is used for frameworks, and it may be veneered with traditional veneer composites (e.g. Visio lign) (Bredent GmbH & Co·KG Senden, Germany).

Another innovative material that was introduced is the Vita ENAMIC® (VITA Zahnfabrik, Bad Säckingen, Germany) is the first hybrid dental ceramic with a dual-network structure. The dominant fine-structure ceramic network (86% by weight) is strengthened by a polymer network, with both networks fully integrated with one another. Its unique balance between strength and elasticity provides high absorption of masticatory forces. ENAMIC delivers significantly lower brittleness than pure ceramic and better abrasion behavior than composite. It is possible to mill restorations with thinner walls.

ENAMIC features a crack-stop function and has enamel-like abrasion properties and antagonist protection achieved by the fine-structure ceramic network. It yields excellent marginal stability, which renders the material very accurate so it can be perfectly milled with diamond instruments, while IPS e-max PRESS is a proven high-strength material for long-lasting clinical results and life-like esthetics (Mörmann et al. 2013).

Digital dentistry CAD/CAM technology has allowed the digital dental team to represent diagnosing, treatment planning, and creating functional esthetic restorations for patients in a new and more productive and efficient manner (see Figure 1.2a–m).

Treatment planning software predominantly ruling the market nowadays, such as The Straumann® Guided Surgery (SGS) system (Straumann Holding AG, Basel, Switzerland), is designed to work with the proprietary standalone virtual implant placement software coDiagnostiX™ (Dental Wings Inc. Montréal, Canada) and in combination with Starumann's goniX™ surgical guide drill unit. CT appliances are fabricated at a laboratory and converted into the actual surgical guide, affording a verified fit of the surgical guide and faster turnaround times. Implants are delivered through the guide, effectively executing precision delivery of the implants as planned through the coDiagnostiX™ virtual implant placement software. Automatic nerve detection, Hounsfield unit detection, intuitive controls, and menus are some of the other key features of the coDiagnostiX™ software or most of the currently available

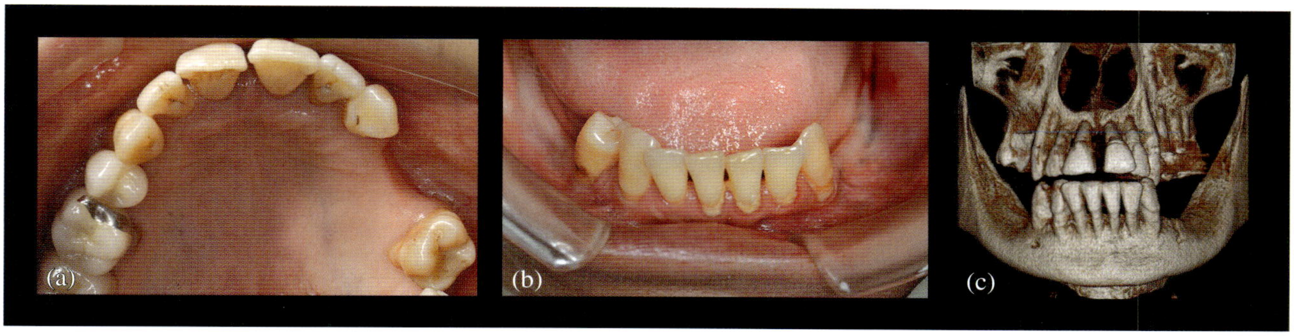

Figure 1.2 (a and b) Pre-operative views of hopeless teeth, due to sever alveolar bone resorption. (c) Pre-operative Cone Beam Computed Tomography (CBCT) showing the alveolar bone deficiency.

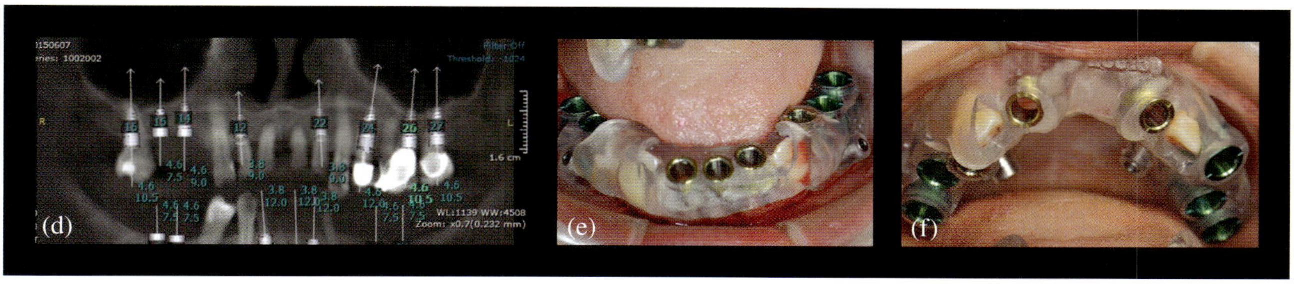

Figure 1.2 (d) Implant planning on the software allowed the use of short implants to support the restoration. (e and f) Maxillary and mandibular surgical cad cam guides are fabricated to place the implants in the best available bone locations.

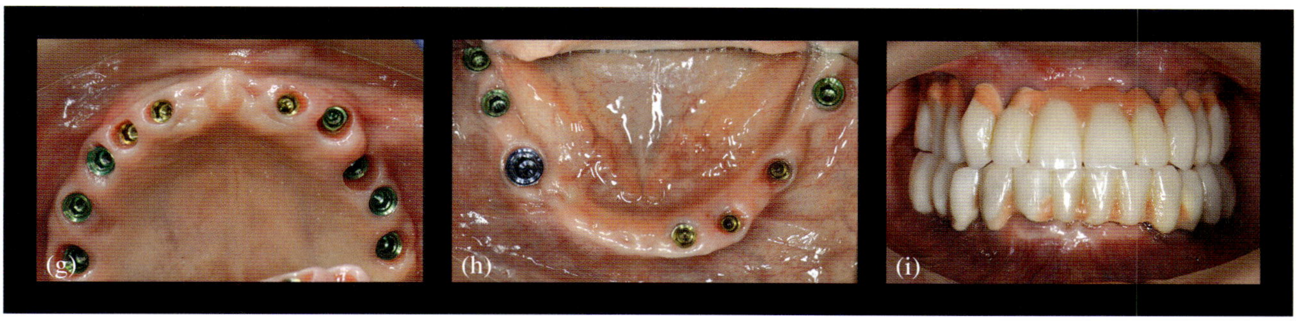

Figure 1.2 (g and h) Showing implant placed and integrated in both mandible and maxilla. (i) Intra oral clinical picture showing the final case restored with two hybrid screw retained implant supported restorations made from peek and vesiolign.

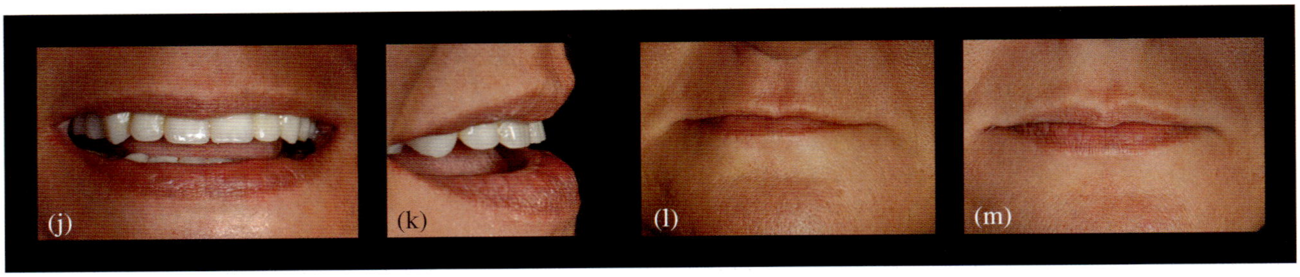

Figure 1.2 (j and k) Frontal and side views showing the facial enhancement of the patient. (l and m) Showing pre and post-operative improvement of the facial tissue support.

planning software. Screw-retained and cementable temporaries can be produced through a goniX™ laboratory before the actual surgery starts. Custom final titanium and zirconia abutments with the accompanying final restoration can be manufactured prior to the surgery to accommodate immediate load situations.

NobelClinician™ (Nobel Biocare, Zürich, Switzerland) is also available for both Windows and MAC OS. DICOM files can be loaded directly into the software for rendering and processing without prior DICOM file conversion. Nobel Guides™ (Nobel Biocare, Zürich, Switzerland) are either dentition or mucosa supported. Each guide will be delivered in a light-blocking pouch along with a detailed drill protocol for each osteotomy site. Mucosa-supported guides are stabilized with auxiliary fixation pins. Specialized guided surgery drills are utilized along with drill keys to achieve osteotomies congruent with the preplanned diameter, position, angulation, and depth of the implants to be installed.

Implant Studio® (3 shape A/S, Denmark, Copenhagen) is a yet another contemporary solution that finally brings implant planning into a single smooth workflow. It is open to any other third-party surface scans. It integrates with a wide range of 3D printers and milling machines and can be used with any implant system, sleeve system, and surgical kit. 3Shape's solution offers a complete digital workflow for clinicians and for laboratories, and it offers implant planning with intuitive tools that merge the benefits of planning, as well as virtual crown functionality, offering optimal implant placement in combination with the intended prosthetic design. There is also the 3Shape Communicate integration, which makes it easy to receive 3D surface scans from TRIOS scanners and from 3Shape desktop scanners and to send the pre-planned implant positions for designing abutments and crowns.

Undoubtedly, digital scanning devices are going to be a significant part of the future of implant dentistry, which is already the case today. In 1994, Jemt and Lie described a technique called 'photogrammetry,' which involves utilizing a series of 3D photographs to record the optimal implant positions for manufacturing implant supported frameworks. They determined that photogrammetry was a valid option for recording implant positions and had a precision comparable to that of conventional impression techniques. Later, it was demonstrated that optical 3D scanning acquisition could be used to determine the position of osseointegrated implants and that image-acquiring technology could be used as an alternative to traditional impression techniques (Karatas and Toy 2014).

Digital scanning technology, a boon to the clinician, is truly changing the face of implant dentistry today and to dental works in general. Compared to the classic impression and its short comings—bubbles and voids; distortion; tray-to-tooth contact; poor tray bond; delamination; sensitivity to temperature; varying shrinkage; stone model pouring; and die trimming discrepancies—digital scanning may offer a less expensive modality, increased productivity, and more efficient clinical workflow, and has proven to be impressive to many clinicians and patients. Digital scanning technology has significantly enhanced clinical accuracy and productivity in comparison to conventional impression techniques (Kamimura et al. 2017). Today in dentistry, implant abutments can be fabricated using its specific scan bodies and the information digitally transferred directly to a five-axis milling center after design. This technology saves time and money for all parties. The introduction of digital impression systems provides clinicians with the opportunity for greater general dentistry productivity (Yuzbasioglu et al. 2014). These digital systems are now being utilized regularly to serve clinicians and patients more effectively. The industry is in continuous development within the digital markets, which will increase market competition, and with more clinicians implementing the technology into their practices, the technology will likely become more affordable.

Digital impression systems have offered the possibility of better-fitting restorations and greater productivity for the general dentist. At the same time, there is minimized the miscommunication between the laboratory technician and the clinician, and the hardship of the prosthetic delivery belongs to the past. These systems offer users the ability to capture a digital image of the preparation or the implant interface or even the edentulous ridge and submit that information electronically in the form of a digital STL file, resulting in fabrication of a working model and die system for fabrication of the restoration. A comparison of crowns made with a digital scan versus those created with a traditional impression found that the scanned restorations showed a greater number of perfect interproximal contacts, better marginal fit, and more accurate occlusion (Rhee et al. 2015).

The iTero™ digital impression device (Align Technology Inc. San Jose, California, USA) developed as an office-based intraoral scanning system, which is connected by the Internet to a centralized milling center and to the partnering dental laboratory. The system's enhanced visualization and real-time analytical tools enable clinicians to adjust measurements before completing the intraoral digital scanning of patients. Digital scanning technology has significantly enhanced clinical accuracy and productivity, consistently displaying highly accurate digital impressions (Derhalli 2013). The iTero digital impression device does not require opaque powder spray to provide uniform light distribution, and the surface registration and accuracy are within 15 μm (Rhee et al. 2015).

Nowadays, clinicians using personal computers at home or at work in conjunction with the advanced computerized techniques provided with modern software, are able to interact with CT scan data combined with the intraoral scans. The state-of-the-art of imaging combined with the intraoral scans, delivers crystal clear planning protocols for accurate implant position and prosthetic designs that are ready for milling and delivery.

Another emerging technology offers a navigation system that allows free guidance of the instrument by the surgeon, analogous to conventional treatment (Mezger et al. 2013). The technology evokes position recognizing sensors that allow the orientation of the instrument and the patient to be calculated in space. Visual and acoustic signals clarify the position of the instrument for the operator, relative to the image data of the patient and the target geometries determined during planning. Then come the Robotic systems that have already paved the way for use in various surgical bone treatment applications. The NaviENT & Micron Tracker (Navident, Toronto, Ontario, Canada) system represents a complete, portable clinical treatment system that can be integrated directly into the operative environment. This system is accomplished through software interfaces with standardized imaging processes and by hardware adaptations of conventional surgical instruments (Shin et al. 2011). The navigation software integrates imaging, virtual implant placement, and the implementation of implant placement. During surgery, the computer calculates the exact position of the patient and instrument, based on data from the infrared camera. Following calculation of the position, the resulting values are visualized on the computer screen and miniature monitor (Dirhold et al. 2012).

In addition, in the navigated systems for oral implantology, the implant position can be transferred precisely to the jaw according to the image-supported design. Image-guided surgery allows for axis-parallelism of the implants, which can be achieved with high precision, requiring a minimal amount of invasive surgery, while avoiding damage to sensitive structures (Widmann 2007).

Another advancement enjoyed in the dental field is readily available microsurgery giving minute dimensional accuracy with microscopes that enhance angular perception during drilling and among other benefits. Dental microsurgery utilizes a dental microscope and a fiber-optic lighting system. Clinicians use a dental operating microscope (DOM) to magnify the area, giving them a more precise view of the procedure. Because magnification spreads light out, making the area appear darker, many dental microscopes also include a fiber-optic light to illuminate the area more thoroughly than traditional overhead light sources. Another modality of microsurgery is the use of dental loupes that magnify the surgical area to 3–6 times its original size; however, dental microscopes provided far greater detail and magnification, enlarging the field of vision up to 20 times. Clinicians can adjust the level of magnification during dental microsurgery, while dental loupes are designed to fit a set distance between the clinician and patient, limiting mobility. One of the benefits of dental microsurgery is the documentation of the ongoing surgical procedure for educational and teaching purposes.

The availability of clinical microscopes and microsurgical lenses has enabled maximum perfection for both the restorative and periodontal surgical aspects that offer long-lasting esthetic restorations. Post-operative complications are also minimized, not to mention the great endodontic benefits of the microscope as well as their use in the documentation of daily surgical and restorative procedures. Powerful laser machines have also been developed to enable painless dental procedures, minimally invasive surgeries, and the whitening of darkened teeth in the same visit. Dental microsurgery can be used to enhance any dental procedure, either surgical or prosthetic, while it transforms outcomes from regular to outstanding due to the ability to see the tiny details that are impossible to see with the naked eye, and so it is considered to be a practice builder.

Lasers are yet to offer a state-of-the-art treatment modality in all fields of dentistry that include implant dentistry. One of the most interesting developments over the past few years has been the introduction of the CO_2 laser, which preserves the tissue with almost no adverse effects at the light microscopic level (Schwarz et al. 2015). The use of photodynamic therapy to treat peri-implant infections with a CO_2 laser also seems to be of more value than conventional methods (Caccianiga et al. 2016). The laser approach is atraumatic; it does not damage the adjacent bone or soft tissue, and does not overheat the surrounding tissues, which would minimize postoperative trauma. Laser energy also has bactericidal properties that virtually eliminate the problems of infection (Jurič and Anić 2014). After removing the implant and debriding the site, the clinician can stimulate the healing of the soft and hard tissues. Another great benefit of laser surgery is that it boosts the wound healing process (Chaves et al. 2014). This in turn reduces the potential complications of wound healing. Laser surgery dramatically reduces or eliminates the inflammatory response by promoting the release of enzymatic inhibitors of the inflammatory process.

The indications for laser surgery are numerous, it is applied in almost every branch of dentistry, it can be used for soft tissue and hard tissue cutting, treating teeth decay, sculpturing gingival margins, bleeding control, disinfecting wounds and infected pockets, sterilizing infected endodontic lesions, treating infected implant fixture related infections, and treating herpetic lesions.

1.4 The Era of Peri-implant Soft Tissue Optimization

A healthy esthetic gingival appearance around dental implant-supported restoration requires the careful assessment of any missing gingival and periodontal defects prior to placing dental implant fixtures, subsequently one should have the technical skills to restore and treat these preexisting defects. Esthetic gingival and periodontal defects can be addressed during the preoperative clinical examination of implant candidates. Examples of gingival and periodontal defects or discrepancies prior to implant therapy are plenty, which may be evident as: loss of attachment levels, loss of the keratinized mucosa, asymmetrical or unbalanced adjacent gingival contours, localized reduction of tissue volume, absence or blunting of the interproximal papillae, and all known types of gingival recession (Elaskary 2008). Suboptimal soft tissue quality or quantity may arise due to many factors, which include aggressive tooth brushing (O'Leary et al. 1971), smoking, plaque accumulation, and tissue injuries due to trauma. Any of these factors that exist at the time of clinical evaluation should be eliminated prior to selecting any clinical approach for dental implant therapy. Esthetics in the anterior region relies heavily on the very existence of healthy keratinized gingival margins; this applies to both natural dentition and implant-supported restorations.

Facilitating long-term maintenance of implant-supported restorations requires a meticulous assessment of the soft tissue status related to the future implant site; this should be established during the clinical examination at the presurgical stage (Kennedy et al. 1985). The gingival form and color should also be evaluated along the course of the presurgical phase. It is valuable to detect the gingival hyperpigmentation, as it can be of a great value to the overall treatment result. Oral pigmentation is most commonly physiologic in nature; however, non-physiologic pigmentations may be encountered. Physiologic pigmentation results primarily from melanin produced by melanocytes present with the stratum basale of the oral epithelium and are typically more generalized than their non-physiologic counterparts; the etiology of these pigmentations may be hereditary, due to pregnancy, or medication-induced. Non-physiologic pigmentations may be pathologic or non-pathologic. Examples of localized pathologic pigmented lesions include hemangiomas, Kaposi's sarcoma, and melanoma, among others. Pathologic pigmented lesions may also be generalized when associated with systemic conditions such as Addison's disease, Peutz-Jeghers syndrome, neurofibromatosis, or heavy metal ingestion. Localized, non-physiologic pigmentations are typically due to implanted material within the oral mucosa, resulting in a clinically evident discoloration. The exogenous pigments may include carbon, iron dust, metallic silver (amalgam tattoos), or graphite (Phillips and John 2005). The existence of pigmented gingival tissues warrants the attention of excercising care to avoid scar tissue formation; this would contribute negatively to the esthetic result, especially in high smile line patients. The continuity of the keratinized band should be preserved by using less invasive therapeutic techniques, such as flapless entries for example (Elaskary 2008).

Gingival components that contribute to an esthetically pleasing implant-supported restoration are the marginal radicular form, the interdental tissue status, and the color and texture of healthy keratinized tissues (Tarnow and Eskow 1995). The original width of attached gingiva in the maxillary anterior area can vary widely from approximately 2–8 mm. The labiolingual dimension of gingival tissue is approximately 1.5 mm at the base of the gingival sulcus. The amount of soft tissue available to achieve predictable implant esthetics and function did not attain any conclusive statements from the authors; some concluded that neither the absence of inflamed soft tissue nor a specific amount of keratinized mucosa is required to ensure a successful osseointegration. On the contrary, some other authors have confirmed that the absence of a keratinized mucosa might jeopardize implant survival. In addition, some authors have stated that a minimum of 2 mm of keratinized tissue width is needed to achieve optimal health of the tissues surrounding natural dentition, while others have suggested that less than 1 mm of keratinized tissue can be adequate when bacterial plaque is well controlled (Zarb and Schmitt 1990).

Generally and logically speaking, the presence of a sufficient band of keratinized mucosa will surely improve the esthetic outcome of the definitive implant-supported restoration. The presence of the keratinized band can minimize the occurrence of postoperative gingival recession, endure the trauma of brushing, resist muscle pull, and reduce the probability of soft tissue dehiscence above implant fixtures. A sufficient amount of healthy keratinized gingival tissue band should exist prior to implant placement (Bengazi et al. 1996). Therefore, optimizing soft tissue quality and quantity during the various treatment stages of implant therapy becomes a vital prerequisite. Diagnosing the type and the reason for intraoral soft tissue defects as well as setting the proper treatment thus becomes an imperative tool to implantology success, but gingival surgery has variable degrees of success.

Currently free gingival grafts or onlay grafts offer great predictability, which has been enhanced by using thicker grafts, butt joints on recipient papillary sites, mattress sutures over the graft, vigorous root preparation, and by etching roots with citric acid. The use of connective tissue grafts has also attained great popularity in implant dentistry recently and offers a fair improvement in deficient soft tissue volume and profile. Apical and coronal repositioning surgeries, either used alone or in combination with other surgeries, offers great predictability whenever the biological width is preserved at its normal known limits.

There is a direct link between an harmonious nonpathologic pre-existing periodontal complex and esthetic and functional implant therapy, because the development or the pre-existence of any periodontopathic organisms can inevitably disrupt the clinician's ability to recreate a long-term healthy environment. This is especially critical in the maxillary anterior region, where the condition of the soft tissue complex and its relationship to the implant restoration and adjacent dentition often determines the implant's success. This influences treatment planning to a great extent. Any existing periodontal condition should be well assessed, diagnosed, and planned for treatment prior to implant therapy; a study by Gouvossis (1997) suggested that transmission of periodontopathic organisms from periodontitis sites to implant sites in the same mouth is a likely event. It calls the attention of the clinician to the potential cross-infection from periodontitis sites to implant sites. This statement was confirmed by the results of cross-sectional microbiologic studies of failing implant sites, where the data suggested similar microbial profiles between these sites and those of periodontitis pockets. This study offered a strong link between a periodontally involved patient and dental implant failure, as an increase in the gram-negative anaerobic flora with high levels of spirochetes was associated with failing implants. The evidence supports the concept that microbiota associated with stable and failing implants are similar to the microbiota of periodontally healthy and diseased teeth, respectively (Gouvossis 1997).

As an interesting confirmation of the previous conclusion, Sanz et al. (1991) reported elevated levels of polymorphonuclear leukocytes (PMNs) associated with disease progression around dental implants and Kao et al. (1995) found gingival crevicular fluid IL-1B levels of diseased implants to be elevated threefold as compared to clinically healthy sites. These findings are similar to a study that evaluated periodontal degeneration around natural teeth caused by inflammatory mediators such as PGE_2, IL-1B, and possibly IL-6 produced by the chronic inflammatory cells of the periodontal tissues. These initiate pathways that stimulate osteoclastic bone resorption, which indicates the similarity in the inflammatory response. In conclusion, existing periopathogenic organisms from intraoral sites have the great potential to colonize at the muco–implant interface through a potential infective process that might lead to loss of the implant and failure of the prosthesis. Therefore, the need for a clinical protocol that includes the elimination of periodontal disease prior to implant placement is mandatory.

1.5 Soft Tissue Bio-characterization and Influence

The composition and structure of the periodontium influences the implant prognosis from an esthetic and a functional perspective. Distinguishing and identifying periodontal phenotypes becomes of great value to the treatment plan and to selection of an appropriate surgical approach and to predicting the long-term success. Identifying the patient phenotype influences not only the surgical technique but also the fate of the clinical procedure. Healthy human periodontium comprises radicular cementum, periodontal ligament, gingival, and investing alveolar bone (Glickman 1972). It can be divided into the gingival unit and the attachment apparatus. The gingival unit consists of the free gingival, attached gingival, and the alveolar mucosa. The gingival unit has a lining epithelium of either masticatory mucosa, which is thick keratinized epithelium with a dense collagenous connective tissue corium, or lining mucosa, which is thin non-keratinized epithelium with a loose connective tissue corium containing elastic fibers. Masticatory mucosa is found in the free and attached gingival, hard palate, and dorsum of the tongue, while lining mucosa is found everywhere else in the oral cavity. Briefly, the free gingiva is that part of the gingiva located above the base of the gingival sulcus. It usually measures less than 3 mm high. The alveolar mucosa is reddish because of the thin nature of the epithelium overlying the vascular corium. The attachment apparatus consists of the alveolar bone, cementum of the tooth, and the collagen fiber attachment. The alveolar bone includes an outer compact bone with an inner trabecular bone: the compact bone that lines the alveolar socket acts as the attachment for collagen fibers incorporated into the compact bone, the bone is known as bundle bone; the cementum, which invests the root structure of the tooth, acts as the origin of the collagen fibers of the principal groups in the periodontal ligament, the principal fiber group being made up of collagen fibers running from the cementum of the root that do not insert in the bone; the dentogingival group runs from the cementum into the free gingival, while the dentoperiosteal group runs from the cementum apically, over the alveolar crest of bone to the mucoperiosteum of the attached gingival. The circular fibers are not attached in cementum but run in the free gingival around the tooth in a circular manner and the transseptal group runs from the cementum, over the alveolar crest bone to the cementum of the adjacent tooth (Ochsenbein and Ross 1973). The value of these groups of fibers to esthetics is immense, as they form the main structure responsible for the shape and position of the interdental papilla. The benefit only applies to natural teeth and not dental implants because dental implants do not possess an insertion place for the fibers unlike the natural root cementum. The periodontal fiber group is also made up of collagen fibers. They are called the dentoalveolar group because they insert in the alveolar bone. They are composed of alveolar crestal fibers, which run from the supra-alveolar cementum down to the alveolar crest. Horizontal fibers run straight across from the cementum to the alveolar bone, and the oblique fibers (the largest group) run from the cementum, apically, from the root to the bone. All of these biological elements maintain the periodontium in a state of harmony that makes it a unique creation (Olson and Lindhe 1991).

The natural morphology of the healthy periodontium is characterized by a rise and fall of the marginal gingiva following the underlying alveolar crest contour both facially and proximally. Two different distinctive periodontal patterns are present in the oral cavity: the thin scalloped phenotype and the thick flat phenotype. The thick flat type is more prevalent, making up almost 85% of the population, while the thin scalloped phenotype makes up 15% of the population. Each type has its own distinctive morphological characteristics in relation to its adjoining structures. Recognizing and distinguishing these basic types is essential for selecting the implant size, implant type, and the surgical approach, and for predicting the overall prognosis to give biological harmony between the dental implants and the existing dentogingival structures. The thick flat phenotype is characterized by abundant amounts of masticatory mucosa; it is dense and fibrous with a minimal height difference between the highest and lowest points on the proximal and facial aspects of the marginal gingiva; therefore, it is called flat (Olson and Lindhe 1991). Larger teeth that are most likely square shaped characterize this type of periodontium. This bulkiness of the tooth shape results in a broader, more apically positioned contact area, a cervical convexity that has greater prominence, and an embrasure that is completely filled with interdental papilla. The root dimensions are broader mesiodistally, almost equal to the width of the crown at the cervix, which causes a diminution in the amount of bone interproximally. The typical reaction of this tissue phenotype to trauma, such as tooth preparation or impression making or endodontic abscess, cracked tooth, or failing endodontic treatment, is inflammation and apical migration of the junctional epithelium with a resultant pocket formation. With the thick flat tissue biotype, marginal inflammation is described in its acute form as marginal redness as magenta-cyanotic in appearance. With chronic inflammation, marginal gingivitis is present with gingiva coloration ranging from red to magenta. The gingiva may range from a normal shape to a boggy, enlarged shape. As inflammation persists, periodontal pocketing tends to occur. In regions with a relatively thick bulk of bone, the pocket formation occurs in conjunction with infrabony defects. The thick flat tissue type is ideal for placing dental implants and restoring it with high esthetic predictability. Here the gingival and osseous scalloping is normally parallel to the cemento-enamel junction (CEJ). The minimal undulation of the CEJ between adjacent teeth, which predictably follows the natural contour of the alveolar crest, makes the gingival tissues more stable. Consequently, this type of periodontium is less likely to exhibit soft tissue shrinkage postoperatively.

On the other hand, the thin phenotype of periodontium exhibits its own distinctive features. These include thin friable gingiva with a narrow band of attached masticatory mucosa and a thin facial bone that usually exhibits dehiscence and fenestration. The tooth crown shape usually exhibits a triangular or thin cylindrical form, and the contact areas are smaller and located in a further incisal location. The cervical convexity is less prominent than that of the thick phenotype, while the interdental papilla is thin and long but does not fill the embrasure space completely, resulting in a scalloped appearance. Additionally, this phenotype possesses a root that is narrow with an attenuated taper, allowing for an increased amount of inter-radicular bone. When inflicted with trauma, this tissue type undergoes gingival recession both facially and interproximally. Both acute and chronic inflammation will result in gingival recession. There are no pockets or infrabony defects that form because the thin bony plate resorbs in advance of the gingival recession. There is at least 0.5–0.8 mm of bone loss. Subsequently the thin labial plate recedes apically, and the soft tissue will follow the bone, causing recession. The extent of this recession is difficult to predict due to the varying thickness of the labial plate of bone among patients (Esposito et al. 1993). Placing dental implants in the esthetic zone becomes a critical task with this particular tissue phenotype because it is difficult to achieve long-lasting symmetrical soft tissue contours, probably due to the proximity of the implant to the natural tooth periodontium next to it and the reduced amount of masticatory mucosa. The resultant recession and bone resorption leave a flat profile between the roots, with marginal exposure of the restoration and subsequent partial loss of the interproximal papilla. Ridge preservation procedures might be carried out for any planned tooth extractions in this tissue phenotype; flapless implant installation will be optimal for this type of bone, provided there is an intact labial plate of bone. However, a mixture of thick and thin tissue types in the same patient can be detected. Areas of thin labial plate are commonly associated with the canine eminencies, the mesial roots of maxillary first molars, and mandibular incisors. These areas tend to have thin gingival as well and, in such cases, can be called thick, thin, or mixed thick–thin gingiva (Gargiulo, Wentz, and Orban 1961).

Evaluating the qualitative nature of the periodontium is of great value and a proper appraisal of the periodontium should be performed prior to commencing any implant therapy in the esthetic zone. The clinician should be able to predict the response of the periodontal apparatus to restorative margins, inflammation, and regular trauma.

In conclusion, a tissue-integrated prosthesis must be placed in a healthy stable environment and any primary or secondary disease process must be resolved before the placement of dental implants. Any localized inflammatory or fibrous processes that require management should be dealt with in advance. Inflammation caused by ill-fitting dentures can often be resolved with tissue-conditioning techniques prior to implant surgery. Any gingival hyperplastic tissues should be excised if it is due to a reactive process. The degree of redundancy of the mucosa covering the residual ridge should be evaluated before fixture placement, if there has been significant resorption of the bone without a corresponding atrophy of the overlying mucosa; a mobile soft tissue ridge crest may be present and should be excised prior to surgery. Muscle pull in conjunction with alveolar mucosa such as that found in the mentalis area should be considered for repositioning. Recent advances in periodontal surgery have made it possible not only to reposition or regenerate tissues to meet esthetic demands, but also to change the tissue quality of the restorative environment for more-predictable treatment outcomes (Kazor et al. 2004).

1.6 Role of Interim Restorations

Immediate loading of dental implants is often not always applicable for several reasons, therefore the fabrication of interim restorations become of great importance to the patient. Establishing an interim esthetic solution remains a critical task because the number of implants used, the condition of the alveolar bone, the location of the implants, and the type of implant design contribute to the length of the healing period for dental implants.

The influence of a successful interim phase has a positive impact from the patient to the clinician. The patient, becomes confident and positively bonded, while unexpectedly high referral rates from patients might be expected.

Within this period, many patients experience apprehension about losing their social image or daily function routine, which could develop into fear or rejection of dental implant therapy. Therefore, clinicians should provide a stable, stress-free, functional, and esthetic provisional restoration to their patients during this critical period. For years, provisionalization was viewed as a thoughtless type of treatment procedure that sought only a rapid, feasible, inexpensive method to obtain disposable crowns and bridges (Shavell 1979). This concept implied that provisional restorations should not be perfected, as it would not serve in the patient's mouth for a very long period. Nowadays, with the wide application of dental implants as a routine tooth replacement therapy, the role of the provisional prosthesis has changed dramatically. Although patients might have stayed edentulous for a long time before implant therapy, those who are especially "esthetically conscious" tend to ask the usual question (Will I stay toothless until the dental implants integrate?), because it is embarrassing for then to be seen in public without teeth or with a temporary tooth that is obviously artificial. Their question is understandable because after they decided to take dental implants as a treatment option, they also started to prepare for a new social and esthetic era in their lives (Balshi and Garver 1986).

The provisional prostheses should be designed to sustain or improve the quality of life for patients undergoing implant therapy. As the word provisional suggests, provisionalization involves something that is used temporarily, to serve briefly, until the permanent service is rendered. When fabricating a provisional prosthesis, several considerations should be applied. The provisional restoration should: (1) not interfere with primary wound closure; (2) provide the patient with harmonious occlusion; (3) restore esthetics and phonetics; (4) protect the underlying gingival tissues, that is, maintain the dentogingival unit health; and (5) not exert any direct biting loads to the underlying implants, in case a delayed method of loading is selected. A properly fabricated provisional restoration can be an important source of biomechanical information. It can be a valuable aid in determining the final tooth position, exact tooth shade, and occlusal scheme of the definitive prosthesis. Moreover, it can reveal some new additional clues for improved esthetics and patient comfort (Balshi and Garver 1986).

After the second stage of surgery, a provisional restoration can also help guide healing of the soft tissues around dental implants to develop the emergence profile until it reaches the original anatomical dimensions; this can minimize the need for further soft tissue manipulation. Therefore, the interim prosthesis acts as a reference in designing the final prosthesis. The type of provisional prosthesis should be determined during the presurgical planning phase by the dental team. When considering a provisional prosthesis for a patient who will receive an implant-supported restoration, there are many available options, including: an existing prosthesis that the patient already uses or a removable partial denture, a resin-bonded bridge, or the use of a modified socket seal template technique, temporary implants, and the use of socket seal methods (natural teeth provisionalization) (Biggs 1996; Soballe et al. 1990).

1.6.1 Using or Modifying an Existing Prosthesis

When the patient seeks implant therapy due to an existing failed prosthesis, the chief complaint usually is not due to the shape or the contour of the prosthesis but due to the functional consequences that have occurred. Therefore, the old prosthesis can be used as a temporary solution because it was already serving the patient on both esthetic and functional levels for a long time. When the patient presents with an old bridge, the following steps should be followed: an overall impression is made with the failed old bridge in place before attempting to remove it from its place; then an indirect or direct provisional bridge is performed and cemented in place after removal of the old bridge takes place. If the old bridge has already been removed from its place, it can be temporarily cemented after relieving pontic areas that touch the soft tissue.

1.6.2 Removable Partial Dentures

One of the easiest ways of provisionalization between Stage I and Stage II implant surgery is the use of a removable prosthesis that is typically fabricated as an interim restoration for partially or fully edentulous patients. It is indicated in bounded and free-end saddles as well as for fully edentulous cases. Being removable can be an advantage by itself: this facility can be valuable for multiple removals during surgical interventions, as the partial denture can be removed and then replaced once the procedure has been completed without clinical complexity. It is simply fabricated by making an impression, casting it, and drawing the design of the saddle; then the laboratory technician constructs a removable partial denture accordingly. Removable dentures might also stimulate bone remodeling around dental implants in totally edentulous patients and can be used to confirm osseointegration before the final prosthesis is constructed. This type of provisional solution provides an inexpensive provisional modality that can be included in any treatment plan, based on the patient's financial status (Leffler 2008). The patient may feel psychologically improved with the edentulous area being temporarily restored and other related facial structures being supported. However, the patient should be reminded that the prosthesis is only a temporary alternative for the missing space. Removable partial dentures can be limiting in their function, especially during speaking or chewing, due to their instability. Furthermore, some clinical precautions need to be observed when removable partial dentures are used as a provisional modality for totally or partially edentulous patients; the appliance should be relieved from its fitting surface on top of the implant heads to avoid any biting load being exerted on the implants during the healing period and to allow undisturbed soft tissue healing. The patient is advised to use the denture primarily for social reasons rather than for masticatory purposes. In addition, when the partial denture is relined, the lining material tends to dry and become stiff over time, usually one to two months. This can be resolved by changing the lining material at monthly intervals to keep the fitting surface of the denture elastic. A removable provisional prosthesis can influence the underlying gingival tissues at the pontic areas to create and simulate a natural gingival architecture of the implant supported restorations. This can be achieved by adding acrylic resin to the fitting surface of the pontic at the specific areas to be stimulated, to press and conform the alveolar mucosa to the required shape and contour.

1.6.3 Adhesive Bridges

This is a highly recommended method for restoring missing teeth and is an alternative conservative treatment option that has been suggested in restoring missing dentition in the esthetic zone. The adhesive bridges eliminate the need for substantial destruction of natural abutments. They were originally introduced by Rochette (1986) for used as periodontal splints. Adhesive fixed prostheses were used successfully as temporary restorations serving the essential objectives of provisionalization (Breeding and Dixon 1995; Rochette 1986). These provisional prostheses help to restore esthetics, maintain occlusion, and free the implant from biting loads. An adhesive bridge, unlike a removable partial denture, does not exert any pressure on the implant area. It is better tolerated by the patient and may be more reassuring than a removable partial denture because of the improved esthetic results, stability, and fixation. However, a resin-bonded bridge can be a deterrent when multiple re-entries to the surgical site are required.

The prosthesis is totally tooth-supported and retained by acid etching the adjacent teeth and by cementing using composite resin. However, adhesive bridges require greater clinical skills than conventional bridges, while another point of consideration is the possibility of recurrent dental caries occurring around the margins and line angles. A debonding tendency occurs with a frequency as high as 25–31%, which requires recementation every time it occurs (Williams et al. 1989). This provisional method can be used when patients are concerned with their social appearance or their work includes speaking in front of the media, so they cannot afford to have any movable devices in their mouths. For those clinicians that use it as the preferred method, acrylic resin-bonded bridges can be used as adhesive bridges temporarily when the load is minimized as a less-expensive alternative, the only drawback being that they tend to break under any direct occlusal load.

1.7 The Value of Patient Records

The dental profession has an ethical and legal responsibility for patient care. A properly maintained patient record is a very important aspect of this patient care system. In general, a "record" can be defined as information generated in the course of an organization's official transactions and one that is documented to act as a source of reference and a tool by which an organization is governed (Devadiga 2014). The dental record is the official office document that records all diagnostic information, clinical notes, treatment performed, and patient-related communications that occur in the dental office, including instructions for home care and consent to treatment. The dental record is hence a legal document owned by the clinician, which contains subjective and objective information about the patient (Waleed et al. 2015).

Accurate and comprehensive clinical records are mandatory, and supplementary high-quality clinical photographic images are often required by many health authorities worldwide (Valenzuela et al. 2000). A properly maintained dental record serves several uses. Clinical records are fundamental to the delivery of good dental care and for ensuring continuity and completeness of treatment. Good records enable monitoring of the patients' state of oral health and can also aid motivation in preventive oral healthcare practices. It is helpful for monitoring the success/failure of any treatment carried out. A detailed and accurate dental record is essential as it serves the clinicians' own best interests in the event of a malpractice suit. A complete record also enables communication with another practitioner who may be required to provide care to the patient in the absence of the primary clinician. Records are essential for dental audit, which is a vital part of quality control. A dental audit critically analyses every aspect of dental care. It begins from initial entry of patient information to assessing competence of the dental professional to diagnose, treat, use resources, and practice evidence-based dentistry. All these factors influence the quality of life as assessed by the patient and the professional. Records can be used in the management and planning of healthcare facilities and services, for healthcare research, and in the production of healthcare statistics (Charangowda 2010). Finally, a person's dental record can play a vital role in forensic dentistry for the identification of a missing person.

As the dental practitioner is solely accountable for complete and accurate patient records, there are certain basic criteria that need to be followed in writing a dental record. A study by Dar-Odeh et al. (2008) on the analysis of clinical records of dental patients attending the Jordan University Hospital found that drug prescriptions and local anesthetic injections were poorly documented by the investigated group of dental specialists. In a study by Osborn et al. (2000) to determine Minnesota clinicians' perception of the adequacy of their dental record documentation, 85% of clinicians felt their record documentation was adequate while, in reality, 9.4–87% of the time information was found to be absent when compared with the American Dental Association (ADA) criteria.

Backup of all records should be performed on a removable medium that will enable data recovery in the event of a systems failure. A breach of confidentiality occurs when private information that the clinician has learned from the patient is divulged to a third party without the patient's consent or a court order. Garbin et al. (2008) found that although clinicians declared to be aware of professional confidentiality, nearly half of the respondents acted unethically by talking about the clinical cases of their patients to their friends or spouses. Violation of professional ethics, no matter how minor, will result in problems for both the clinician and the patient (Devadiga 2014; Garbin et al. 2008).

Adequate dental records might be given to another clinician either for consultation or treatment; or used for medicolegal issues, or tax reasons. A clinician leaving or selling a practice should ideally give patients advance written notice about the change of ownership. If the outgoing clinician is unable to do so, the incoming clinician should notify patients that he or she is now the new owner of the practice and is therefore in possession of their records (Devadiga 2014; Lawney 1998).

Morgan (2001) emphasized the value of keeping prompt dental records, as well as the principles of executing it. Furthermore, in addition to using an accurate dental record, informed consent should be obtained from the patient together with the all possible treatment options and possible complications of the treatment options, and the advantages and disadvantages of each proposed treatment modality (Nelson 1989).

Digital dental photography can also add value to the record with fidelity, it can be used for documentation, education, communication, portfolios, and marketing. While most patients will not usually object to dental documentation for the purpose of recording pathology and treatment progress, they may be more reticent to offer full face pictures or to agree to their images being used for marketing, such as on practice brochures or newsletters for distribution by a mailshot (Osborn et al. 2000).

Printed photographs are no longer needed for patient education as proposed earlier (Oberbreckling 1993) because the era of digitized images and the use of multimedia devices has made these printed images obsolete (see Figures 1.3a–c, 1.4a, b, and 1.5a–c).

1.8 The Value of Team

Collaboration is a modern discipline in the medical field; each treatment plan usually involves more than one member so many qualified members may be needed to fulfill an accurate plan. It is important to demonstrate professional expertise by recognizing and applying relevant information to create a logical conclusion consistent with reality. This view of professionalism is existentialist. The professional rejects dogma and does not accept conclusions drawn from another person until that professional verifies those conclusions. This existential attitude is consistent with the philosophy of evidence-based care, which Chichester et al. (2002) regarded as applying scientific evidence and personal resources to each patient's needs and expectations. Thus, a collaborative practice must have practitioners who appraise one another's diagnosis and treatment plans for the purpose of either corroborating or improving those decisions (Atkins and Walsh 1997). In a study that explored the current understanding about inter-professional collaborative client-centered practice and nursing's role in this form of care delivery, they have emphasized the role of the dental nurse and concluded that all professionals, including nurses, must move away from a service-oriented delivery to a patient-centered collaborative approach to care (Orchard 2010).

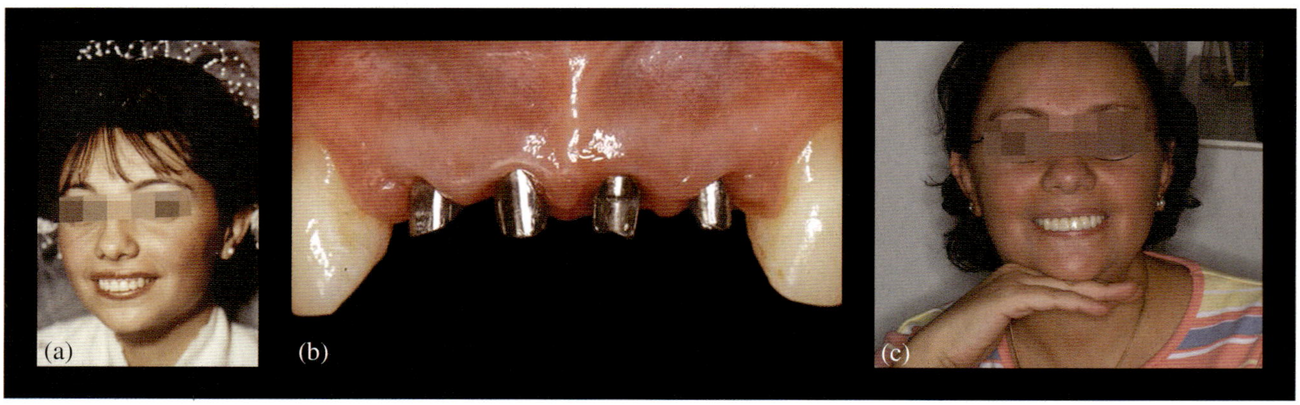

Figure 1.3 (a) A female patient scheduled for extraction of her maxillary four front teeth (15 year old picture). (b) Dental implants showing where placed and with abutments connected. (c) The patient finally restored. Note the similarity between the teeth shape and revealed pre- and post-teeth loss.

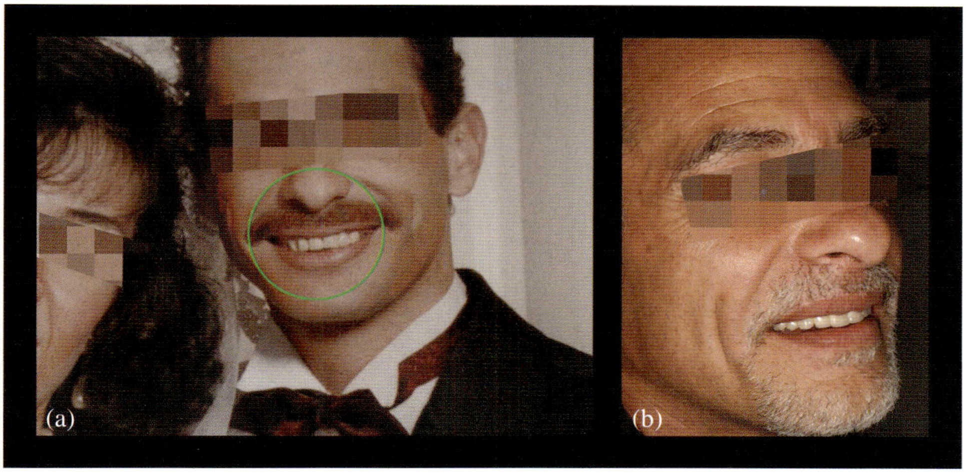

Figure 1.4 (a) Ten year old picture of a male patient. (b) Immediate postoperative picture of the patient being restored. Note the duplication of the amount of teeth display and shape, which preserves the patient's own physical character.

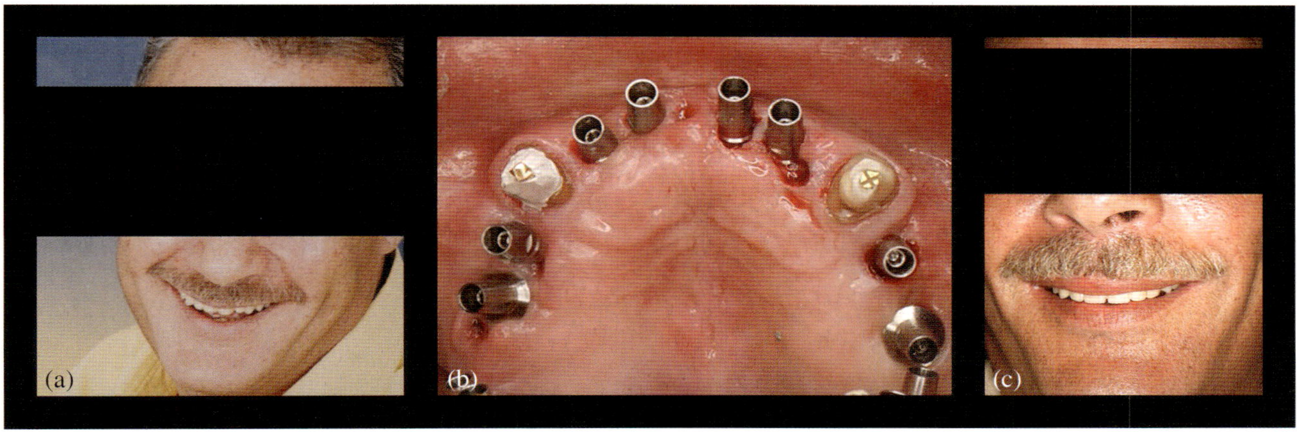

Figure 1.5 (a, b, and c) Pre- and post-operative pictures that show the duplication of the old teeth anatomy and smile arch to the new restoration; the pictures are taken 12 years apart.

In 2011, the Interprofessional Education Collaborative comprising the American Association of Colleges of Nursing, the American Association of Colleges of Osteopathic Medicine, the American Association of Colleges of Pharmacy, the American Dental Education Association, the Association of American Medical Colleges, and the Association of Schools of Public Health sponsored an expert panel of their members to identify and develop four domains of core competencies needed for a successful interprofessional collaborative practice: (1) Values/Ethics for Interprofessional Practice; (2) Roles/Responsibilities; (3) Interprofessional Communication; and (4) Teams and Teamwork (Swihart 2016). Ideally, nowadays practitioners can create synergistic case management plans by identifying risks, preventing disease, and addressing disorders early, thereby reducing the need for expensive remedies (Barnsteiner et al. 2007). By far the most effective communication is the face to face communication between the clinician and the patient; authentically focused communication is definitely enjoyable and trustful. The way team members communicate is yet another important issue (Barrington et al. 1998), which should be addressed by continuous training and motivation of the working team (Barnard et al. 2007). Clear guidelines and effective systems allow teammates to empower each other and strengthen the level of trust within an office. For a team to function well together, each member must have faith that tasks will be completed accurately and in a timely manner (Cooper et al. 2005). Each member of the team should have his or her designated responsibilities, which often requires the continuous development of decision-making skills (Jiffry 2002).

1.9 Fulfilling Patient Expectations in Esthetic Implant Therapy

Oral implantology indeed offers safe, effective, and predictable results for patients with complete or partial edentulism and it also offers a permanent long-term functional and esthetic solution to many clinical circumstances that previously had no solution. The high success rates of treatment involving implant-supported prosthesis are based on different parameters, the most common of which is clinical. However, results based on patient satisfaction are an important aspect in determining treatment success.

Patient satisfaction according to the treatment outcome has a high significance. A patient's perception of treatment has been recognized as important for the assessment of healthcare quality for several decades (Fong Ha, Ana, and Lomgnecker 2010). What a patient expects from their treatment is thought to have an impact on their satisfaction with the outcome. Expectations from dental implants have been investigated by a diversity of approaches within the available literature (Waitzkin 1984) (see Figure 1.6a and b).

Unrealistic patient expectations are often found among many patients, which may lead mostly to dissatisfaction with the final treatment outcome. A balance between expectations and satisfaction should be attained.

1.9.1 Ideal Patient–Clinician Relation

Patient's satisfaction toward the esthetic outcome of implant therapy is a cornerstone of the outcome of implant therapy. Apparently, any successful implant therapy should primarily focus on patient satisfaction from the overall treatment experience and should be tested throughout the treatment stages, not only at the final stage. One of the principal criteria of appraisal is the level of patients' expectations (Elaskary 2008). Patients with realistic expectations will be more easily satisfied than those with unrealistic expectations. When patients are duly informed and aware that immediately after the operation they may experience personal inconvenience for a short time, the occurrence and discomfort may be easily overcome. More information is always better than less; when patients know the reason that explains their condition, they adjust their expectations and react accordingly. An accurate appraisal of a patient's psychological profile at the time of treatment planning is mandatory. There must be no discrepancy between a patient's own perception of his or her body image and the esthetic appraisal of the clinician. Solid communication between the patient and the clinician is certainly fundamental. It allows the patient to obtain complete information about the relationship between the cost of treatment, its benefits, and its risks. Good communication allows the clinician to identify any pre-existing psychological disorders, whether the patient's motives for undergoing surgery are real, and whether the patient's expectations are realistic or unrealistic (De Bruyn et al. 1997; Levi et al. 2003; Rittersma, Casparie, and Reerink 1980).

The nature of the clinician–patient relationship is somehow critical and requires a special emphasis as the relationship with a patient who seeks a rehabilitative esthetic job often starts by word of mouth via a former patient or a colleague. Patients usually do not have clear preconceived notions about oral reconstructive surgeries. A patient's expectations are considered to be the first valuable information collected prior to clinical examination; many patients have been disappointed with their clinicians because their unrealistic expectations were not fulfilled. Therefore patient's expectations should be first detected and identified prior to the treatment commencement. Another important issue is the financial

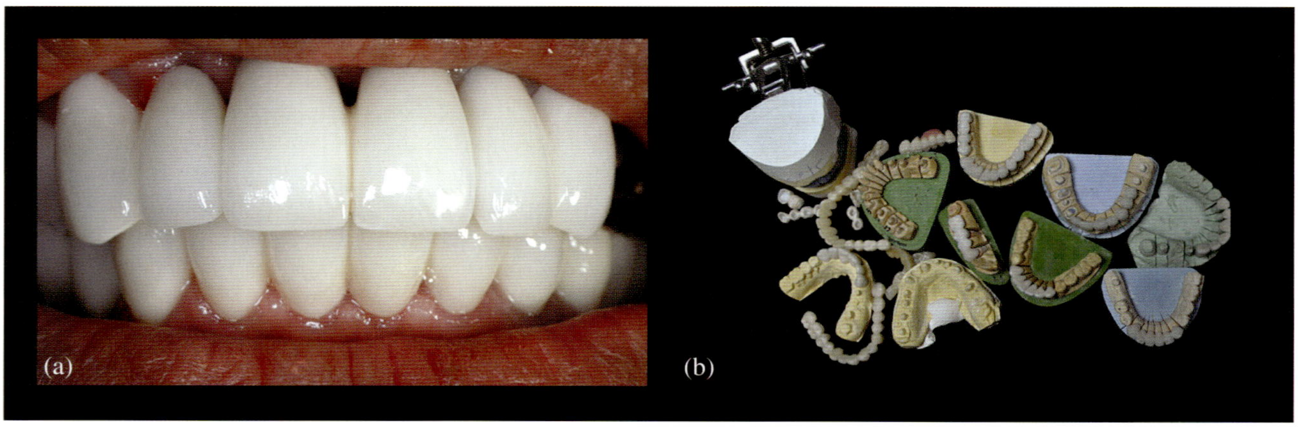

Figure 1.6 (a and b) Faulty selection by the patient might lead to loss of patient confidence, staff frustration, and financial losses.

one; cost should be fully explained and detailed to the patient as well as any possibility of exceeding the preset expense for esthetic major reconstructive cases that sometimes require additional corrective surgeries. The risk and possible treatment complications should be well addressed and explained to the patient prior to surgery, not only for financial reasons but also for discomfort and assurance reasons, because it has been found that patients tend to accept any postoperative complications, such as swelling, bruising, etc., if they have been forewarned. Rushing treatment commencement did not prove to have any greater acceptance from the patients (Karunakaran et al. 2011); on the contrary, it sometimes made patients uncomfortable and suspicious of the need to rush the start of their treatment. Apprehensive and anxious patients should be dealt with carefully and slowly to gain their confidence. It has been concluded that most pretreatment apprehension is due to the faulty information that the patients have gathered from sources other than the clinician. Such patients require more pre- and postoperative assurance than other patients; they may want to be able to reach you or any of your staff at any time to have their inquiries or complaints answered. Usually, they simply want to be reassured that they are improving and that they are on the right treatment track (Newsome and Wright 1999).

Many factors might influence patient satisfaction with the execution of the overall dental implants treatment plan. Literature lacks valid studies of the relationship between satisfaction and personality profiles, and their impact on the success of this treatment modality. Determining the prosthodontic protocol that has a better impact on the quality of life and satisfaction is often a balance between esthetics and function. Patient satisfaction and improved quality of life assessments are among the most critical factors that govern such success, as most of the related studies showed that dental implants provided promising and predictable results regarding patient satisfaction and various aspects of life assessment (Al-Omiri, Hantash, and Al-Wahadni 2005). Any foreseen or unforeseen treatment complications should be well addressed, advising the patient of a plan for resolution rather than denial because the most people welcome and admire truthfulness and straightforward statements. Often, consultation with another clinician has proven to have a highly positive impact on the patient's own state of mind. For possible treatment hardships it can be a valuable aid by soothing the patient's inner worries, as the patient is usually reassured that every avenue id being explored to solve the problem. Almost invariably the patient returns to his/her original clinician with restored confidence. If the request for a second opinion comes from the patient, the doctor should welcome the request with an open heart and mind by showing sincere concern for the patient's welfare (Terry and Geller 2013). In those circumstances, when receiving a new patient who left his/her original treating office to seek another clinician's assistance, then (with the patient's permission) contacting the patient's original clinician in the presence of the patient can make the patient feel that all efforts are being made in a positive and constructive direction. This open approach has been shown to be more efficient than a covert or a philosophical manner; it is also the clinician's responsibility to be willing to accept this patient if all parties agree (Somani et al. 2010).

1.9.2 Hazardous Effects of Poor Dental Practice

Qualitative methods can complement qualitative data by providing a deeper exploration of patients' psychological and social experiences both before and after treatment (Sutton 2015), which can throw some light on their treatment choices and resultant outcomes including oral hygiene behaviors. Since pretreatment expectations strongly predict satisfaction with dental treatment outcomes, it is empirical to identify and understand what a patient expects from different types of replacements and take steps to correct any confounding or misguided expectations.

Given the plethora of advancements and awareness among the population as a whole, treatments are increasingly patient driven rather than entirely clinician directed. The focus and scope of dentistry has also undergone a metamorphosis. Society is more aware of appearance and globalized the perception of what is attractive, desirable, and appealing to the general public. The dramatic development and improvement in restorative materials and techniques in recent decades has led to an impressive range of capabilities and techniques for restoring and enhancing esthetically impaired smiles. In the present consumer-driven society, patients may ask their clinician not only for conventional dental therapy to restore oral health but also for newer esthetic procedures that create 'beauty' and enhance appearance. The trend toward commercialization has the potential to tilt the balance or focus of services more toward business interests and profits rather than the patient's best interest. This trend, driven by the media and by public demand, has begun to foster a practice model of commercialization previously unseen in dentistry.

Clinicians are taking advantage of the ever-increasing demand for esthetic procedures by developing their skills and knowledge in this field and promoting esthetic parameters in their practice. This places a burden on the clinician to present the most appropriate treatment option for each individual case. Dental clinicians are obligated to upgrade their knowledge and skills on available treatment options so that patients can be appropriately and adequately informed about alternative options, possible complications, and associated risks, and so that the clinicians are able to perform such procedures. However, the continuous attention to tiny details, the continuous dealing with fearful and apprehensive patients in the daily life of clinicians as they strive for perfection, often leads to stress-related symptoms (increased heart rate, high blood pressure, sweating, etc.). This in turn might lead to an early heart attack for the clinician (Ahmad 2010; Bellini et al. 2009; Critchlow and Ellis 2010). Studies have detailed the reasons behind the physicosomatic symptoms that dental practitioners present as a result of: (1) compulsive attention to detail; (2) extreme conscientiousness; (3) careful control of emotions; (4) unrealistic expectations of himself or herself and others (i.e. employees and patients); and (5) a marked dependence on individual performance and prestige. Although stress can never be totally eliminated from dental practice, it must be minimized as much as possible to avoid the many stress-related physical and emotional problems that it causes (Soldz and Vaillant 1999; Somani et al. 2010).

1.9.3 Financial Resolution

Dentistry has historically been a caring profession with a core ethical obligation that centers on the obligation to treat and prevent disease and ultimately promote well-being (Simonsen 2007). The achievement of esthetic enhancement goals in an ethical manner is only possible through active patient participation, a multidisciplinary treatment approach, and excellence in treatment performance (Nash 1988). Our clinical decision-making, behavior, and standard of care is guided by a professional or ethical code of conduct, which is based on four fundamental ethical principles. The four fundamental principles of ethics that set the moral boundaries and ethical guidelines and duties that drive treatment decisions are: (1) *beneficience* (promoting good or doing good), (2) *non-maleficience* (preventing harm), (3) *autonomy* (patient's right to make or participate in decision-making and make their own choices), and (4) *justice* (fairness in treating each other justly). Among these guidelines, the principle of autonomy expresses the concept that dental clinicians have province to respect the patient's right to select or refuse treatment according to their desires, within the bounds of accepted treatment.

A clinician's primary obligations include involving the patient in treatment decisions in a meaningful way with due consideration being given to patient's needs, desires, and abilities, facilitated by the process of informed consent (Leffler 2008). Informed consent is obtained by conducting a structured, formal consultation with a patient to explain the goals of treatment, alternative options, the probable benefits and risks associated with the treatment and the alternative options, prognosis or treatment outcome, costs, and the risks of non-treatment (Nash 1988). Clinicians are obligated to tell the truth, protect confidentiality, and respect privacy (Jessri and Fatemitabar 2007). By communicating relevant information effectively, openly, and truthfully, clinicians assist patients to make informed choices from all the treatment options available and to participate in achieving and maintaining optimum oral health, rather than promoting the most profitable option. Dental clinicians should embrace this changing market as long as they leave their patients in as good as, or better, health than they found them, while also meeting their demands.

Prior to the final selection of the course of treatment to be undertaken, the patient must be made aware of the overall approximate financial cost of the treatment and the treatment time involved. One reason for patient dissatisfaction during the course of any treatment is a change to the financial plan, which leads to mistrust and raises questions in the patient's mind. Therefore, a clear financial statement prior to the treatment is important. The financial budget should include all the treatment elements in a detailed description, so the patient can be made aware of the forecast of the procedure as well. The patient should be also be aware of the possibility of altering the course of treatment at any time and its financial consequences and implications. One of the most crucial financial aspects in implantology is the financial implications of dental implant failure. A resolution plan should be made and signed by the patient that details the rights of the patient should implant failure occur. This exit plan minimizes to a great extent the medicolegal problems that would arise and sets the basis for post-failure management. One example of this resolution plan is that when an implant fails, a new implant will be placed at no cost to the patient (one-time replacement only). Another example is a refund made to the patient that is half of the amount paid previously, while another example is no compensation at all. All of these resolutions are acceptable provided that both parties have agreed prior to the start of the treatment.

Some clinicians prefer to cover the cost of the implant failure totally for failure during the first year post-restorative (if they have the prostheses completed in their office), while some prefer to include the patient in the responsibility for the failure on a split share basis, while others give a lifetime warranty for their work. The common chronic dilemma occurs when the surgical part of the dental implant service is carried out in one office and the prosthetic work is performed in another office. Fabricating an esthetic implant-supported prosthesis is unlike fabricating a merely functioning implant-supported prosthesis, as the first may involve a higher treatment cost, due to the possibility of using tooth-colored abutments, laser-milled abutments, or performing extra corrective surgeries. The fact that there are clinicians who charge higher fees for their esthetic rehabilitative cases than for regular cases is then explained. An anterior implant-supported prosthesis invariably requires the clinician to spend more time, effort, and skill than replacements in the posterior zone. Such clinicians probably undertook educational courses to learn more about restoring patients to give esthetically predictable results. Consequently they increase the overall cost of a single anterior implant-supported restoration by up to one-third of the total cost; the time required for treatment completion eventually may be doubled. Therefore, the approximate time and cost required for each treatment option should be a distinctive part of the doctor–patient preoperative communication, which is then confirmed with a signed consent by the patient. It is also possible that the clinician selects a particular treatment plan, rather than following an objective approach, because he/she is capable of performing some procedures better than others. It is the clinician who is ultimately responsible for the treatment choice and its consequent results. Therefore, the clinician is urged to select a reasonable treatment option that both suits the patient's best interest and exploits the clinician's skills and training background. This indicates an individualized approach for each patient's treatment plan.

Treatment planning and acceptance of a plan are influenced to a large degree by the cost of treatment and the corresponding insurance coverage in some countries. The proposed treatment plan must be affordable to the patient and remunerative to the provider. In many situations, the sequencing of treatment is staged to maximize insurance coverage. While staged or quadrant dentistry has become the normal factor for treating patients who want to maximize insurance benefits, it does not always reflect the ideal approach or proper treatment sequence. For example, a patient with extensive dental needs and limited insurance benefits may desire to have the more visible anterior crowns completed first, although the posterior crowns may have a higher functional priority. Treating the anterior teeth first may be a mistake, especially if the patient does not follow through with the posterior crowns. A rational treatment plan cannot be subverted to meet unrealistic patient demands or to maximize insurance benefits. The public perception is that dental insurance should pay for the treatment of dental diseases; however, the reality is that most insurance plans provide inadequate benefits for effective treatment of dental diseases, whether the treatment is innovative or even considered the standard of care. The increase in the number of insurance plans and third-party payers clearly influences (and will continue to influence) the treatment planning process. A study by Brägger, Krenander and Lang (2005) assessed and compared the economic parameters of two treatment options in patients requiring single-tooth replacements. Thirty-seven patients received 41 conventional three-unit fixed partial dentures (FPDs). Fifty-two patients received 59 single crowns on implants. The treatment assignments for patients were not random. Economic parameters were noted for the preparatory phase, the actual reconstruction, and for treatment of biological and/or technical complications thereafter in a period from one to four years: number of visits, chair-side time, treatment costs, costs for implant components, and laboratory work. Results showed that the total treatment times were similar, laboratory costs were higher for FPD, and costs for treatment of technical and biological complications were similar. Even when considering opportunity costs for each visit, the implant solution was less expensive and costs for treatment of complications were similar in both situations.

References

Ahmad, I. (2010). Risk management in clinical practice. Part 5. Ethical considerations for dental enhancement procedures. *Br. Dent. J.* 209: 207–214.

Al-Omiri, M., Hantash, R.A., and Al-Wahadni, A. (2005). Satisfaction with dental implants: a literature review. *Implant. Dent.* 14 (4): 399–406.

Atkins, J.M. and Walsh, R.S. (1997). Developing shared learning in multiprofessional health care education: for whose benefit? *Nurse Educ. Today* 17: 319–324.

Balshi, T.J. and Garver, D.G. (1986). Osseointegration: the efficacy of the transitional denture. *Int. J. Oral Maxillofac. Implants* 1: 113–118.

Barnard, A., Greenfield, D., Corbett, A. et al. (2007). An action research protocol to strengthen system-wide interprofessional learning and practice. *Health Serv. Res.* 7: 144–154.

Barnsteiner, J.H., Disch, J.M., Hall, L. et al. (2007). Promoting interprofessional education. *Nurs. Outlook* 55: 144–150.

Barrington, D., Rodger, M., Gray, L. et al. (1998). Student evaluation of an interactive multi-disciplinary clinical learning model. *Med. Teach.* 20: 530–535.

Basten, C. (1995). The use of radiopaque templates for predictable implant placement. *Quintessence Int.* 26 (9): 609–612.

Bellini, D., Dos Santos, M.B., De Paula Prisco Da Cunha, V., and Marchini, L. (2009). Patients' expectations and satisfaction of complete denture therapy and correlation with locus of control. *J. Oral Rehabil.* 36: 682–686.

Bengazi, F., Wennstrom, L., and Lekholm, U. (1996). Recession of the soft tissue margin at oral implants: a 2-year longitudinal prospective study. *Clin. Oral Implants Res.* 7: 303–310.

Besimo, C. and Kempf, B. (1995). *In vitro* investigation of various attachments for overdentures on osseointegrated implants. *J. Oral Rehabil.* 22 (9): 691–698.

Biggs, W.F. (1996). Placement of a custom implant provisional restoration at the second-stage surgery for improved gingival management: a clinical report. *J. Prosthet. Dent.* 75: 231–233.

Brägger, U., Krenander, P., and Lang, N.P. (2005). Economic aspects of single-tooth replacement. *Clin. Oral Implants Res.* 3 (16): 335–341.

Brånemark, P.I., Adell, R., Breine, U. et al. (1969). Intra-osseous anchorage of dental prosthesis. I. Experimental studies. *Scand. J. Plast. Reconstr. Surg.* 3 (2): 81–100.

Breeding, L.C.I. and Dixon, D.L. (1995). A bonded provisional fixed prosthesis to be worn after implant surgery. *J. Prosthet. Dent.* 74 (1): 114–116.

Buser, D., Bragger, U., Lang, N.P., and Nyman, S. (1990). Regeneration and enlargement of jaw bone using guided tissue regeneration. *Clin. Oral Implants Res.* 1 (1): 22–32.

Caccianiga, G., Rey, G., Baldoni, M., and Paiusco, A. (2016). Clinical, radiographic and microbiological evaluation of high level laser therapy, a new photodynamic therapy protocol, in Peri-implantitis treatment; a pilot experience. *Biomed. Res. Int.* 2016: 6321906.

Charangowda, B.K. (2010). Dental records: an overview. *J. Forensic Dent. Sci.* 2 (1): 5–10.

Chaves, M., Araújo, A., Piancastelli, A., and Pinotti, M. (2014). Effects of low-power light therapy on wound healing: LASER x LED. *An. Bras. Dermatol.* 89 (4): 616–623.

Chichester, S.R., Wilder, R.S., Mann, G.B., and Neal, E. (2002). Incorporation of evidence based prnciples in baccalaureate and non-baccalaureate degree dental hygiene programs. *J. Dent. Hyg.* 76 (1): 60–66.

Cooper, H., Spencer-Dawe, E., and McLean, E. (2005). Beginning the process of teamwork: design, implementation and evaluation of an inter-professional education intervention for first year undergraduate students. *J. Interprof. Care* 19: 492–508.

Critchlow, S.B. and Ellis, J.S. (2010). Prognostic indicators for conventional complete denture therapy: a review of the literature. *J. Dent.* 38: 2–9.

Dar-Odeh, N., Ryalat, S., Shayyab, M., and Abu-Hammad, O. (2008). Analysis of clinical records of dental patients attending Jordan University Hospital: documentation of drug prescriptions and local anesthetic injections. *Ther. Clin. Risk Manag.* 4: 1111–1117.

David, A., Garber, A., and Salama, M.A. (2000). The aesthetic smile: diagnosis and treatment. *Periodontology* 11 (1): 18–28.

De Bruyn, H., Collaert, B., Linden, U. et al. (1997). Patient's opinion and treatment outcome of fixed rehabilitation on Branemark implants. A 3-year follow-up study in private dental practices. *Clin. Oral Implants Res.* 8 (4): 265–271.

Deeb, G.R., Allen, R.K., Hall, V.P. et al. (2017). How accurate are implant surgical guides produced with desktop stereolithographic 3-dimentional printers? *J. Oral Maxillofac. Surg.* 75 (12): 2559.

Derhalli, M. (2013). The digitalizing of implant dentistry: a clinical evaluation of 15 patients. *Compend. Contin. Educ. Dent.* 34 (3): 192–196.

Devadiga, A. (2014). What's the deal with dental records for practicing dentists? Importance in general and forensic dentistry. *J. Forensic Dent. Sci.* 6 (1): 9–15.

Dirhold, B., Citak, M., Al-Khateeb, H. et al. (2012). Current state of computer-assisted trauma surgery. *Curr. Rev. Musculoskelet. Med.* 5 (3): 184–191.

Elaskary, A.S. (2003). Introduction. In: *Reconstructive Aesthetic Implant Surgery*. Iowa State press, Black well Science 3–5.

Elaskary, A.S. (2008). Contemporary Facial Evaluation. In: *Fundamentals of Esthetic Implant Dentistry*. Blackwell publishing –John Wiley 79–108.

Elaskary, A.S. (1999). Esthetic considerations in anterior single tooth replacement. *Implant. Dent.* 8: 61–67.

Elaskary, A.S., Meffert, R.M., and Griffin, T. (1999). Identifying the reasons for implant failure. *Dent. Abstr.* 44 (5): 202.

Engelman, M.J., Sorensen, J.A., and Moy, P. (1988). Optimum placement of osseointegrated implants. *J. Prosthet. Dent.* 59: 467–473.

Esposito, M., Ekestubbe, A., and Gröndahl, K. (1993). Radiogical evaluation of marginal bone loss at tooth surfaces facing single Brånemark implants. *Clin. Oral Implants Res.* 4: 151–157.

Fong Ha, J., Ana, D., and Longnecker, N. (2010). Doctor-patient communication: a review. *Ochsner J.* (1): 38–43.

Garber, D.A. (1995). The esthetic dental implant: letting the restoration be the guide. *J. Am. Dent. Assoc.* 126: 319–325.

Garbin, C.A., Garbin, J.A., Saliba, N.A. et al. (2008). Analysis of the ethical aspects of professional confidentiality in dental practice. *J. Appl. Oral Sci.* 16: 75–80.

Gargiulo, A.W., Wentz, F.M., and Orban, B. (1961). Dimensions and relations of the dentogingival junction in humans. *J. Periodontol.* 32: 261–267.

Glickman, I. (1972). *Clinical Periodontology*, 4e. Philadelphia: W.B. Saunders.

Gouvossis, J. (1997). Cross infection from periodontitis site to failing implants sites in the same mouth. *J Oral Maxillofac. Implants* 12: 666–673.

Grunder, U. (2000). Stability of the mucosal topography around single tooth implants and adjacent teeth: 1 year results. *Int. J. Periodontics Restorative Dent.* 20: 11–17.

Han, K.H., Lee, J.Y., and Shin, S.W. (2016). Implant- and tooth-supported fixed prostheses using a high-performance polymer (Pekkton) framework. *Int. J. Prosthodont.* 29 (5): 451–454.

Israelson, H., Plemons, J.M., Watkins, P., and Sory, C. (1992). Barium coated surgical stents and computer assisted tomography in the preoperative assessment of dental implant patients. *Int. J. Periodontics Restorative Dent.* 12 (1): 52–61.

Jemt, T. (1997). Regeneration of gingiva papillae after single implant treatment. *Int. J. Periodontics Restorative Dent.* 17: 327–333.

Jemt, T. and Lie, A. (1994). Mucosal topography around implants in edentulous upper jaws. Photogrammetric three-dimensional measurements of the effect of replacement of a removable prosthesis with a fixed prosthesis. *Clin. Oral Implants Res.* 5: 220–228.

Jessri, M. and Fatemitabar, S.A. (2007). Implication of ethical principles in chair-side dentistry. *Iran. J. Allergy Asthma Immunol.* 6 (Suppl. 5): 53–59.

Jiffry, M.T. (2002). Multiprofessional and continuing education of health professionals. *Asia Pac. J. Public Health* 14: 40–43.

Jivraj, S. and Chee, W. (2006). Treatment planning of implants in the aesthetic zone. *Br. Dent. J.* 201: 77–89.

Jurič, I. and Anić, I. (2014). The use of lasers in disinfection and cleanliness of root canals: a review. *Acta Stomatol. Croat.* 48 (1): 6–15.

Kamimura, E., Tanaka, S., Takaba, M. et al. (2017). In vivo evaluation of inter-operator reproducibility of digital dental and conventional impression techniques. *PLoS One* 12 (6): e0179188.

Kao, R.T., Curtis, D.A., Richards, D.W., and Preble, J. (1995). Increased interleukin B in the cervicular fluid of diseased implants. *Int. J. Oral Maxillofac. Implants* 10: 696–701.

Karatas, O. and Toy, E. (2014). Three-dimensional imaging techniques: a literature review. *Eur. J. Dent.* 8 (1): 132–140.

Karunakaran, T., Gilbert, D., Asimakopoulou, K., and Newton, T. (2011). The influence of visible dental caries on social judgements and overall facial attractiveness among undergraduates. *J. Dent.* 39: 212–217.

Kassem, S. (2011). *Rise Up and Salute the Sun: The Writings of Suzy Kassem*. Dubai: Awakened Press.

Kazor, C.E., Al-Shammari, K.,.a., Sarment, D.P. et al. (2004). Implant plastic surgery: a review and rationale. *J. Oral Implantol.* 30 (4): 240–254.

Kennedy, J., Bird, W., Palcanis, K., and Dorfman, H. (1985). A longitudinal evaluation of varying widths of attached gingiva. *J. Clin. Periodontol.* 12: 667–675.

Lawney, M. (1998). For the record. Understanding patient recordkeeping. *NY State Dent. J.* 64: 34–43.

Leffler, W.G. (2008). How do I justify my views on what I consider unnecessary treatment. *J. Am. Dent. Assoc.* 139: 1546.

Levi, A., Psoter, W.J., Agar, J.R. et al. (2003). Patient self-reported satisfaction with maxillary anterior dental implant treatment. *Int. J. Oral Maxillofac. Implants* 18: 113–120.

Mecall, R.A. and Rosenfeld, A.L. (1996). Influence of residual ridge resorption patterns on fixture placement and tooth position, part III: presurgical assessment of ridge augmentation requirements. *Int. J. Periodontics Restorative Dent.* 16 (4): 322–327.

Mezger, U., Jendrewski, C., and Bartels, M. (2013). Navigation in surgery. *Langenbeck's Arch. Surg.* 398 (4): 501–514.

Minoretti, R., Merz, B.R., and Triaca, A. (2000). Predetermined implant positioning by means of a novel guide template technique. *Clin. Oral Implants Res.* 11: 266–272.

Misch, C.M. (1997). Comparison of intraoral donor sites for onlay grafting prior to implant placement. *Int. J. Oral Maxillofac. Implants* 12 (6): 767–776.

Morgan, R.G. (2001). Quality evaluation of clinical records of a group of general dental practitioners entering a quality assurance programme. *Br. Dent. J.* 191: 436–441.

Mörmann, W., Stawarczyk, B., Ender, A. et al. (2013). Wear characteristics of current aesthetic dental restorative CAD/CAM materials: two-body wear, gloss retention, roughness and Martens hardness. *J. Mech. Behav. Biomed. Mater.* 20: 113–125.

Nash, D.A. (1988). Professional ethics and esthetic dentistry. *J. Am. Dent. Assoc.* 117 (4): 7E–9E.

Nelson, G.V. (1989). Guidelines to the prevention of problems in recordkeeping. Part 1. *Pediatr. Dent.* 11: 174–177.

Nemcovsky, C.E., Moses, I., and Artzi, Z. (2000). Interproximal papillae reconstruction in maxillary. *J. Periodontol.* 71: 308–314.

Newsome, P.R. and Wright, G.H. (1999). A review of patient satisfaction: 2. Dental patient satisfaction: an appraisal of recent literature. *Br. Dent. J.* 186: 166–170.

Oberbreckling, P.J. (1993). The components of quality dental records. *Dent. Econ.* 83: 29–38.

Ochsenbein, C. and Ross, S. (1973). A concept of osseous surgery and its clinical applications. In: *A Periodontal Point of View* (ed. H.L. Ward and C. Chas). Springfield, IL: Charles C. Thomas.

O'Leary, T.J., Drake, R.B., Crump, P.P., and Allen, M.F. (1971). The incidence of recession in young males: a further study. *J. Periodontol.* 42: 264–267.

Olson, M. and Lindhe, J. (1991). Periodontal characteristics in individuals with varying forms of the upper central incisors. *J. Clin. Periodontol.* 18: 78–82.

Olson, M., Lindhe, I., and Marinello, C.P. (1992). On the relationship between crown form and clinical features of the gingiva in adolescents. *J. Clin. Periodontol.* 20: 570–577.

Orchard, C.A. (2010). Persistent isolationist or collaborator? The nurse's role in interprofessional collaborative practice. *J. Nurs. Manag.* 18 (3): 248–257.

Osborn, J.B., Stoltenberg, J.L., Newell, K.J., and Osborn, S.C. (2000). Adequacy of dental records in clinical practice: a survey of dentists. *J. Dent. Hyg.* 744: 297–306.

Palacci, P. (2000). Optimal implant positioning. In: *Esthetic Implant Dentistry. Soft and Hard Tissue Management* (ed. P. Palacci and I. Erecsson), 101–111. Berlin: Quintessence.

Pesun, I.J. (1997). Fabrication of a guide for non-radiographic evaluation of bone contour. *J. Prosthet. Dent.* 77: 621–623.

Phillips, G.E. and John, V. (2005). Use of a subepithelial connective tissue graft to treat an area pigmented with graphite. *J. Periodontal.* 76: 1572–1575.

Rhee, Y., Huh, Y., Cho, L., and Park, C. (2015). Comparison of intraoral scanning and conventional impression techniques using 3-dimensional superimposition. *J. Adv. Prosthodont.* 7 (6): 460–467.

Rittersma, J., Casparie, A.F., and Reerink, E. (1980). Patient information and patient preparation in orthognathic surgery: a medical audit study. *J. Oral Maxillofac. Surg.* 8: 206–209.

Rochette, A.L. (1986). Attachment of a splint to enamel of lower anterior teeth. *J. Prosthet. Dent.* (56): 416–421.

Rustemeyer, J. and Martin, A. (2013). Soft tosdur response in orthognathic surgery patients treated by bimaxillary osteotomy: cephalometry compared with 2D photogrammetry. *Oral Maxillofac. Surg.* 17 (1): 33–41.

Sanderink, G.C.H., Dula, K., Huiskens, R. et al. (1997). *The Loss of Image Quality in Digital Panoramic Radiography Using Image Compression*, 299–305. Elsevier.

Sanz, M., Alandez, J., Lazaro, P. et al. (1991). Histopathologic characteristices of peri-implant soft tissues in Branemark implants with 2 distinct clinical and radiological patterns. A histometric and ultrastructural study. *Clin. Oral Implants Res.* 128–134.

Schwarz, F., Schmucker, A., and Becker, J. (2015). Efficacy of alternative or adjunctive measures to conventional treatment of peri-implant mucositis and peri-implantitis: a systematic review and meta-analysis. *Int. J. Implant. Dent.* 1 (1): 22.

Shavell, H.M. (1979). Mastering the art of provisionalization. *CDA J.* 44–51.

Shin, S., Kim, Y., Kwak, H. et al. (2011). 3D tracking of surgical instruments using a single camera for laparoscopic surgery simulation. *Stud. Health Technol. Inform.* 163: 581–587.

Simonsen, R. (2007). Commerce vs care: troubling trends in ethics of aesthetic dentistry. *Dent. Clin. N. Am.* 281–287.

Soballe, K., Hansen, E.S., Brockstedt-Rasmussen, H. et al. (1990). Hydroxyapatite coating enhances fixation of porous coated implants. *Acta Orthop. Scand.* 61 (4): 299–306.

Soldz, S. and Vaillant, G.E. (1999). The big five personality traits and the life course: a 45-year longitudinal study. *J. Res. Pers.* 33: 208–232.

Somani, A., Newton, J.T., Dunne, S., and Gilbert, D.B. (2010). The impact of visible dental decay on social judgements: comparison of the effects of location and extent of lesion. *Int. Dent. J.* 60: 169–174.

Sutton, S. (2015). Qualitative research: data collection, analysis, and management. *Can. J. Hosp. Pharm.* 68 (3): 226–231.

Swihart, D. (2016). Finding common ground: interprofessional collaborative practice competencies in patient-centered medical homes. *Nurs. Adm. Q.* 40 (2): 103–108.

Tarnow, D. and Eskow, R.N. (1995). Preservation of implant esthetics: soft and restorative considerations. *J. Esthet. Dent.* (8): 12–19.

Tarnow, D., Elian, N., Fletcher, P. et al. (2003). Vertical distance from the crest of bone to the height of the interproximal papilla between adjacent implants. *J. Periodontol.* 74 (12): 1785–1788.

Terry, D.A. and Geller, W. (2013). *Esthetic and Restorative Dentistry: Material Selection and Technique.* Hanover Park, IL: Quintessence Publishing.

Valenzuela, A., Martin-de las Heras, S., Marques, T. et al. (2000). The application of dental methods of identification to human burn victims in a mass disaster. *Int. J. Legal Med.* 113: 236–239.

Verdi, M.A. and Morgano, S.M. (1993). A dual-purpose stent for the implant-supported prosthesis. *J. Prosthet. Dent.* 69: 276–280.

Waitzkin, H. (1984). Doctor-patient communication. Clinical implications of social scientific research. *JAMA* 252 (17): 2441–2446.

Waleed, P., Baba, F., Alsulami, S., and Tarakji, B. (2015). Importance of dental records in forensic dental identification. *Acta Inform Med.* 23 (1): 49–52.

Widmann, G. (2007). Image-guided surgery and medical robotics in the cranial area. *Biomed. Imaging Interv. J.* 3 (1): e11.

Williams, V.D., Thayer, K.E., Denehy, G.E., and Boyer, D.B. (1989). Cast metal, resin bonded prosthesis: a 10-year retrospective study. *J. Prosthet. Dent.* 61: 436–441.

Yuzbasioglu, E., Kurt, H., Turunc, R., and Bilir, H. (2014). Comparison of digital and conventional impression techniques: evaluation of patients' perception, treatment comfort, effectiveness and clinical outcomes. *BMC Oral Health* 14: 10.

Zarb, G.A. and Schmitt, A. (1990). The longitudinal clinical effectiveness of osseointegrated dental implants: the Toronto study. Part III: problems and complications encountered. *J. Prosthet. Dent.* 64: 185–194.

2

Extraoral Clinical Reflections

2.1 Value of a Smile to Human Beings

Smiles…

> There is a Smile of love, and there is a smile of deceit, and there is a smile of smiles, in which these two smiles meet. It only once smiled can be. But when it once is smiled, there's an end to all misery.
>
> *Blake (1908)*

> A smile is a frown turned upside down. A smile is painted on the face of a clown. A smile brightens a dreary day. A smile chases tears away. A smile is a gift that shows you care. A smile is priceless no matter where. A smile is the key to happiness. A smile is a sure sign of success. If there is any real magic around. It's the silent magic of smile's sound.
>
> *Hearth (1986)*

> The smile that is worth the praises of earth is the smile is the smile that shines through the tears.
>
> *Ella Wheeler Wilcox (1995)*

> An important aspect of social behavior, a smile, is facial expression, as it contains valuable information that may influence an interaction.
>
> *Fridlund (1994)*

From the facial expression of an opponent, one may infer not only emotional states (Ekman, Friesen and Ellsworth 1982) but also information regarding intentions, personality, and complex social characteristics (Horstmann, Lorenz and Egelhaaf 2003). A smiling expression of an opponent infers intentions such as trust, cooperation, or affiliation, therefore facilitating an approach behavior. By contrast, an angry facial expression might be interpreted as threatening, spiteful, or malicious and associated with intentions such as rejection or causing damage, which subsequently might facilitate avoidance behavior (Horstmann et al. 2003). Therefore, we expect that facial expressions have a direct influence on decision-making, as seen in Figure 2.1a and b.

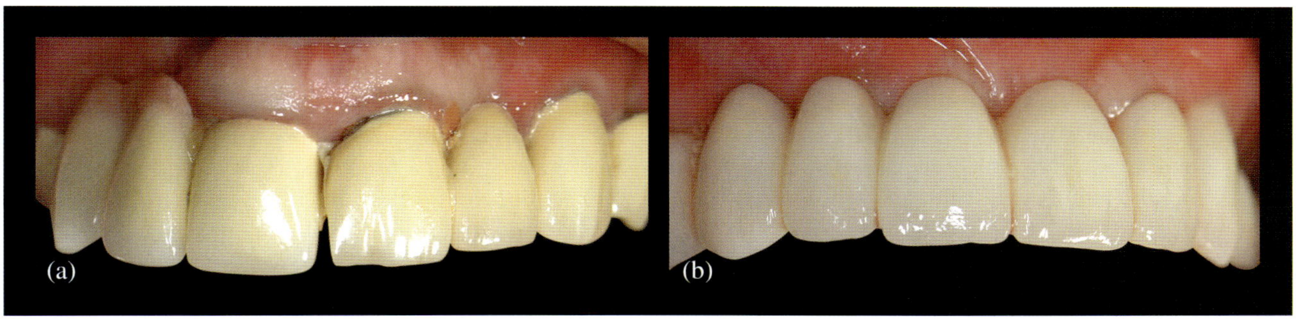

Figure 2.1 (a) Preoperative and (b) and postoperative result using dental implant knowledge (regenerative and restorative) to repair lost smile and contours to enhance the patient's own smile.

Advances in Esthetic Implant Dentistry, First Edition. Abdelsalam Elaskary.

Companion website: www.wiley.com/go/elaskary/esthetic

A smile begins in our sensory nerves. The emotional data funnels to the brain, exciting the left anterior temporal region in particular, then smolders to the surface of the face, where two muscles, standing at attention, are roused into action: the zygomatic major and the orbicularis oculi (Abel and Kruger 2010). Other muscles can simulate a smile, but only the peculiar tango of the zygomatic major and the orbicularis oculi produces a genuine expression of positive emotion (Bernstein et al. 2010). Psychologists call this the "Duchenne smile," and most consider it the sole indicator of true enjoyment. The name is a nod to French anatomist Guillaume Duchenne, who studied emotional expression by stimulating various facial muscles with electrical currents (Duchenne 1990).

Variables such as age, gender, culture, and social setting influence the smile pattern, while scientists have learned that one of humanity's simplest expressions is beautifully complex (Mehua, Grammerb and Dunbara 2007) as seen in Figures 2.2 and 2.3a, b.

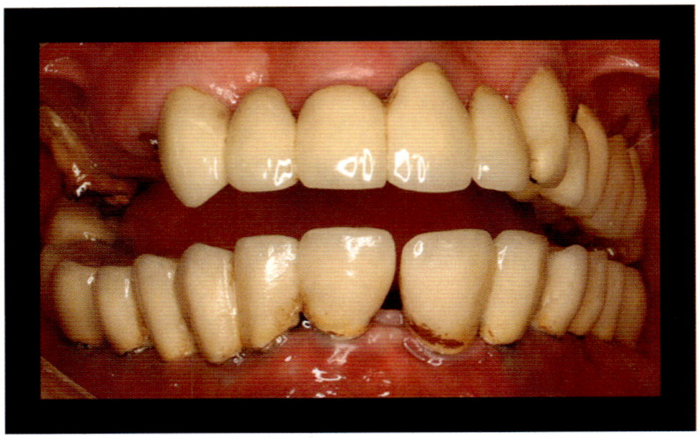

Figure 2.2 An example of poor prosthetic design that lacks the duplication of natural tooth anatomy and distorts the overall esthetic appearance.

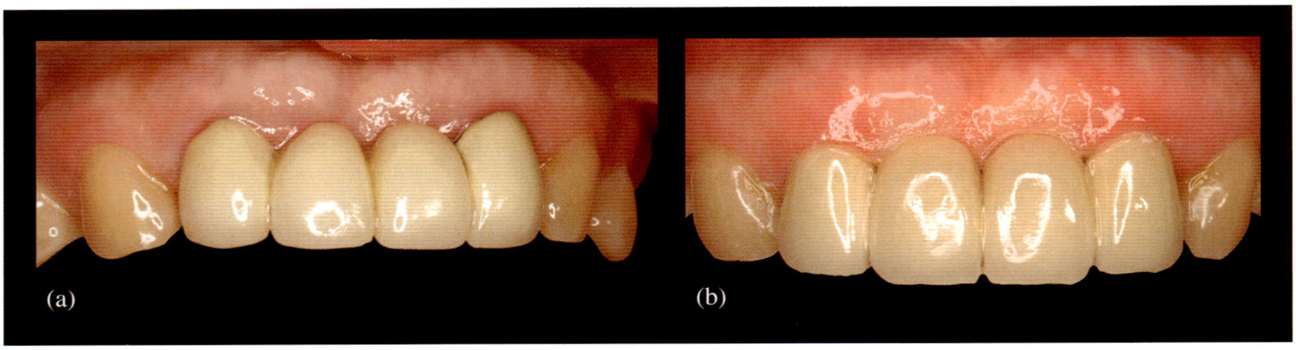

Figure 2.3 (a) Poor implant supported restoration anatomy as well as pontic design. (b) Restoration replaced that enhances the patient's overall appearance, teeth display, smile arch, and pontic ridge relation.

2.1.1 Human Face

The human face is a unique part of the human body; it is created miraculously with a very delicate unique perfection and is made from a gathering of balanced proportionate elements of various sized parts put together in harmony. The proportional relationships between the dental anatomy and the morphological features of the face deserve the attention of clinicians who seek perfect intraoral esthetic restorative therapy. However, the infinite variations of the human face usually become a limiting factor because there are no limits to the available facial classes and the variations are numerous and unlimited (a true miracle in life), and emotional drives come on top of that to make the assessment more complex. The facial organs that constitute a human smile are also in abundance; the cheeks, nose, nasal bridge, chin, eyes, eyebrows, forehead, zygomatic arch, lips, and displayed teeth are considered to be the variables that govern facial appearance. In addition, race, skin color, and character contribute to the final overall picture. That makes the overall clinical assessment for any smile a mere personal perception rather than a step-by-step methodology (Elaskary 2008).

Many attempts have been made to relate a proportional relationship between dental anatomy and facial anatomy before concluding a proportional relationship. Although these ratios were often practically applied, they sometimes deviate from reality in many clinical instances, probably due to the numerous variations of facial patterns (Rufenacht 1990a). Until now, the orofacial complex has been a prime challenge for both dentists and cosmetic surgeons. Many clinicians consider the facial complex as a separate entity from the dental complex, although they are linked together, because many dentists performing major esthetic reconstruction jobs focus on the intraoral parameters only, while, on the other hand, cosmetic surgeons focus only on the extraoral clinical parameters and the facial structure, which makes the overall cosmetic job incomplete. Therefore, the demand for combining the two entities in one treatment plan becomes a logical request, and in fact any treatment plan should be able to achieve the delicate balance and harmony of the relationship between the extraoral and the intraoral features.

Usually patients that seek major reconstructive esthetic rehabilitation have certain personal expectations; these expectations revolve around the improvement in the way they look, specifically the way they smile and how their smile can become prettier, younger, and healthier. They do not particularly pay attention to the quality or the precision of manufacturing of the new dental restoration itself, but rather on how it affects their overall appearance (A. Ameed (2001), Personal communication, London, United Kingdom). This becomes a valuable vision for performing a successful comprehensive treatment plan. Therefore, achieving patients' desires requires meticulous assessment of the face and smile and its inclusion in the original treatment plan, as any treatment plan that seeks comprehensive esthetics cannot omit the role of the facial balance within it. Subsequently, evaluation of smile patterns becomes a prime concern in the treatment of major oral rehabilitation procedures. An in-depth analysis of facial morphology as related to the future dental assembly should be performed, that is, lip anatomy (Hulsey 1970), thickness, line, and curvature. Other related landmarks like the nasolabial angle, intercommissure line, smile arc, Burstone line (Burstone 1967), Steiner line (Weickersheimer 1995), and the Ricketts E plane (Viazis 1991) should also be evaluated and included in the treatment plan.

Other elements that complement facial beauty and contribute to its character include: the size of the cheeks, nasal bridge continuity, overall nose size, the shape and size of the chin, eye width, color, and volume, the extent of eye brow elevation, forehead size, and zygomatic arch prominence. Therefore, learning about the facial landmarks, identifying smile patterns, detecting the extent of teeth display, and observing the details of the patient's facial composition become valuable for esthetic restorative therapy. Most of this information should be gathered during verbal communication with the patient and preferably surreptitiously during the assessment procedure, to avoid patients exaggerating their facial reactions when they are asked to reveal it.

Other factors like patient character, profession, social standard, and treatment expectations should be also noted; this information should assist in the overall assessment of the treatment protocol. The evidence that relates the intraoral condition to the extraoral condition is the effect of teeth loss on the facial features: the consequences of teeth loss on the face have been described by Misch (2005a) as a decrease in facial height, loss of the labiomental angle, deepening of vertical lines of the face, the chin rotating forward and creating a prognathic facial appearance, a decrease in the horizontal labial angle at the corner of the lips, thinning of the vermillion border of the lips, the loss of overall tonicity of the muscles involved in facial expression, deepening of the nasolabial groove, an increase in the depth of the columella philtrum angle that usually accompanies these changes, which can make the nose appear larger in size, the loss of muscle attachments leading to ptosis of the chin (witch's chin) and a reversed lip line, and an increased lip angle under the nose. The effect of the teeth loss is also accumulative startings with teeth loss, then by bone loss, then alteration of muscle attachments, and consequent soft tissue loss (see Figure 2.4a and b).

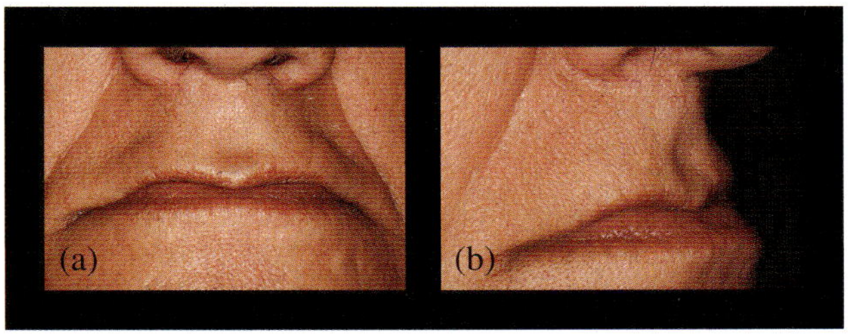

Figure 2.4 (a) and (b) The effect of the lost dentition on the human face.

2.2 Smile Art

The human smile does not possess any financial burden to any one, although it has a lot to celebrate; it enriches the soul of people through its tremendous effect, its effect consumes a moment, but it can last for many years engraved in someone's memory. A true smile creates happiness that does not differentiate between the intelligence and financial categories of the recipients and melts barriers among humankind. It is one of the mercies that we have been given and acquired in the fetus stage. Its value can be felt when it fades away. The human smile is defined in the literature as the changes in the facial musculature that occur as a result of the incumbent emotional state to the smile effect and the manner in which the lips, teeth, and silhouettes blend to create harmony that gives a smile its own unique magical character. The smile has many valuable benefits to people; its profound psychological effect on human beings explains its value. The most vivid of all our facial features is the smile, as it is an extension and expression of the person as a whole and is the way that facial expressions reveal a part of our daily basic non-verbal communication. The smile magnifies the beauty of the human face and gives the face its glamour. How many times have you seen faces that lack vitality but when a smile appears, it fills it full of life? The smile also reflects the virtues of the person's character. The smile can convey countless emotions, from the small grin of embarrassment to the wider smile of happiness and enchantment to the full-teeth dazzling smile of exhilaration. It may last for a fleeting moment or remain intense for quite a while, as it reveals the emotions of happiness and joy (Elaskary 2008).

During our daily patient's clinical assessment, the competent smile should be evaluated or reconstructed to attain four major components that complement each other, as stated by Morley (1997): (1) facial esthetics, which concerns evaluating the lips and facial muscles during speech, smiling, and laughter; (2) gingival esthetics, which concerns evaluating gingival health in terms of asymmetry or inflammation or blunted papillae; (3) microesthetics, which concerns evaluating tooth anatomy and their location within the arch as well as shade and characterization; and (4) macroesthetics, which concerns evaluating the relationship between the teeth and the orofacial structures. When someone expresses joy internally, the joyful feeling is expressed by the muscles of the face accordingly. The smile is expressed by muscular action around the lips in the inferior third of the face. Duchenne (1990) noted that the emotion of frank joy is expressed on the face by the combined contraction of the zygomaticus major muscle and the inferior portion of the orbicularis oculi muscle. The first muscle obeys the will, but the second is put into play only by the appropriate emotions. Fake joy or a deceitful laugh cannot provoke the contraction of the latter muscle. The muscles that are mainly responsible for the smile are: levator labii superioris, which is responsible for raising the upper lip; the zygomaticus major and levator anguli, which are responsible for lifting the corners of the mouth up; the depressor anguli oris, which pushes down the corners of the mouth; the risorius, which pulls the corners of the mouth sideways while laughing; the buccinator muscle, which pushes the cheeks against the teeth medially; the orbicularis oris, which provides the basis for the structure of the lips and functions as the opening-and-closing mechanism of the mouth; the mentalis muscle, which is responsible for elevating the chin skin upwards while laughing; and the depressor labii infreriors, which pushes the lower lip down.

It is worth mentioning that Gibson (1989) has developed a smile exercise program to develop and control facial muscles to improve someone's smile. In Gibson's first smile exercise, the patient stands or sits in front of a mirror and goes through the process of smiling. The patient progresses from a narrow smile to a larger one and then reverses the process. Each position is to be held for 10 seconds and repeated several times. In this isotonic exercise, the muscles are taken repeatedly through their entire range of movement. Another exercise is an isometric exercise that involves closing the smile against the resistance of the fingers, which increases the tone and strength of the muscles around the mouth. The patient makes a full smile and holds the corners of the mouth firmly with the fingers, then slowly closes the lips back to no smile, against the resistance of the fingers.

2.3 Smile Pattern

The amount of teeth displayed during smiling determines the type of smile. This statement fits all classification systems available for the smile, so this statement should probably be kept in mind while evaluating someone's smile. The clinician should learn how to detect the teeth revealed for any smile, thus distinguishing the type of smile. A group of people can share a smile upon any stimulus, but they might differ in the amount of teeth displayed during the smile itself. This characterizes each individual smile as a separate entity. Many factors control teeth display during the smile, including age, the tonicity of the facial muscles, the depth of the stimulant, length of the maxillary incisors, length of the lip, thickness of the lip, and the class of skeletal and dental occlusion. Ackerman et al. (1998) have classified the smile according to its very nature, as shown in Figure 2.5a and b. An enjoyment smile, which is used when experiencing real pleasure, is involuntary, attains maximum muscle contraction of the lips, and attains maximum gingival and tooth display. A social smile, which is used in greeting, is voluntary, unstrained, and a static facial expression, with moderate lip muscle contraction, and attains a slight amount of teeth and gingival display (Elaskary 2008).

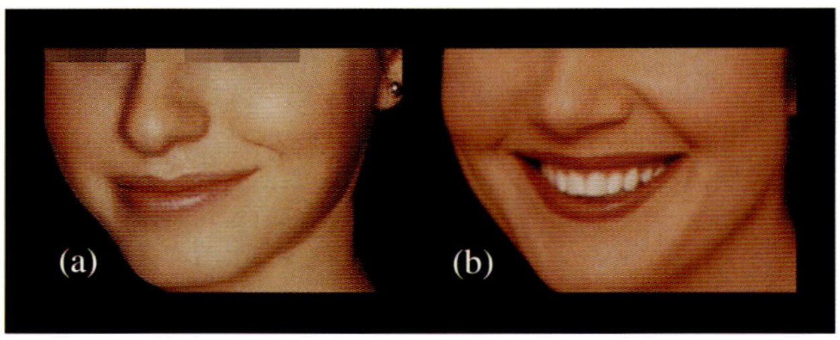

Figure 2.5 The difference between (a) social smile and (b) an enjoyment smile.

Another classification by Rubin (1974) was introduced to identify the smile according to the amount of teeth display: a maxillary smile showing only the maxillary teeth; a maxillary smile showing more than 3 mm of gingiva, also often referred to as a gummy smile; a solely mandibular smile; a smile with both maxillary and mandibular teeth appearing; and, lastly, a smile that shows neither maxillary nor mandibular teeth, as seen in Figure 2.6a–e.

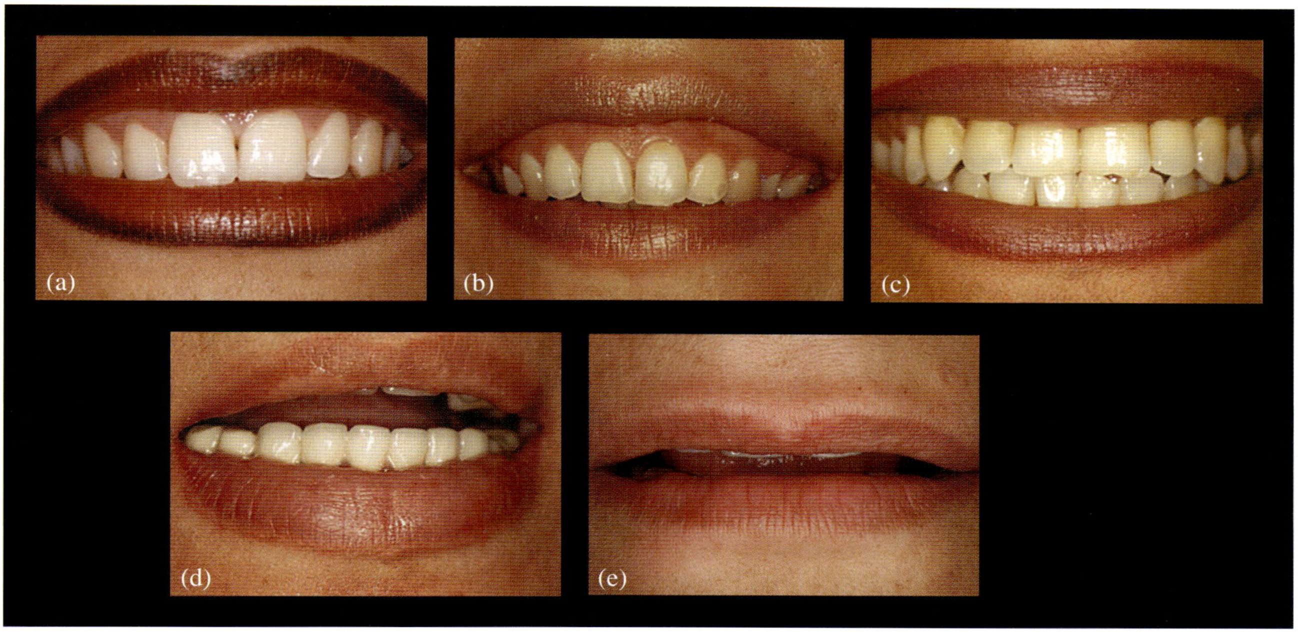

Figure 2.6 (a) Solely maxillary smile. (b) Maxillary smile with 3 mm of the gingiva. (c) Both maxillary and mandibular smile. (d) Solely mandibular smile. (e) Neither maxillary nor mandibular smile.

A smile line is defined by Philips (1990) as a line that shows a dark or negative space when both jaws separate. In other words, the silhouettes of the incisal edges of the maxillary teeth in comparison to the mandibular incisal edges can also define the smile line. The smile line can vary in shape; it is thought that it is frequently seen to be convex in females. The development of the smile, from the quarter smile, to the half-smile, to the full smile, in relation to the amount of tooth displayed will suggest to the clinician whether to display or hide the morphological deviation in tooth–gingival relationships (Hulsey 1970; Tjan and Miller 1984). In practice, the smile line is the lower margin of the upper lip that limits the visibility of the teeth; it follows the edges of the maxillary anterior teeth and the curvature of the inner border of the lower lip. Rufenacht (1990b) described the ideal smile line as one that is achieved when the angles of the mouth are parallel to the bipupillary line and the occlusal plane, with the tips of the canines barely touching the lower lip. When the lower lip curves upward and posteriorly to the corner of the mouth where it meets the upper lip, the viewer's attention is drawn to the dentition that is framed in the upward curve of the lips. As the viewer's eye is attracted to the elevation of the lower lip, it is focusing on the occlusal and incisal planes. Frush and Fisher (1985) have directed attention toward the smile line as the harmony between the curvature of the incisal edges of the maxillary anterior teeth and the upper border of the lower lip while Hulsey (1970) found that the smile line ratio – the congruency of the arc of curvature of the upper border of the lower lip and the arc of curvature of the incisal edges of the maxillary anterior teeth – appeared to be important in an attractive smile, and the most attractive smile displayed a smile line ratio of 1.00 : 1.25. Tjan and Miller (1984) reported that an average smile exhibits the full length of the maxillary anterior teeth, displays an incisal curve of the maxillary teeth that is parallel to the inner curvature of the lower lip, and displays the six maxillary anterior teeth and the premolars. Prior to any esthetic comprehensive therapy, the information about the position, shape, and size of the original dentition and its surrounding facial tissues is vital in restoring a patient's smile and should be collected. Rubin (1974) stated that there are three basic styles of smiles. A commissure smile is the most common type (67%); the corners of the mouth are initially pulled upward and outward, followed by rising of the upper lip to exhibit only the maxillary teeth. A cupid smile, occurring in 31% of the population, exposes the canines and then the corners of the mouth. A complex smile, however, appears in only 2% of the population; it shows all the maxillary and mandibular teeth simultaneously during elevation of the upper lip and contraction of the lower lip (Elaskary 2008).

Prior to esthetic comprehensive therapy, the information about the position, shape, and size of the original dentition and its surrounding facial tissues that is vital in restoring a patient's smile should be collected. The role of the clinician in smile analysis is to comprehend the patient's desire and expectations from the treatment, then to gather information about the cause of an esthetic or functional problem, such as trauma, faulty dentistry, pathological reasons, or others. Photography can be of great assistance in examining the facial features during speech and laughter in paused positions. A complete understanding of the patient's desires, personality, and psychological state will result in greater patient satisfaction (Levin 1988).

2.4 Smile Design

Smile design is a recent term that was introduced by Morley (1997). He defined the smile design as a discipline involving the diagnosis and subsequent planning primarily for the esthetic component of the overall dental treatment. In other words, smile designing is the enhancement of the amount of tooth display during smiling, using the available tools and applying the principles of design to anterior dental esthetics. This approach can turn an average restorative job into an outstanding one, while at the same time preserving the existing natural beauty (Golub-Evans 1994) (see Figure 2.7a–d).

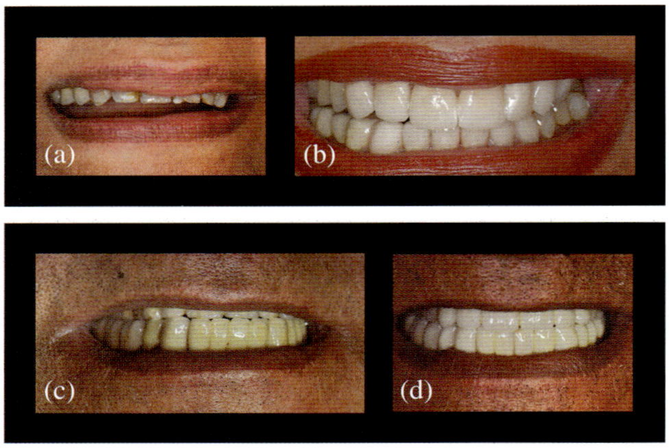

Figure 2.7 (a) and (b) An example of enhancing a patient's smile using the smile design concept. (c) and (d) Another example of enhancing a patient's smile using the smile design concept.

Esthetic factors that contribute to smile design and can be influenced in the treatment include the incisal and occlusal plane, size and inclination of the central incisors, midline position, axial alignment of the remaining teeth, size and form of the arch, lip line to the incisal edge position, form and morphology of the dentition, position of the contact points, and gingival height, zenith color, and contour (Dickerson 1996; Moskowitz and Nayyar 1995; Rufenacht 1990c). The patient's character and their life-style also can influence the treatment to some extent.

The clinician's own personal artistic abilities and subjective tools to individualize each treatment plan distinguish an excellent clinician from an average one. Therefore, smile design should focus more on an individualized approach that allows each restoration to be designed according to a particular individual's needs and that provides balance and harmony with the functional demands. Smile harmony can be achieved when the various lines, proportions, and structures are in visual balance with each other (Gwinnett 1992). A smile can be changed slightly by altering these proportions, creating illusions, and minimizing the negative visual tension produced by improperly aligned teeth, gingiva, and the lips (Moskowitz and Nayyar 1995). When attempting to perform smile design, one must consider teeth not as a separate component but rather as a part of the entire facial structure.

The concept of esthetics has been explored by various authors and discussed by eminent philosophers. While their definitions are subjective, they all agree on the natural origin of the term "esthetics." For this reason, it is believed that the real objective of esthetic dentistry must be imitating nature, which is so simple to perceive yet so difficult to copy, particularly as regards the esthetics of the lower third of the face. The skill and visual perception of the dental team are essential in pursuing this goal, and the dentist acts as architect and artisan of the oral and periodontal tissue by molding the physiology of the smile.

Dental surgery is increasingly being forced to adopt a multidisciplinary approach to treating the face and smile, in which the clinician plays an influential role. A balance between the teeth, interoral, and perioral tissue, face, smile, and person creates an esthetic ideal, and synergizes the artistic capacities and the expertise necessary to see the design in the context of the face. At present esthetics is increasingly linked to measure, proportion, and symmetry, which were already present in ancient civilizations but today have been considerably perfected by the digital age. Modern scientific knowledge puts various therapeutic options at the disposal of professionals. This along with collaboration between different specialists (orthodontists, implantologists, periodontologists, dental technicians, maxillofacial surgeons, and plastic and cosmetic surgeons) enables a treatment plan to be developed with ever-greater precision (see Figure 2.8).

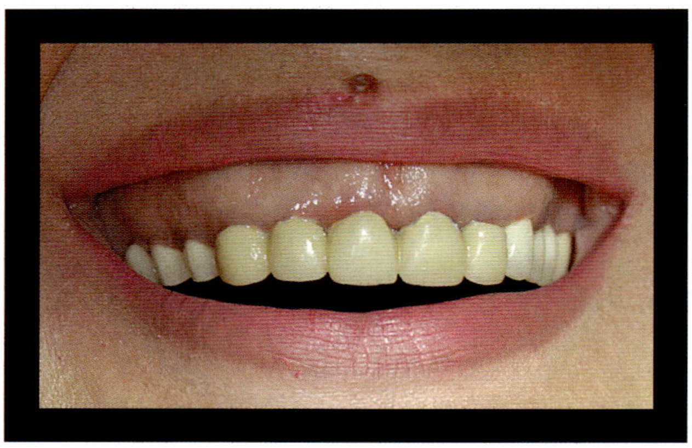

Figure 2.8 Excessive gingival display treated showing reduction of the excessive teeth display.

Digital dentistry had added a new horizon to smile design, often called digital smile design. Today, the use of 2D and 3D software for editing photographs and digital images allows us to process data and customize parameters for each specific clinical and esthetic requirement of the smile makeover. Modern digital technology that is implemented daily into the life of the clinician, is fundamental to the success of digital smile design. *The Digital Smile Design* is a multi-use tool that can assist the restorative team throughout treatment, improving the dental team's understanding of the esthetic issues and increasing patient acceptance of the result (Coachman et al. 2012). Digital smile design offers a more predictable outcome for the patient, for both the final esthetic results and the course of therapy agreed upon to acheive it. The combination of terms such as "esthetic dentistry," "interdisciplinary vision," "digital dentistry," and "predictability" even led to the consideration of a new professional figure, "the smile designer," whose fundamental role would be communicating with the patient and the esthetics medical team, whose members are crucial in virtual planning (Coachman, Calamita and Sesma 2017), as shown in Figure 2.9a–d. Using various software platforms, clinicians have pursued the development of a protocol for Aesthetic Digital Smile Design (ADSD) (Tak On and Kois 2016) to be used alongside other important diagnostic elements useful for diagnosis and prognosis, ultimately to improve the health and well-being of the patient. Explaining to the patient detailed images, on the monitor, the before and after photographs allow an index of predictability and a point of comparison for the patient.

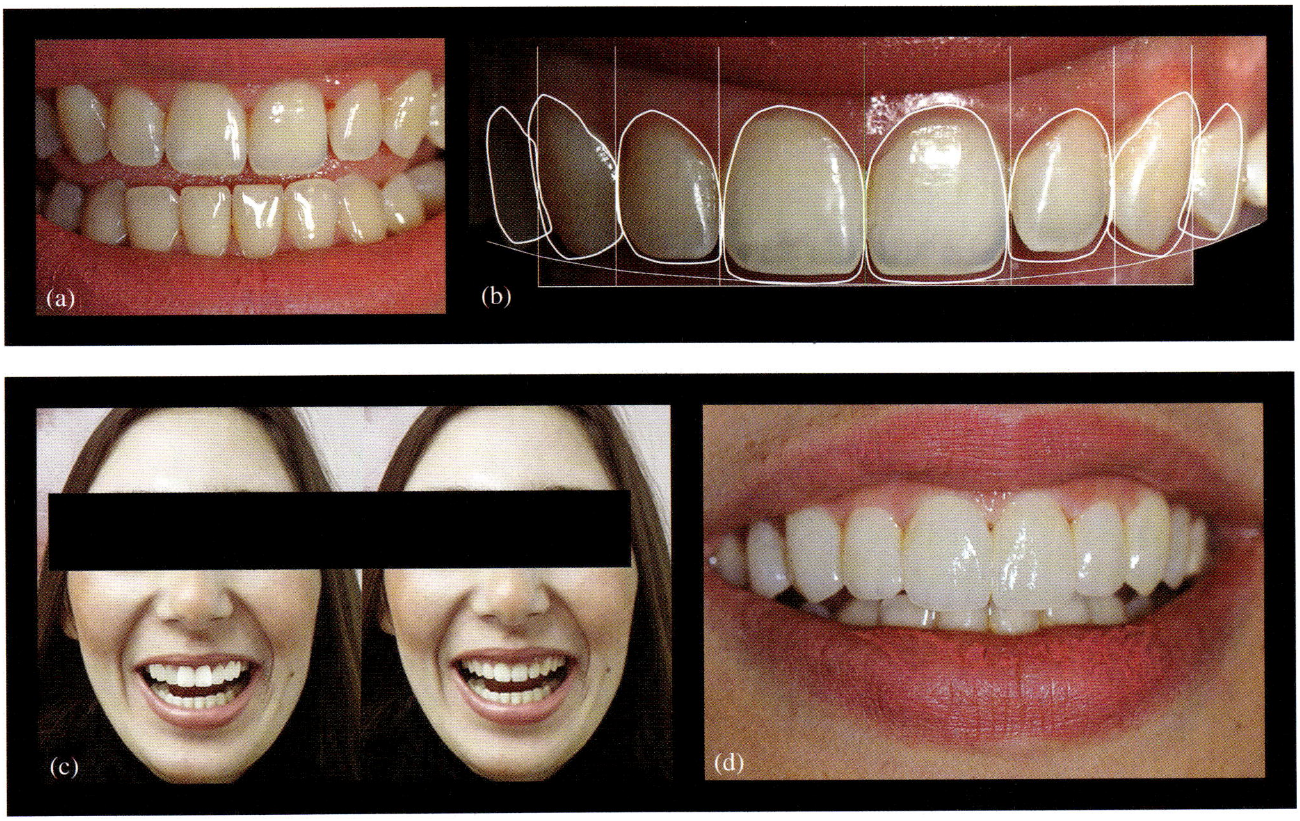

Figure 2.9 (a) Preoperative view of a patient who will receive smile design treatment. (b) The smile design is applied. *Source:* By courtesy of Dr. A. Radwan, Mansoura, Egypt. (c) Mock up trial intraorally. (d) Final case restored showing great enhancement of the patient overall looks.

The digital smile design protocol starts with the acquisition of full-frame digital images with specific views and video recordings of the patient (Coachman and Paravina 2016). A video recording is especially capable of capturing the dynamic phases of the smile linked to its physiology (mimicry, phonetics, relationship between the teeth and lips). Three basic photographic views are necessary: full face with a wide smile and the teeth apart, full face at rest, and retracted view of the full maxillary arch with teeth apart. A short video is also recommended in which the patient is prompted by the clinician to explain his or her treatment concerns and expectations. Simultaneously, the video should capture all possible dental and smile positions, including 45° and profile views (Coachman et al. 2017). Photographs should be taken with a regular SLR camera with semiprofessional features and with a good illumination system. The photographs and videos are downloaded and inserted into the slide presentation. Importing this vital data into the digital clinical file of the patient is an integral part of the intra- and extraoral objective examination and will subsequently be the subject of esthetic analysis along with the main guiding principles. Then comes the sketching phase, which involves drawing the facial reference lines and preferred teeth shapes on the digital photographs; at this phase the asymmetries, disharmonies, and violations of esthetic principles will be managed and corrected (Coachman et al. 2012).

The next phase in digital data processing is virtual planning using digital image editing, which can be implemented on either power point file or key note file, then the sketching phase that starts with the intraoral photograph adjusted to the three reference lines. Central incisor length/width proportion is measured followed by drawing the tooth outline, as guided by the rectangle proportion of the desired central incisor height. Other drawings can then be made, such as the smile arc formulation, to complete the esthetic plan. A digital ruler helps detect the exact size of the original teeth preoperatively, and the new shape of the future restoration in its actual size that will be transferred to the cast for wax up. More accurate and detailed measurements of the teeth and gingival parameters can be obtained by digital caliper, or digital ruler, whose tips are placed at the cervical margin and incisal edge (the length of the tooth) or at the mesial and distal margins relative to the dental line (width of the tooth). The measurements replicated to the wax-up are produced on the models to make the mock-up then tried in; this procedure ensures a high accuracy until the provisional and definitive restorations are fitted. The digital methodology used for photograph and image editing is very reliable, especially for communicating information during the ongoing clinical case to the dental laboratories.

2.5 Smile Landmarks

The specific areas of objective analysis that are pertinent to the clinical evaluation of the esthetics of the smile from that provided by various authors are:

- Facial analysis; frontal/lateral, determining morphological features, horizontal/vertical reference lines, vertical/horizontal facial proportions, golden ratio, horizontal/vertical dimensions, analysis of the facial profile, and analysis of the lips, nose, and eyes as regards position and size.
- Dental analysis; dental composition, dental arrangement and position, dimensions, proportions, shapes, contours, margins, textures, surfaces, axial inclinations, interincisal angles, interproximal contacts, and color.
- Dentolabial analysis; labial dynamics, smile line, width of smile, labial corridors, occlusal plane, midline, and interincisal and commissural lines.
- Phonetic analysis; this is complementary to the dentolabial analysis and involves recording the phonetics with particular attention to consonants and their combinations. In addition, the analysis of the phonemes "/m/" and "/i/" (sometimes also the phoneme "/e/") is of great importance for detecting and determining the position of the lips and the maxillary incisors relative to the age and sex of the subject being analyzed.
- Gingival analysis; architecture, shape parallelism, symmetry, zenith, papillae, biotype, and color.

Several clinical orofacial landmarks should be diagnosed and assessed when constructing a new smile or performing a smile design operation. These landmarks greatly influence the treatment outcome and the achievement of a natural smile, while avoiding the misbalance between intraoral and extraoral relationships. In any major reconstructive cases, these landmarks should be regarded if the clinician is willing to make a harmonious esthetic prosthesis (Elaskary 2008).

2.5.1 Intercommissure Line

The intercommissure line (ICL) is an imaginary line that is drawn through the corners of the mouth. It connects the two corners of the mouth in a paused smile. The amount of maxillary teeth that are revealed below the ICL can give information on the patient's age. In youthful smiles, 75–100% of teeth structure shows below this line and the amount of display can reach up to 10–13 mm from the incisal edge to that line. In aged patients, fewer maxillary teeth show below this line, which is attributed to: (1) losing muscle tone of the face and (2) attrition of the teeth (Elaskary 2008).

The value of this line is that it highlights the age of the patient and their youthfulness. The more teeth–gingiva displayed, the younger a patient looks. Therefore, this line may be important, especially in totally edentulous reconstructive procedures (see Figure 2.10a and b).

An interesting study (Choi and Demf 1991) has evaluated changes in the smile caused by aging.

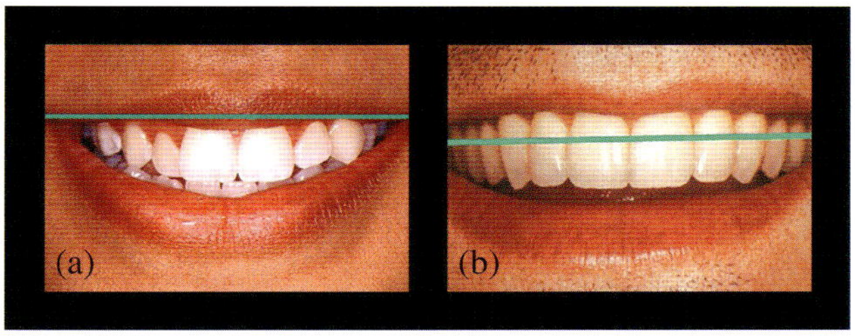

Figure 2.10 (a) Intercommissure line revealing a youthful smile. (b) Intercommissure line of an older smile with less teeth structure beneath it.

It measured the exposure of the maxillary and mandibular central incisors in both resting and smiling positions in 230 subjects (103 male, 127 female) that were 20–69 years of age. It reported that the amount of maxillary incisal exposure gradually decreased with age; this was accompanied by a gradual increase in mandibular incisal exposure in the smiling position. The mean amount of incisal exposure was 5.92 mm in the maxilla and 2.78 mm in the mandible. Another study (Robinson 1969) regarding the amount of teeth revealed in relation to age stated that a 30-year-old patient exposes more than 3 mm of the maxillary central incisors when the maxillary lip is at rest or repose. A 40-year-old shows 1.5 mm of maxillary central incisors, a 50-year-old exposes less or equal to 1 mm, and a 60-year-old exposes 0.5 mm, while at the age of 80, the lip margin is leveled with the incisal edges of the maxillary teeth. These rates are reversed with the relationship of the lower lip to the maxillary incisal edges.

2.5.2 Smile Arc

The relationship of the incisal edges of the maxillary incisor and canine tips to the curvature of the lower lip in the posed smile is called the 'smile arc' (Golub-Evans 1994). An ideal smile arc occurs when a line drawn touching the incisal edges and the tips of the canines and another line that touches the lower lip curvature, and these two lines are parallel to the infraorbital line and perpendicular to the facial mid-line. In other words, the ideal smile arc has the maxillary incisal edge curvature parallel to the curvature of the lower lip (Moskowitz and Nayyar 1995; Sarver 2001) (see Figure 2.11a–c).

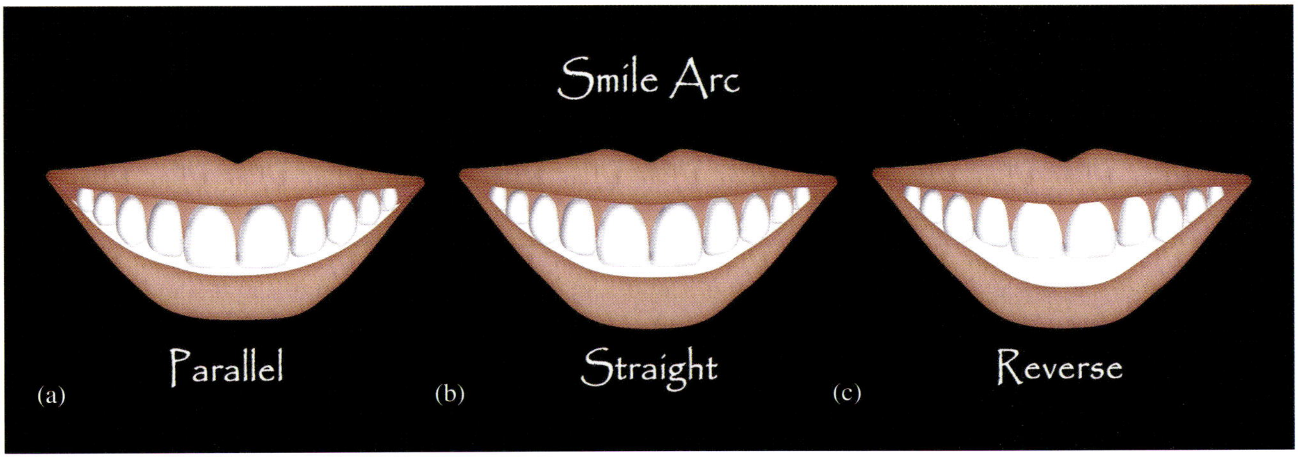

Figure 2.11 (a–c) Drawing showing the different smile arc variations.

The parallelism of the maxillary anterior incisal curve with the lower lip was divided into three categories: (1) *parallel* when the incisal edges of the maxillary anterior teeth are parallel to the upper border of the lower lip, (2) *straight* when the incisal edges of the maxillary anterior teeth are in a straight line, and (3) *reverse* when the incisal edges of the maxillary anterior teeth curved in reverse to the upper border of the lower lip (Elaskary 2008).

A study by Dong et al. (1999) concluded that there were many subjects with a parallel smile (60%), some with a straight smile (34%), and only a few subjects with a reverse smile (5%). Parallel and straight smiles received higher esthetic ranks than reverse smiles ($P < 0.05$), as shown in Figure 2.12.

The ideal smile has been described by another study (Yoon and Dong 1992) as one in which the upper lip

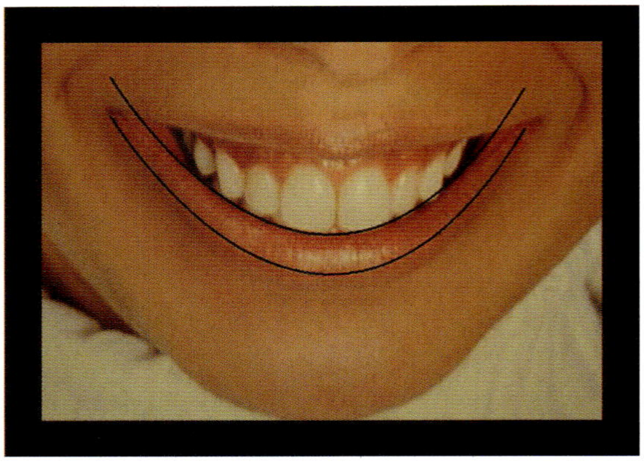

Figure 2.12 Ideal smile arc.

curved upward or was straight when the full shape of the maxillary anterior teeth was displayed between the upper and lower lip, the maxillary anterior incisal curve was parallel to the lower lip, and the teeth were displayed to the first molar (see Figure 2.13a and b).

2.5.3 Vestibular Reveal

The vestibular reveal is the amount of teeth and/or gingival structure that shows in various lip positions through the buccal corridor when the teeth are viewed from the front. The amount of posterior teeth that show during smiling can be called the vestibular reveal. In natural teeth, the maxillary teeth after the canine starts to look smaller, darker, and become blurred. When fabricating any prostheses in the maxillary arch, this reveal should be duplicated and not violated. When there is excessive teeth show within the buccal corridors, this condition is called the deficient vestibular reveal (DVR) or the excessive vestibular reveal (EVR) (Morley 1999) (see Figures 2.14a, b and 2.15a–c). The assessment of the vestibular reveal before any esthetic plan starts will be inspiring and it will be very useful in digital smile design cases. The vestibular reveal is considered to be the cornerstone of delivering a naturally looking and harmonious esthetic restoration (Elaskary 2008).

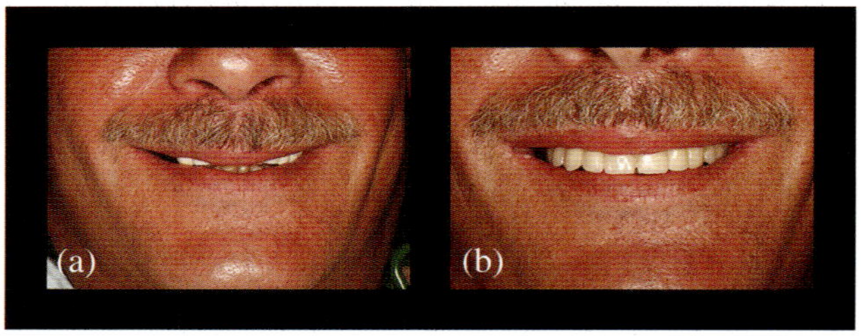

Figure 2.13 (a) Reverse smile arc as a result of applying faulty prosthetic anatomy. (b) Smile arc being corrected.

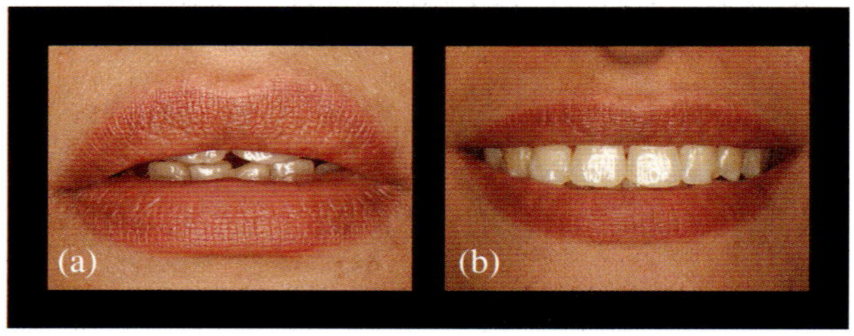

Figure 2.14 (a) Minimum and (b) maximum teeth revealed at a posed smile.

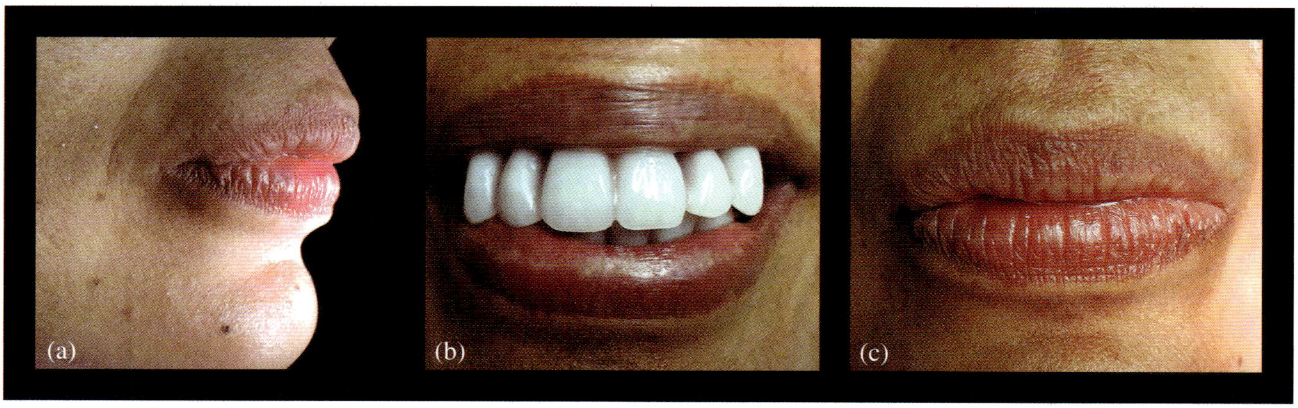

Figure 2.15 (a–c) Faulty implant supported restoration due to excessive teeth reveal.

For the clinical detection of the amount of teeth reveal, ask the patient to sit in an upright position and pronounce the letter "M" several times. After pronunciation ceases, the lips return to the relaxed rest position for evaluation, and a picture can be taken to detect the minimum tooth reveal. The patient is then asked to pronounce the letter (E) and pause, to detect the maximum teeth reveal. By detecting these parameters, the clinician will form an idea or a vision of the amount of teeth reveals for the patient and can duplicate it in the final prostheses (see Figure 2.16a–c).

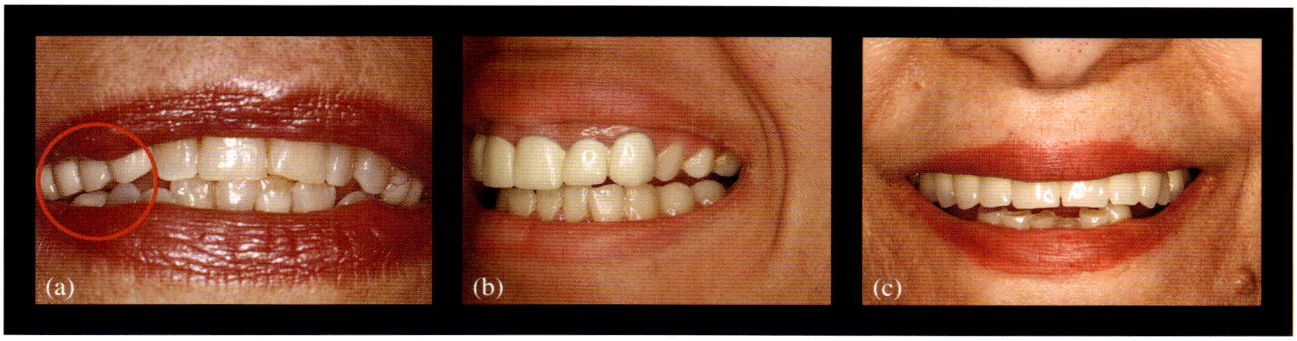

Figure 2.16 (a–c) Three examples with faulty excessive teeth vestibular revealed.

The relationship between the opposing dental arches determines the length of the maxillary incisors; this extent of the maxillary incisors plays an important role in the anterior guidance and phonetics of the patient. Some factors should be considered when detecting the extent of the maxillary incisors in fully edentulous cases: the length of the upper lip, the age of the patient, and maximum and minimum teeth reveal. The maxillary teeth should be displayed halfway between the upper and lower lip lines in the maximum teeth reveal position (Vig and Brundo 1978).

The lingual tilt of the maxillary central incisor (the incisal third) determines the correct pronunciation of the letters "F" and "V." The maxillary central incisor should slightly press against the lower lip inner edge of the vermilion border, blocking the remaining air from coming out of the mouth (Dawson 1983).

In fully edentulous cases, determination of the optimal incisal edge position becomes randomized by many clinicians. Misch (2005b) has set his original methodological maxillary incisal edge position guidelines, noting that the canine position is more consistent and less affected by age than the other natural teeth within the arch in the frontal area. In general, the canine tip is in the lateral position to the lip bow and is usually 1 mm longer than the maxillary lip in repose (letter "M") at the ages of 20–40 years. The canine is in an even position with the lip line from 40 to 60 years, and the lip is 1 mm longer than the canine position at 60–80 years. Once the position of the canine tip is set, then the other teeth can follow. Speech then can be checked with the pronunciation of the letter "F" to set the length of the labiolingual position. The pronunciation of the letter "N" can be used to set the incisal edge touching point with the lower border of the lip, as it should lightly touch the wet–dry border of the lower lip, similar to the lower lip position during a broad smile position (Heinlein 1980). He also stated that when the patient says "E," 50–70% of the space between the maxillary and mandibular lip should be occupied by the maxillary central incisors. If less than 50% of the space is occupied, the teeth usually can be lengthened, but if more than 70% of the space is occupied by maxillary centrals, lengthening the teeth usually is not indicated.

2.6 The Lip Influence

The lip value refers to both the face and the oral cavity. As both upper and lower lips compose the frame of the mouth, they are considered to be the curtains that reveal what is behind when moved in any direction. Generally speaking, both lips contribute to the shape of the face and to the pronunciation of words and they complement the facial composition to a great extent. The lip frame, which surrounds natural dentition, is a major facial element that contributes dramatically to dental esthetics. Consequently, it demands careful inspection and assessment (Hulsey 1970). The anatomy of the lips enclosing the orbicularis oris muscle that joins the lips superiorly to the base of the nose, laterally by the nasolabial sulci and inferiorly by the mentolabial sulcus, the vertical depression called the "philtrum," is located on the upper lip. It proceeds superiorly on the facial skin from the tubercle of the upper lip and runs to the base of the nose. The philtrum is one of the most important landmarks when the placement of the dental mid-line is of concern (Vig and Brundo 1978). Different positions of head posture can easily change the vertical or horizontal display of lips owing to the weaker muscle tone. The difference between a normal lip and a cleft lip can give an indication of the importance of the upper lip to the facial composition (Elaskary 2008).

In early teeth loss, the lips lose support and drop medially toward the oral cavity. This can be a starting point for facial deformity and subsequent skin wrinkles. In such conditions the clinician should be able to restore the missing lip support by returning it to its original place prior to teeth loss. Restoring missing teeth has proven to greatly improve facial appearance. Teeth loss not only affects lip support but also cheek support, because the posterior support (the buccinator muscle) is lost.

In severe alveolar ridge resorption, a carefully fabricated wax-up on the study cast will indicate the amount of osseous structure required facially to support the lip and return it to its original position along with the prosthetic contours, taking into consideration the fact that the cervical and middle thirds of the crown contour are mainly responsible for determining lip support (Maritato and Douglas 1964) (see Figure 2.17a–d).

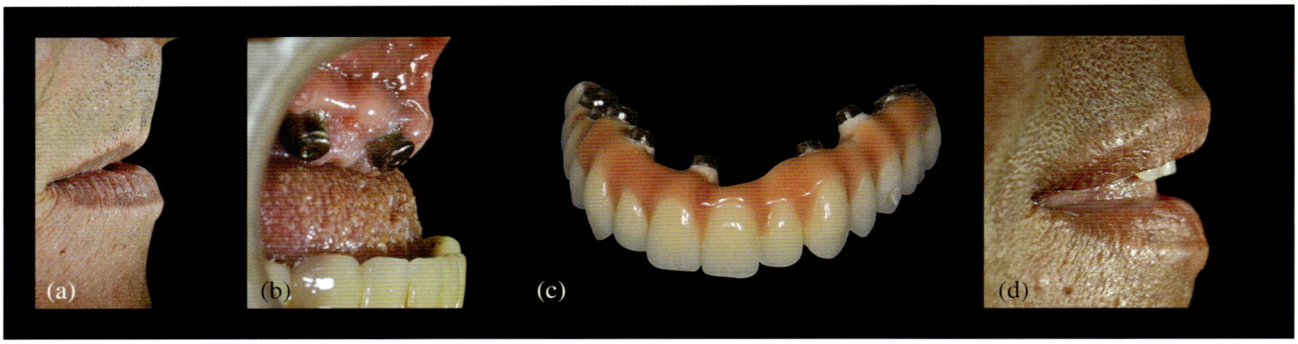

Figure 2.17 (a) Insufficient support of the upper lip as a result of long-term edentialism. (b) Dental implants being placed. (c) Hybrid implant supported prosthesis milled BioHPP bar with visiolign teeth (Bredent, Germany). (d) Improved support of the upper lip with the implant-supported restoration.

The lower lip has a tendency to be wider, fuller, longer, and more elastic (Renner 1985). The relationship between the upper and lower lips varies according to the skeletal class of the occlusion. The relationship plays an important role in determining tooth spatial alignment, while the degree of lip protrusion or retrusion has an important affect on the facial profile (Tweed 1991).

Several authors have described the anatomical landmarks of the lip in order to diagnose facial deformities within the treatment plan. The Burstone line is a reference line that connects the subnasale point to the pogonion point. The upper and lower lips are compressed by this reference line (ideally +3.5 and +2.2 mm, respectively, above this line) (Burstone 1967). The Steiner S line is a line joining the midpoint of the nose to the chin, where the patent's lips touch this line (Weickersheimer 1995). The Ricketts E-plane describes a line that extends from the tip of the nose to the chin, in which the maxillary and mandibular lip positions measure 4 and 2 mm, respectively (Viazis 1991). For the most favorable facial esthetics, the distance between the subnasale point (base of the nose) and the upper lip should be approximately half the distance measured from the lower lip to the menton (lowest chin) point (Rifkin 2000).

The upper lip position can be divided into three categories, where all of these positions were recorded in a full smiling position (Dong et al. 1999):

1) a higher lip position that reveals the total length of the maxillary anterior teeth and a contiguous band of gingiva.

2) an average lip position that reveals 75–100% of the maxillary anterior teeth length and the interproximal gingiva only (which is equal to the maxillary smile).
3) a low lip position that reveals less than 75% of the anterior teeth height with no gingival tissues revealed.

Another classification for the lip lines comprises the following three categories (Touati, Miara and Nathanson 1999):

1) A low lip line hides the gingiva and a considerable portion of the anterior teeth where it is difficult to show the incisor tips when the lips are at rest position. The anterior teeth may be displayed when the patient is in full smile. In this class, it may be necessary to perform crown lengthening to establish a balance between the lengths of the lip line when at rest and when smiling.
2) A medium lip line applies where 1–3 mm of the maxillary incisal edges are shown at the rest position.
3) A high lip line can be seen when more than 4–5 mm of the gingiva are displayed during a posed smile.

A medium lip line is considered to be the most preferable type in several oral rehabilitation procedures (see Figure 2.18a–c).

The upper lip curvature influences the smile directly and can be divided into three categories, as seen in Figure 2.19a–c.

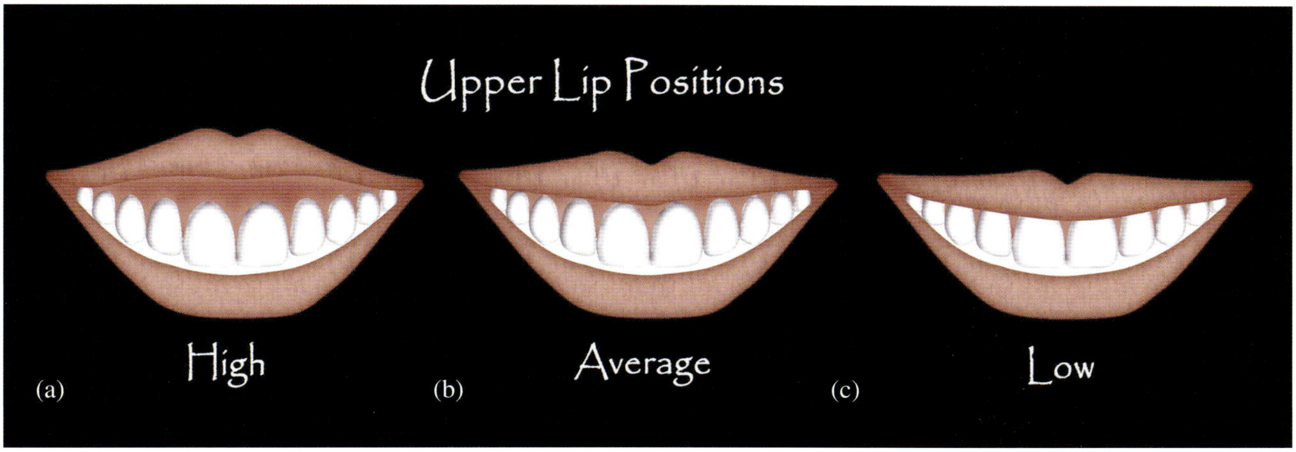

Figure 2.18 (a–c) An illustration showing various upper lip positions.

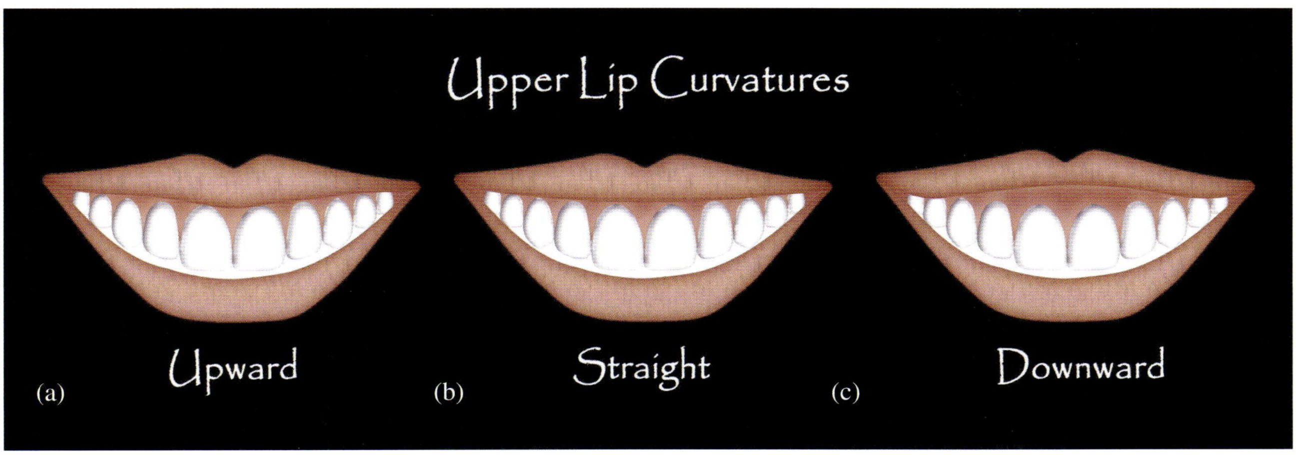

Figure 2.19 (a–c) An illustration showing various upper lip curvatures.

1) Upward curvature (12%), when the corner of the mouth is higher than the center of the lower border of the upper lip.
2) Straight orientation (45%), when the corner of the mouth and the center of the lower border of the upper lip are in a straight line.
3) Downward curvature (43%), when the corner of the mouth is lower than the center of the lower border of the upper lip.

The size of lips can influence the treatment plan when terms of defining the amount of the teeth display as well as the artificial teeth selection in most of the major oral rehabilitation procedures. A thick lip often does not reveal much of the tooth–gingiva structure because lip tissues hide the teeth behind it.

It is worth mentioning that thick lips can be more favorable than thin lips in cosmetic dental reconstruction because thick lips may hide any marginal prosthetic artifact (if it exists). On the other hand, when a thin lip contracts, it reveals most of the dentogingival complex. A thin lip requires meticulous attention to the marginal details of the prosthesis. With short and thin lips, the natural teeth behind usually possess a lingual inclination (Martone and Edwards 1978) (see Figure 2.20a–c). For defects that might affect the teeth display, a wise use of lip augmentation therapy may help improve the teeth display, as shown in Figure 2.21a and b.

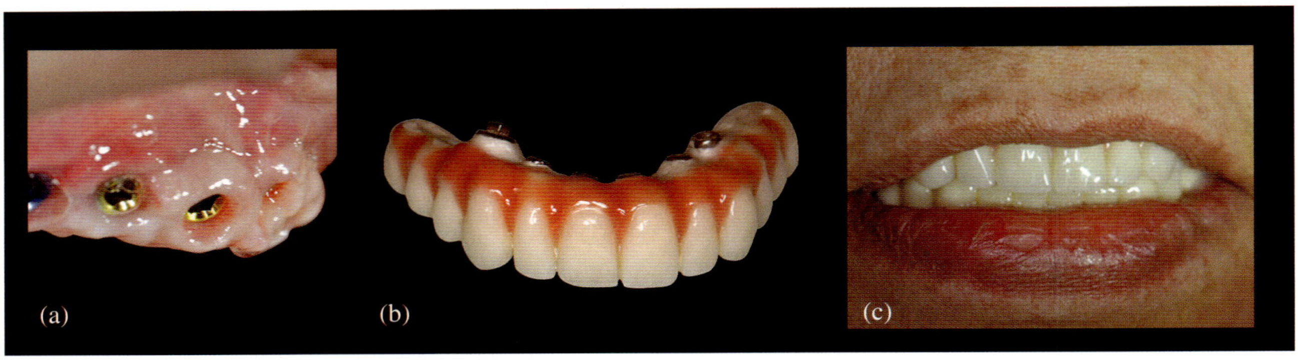

Figure 2.20 (a) Preprosthetic insertion of an implant-supported hybrid bridge. (b) and (c) Screw-retained hybrid bridge that is used to overcome both soft and hard tissue deficiency that possess lingually inclined edges to match the thin upper lip architecture.

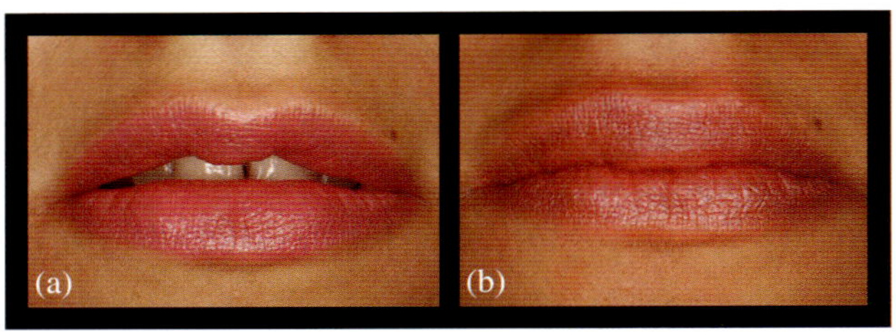

Figure 2.21 (a) and (b) Using lip augmentation therapy to enhance lip size.

Because teeth are not well displayed in patients with thick upper lips, a lighter teeth shade selection may be required to enhance and improve the amount of tooth display. It is suggested that the upper lip takes more responsibility for controlling teeth display, while the lower lip plays a major role in pronunciation. Treatment of patients with a high upper lip line is often more complex and unpredictable. Therefore, a careful evaluation of lip size, thickness, and character will determine how much of the restoration should be displayed while smiling or with the lip in any other position.

2.7 Teeth Morphology

Attempts to solve esthetic problems in an age of scientific revolution led clinicians to seek an evidence-based concept. This search for esthetic success with dental restorations was led by Williams (1914) but involved many other ideas and authors as well (Wavrin 1920; Young 1954). Credit is often given to William Hall (1986) who was the first to describe what he believed was a correlation between face form and tooth form. He stated that three basic forms of teeth existed: square, tapering, and ovoid (Stein 1936). The correlation succeeded due to its practicality and manufacturer support and not because of any actual relationship (Young 1954). However, most research has shown that no significant correlation exists between facial form and tooth form (Sellen, Jagger and Harrison 1998) because it is clinically complicated by alterations in facial form appearance due to age, hairstyle, eyewear, and body mass changes. Furthermore, no significant correlation exists because of the vast variety of facial forms and because an amazing face creation cannot be confined within any forms and formulas. In all cases, the guidelines overviewed within this topic are considered to be only secondary guidance to the overall appearance and not rules to be followed (Elaskary 2008).

The correct understanding of the dental morphology of humankind allows naturally looking implant-supported prostheses to be obtained. Lombardi (1973) detailed artificial teeth characters and their impact on the smile design and final treatment results. Learning from the standard anatomical object characters of natural teeth has led to a wealth of knowledge and information that can be in valuable in any esthetic reconstructive procedure. Many factors that influence teeth characters – age, gender, personality, habits, tooth position, shade, illumination, and illusion – are all factors that influence the selection of the shape of the anterior maxillary teeth either for fully or partially edentulous patients. For restoring missing maxillary teeth in the esthetic zone with or without dental implants, the clinician should strive to fabricate identical restorations that are almost a replicate of the natural missing dentition. If the missing teeth cannot be used as a reference due to their absence, then other references may be used as a guide. Therefore, the relationship between form and the human face becomes poorly evidenced whereas the relationship between teeth, characters, and extraoral or intraoral factors become more logical (Elaskary 2008).

2.7.1 Age

A thorough understanding of the relationship between age and teeth morphology will ensure a great esthetic out come from any esthetic plan, because the morphological characters of the anterior maxillary teeth are strongly influenced by a patient's age. In young individuals, the central and lateral incisors are long and rectangular, which emphasizes youthfulness (see Figures 2.22a, b and 2.23a, b).

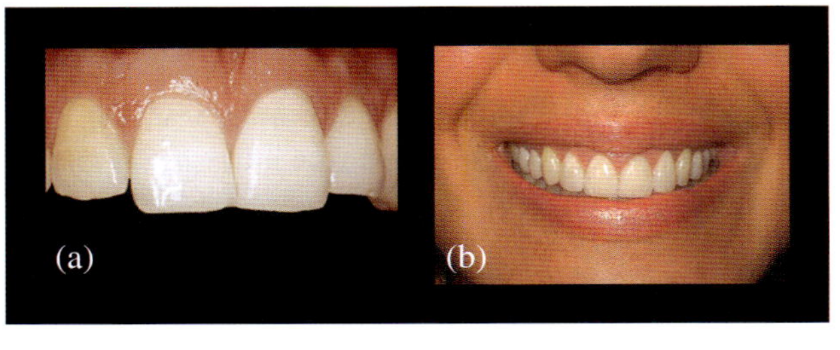

Figure 2.22 (a) and (b) The longer the central incisor length the more youthful effect it gives.

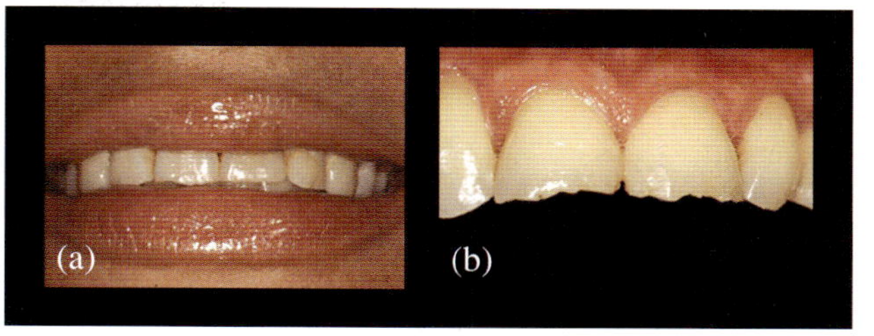

Figure 2.23 (a) and (b) Both central incisors exhibit wear that led to an elderly looking smile.

In older individuals, the front teeth often become worn and lose their rectangular shape, become square in shape with some incisal micro- or macrocracks, and sometimes attain up-fractions. The central incisors grow shorter due to parafunction, gingival recession, enamel cracks, and faulty dentistry. Less tooth structure will be visible when smiling. Small incisal embrasures occur while the gingival embrasures widen owing to the recession of the gingiva (Goldstein 1998). Flat broad incisal edges and functional or parafunctional generalized attrition results in posterior wear of the dentition. This excessive wear can eventually lead to narrowing of the teeth and the incisal edges of the maxillary central incisors tend to wear more cervically, affecting the lingual rather than the labial enamel. Eventually, the maxillary central and lateral incisors will exhibit the same incisogingival length (Yamamoto, Miyoshi and Kataoka 1990/1991).

When the mouth is slightly open, approximately 3.5 mm of the incisal portion of the maxillary teeth are visible in a 20-year-old person, while the mandibular teeth are barely visible. Between the ages of 30 and 40 years, mandibular incisor exposure increases while the maxillary tooth length exposure decreases (Vig and Brundo 1978).

The maxillary central incisor is the key tooth in the oral cavity, it dominates the composition of the oral cavity by its size and location, and it brings order and coherence to the oral cavity (Frush and Fisher 1956). Sometimes the central incisors are not visible when the lips are at rest but can be seen when smiling. This tends to render an older appearance to the dentition. Should any morphological deviation exist in the original dimensions and contours, then an interdisciplinary approach might be taken (see Figure 2.24a and b).

Hence, the importance of selecting the correct shape of the central incisor in major or minor implant-supported prosthetic cases becomes apparent. Many factors influence the selection of the shape of the central incisors for the restorative plan, including: (1) the amount of gingival display required, (2) the lip,

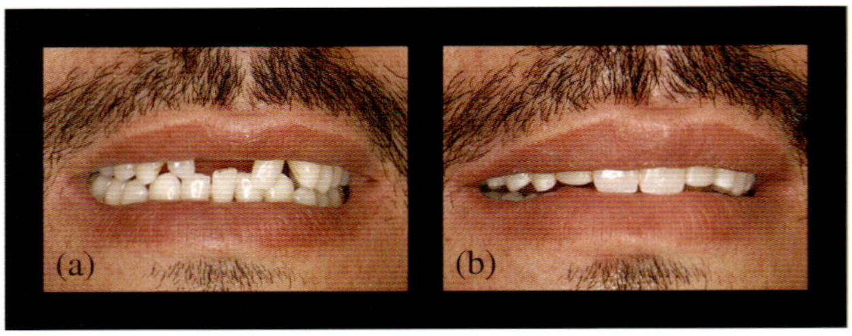

Figure 2.24 (a) and (b) Pre-operative view of lost two central incisors, trying in different teeth height to match the best height possible that enhances the smile.

line, (3) the type of smile, (4) the age of the patient, (5) the amount of available interarch space, (6) the golden proportion, (7) the existing occlusion, and (8) the length and curvature of the upper lip. Other factors that contribute to the selection of the shape of the maxillary central incisors are the lip muscle tone and skeletal build-up, and the incisal edge to the anterior guidance relationship (Qaltrough and Burke 1994).

When performing major esthetic implant-supported restorations in totally edentulous patients, the selection of the right shape of the anterior maxillary teeth and the amount of teeth display during smiling becomes of extreme importance to the overall prognosis of the treatment plan. The incisal edge of the maxillary central incisor is the most important determinant factor in the fabrication of the artificial teeth set-up. Once it is set, it determines the correct teeth proportion to follow and their related gingival levels; therefore, the improper placement of the central incisor can lead to an inadequate tooth display or a displeasing tooth or crown proportion (see Figure 2.25a–d).

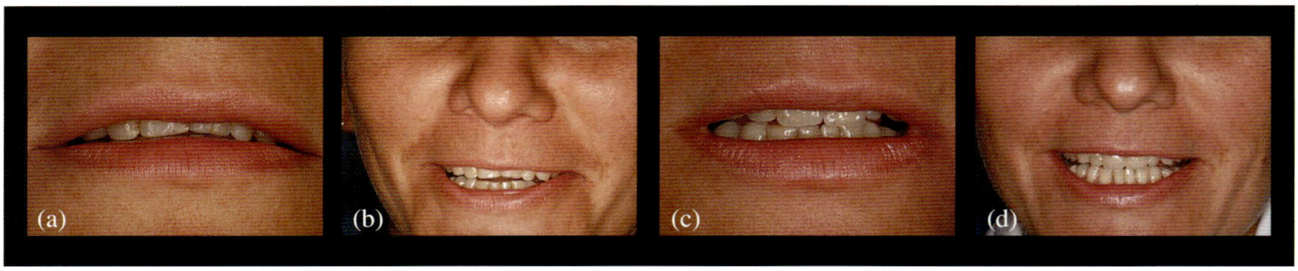

Figure 2.25 (a) and (b) Poor smile as a result of deficient anatomy of the central incisor. (c) and (d) The two central incisors are restored to their original anatomy, thus providing the total smile improvement of the patient.

In a few clinical instances, shortening the incisal edge may be required to compensate for excessive display resulting from generalized gingival recession, especially in high smile line patients.

The self-image of the patient and the patient's desire for a dynamic and youthful appearance can help determine how prominent the dental arch can be. The average anatomic crown length for the maxillary central incisor ranges from 10.4 to 11.2 mm. Treatment records might help to determine the original shape and height of the future prosthesis. Without this reference, determining the original shape and morphology of the missing teeth becomes a difficult task. When the treatment records do not exist, the clinician can use the upper lip position, the smile arc, and the remaining teeth as reference points. Therefore, determination of the relationship between the lost central incisors and the lips mainly falls on the clinician's skills and prosthodontic experience, in addition to the factors already mentioned (see Figure 2.26a and b).

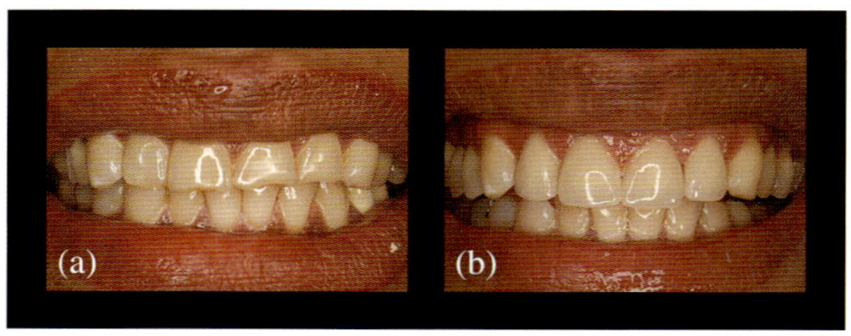

Figure 2.26 (a) and (b) Pre- and postoperative views of restoring the anatomy of the four anterior teeth to enhance the smile of the patient.

The optimal position of the incisal edge of the maxillary teeth influences not only esthetics but also phonetics, because the lips and teeth attain a different position and relationship for each sound that is made. The clinician should ask the patient to pronounce the letter "V" to determine the length and lingual tilt of the incisal third of the maxillary central incisors and the letter "F" to determine the relationship between the maxillary teeth and the lower lip position.

To emphasize a younger look to the artificial teeth, the cervical line can be set below the gingival margin, and the use of cylinder-shaped incisors may also help. The enamel surface of a youthful dentition is semi translucent, hard, and shiny with a slightly irregular surface. Younger teeth often have white hypoplastic lines and have a lower saturation and less characterization, owing to lower chroma, with a more textured, lighter, brighter, and higher value (Heymann 1987).

2.7.2 Gender

The female tooth shape characters are different from the male ones. The general teeth line angles in feminine dentition are rounded and not square. Femininity can be expressed in terms of delicacy and softness, whereas masculinity can be expressed in terms of vigor and angularity. The character in the female form appears as the roundness, smoothness, and softness that is typical in a woman. Masculinity, on the other hand, according to Frush and Fisher (1956), is the "cuboidal, hard, muscular, vigorous appearance, which is typical of men." For example, the shape of maxillary lateral incisors characterizes femininity to a certain extent. The feminine lateral incisor has rounded edges and possesses a constricted neck. On the other hand, the shape of the masculine lateral incisor is more rectangular, wider, and possesses sharp line angles (Lombardi 1973). The rotation of the lateral incisor's mesial surface, outward, and beyond the distal surface of the central incisor, can create a more delicate or softer position of the lateral when observed. In contrast, the masculine lateral incisor appears square, with a flat surface and sharper line angles, as shown in Figure 2.27a and b.

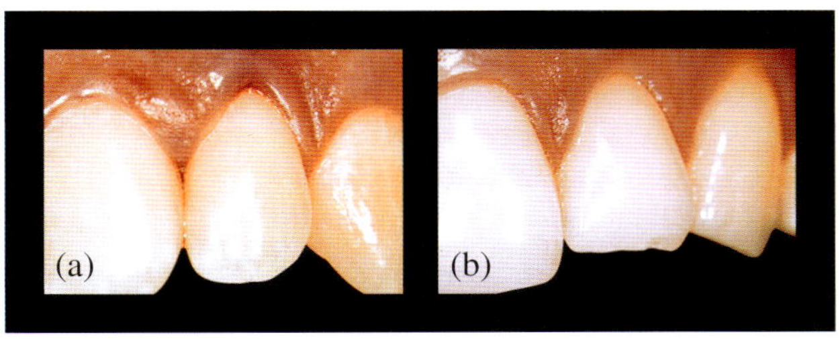

Figure 2.27 (a) Feminine looking lateral incisor (rounded in shape with constricted neck). (b) Masculine shaped lateral incisor (flat with sharp angles).

2.7.3 Personality

Major worries about physical attraction are concentrated on the face. Adults who are highly satisfied with their own face normally feel more confident than others. Despite the lack of research supporting the fact that personality is connected to facial features, it is a common perception that beautiful adults and children have a better advantage for social qualification and intelligence than those that are not considered to be beautiful (Adams 1977, 1978; Dion, Berscheid and Walster 1972). According to Proffit and White (1990), the psychological response of the patient to the malformation may be classified as follows: (1) a response of compensation (the patient takes on an attitude that allows him/her to overcome a disfigurement); (2) an inadequate response (the patient blames the malformation for certain difficulties in his/her life and relationships); and (3) a pathological response (the patient appears to have some definite traits of neurosis and prepsychosis). A negative body image may cause some serious defensive personal complexes that might slowly regress after correction and may modify psychological problems related to body image (Belfer et al. 1982). Early detection and handling of the facial deformities might improve the psychological and social welfare of patients. In less extreme situations, such as those of patients with common dentoskeletal deformations, there are some psychological problems, often unmentioned, which can be solved when a better harmony of the face is attained (Arndt et al. 1987; Strauss et al. 1988).

Kiyak and Bell (1990) studied 977 teenagers to appraise the influence of dental esthetics on body image and social factors. There was a remarkable difference between those who had an intermaxillary discrepancy and those who did not. The more serious cases of intermaxillary discrepancy considerably affected self-esteem and body image. However, Kenealy, Frude and Shaw (1989) examined 1918 children aged from 1 to 12 and did not find any psychological problems among children with intermaxillary discrepancy.

In general, patients are more satisfied with the improvement in their personality and appearance than they were with the improvement in their oral functions. In a longitudinal study, Wictorin, Hillstrom and Sorenson (1969) examined 95 patients before the operation and 49 patients one year after surgery: 96% were satisfied, 74% reported improvement in their social relationships, and 60% were found to be more confident. Laufer et al. (1976) studied 25 patients from two to six years after the surgical correction of facial deformities. They found 84% to be satisfied and pointed out an improvement in personality. Despite favorable outcomes, some patients are not satisfied. It is often difficult to understand the true reason, even if possible causes are known. Some patients have previous psychological or psychiatric problems, which were not openly declared to the surgeon.

Kim et al. (1995) investigated the correlation between personality factors and the smile, assuming that smile esthetics is closely related to an individual's physical condition and psychological state. The 30 male and 30 female students selected had no missing teeth, no experience of orthodontic or prosthodontic treatments, and good dentition. The personalities of the subjects were assessed using a 16 personality factor questionnaire. The authors took standardized frontal photographs of the each subject's face during a full smile and estimated the smile score. Then they assessed the statistical relation between smile score and personality. Warm, calm, enthusiastic, venturesome, self-assured, group-oriented, and relaxed personality traits are correlated to an attractive smile. Of the second-order personality factors derived from the primary personality traits, extroversion, and low anxiety are correlated to an attractive smile. Interestingly, women's personalities are correlated to attractive smiles but men's personalities are not. The esthetic levels of women's smiles were correlated at statistically significant levels to four primary and two second-order personality traits. However, for men, there were no statistically significant relationships between personality trails and smile esthetics.

Maxillary canines are the key teeth that provide the vigor of the personality effect because they may emphasis vigor of the personality (Lombardi 1973). A sharp and a pointed incisal tip canine will appear and add more vigor while a passive cuspid may show no aggression at all in the personality. The passive cuspid may have a blunt rounded tip and a convex profile, often exhibiting large incisal embrasures between the laterals and canines that create a passive appearance (Morley 1997), as shown in Figures 2.28a, b and 2.29.

The shade of the teeth also can give an impression of the personality of a person. In general, light teeth characterize a young, strong, and/or sharp personality, while darker teeth sometimes characterize a workaholic, stressed, or loaded personality. Placing the maxillary anterior teeth slightly in a labial position can give an effect of youthfulness and optimistic look, while a slight increase in the incisal edge of the front teeth (in very limited micrometers) can improve the personal impact (see Figure 2.30a–f).

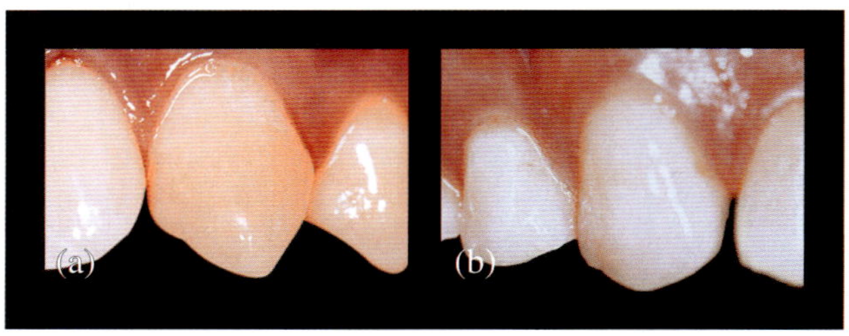

Figure 2.28 (a) Sharp tipped canine emphasizing the vigor of the personality. (b) Rounded tipped canine emphasizing an average personality.

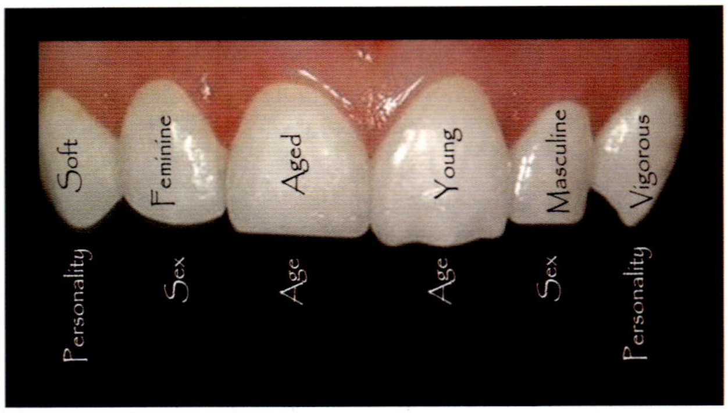

Figure 2.29 A conclusion of the impact of the teeth shape.

Using sharp teeth line angles sharpening the look of the face, a consistent arch form, and correct proportion to the facial morphology are essential factors in achieving pleasing dentition with a strong personal impact. The proportion must be in harmony with the strong or weak features of the face; this might be applied successfully to the central incisor length (Rufenacht 1990b).

2.8 Symmetry

Symmetry is an important biologically based determinant of facial attractiveness, and assessment of symmetry in a patient's face is paramount to the development of a complete dentofacial diagnosis. Symmetry and balance are two conjoined requirements in any esthetic intraoral restoration that involves the extraoral tissues; when optimal or, in other words, harmonious, they provide visual comfort and do not disturb or obscure the feeling of natural facial beauty. Among the factors that influence balance and symmetry in oral rehabilitation with dental implants is the determination of the correct occlusal or incisal plane and mid-line; this helps achieve balance and symmetry of the oral mechanism and appearance (Strub and Turp 1999). Symmetry of the oral cavity indicates that the different elements are being put together with respect to each other and with harmony. Any deviation from the natural known and created symmetry may not only lead to esthetic problems but also to functional ones.

Balance can be defined as the stabilizing result obtained from the exact adjustment of opposing forces (Goldstein 1984). Balance can be differentiated from symmetry; balance is observed while the eyes move distally starting

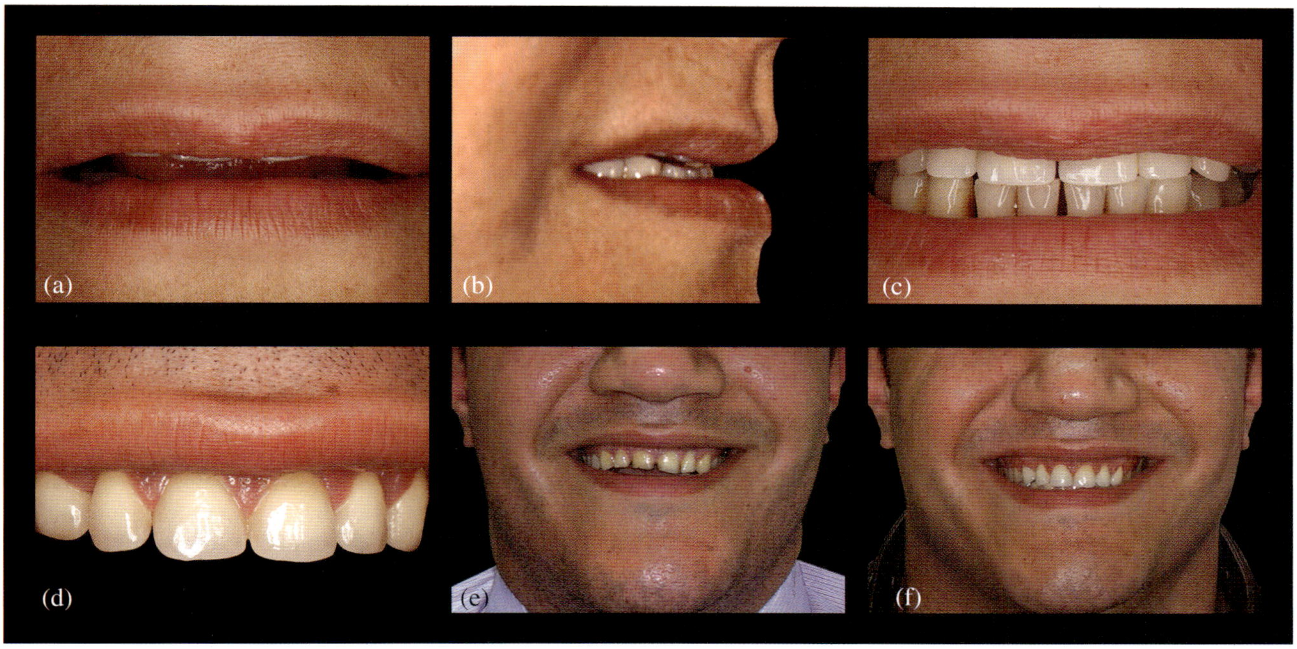

Figure 2.30 (a) Patient with defective teeth revealed. (b) Lateral profile. (c) Teeth revealed as enhanced by using the smile design concept. (d–f) Enhancing the teeth revealed by redesigning the shape of the front teeth.

from the center of an object, whereas symmetry is centrally located (Goldstein 1984). A good example of poor symmetry is the disproportionate size of two adjacent central incisors or where one of them is rotated facially or lingually, and a good example of poor balance is a deviated mid-line, or an uneven implant supported over the denture height. Lombardi (1973) noted that proper location of the dental mid-line is necessary for stability of the dental composition, as improper placement of the mid-line makes it impossible to balance the elements on either side of it. Tension is produced because of induced forces that make the viewer feel that the line must move to its proper place to produce stability and permanence (Elaskary 2008) (see Figure 2.31a–d).

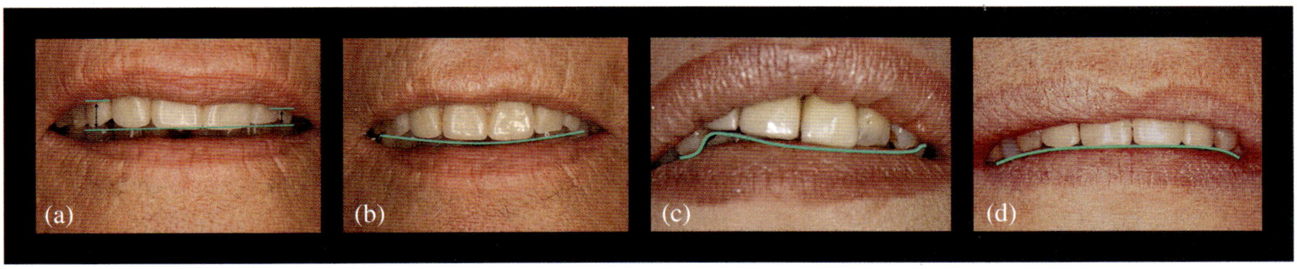

Figure 2.31 (a–d) Pre- and postoperative pictures enhancing the incisal plane to provide both sides with symmetry.

Functional asymmetries in human faces have been reported for emotions (Richardson et al. 2000; Wylie and Goodale 1988; Zaidel et al. 1995), both positive and negative (Benson and Laskin 2001), resemblance (Chen et al. 1997), and attractiveness (Zaidel et al. 1995). Structural asymmetries have long been described by craniofacial and dental researchers (Ferrario et al. 2003; Peck et al. 1991; Skvarilova 1994; Vig and Brundo 1978), and have been depicted in the realistic art of ancient Greece and Egypt (Peck et al. 1991; Peck and Peck 1995).

The specific phenotypic facial features of beauty remain to be identified and their spatial relationship within the facial frame should be clarified with future research. However, left–right bilateral symmetry has always been assumed to be a major contributing feature in the perceptual assessment of beauty. The invisible demarcating line, or even range, separating beautiful from non-beautiful is also unknown. Such an imaginary cut-off nevertheless does seem to play a role when participants compare the attractiveness of bilaterally symmetric laboratory constructed left–left and right–right faces. This is seen when comparing the results from the present study with the strong asymmetric appearance of attractiveness in earlier reports from this laboratory with ordinary faces (Zaidel et al. 1995).

The rule of thirds might be a fair way to determine the correct occlusal plane. The rule divides the lower third of the face into three thirds, the ideal position of the occlusal plane being located at the junction of the upper and middle thirds, as shown in Figure 2.32.

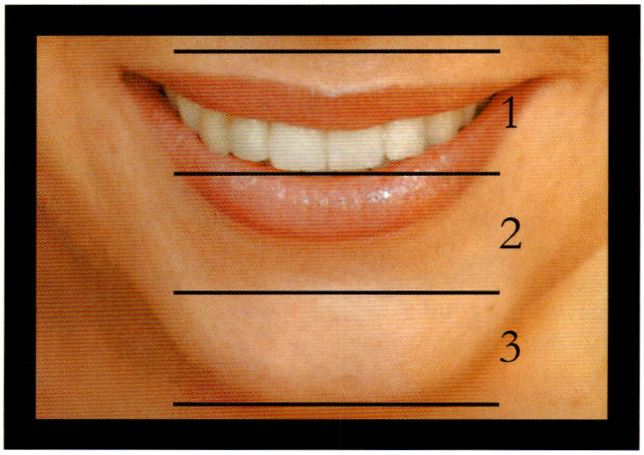

Figure 2.32 Rule of thirds.

In regard to the mid-line, the dental mid-line is an imaginary vertical line that does not necessarily coincide with the facial mid-line. Ideally, the papilla between the maxillary central incisors coincides with the mid-line of the face. However, it is not necessary that the dental mid-line coincides with the facial mid-line (Johnston, Burden and stevenson 1999), as not all patients have symmetrical faces. It may be that their chins or noses are not always centered, although they do not look disfigured, or sometimes the right and left sides of the cheeks do not coincide. Hence, it is impossible to use them as landmarks for the facial mid-line (Rufenacht 1990d).

The natural appearance of the face as a whole does not influence the visual perception of the dental mid-line, which should be right in line with the precise mid-line of the smile, which is located in the center and coincides with the symmetry of the dental composition. In those cases where the dental and facial mid-lines do not coincide, the dental mid-line should be made perpendicular to the pupillary or horizontal lines, to prevent the illusion of asymmetry. Once it is vertical, the composition will appear symmetrical or at least pleasing (Latta 1988) (see Figure 2.33a and b).

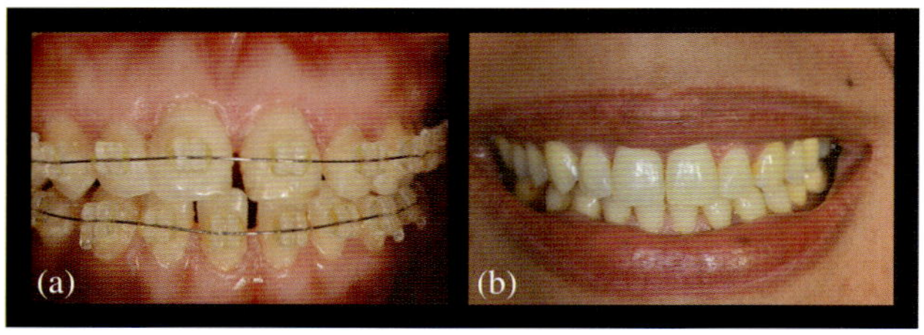

Figure 2.33 (a) and (b) Using orthodontic treatment to restore symmetry.

References

Abel, E. and Kruger, M. (2010). Smile intensity in photographs predicts longevity. *Psychol. Sci.* 21: 542–544.

Ackerman, J., Ackerman, M., Brensinger, C., and Landis, J. (1998). A morphometric analysis of the posed smile. *Clin. Orthod. Res.* 1: 2–11.

Adams, G.R. (1977). Physical attractiveness research: toward a developmental social psychology of beauty. *Hum. Dev.* 20: 217–230.

Adams, G.R. (1978). Racial membership and physical attractiveness effects on preschool teacher's expectations. *Child Study J.* 8: 29.

Arndt, E.M., Travis, E., Lefebvre, A., and Munro, I.R. (1987). Psychosocial adjustment of 20 patients with Treacher Collins syndrome before and after reconstructive surgery. *Br. J. Plast. Surg.* 40: 605–609.

Belfer, M.L., Harrison, A.M., Pillemer, F.C., and Murray, J.E. (1982). Appearance and the influence of reconstructive surgery on body image. *Clin. Plast. Surg.* 9: 307–315.

Benson, K.J. and Laskin, D.M. (2001). Upper lip assymetry in adults during smiling. *J. Oral Max. Fac. Surg* 59: 396–398.

Bernstein, M.J., Sacco, D.F., Brown, C.M. et al. (2010). A preference for genuine smiles following social exclusion. *J. Exp. Soc. Psychol.* 46: 196–199.

Blake, W. (1908). *The Poetic Works of William Blake.* London and New York: Oxford University Press.

Burstone, C.J. (1967). Lip posture and its significance in treatment planning. *Am. J. Orthod.* 53: 262–284.

Chen, A.C., German, C., and Zaidel, D.W. (1997). Brain asymmetry and facial attractiveness: Beauty is not simply in the eye of the beholder. *Neuropsych.* 35: 471–476.

Choi, T.R. and Demf, I.K. (1991). A study on the exposure of maxillary and mandibular central incisor in smiling and physiologic rest position. *J. Wonkwang Dent. Res. Inst.* 5 (371): 79.

Coachman, C., Calamita, M.A., and Sesma, N. (2017). Dynamic documentation of the smile and the 2D/3D digital smile design process. *Int. J. Periodontics Restorative Dent.* 37 (2): 183–193.

Coachman, C. and Paravina, R.,.D. (2016). Digitally enhanced esthetic dentistry – from treatment planning to quality control. *J. Esthet. Restor. Dent.* 28 Suppl 1: S3–S4.

Coachman, C., Van Dooren, E., Gürel, G. et al. Smile design: from digital treatment planning to clinical reality. In: *Interdisciplinary Treatment Planning. Volume 2: Comprehensive Case Studies* (ed. M. Cohen), 119–174. Chicago: Quintessence.

Dawson, P.E. (1983). Determining the determinants of occlusion. *Int. J. Periodontics Restorative Dent.* 3: 9.

Dickerson, W. (1996). Trilogy of creating on esthetic smile. *Tech Update* 1: 1–7.

Dion, K., Berscheid, E., and Walster, E. (1972). What is beautiful is good. *J. Pers. Soc. Psychol.* 24: 285–290.

Dong, K., Ho, T., Cho, H. et al. (1999). The esthetics of the smile: a review of some recent studies. *Int. J. Prosthodont.* 72: 9–19.

Duchenne, G.B. (1990). *The Mechanism of Human Facial Expression*. New York: Cambridge University Press.

Ekman, P., Friesen, W.V., and Ellsworth, P.C. (1982). *Emotion in the Human Face*. Cambridge, UK: Cambridge University Press.

Elaskary, A.S. (2008). *Fundamentals of Esthetic Implant Dentistry*. Blackwell publishing –John Wiley.

Ferrario, V.F., Sforza, C., Dellavia, C. et al. (2003). A quantitative three-dimensional assessment of soft tissue facial symmetry of cleft lip and and palate adult patients. *J. Cranio. Fac. Surg.* 14: 739–746.

Fridlund, A.J. (1994). What do facial expressions express? *J. Pers. Soc. Psychol.* 229–231.

Frush, J.P. and Fisher, R.D. (1956). How dentogenic restorations interpret the sex factor. *J. Prosthet. Dent.* 6: 160–171.

Frush, J.P. and Fisher, R.D. (1985). The clynasthetic interpretation of the clentogenic concept. *J. Prosthet. Dent.* 8: 518–531.

Gibson, R. (1989). Smiling and facial exercise. *Dent. Clin. N. Am.* 33: 139–144.

Goldstein, R.E. (1984). *Change Your Smile*, 1e. Chicago: Quintessence.

Goldstein, R.E. (1998). *Esthetics in Dentistry*, 2e, 133–186. Hamilton, Canada: Decker Inc.

Golub-Evans, J. (1994). Unity and variety: essential ingredients of a smile design. *Curr. Opin. Cosmet. Dent.* 2: 1–5.

Gwinnett, A.J. (1992). Moist vs dry dentin: its effect on shear bond strength. *Am. J. Dent.* 5: 127–129.

Hall, W.R. (1986). Temperament in mechanical dentistry. *Dent. Pract.* 4: 49–54.

Hearth, K. (1986). *A Smile*. Warrior Reflections Publications Self-Published March 1986.

Heinlein, W.D. (1980). Anterior teeth: esthetics and function. *J. Prosthet. Dent.* 44: 389–393.

Heymann, H.O. (1987). The artistry of conservative esthetic dentistry. *J. Am. Dent. Assoc.* 115 (Special Issue): 14E–23E.

Horstmann, W., Lorenz, S., and Egelhaaf, M. 2003. Educational simulations for the neural and cognitive sciences. European Cognitive Science Conference 2003.

Hulsey, C.M. (1970). An esthetic evaluation of lip–teeth relationships present in the smile. *Am. J. Orthod.* 57: 132–144.

Johnston, C.D., Burden, D.J., and Stevenson, M.R. (1999). The influence of dental midline discrepancies on dental attractiveness ratings. *Eur. J. Orthod.* 21: 517–522.

Kenealy, P., Frude, N., and Shaw, W. (1989). An evaluation of the psychological and social effects of malocclusion: some implications for dental policy-making. *Soc. Sci. Med.* 6: 583–591.

Kim, H.S., Kim, I.P., Oh, S.C., and Dons, J.K. (1995). The effect of personality on the smile. *J. Wonkwang Dent. Res. Inst.* 29: 311–314.

Kiyak, H.A. and Bell, R. (1990). Psychosocial considerations in surgery and orthodontics. In: *Surgical-Orthodontic Treatment* (ed. W.R. Proffit and R.P. White), 71–93. St Louis: CV Mosby Co.

Latta, G.H. (1988). The midline and its relation to anatomic landmarks in the edentulous patient. *J. Prosthet. Dent.* 59: 681–683.

Laufer, D., Glick, D., Gutman, D., and Sharon, A. (1976). Patient motivation and response to surgical correction of prognathism. *Oral Surg. Oral Med. Oral Pathol. Oral Radiol.* 41: 309–313.

Levin, R.P. (1988). Patient personality assessment improves the presentation. *Dent. Econ.* 78: 49–50. 52, 54–55.

Lombardi, R.E. (1973). The principles of visual perception and their clinical application to denture esthetics. *J. Prosthet. Dent.* 29: 358–382.

Maritato, F.R. and Douglas, J.R. (1964). A positive guide to anterior tooth placement. *J. Prosthet. Dent.* 14: 848.

Martone, A.L. and Edwards, L.F. (1978). Anatomy of the mouth and related structures. Part 1. The face. *J. Prosthet. Dent.* 39: 128–134.

Mehua, M., Grammerb, K., and Dunbara, R.I.M. (2007). Smiles when sharing. *Evol. Hum. Behav.* 28: 415–422.

Misch, C.E. (2005a). Rational for dental implants. In: *Dental Implant Prosthodontics* (ed. C.E. Misch), 10–12. St Louis: Elsevier Mosby.

Misch, C.E. (2005b). Maxillary denture opposing implant prosthesis and modified occlusal concepts. In: *Dental Implant Prosthodontics* (ed. C.E. Misch), 568–586. St Louis: Elsevier Mosby.

Morley, J. (1997). Smile design – specific consideration. *J. Calif. Dent. Assoc.* 25: 633–637.

Morley, J. (1999). The role of cosmetic dentistry in restoring a youthful appearance. *J. Am. Dent. Assoc.* 130: 1166–1172.

Moskowitz, M. and Nayyar, A. (1995). Determinants of dental esthetics: a rational for smile analysis and treatment. *Compend. Cont. Educ. Dent.* 16: 1164–1186.

Peck, S. and Peck, L. (1995). Selected aspects of the art of facial esthetics. *Sem. in Ortho.* 1: 105–126.

Peck, S., Peck, L., and Kataia, M. (1991). Skeletal asymmetry in esthetically pleasing faces. *Ang. Ortho.* 61: 43–48.

Philips, E.D. (1990). The classifications of smile patterns. *J. Can. Dent. Assoc.* 65: 252–254.

Proffit, W.T.R. and White, R.P. (1990). *Surgical Orthodontic Treatment.* St. Louis: CV Mosby Co.

Qaltrough, A.J.E. and Burke, F.J.T. (1994). A look at dental esthetics. *Quintessence Int.* 25: 7–14.

Renner, R.P. (1985). *An Introduction to Dental Anatomy and Esthetics*, 125–166. Chicago: Quintessence 187–233, 241–272.

Richardson, C.K., Bowers, D., Bauer, R.M. et al. (2000). Digitizing the moving face during dynamic displays of emotion. *Neuropych.* 38: 1028–1039.

Rifkin, R. (2000). Facial analysis: a comprehensive approach to treatment planning in aesthetic dentistry. *Pract. Periodontics Aesthet. Dent.* 12: 865–871.

Robinson, S.C. (1969). Physiological placement of artificial anterior teeth. *Can. Dent. J.* 35: 260–266.

Rubin, L.R. (1974). The anatomy of a smile: its importance in the treatment of facial paralysis. *Plast. Reconstr. Surg.* 53: 384–387.

Rufenacht, C.R. (1990a). *Fundamentals of Esthetics*, 9–31. Chicago: Quintessence.

Rufenacht, C.R. (1990b). *Fundamentals of Esthetics*, 13–48. Chicago: Quintessence.

Rufenacht, C.R. (1990c). *Fundamentals of Esthetics*, 67–134. Chicago: Quintessence.

Rufenacht, C.R. (1990d). *Fundamentals of Esthetics*, 77–126. Carol Stream: Quintessence.

Sarver, D. (2001). The importance of the incisor positioning in the esthetic smile: the smile arc. *Am. J. Orthod. Dentofac. Orthop.* 120: 98–111.

Sellen, P.N., Jagger, D.C., and Harrison, A. (1998). Computer-generated study of the correlation between tooth, face, arch forms, and palatal contour. *J. Prosthet. Dent.* 80: 163–168.

Skvarilova, B. (1994). Facial asymmetry: an x-ray study. *Acta Chirurgiae Plasticae* 36: 89–91.

Stein, M.R. (1936). Williams' classification of anterior tooth forms. *J. Am. Dent. Assoc.* 23: 1512–1518.

Strauss, R.P., Mintzker, Y., Fenerstein, R. et al. (1988). Social perceptions of the effects of down syndrome: school-based study of ratings by normal adolescents. *Plast. Surg. Reconstr.* 81: 841–851.

Strub, J.R. and Turp, J.C. (1999). Esthetics in dental prosthetics. In: *Esthetics and Prosthetics* (ed. J. Fischer), 11. Chicago: Quintessence.

Tak On, T. and Kois, J.C. (2016). Digital smile design meets the Dento-facial analyzer: optimizing esthetics while preserving tooth structure. *Compend. Contin. Educ. Dent.* 37 (1): 46–50.

Tjan, A.H.L. and Miller, G.D. (1984). Some esthetic factors in a smile. *J. Prosthet. Dent.* 51: 24–28.

Touati, B., Miara, P., and Nathanson, D. (1999). *Esthetic Dentistry and Ceramic Restorations*, 139–161. New York: Martin Dunitz.

Tweed, C.H. (1991). The diagnostic facial triangle in the control of treatment objectives. *Am. J. Orthod.* 55: 651.

Viazis, A.D. (1991). A new measurement of profile esthetics. *J. Clin. Orthod.* 25: 15–20.

Vig, R.G. and Brundo, G.C. (1978). The kinetics of anterior tooth display. *J. Prosthet. Dent.* 39: 502–504.

Wavrin, J.A. (1920). A simple method of classifying face forms. *Dent. Dig.* 26: 331–335.

Weickersheimer, P.B. (1995). Steiner analysis. In: *Radiographic Cephalometry* (ed. A. Jacobson), 83–85. Carol Stream: Quintessence Publishing.

Wheeler Wilcox, E. (1995). *Custer and Other Poems.* University of Michigan Humanities Text Initiative.

Wictorin, L., Hillestrom, K., and Sorensen, S. (1969). Biological and psychosocial factors in patients with malformation of the jaws. *Scand. J. Plast. Reconstr. Surg.* 3: 138–143.

Williams, J.L. (1914). The temperamental selection of artificial teeth fallacy. *Dent. Dig.* 20: 63–75.

Wylie, D.R. and Goodale, M.A. (1988). Left sided oral asymmetries in spontaneous but not posed smiles. *Neuropsych.* 26: 823–832.

Yamamoto, M., Miyoshi, M., and Kataoka, S. (1990/1991. Special Discussion). Fundamentals of esthetics: contouring techniques for metal ceramic restorations. *Quintessence Dent. Technol.* 14: 10–81.

Yoon, M.E. and Dong, I.K. (1992). A study on the smile in Korean youth. *J. Korean Aciad. l'Rosthoc Jont.* 30: 259–270.

Young, H.A. (1954). Selecting the anterior tooth mold. *J. Prosthet. Dent.* 4: 748–760.

Zaidel, D.W., Chen, A.C., and German, C. (1995). She is not a beauty even when she smiles: Possible evolutionary basis for a relationship between facial attractiveness and hemispheric specialization. *Neuropsych.* 33: 649–655.

3

Esthetic Outcome of Immediately Implanted and Loaded Implants in the Esthetic Region

A Discussion of Preclinical and Clinical Evidence

Arthur Belém Novaes, Jr.[1], *Raquel Rezende Martins de Barros*[1], *Flavia Adelino Suaid Malheiros*[1], *and Valdir Antonio Muglia*[2]

[1] Department of Oral and Maxillofacial Surgery and Traumatology and Periodontology, School of Dentistry of Ribeirão Preto, University of São Paulo, São Paulo, Brazil
[2] Department of Prosthodontics, School of Dentistry of Ribeirão Preto, University of São Paulo, São Paulo, Brazil

3.1 Preclinical Evidence

The outcome of placing implants at the time of tooth removal has been reported to be as predictable as placing implants into healed sites (Chen et al. 2009) when considering the rates of osseointegration.

Immediate implants are better accepted by the patients, reduce the period of edentulism, and reduce the overall treatment time. They are advocated to preserve soft tissue form and contour and preserve bone dimensions; turning them into the first option to treat esthetic regions. However, to achieve these desirable esthetic outcomes when placing immediate implants, the diagnosis and planning of the case must be precise.

During recent years a wide knowledge from this therapy was achieved with the contribution of preclinical studies. They provide unique information about histological, histomorphometrical, and, more recently, microtomographical features of peri-implant tissues. Thus, a series of key aspects was evidenced to help the decision-making process of treating esthetic regions with immediately placed and loaded implants. The following topics include: (1) delicate flapless extraction surgeries, (2) implant positioning, (3) implant surface, (4) filling of the gap between the buccal plate and the implant, and (5) the presence and thickness of the buccal bone plate (BBP) (tissue biotype).

3.1.1 Flapless Extraction Surgeries: Basis for Its Use

One of the first justifications to use immediate implants is to counteract the progressive involution of the alveolar bone resulting from the tooth loss (Pietrokovski and Massler 1967; Schropp et al. 2003). However, some studies in animals have shown a marked reduction of the buccal hard tissue height after implant placement in fresh extraction sockets (Araujo et al. 2006a, 2006b). Such a tragic outcome elicited the importance that anatomical and microstructural characteristics of the bone plates can have for implant success. In order to better understand this biological basis, the anterior mandibular region of dogs was histologically evaluated (Novaes et al. 2011b). It was observed that the width of buccal and lingual bone plates increased from the coronal third to the most apical third, but all the buccal thirds were significantly thinner when compared to the lingual thirds (Figure 3.1). Furthermore, the bone density of the coronal and middle thirds of BBPs presented statistically significant higher values than the lingual bone plates, which signifies that

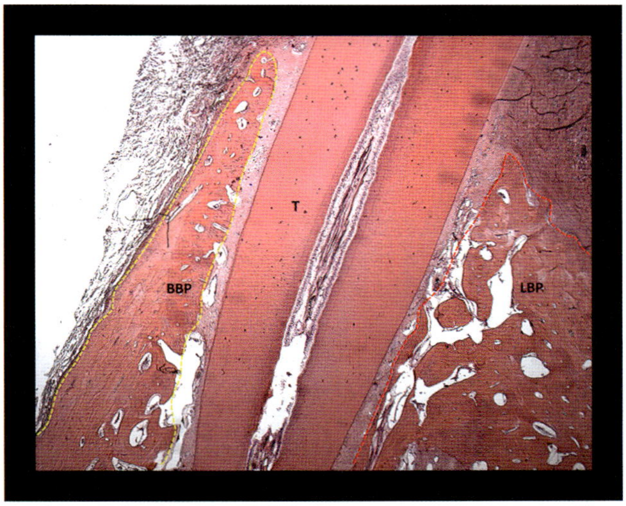

Figure 3.1 The width of buccal (BBP – yellow dashed line) and lingual bone (LBP – red dashed line) plates increased from the coronal third to the most apical third, but the buccal thirds were significantly thinner when compared to the lingual thirds.

Advances in Esthetic Implant Dentistry, First Edition. Abdelsalam Elaskary.

Companion website: www.wiley.com/go/elaskary/esthetic

these areas were composed of scarce or no marrow spaces (Figure 3.2). One of the main functions of the periosteum and periodontal ligament (PDL) blood vessels is to supply the osteoblasts (OB) in the alveolar bone with nutrients (Matsuo et al. 2000). Additionally, the marrow spaces should also be recognized as a source of blood supply. In accordance with this, some interesting images showed a direct link between the periosteum and the marrow spaces in the BBP as shown in the Novaes et al. (2011b) study (Figures 3.3–3.5). This information underlies the Nobuto et al. (2005b) study, which investigated the microvascular responses after mucoperiosteal flap surgery in dogs and concluded that the periosteum detachment may cause circulatory insufficiency, resulting in bone resorption. In general, the bone surface that is temporarily exposed usually undergoes a necrotic process that finishes with bone resorption, but it is important to emphasize that a thick bone plate containing marrow spaces could have lower bone height loss at the end of the healing period (Wilderman, Wentz and Orban 1960).

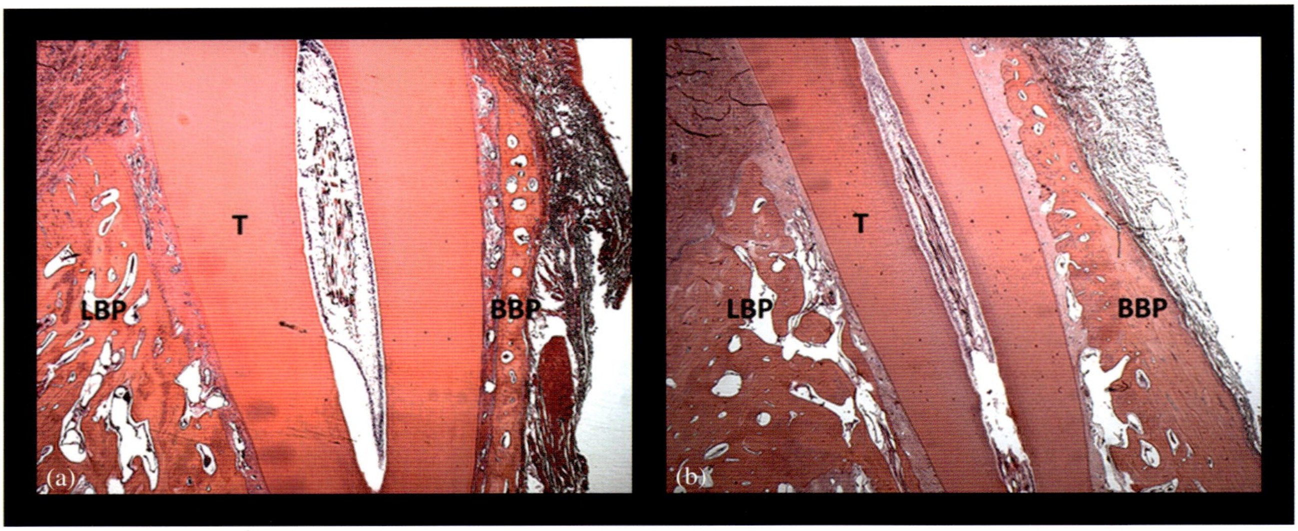

Figure 3.2 (a) and (b) Images showing the lingual bone plates (LBP – on the left of the tooth) and the buccal bone plates (BBP – on the right of the tooth) of anterior mandibular teeth of dogs studied by Novaes et al. (2011b). Note the microstructural differences between them, like the thickness, the number, and volume of the marrow spaces.

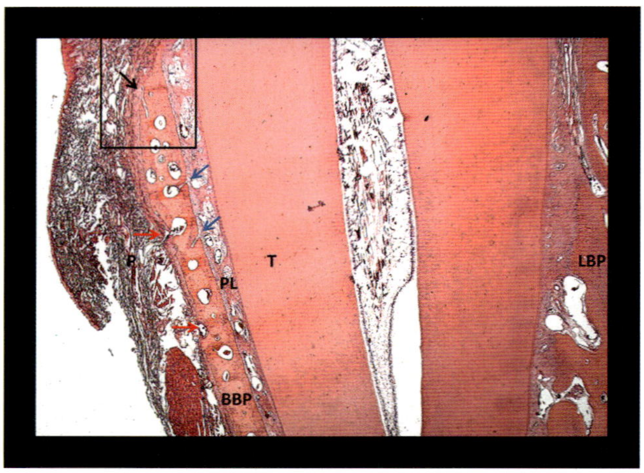

Figure 3.3 Image showing a dog anterior mandibular tooth (T) inserted in the alveolus. Note that the coronal third of the buccal bone plate (BBP), detached by the black rectangle, is very thin and composed of scarce marrow spaces. One of these marrow spaces (black arrow) is directly linked to the periosteum (P). Other similar situations were observed in the middle third of the buccal bone plate (red arrows). Additionally, direct connections between the marrow spaces of the BBP and the periodontal ligament (PL) were also detected (blue arrows).

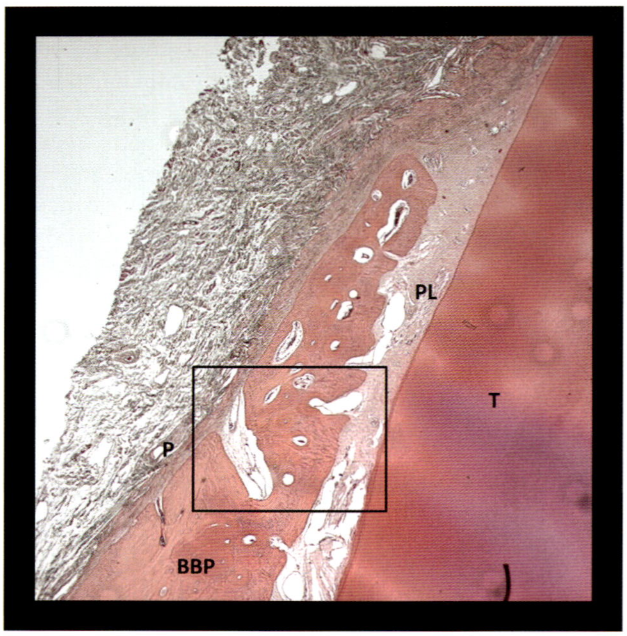

Figure 3.4 Image of the buccal bone plate (BBP) of a dog anterior mandibular tooth (T). The black rectangle highlighted the direct link between the periosteum (P) and a marrow space of the BBP, and also between the periodontal ligament (PL) and another marrow space.

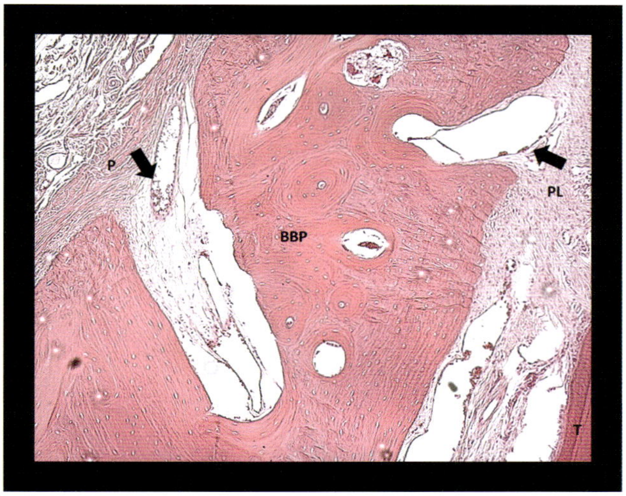

Figure 3.5 A higher magnification of the image highlighted in Figure 3.4.

These observations have implications for implant therapy in general, and even more for immediate implants. Based on these studies, the flapless approach concept, a minimally invasive surgical procedure based on the non-detachment of the periosteum, has emerged. The benefits, esthetics, and comfort have been described (Rocci, Martignoni and Gottlow 2003; Zeren 2006) but the preservation of the integrity of the bone plates to provide a self-contained defect around the implant with a higher potential of regeneration is the main reason behind them.

Different studies (Fickl et al. 2008; Novaes et al. 2011a) investigated the effectiveness of the flapless procedure as an alternative to buccal bone preservation, at least to some extent. Considering that tooth extraction eliminates the alveolar bone blood supply that comes from the PDL, only the vascularization that remains is provided by the periosteum. Thus, raising mucoperiosteal flaps in this situation may strongly compromise the blood supply that comes from the periosteum, directly affecting the regions that are anatomically thin and microstructurally composed of cortical bone.

Novaes et al. (2011b) evaluated buccal bone remodeling in dogs after immediate implantation with the flap or a flapless approach. They found a strong association between the surgical flap and the extent of bone resorption around immediate implants. In this study, the only difference between the groups was the flap elevation in the control group, and this group exhibited at least twice the buccal bone height loss when compared to the flapless group (Figure 3.6).

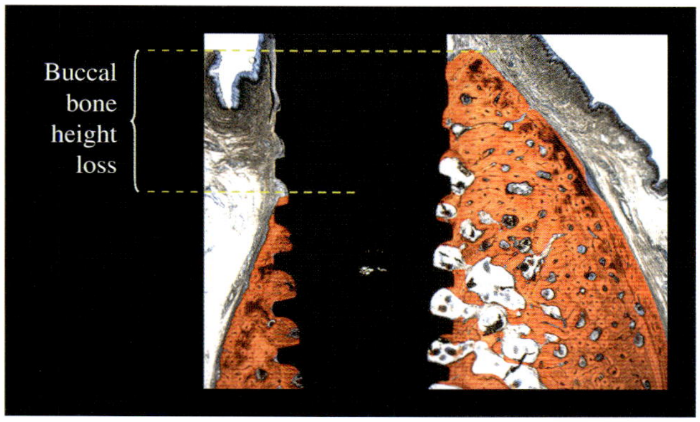

Figure 3.6 Buccal bone resorption evaluation. Note the difference in the height of the buccal bone plate (on the left) and the lingual bone plate (on the right) around an immediately placed implant during a flap surgical intervention.

Similar to the anatomical and microstructural characteristics of the bone plates surrounding the mandibular teeth of dogs described above (Novaes et al. 2011b), the histological specimens of this sequential study (Novaes et al. 2011b) evidenced the BBPs around the immediate implants to be significantly thinner when compared to the lingual components (Figures 3.7 and 3.8). When comparing their bone densities, while the buccal plates were constituted by a cortical bone type with sparse and decreased numbers of marrow areas, the lingual bone plates exhibited numerous and large marrow areas (Figures 3.7 and 3.8). These differences between the buccal and lingual bone densities achieved statistical significance in the apical portion of flapless and flap groups, and in the coronal portion of the flap group (Table 3.1). This last finding could mean that this portion exhibited insufficient bone marrow spaces and source of blood vessels, and consequentially a compromised angiogenesis that used to be related to bone loss (Nobuto et al. 2005).

3.1.2 Implant Buccolingual Positioning

Technically, immediate implants have to be allocated in the confines of the alveolus (Blanco et al. 2008) and 5 mm in host bone apically to obtain primary stability (Nemcovsky et al. 2002). Nevertheless, it has to be considered that the variations in buccolingual positioning of an immediate implant can also interfere with the level of crestal bone resorption.

Qahash et al. (2008) demonstrated a significant association between the width of the buccal alveolar ridge and the extent of bone resorption evaluated by light microscopy. They suggested that the width of the buccal alveolar ridge

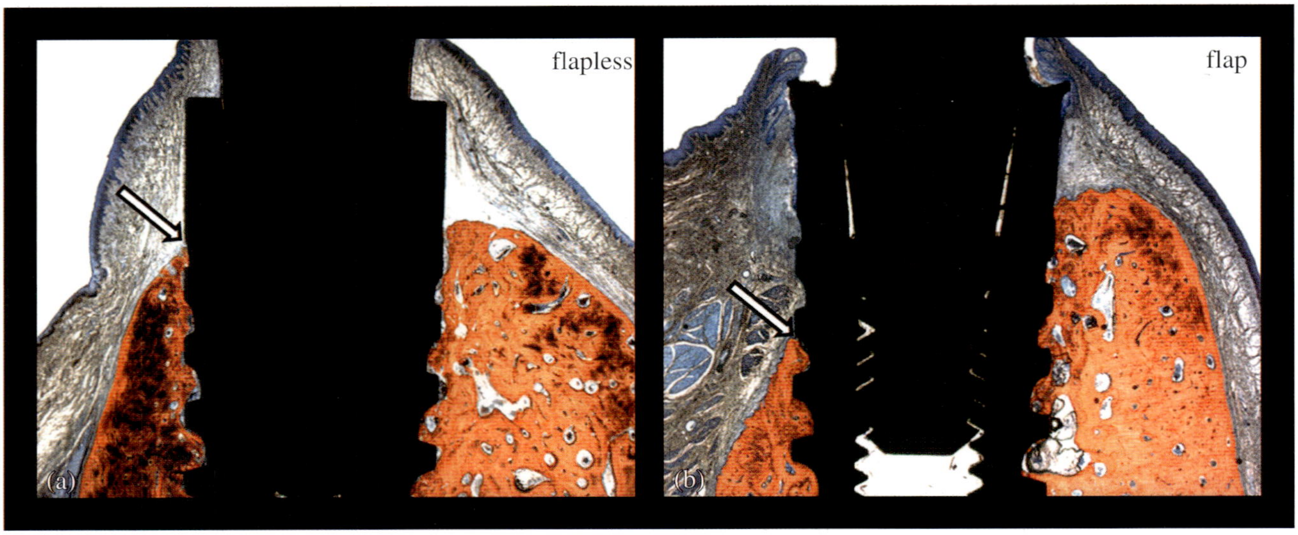

Figure 3.7 Evidence the buccal bone plates (on the left of the implants) being significantly thinner when compared to the lingual components (on the right of the implants). In terms of bone density, while the buccal plates presented a cortical bone type with a sparse and decreased number of marrow areas, the lingual bone plates exhibited numerous and large marrow areas. In (a), the implant was immediately placed during a flapless intervention and modest buccal bone resorption was observed when compared to the lingual bone plate; however in (b), in which a flap surgical approach was used, a significantly higher buccal bone resorption can be noted.

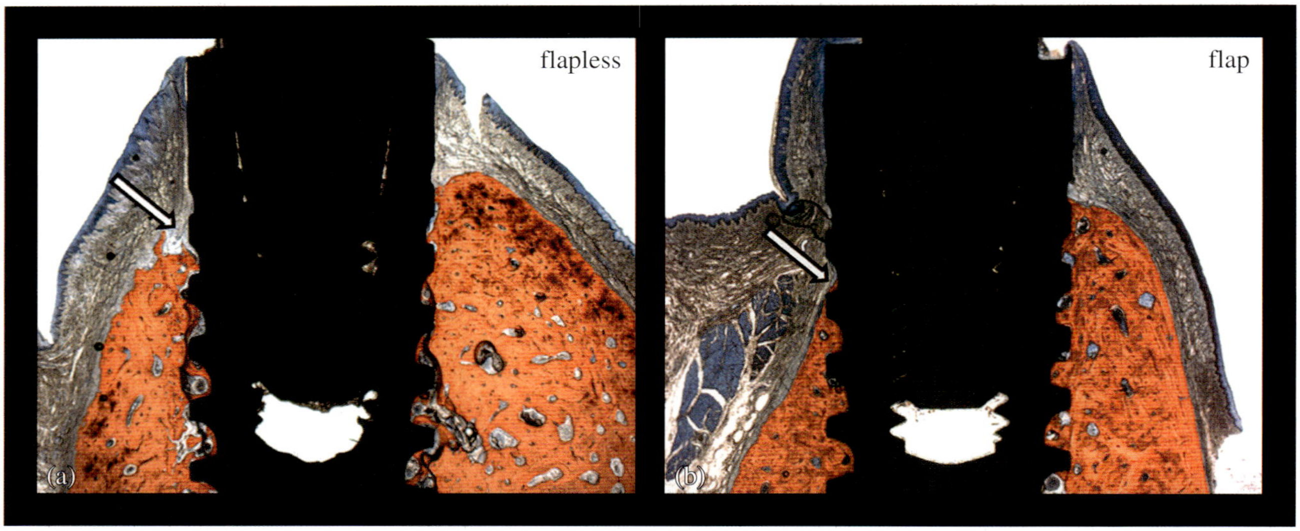

Figure 3.8 Again the buccal bone plates appeared very different from the lingual bone plates, considering the thickness, bone density, number, and volume of the marrow spaces. In (a), another example of an implant installed during a flapless procedure versus an implant placed during a mucoperiosteal flap raising in (b). Observe the difference in buccal bone height between them.

Table 3.1 Bone densities in flapless and flap groups in the different thirds of the implants described as mean ± SD.

	FLAPLESS		FLAP	
	coronal	apical	coronal	apical
BUCCAL	90.37 ± 6.12	85.80 ± 13.87[a]	93.42 ± 4.43[b]	94.39 ± 5.29[c]
LINGUAL	87.13 ± 7.99[d]	59.88 ± 13.19[a,d]	84.55 ± 4.97[b,e]	50.69 ± 9.90[c,e]

[a] $p = 0.0070$.
[b] $p = 0.0070$.
[c] $p = 0.0006$.
[d] $p = 0.0023$.
[e] $p = 0.0006$.

should be at least 2 mm to maintain the alveolar bone level. This information was reinforced by Polimeni et al. (2004) and Wikesjo et al. (2006), who studied the alveolar bone healing potential in peri-implant critical-size defects. They demonstrated that a thicker bone plate could provide a large wound space that was correlated to enhanced bone regeneration, whereas implants placed closer to thin buccal plates, usually evidenced in immediate implants procedures, were associated with increased crestal bone loss. Such results can sustain one other explanation for a higher BBP resorption found after immediate implants placement in fresh extraction sites by Araujo et al. (2005). They installed 4.1 mm wide implants in premolar extraction sites that exhibited a mean buccal-lingual entrance width of 3.8 ± 0.2 mm, which signifies that the diameters of the implants were greater than the alveoli themselves, probably invading the BBP space during the implant placement.

The recession of the marginal mucosa was also correlated to the buccolingual implant positioning. Buser, Martin and Belser (2004) recommended that the implant shoulder must be placed 1–2 mm lingual to the emergence of the adjacent teeth to ensure maintenance of an adequate width of buccal bone and to stabilize the mucosa over the buccal implant surface. Additionally, Evans and Chen (2008) recorded three times more recession of the marginal mucosa for implants with a buccal shoulder position than for implants with a lingual shoulder position.

In our first flapless study (Novaes et al. 2011a), the implants were placed 1 mm away from the buccal marginal bone wall, preserving its integrity but also leaving a gap between this plate and the implant. After 12 weeks of healing, no residual defect was observed on the histological specimens and the formation of new bone could be a possible explanation, as evidenced by the "jumping gap distance" studies (Botticelli et al. 2003).

3.1.3 Jumping Gap and Implant Surface

An important difference between installing implants in a healed bone and in fresh extraction sockets is the gap frequently observed between the walls of the extraction socket and the implant, which is usually widest in the coronal part of the recipient site (Botticelli et al. 2003). One way to explain this lack of adaptation is that fresh extraction sockets vary drastically in configuration, health of the bony walls, size, and shape. "Jumping gap" was defined as the ability of a defect surrounding an immediate implant to regenerate without the use of additional biomaterials such as membranes, grafts, or combinations. Even though a "self-contained" bone defect may heal properly with new bone formation by the presence of the coagulum itself, this is highly dependent on the gap dimension, the implant surface, and the time of healing after implant installation (Barros et al. 2012). The benefits of the association of biomaterials to encourage bone growth within these defects are still controversial (Araujo, Linder and Lindhe 2011; Hsu et al. 2012).

Historically, data derived from experiments in different animal models (Akimoto et al. 1999; Carlsson et al. 1988; Caudill and Meffert 1991; Knox, Caudill and Meffert 1991) showed that defects wider than 0.5 mm at the time of implant installation might compromise its osseointegration when bone regeneration techniques are not used. Residual gaps and bone-to-implant contact established at a more apical level were described in those studies. In contrast, the histomorphometric results of Barros et al. (2012) demonstrated that circumferential defects varying from 1.0 to 2.0 mm wide and 5.0 mm deep may allow complete bone fill around microrough and nanomodified implant surfaces (Figures 3.9–3.13). However, in a general, as the gap widened, the bone-to-implant contact decreased, the bone density also decreased, and the vertical bone resorption increased; in other words, the gap resolution potential decreased.

This trend was previously demonstrated, but some important differences need to be highlighted. Akimoto et al. (1999) investigated the amount of bone fill that occurred in gaps ranging from 0.5 to 1.4 mm wide. They used a similar methodology in a dog model and observed statistically significant differences for bone-to-implant contact between all experimental groups (control = 38.8%; 0.5 mm defect = 22.9%; 1.0 mm defect = 11%, and 1.4 mm defect = 2.7%). In the Barros et al. (2012) study, the differences between the groups were not so drastically evident and even the larger circumferential gaps of 2 mm achieved the indices of 18.97 or 21.36% of bone-to-implant contact (Figure 3.13). These could be ascribed to the implant surface characteristics, because Akimoto et al. (1999) tested implants designed with a machined surface, whereas Barros et al. (2012) compared nano- and microstructured surfaces. Confronting the vertical bone resorption of the buccal plates of both studies, relevant differences were noted between the test sites, but not when comparing the control sites. Akimoto et al. (1999) showed a mean distance from the implant shoulder to the highest point of the buccal bone contact of 0.9 mm in control sites, 2.4 mm in the 1.0 mm defect sites and 3.1 mm in the 1.4 mm defect sites, while Barros et al. (2012) found that the vertical bone resorption was 0.8–0.6 mm in the control sites, 1.5–1.4 mm in the 1.0 mm defect sites and 1.6 mm in the 1.5 mm defect sites, respectively, for nano- and microstructured surfaces. Thus, it seems that turned implant surfaces can impair the quality of osseointegration and make the crestal bone resorption more likely to happen when dealing with circumferential defects around immediate implants. Modified implant surfaces may partly counteract these undesirable results, especially when the gaps became wider. However, in those circumstances, the association of bone regenerative procedures has to be considered.

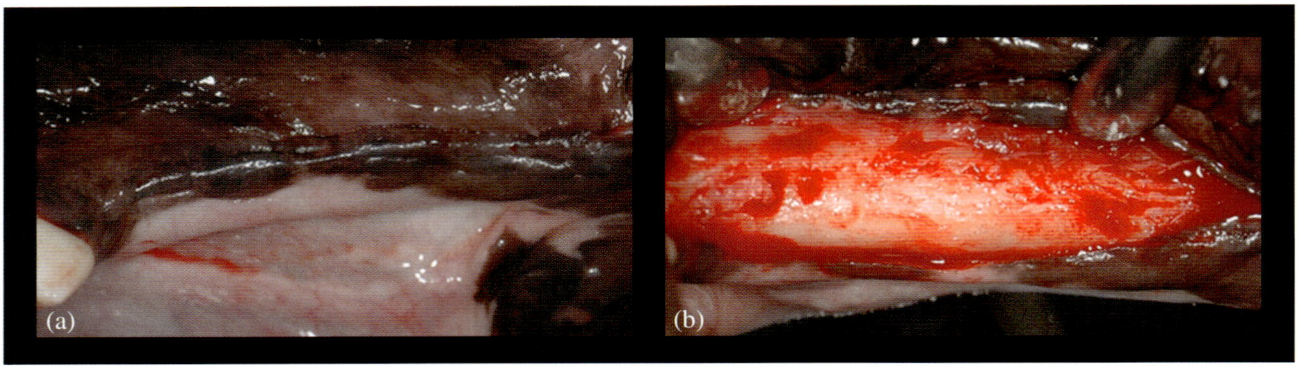

Figure 3.9 Clinical images of a Barros et al. (2012) study developed in dogs. (a) and (b) Eight weeks after the extraction of the four mandibular premolars, note the alveolar ridge completely healed.

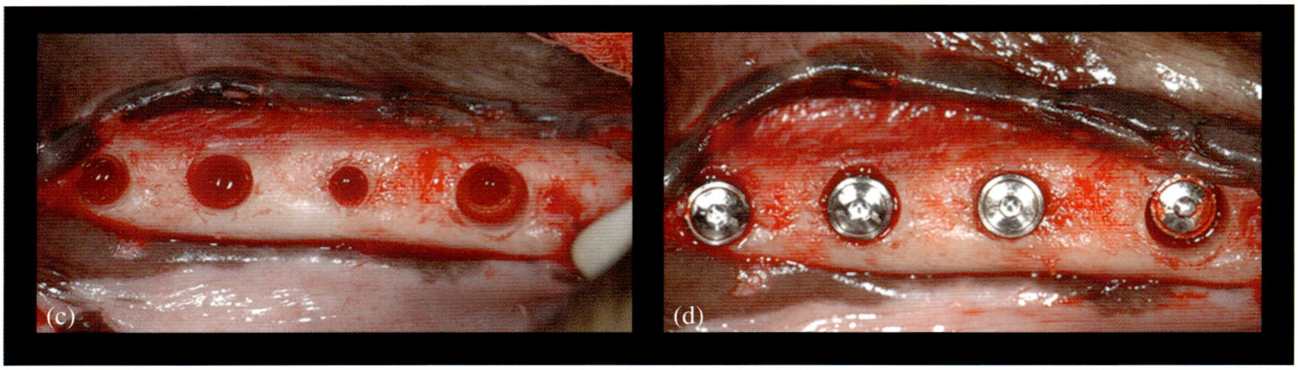

Figure 3.9 (c) The position of the different gap defects and control sites were randomly determined in each animal. The control preparation remained without a gap, while the three different circumferential gap defects of 1.0, 1.5, or 2.0 mm wide were created using other incremental drills. (d) In one hemiarch of each dog, four 3.25 × 10 mm implants with a nanomodified surface with a discrete crystalline deposition of nanometer-sized CaP (Nanotite™ Biomet 3i, Palm Beach Gardens, Florida, USA) were installed, while the other side received the other four 3.25 × 10 mm implants with a microrough surface (Osseotite® Biomet 3i, Palm Beach Gardens, Florida, USA).

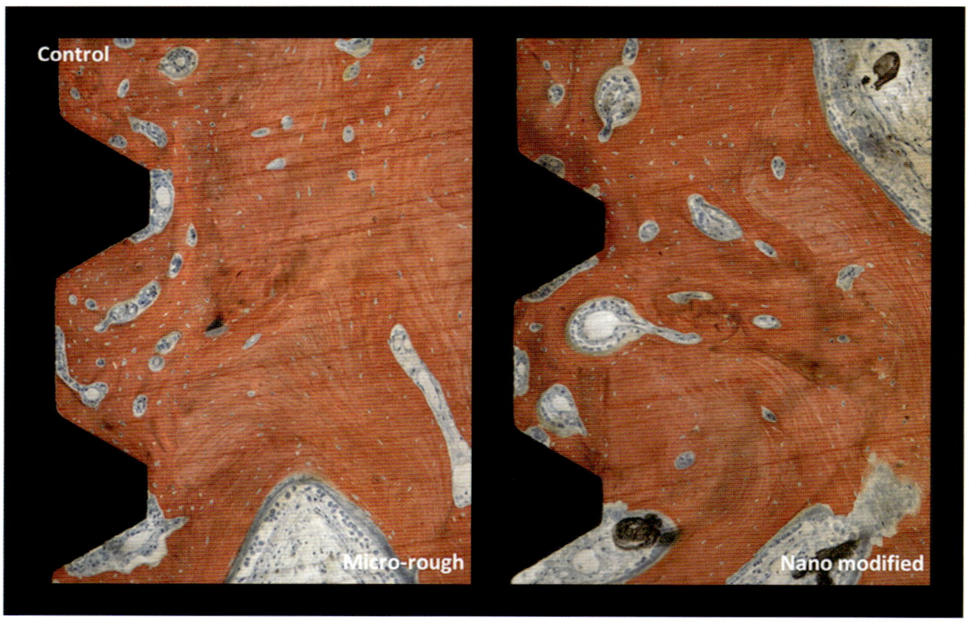

Figure 3.10 Histological images of the control sites of microrough and nanomodified implant surfaces (Barros et al. 2012). Note the very high adjacent density in both specimens. Stevenel's blue and Alizarin red stain. Magnification × 100.

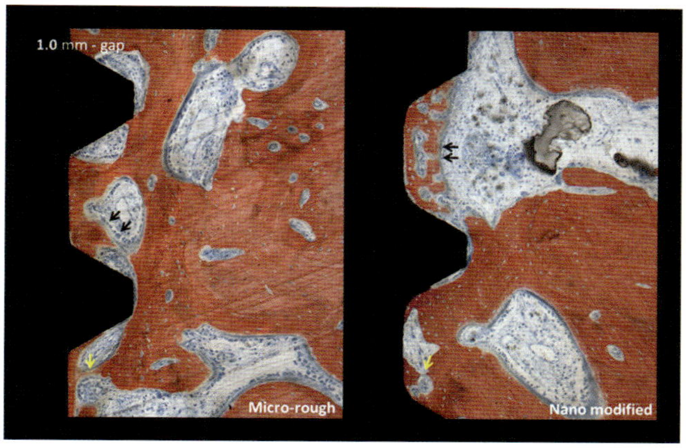

Figure 3.11 Histological images of the 1.0 mm gap sites of microrough and nanomodified implant surfaces (Barros et al. 2012). The number and volume of the marrow spaces of both images are not relative to a cortical bone; a decrease in bone density can be observed. The black arrows evidence the osteoblasts lining an active bone formation and the yellow arrows highlight new bone forming bridges to the implant surface, establishing a good level of bone-to-implant contact. Stevenel's blue and Alizarin red stain. Magnification × 100.

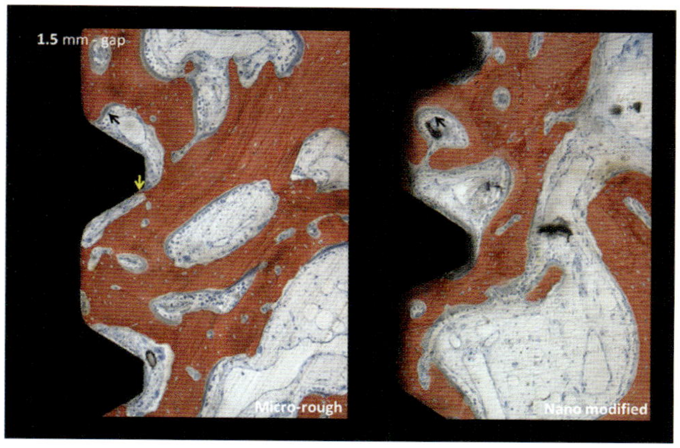

Figure 3.12 Histological images of the 1.5 mm gap sites of microrough and nanomodified implant surfaces (Barros et al. 2012). Note that both images evidence many marrow spaces, constituting a bone with inferior density when compared to those exhibited by the images representative of the control group in Figure 3.10. Again the black arrows evidence the OB lining an active bone formation and the yellow arrow exhibits new bone forming a bridge to the implant surface. Stevenel's blue and Alizarin red stain. Magnification × 100.

3.1.4 Gap Filling and Implant Coronoapical Positioning

In an attempt to optimize the osseointegration in a critical size gap, many bone-replacing materials have been used to encourage bone growth within these defects. These materials exhibit osseoconducting properties and act as a scaffold for cell adhesion and proliferation, thus facilitating gap fill (Karring et al. 2005; Molly et al. 2008; Schopper et al. 2005). Several biomaterials have been used in conjunction with immediate implantation, with many of them showing successful results (Gher et al. 1994; Molly et al. 2008; Schwartz-Arad and Chaushu 1997).

As bone tissue undergoes constant remodeling, both vertically and horizontally during the healing process, all dimensions must be carefully taken into consideration for adequate implant positioning. The bone loss that can occur after implant placement is justified by the formation of biological spaces in the peri-implantar tissue, implant–abutment connection, and implant design and position (Oh et al. 2002). However, when an implant is performed utilizing Morse Cone connections, reduced bone loss was observed and can be explained by the specific characteristics of the inner connection between abutment and implant and also by the external profile of such a connection (Barros et al. 2010; Doring, Eisenmann and Stiller 2004).

To continue our line of immediate implant research and again highlighting the importance of the preservation of the BBP on the esthetic and long-term success of such therapy, Suaid et al. (2014) evaluated the BBP remodeling following immediate implantation, using flapless procedures. In particular, this study compared sites that received or did not receive synthetic bone grafts (BCP) in the gap between the implant and the BBP, and also verified the effect of two different vertical implant positions in the bone level changes. From the combination of study variables, four groups were formed: equicrestal with synthetic bone graft (biphasic calcium

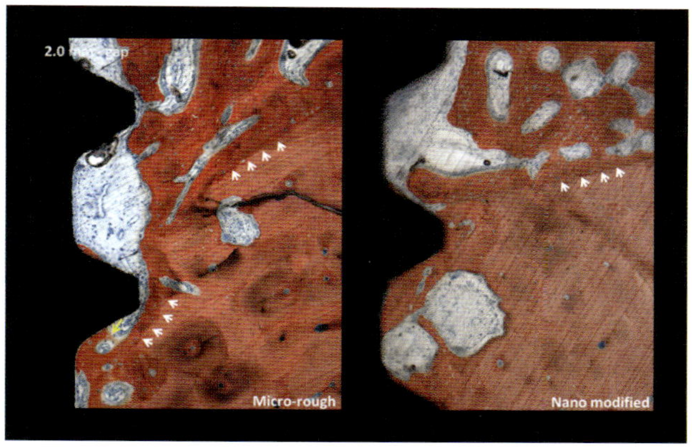

Figure 3.13 Histological images of the 2.0 mm gap sites of microrough and nanomodified implant surfaces (Barros et al. 2012). Yellow arrows show the new bone forming a bridge to the implant surfaces. White arrows highlight the difference between the pre-existent bone and the new bone (strong red). Note that in the more coronal third of the implants, surrounded by the new bone, the bone-to-implant contact was compromised. Stevenel's blue and Alizarin red stain. Magnification × 100.

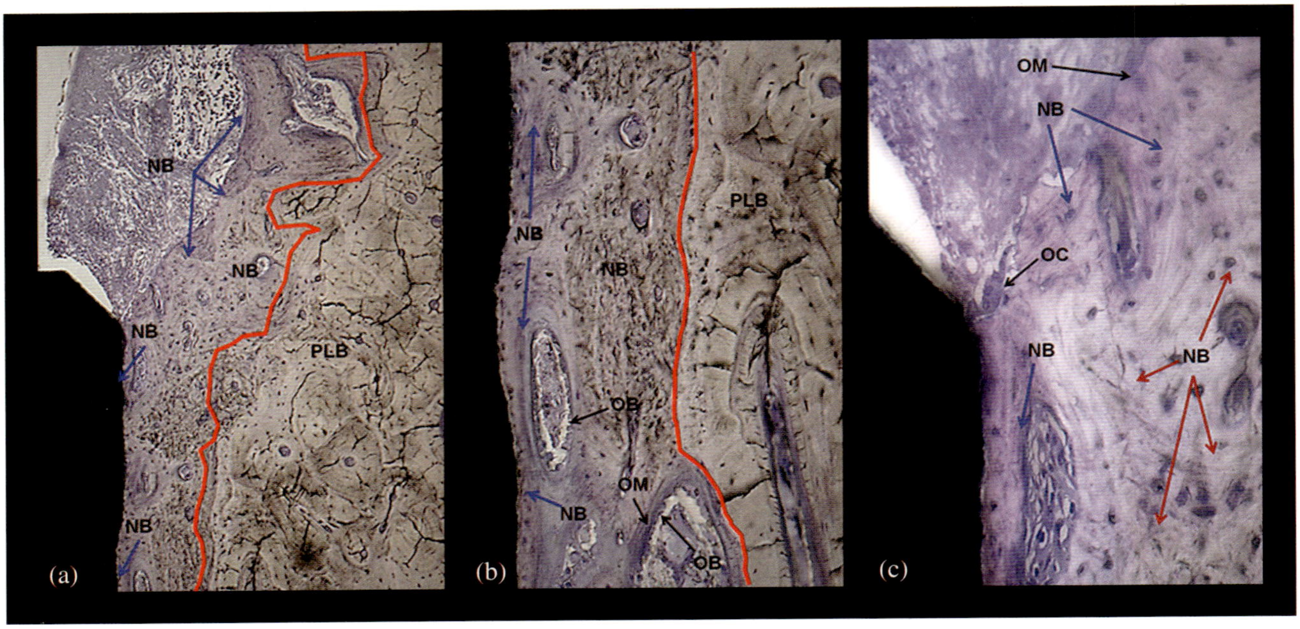

Figure 3.14 Histological images of the control sites. (a) The presence of the two types of bone tissue: parent lamellar bone (PLB) representing the "old bone" and newly formed bone (NB). Note the red line separating the "old" and "new" structures (magnification × 10). (b) This specific area of the new bone shows immature aspects of bone with some concentric lamellae (blue arrows) and the presence of osteoblasts (OB) and osteoid matrix (OM) (magnification × 20). Blue arrows: the new bone appeared in direct contact with the implant surface and sometimes circumscribing the lamellae. (c) The blue and red arrows indicate the details of the new bone (NB) structures. The osteoid matrix on the external surface of the NB and osteoclast (OC) activity (magnification × 40). Toluidine blue stain.

phosphate: BCP) (test ECTG); equicrestal with coagulum (control ECCG); subcrestal (2 mm) synthetic bone with graft (BCP) (test SCTG); and subcrestal with coagulum (control SCCG). In the histologic analysis, the newly formed bone (NB) was observed mostly in the gap area, and the surface between this structure and the parent lamellar bone ("old bone") was evident (Figures 3.14a, b, 3.15a, b, and 3.16a). An osteoid matrix (OM) was also identified in some areas of the newly formed bone (Figures 3.14b, c and 3.16c); it was paved with OB and represented the bone formation process (Figures 3.14b, c and 3.16c). It was possible to observe the presence of residual graft particles (RGP) in the test groups, and these particles were dispersed in the non-mineralized and mineralized matrices in the region corresponding to the gap area (Figure 3.16a–c).

In relation to the vertical positioning of the implants, histomorphometric evaluation of vertical crestal bone resorption (VCBR) that analyzed the crestal bone loss in relation to the implant shoulder showed a very small loss between 0.08 mm (mean) and 0.20 mm (mean) in the grafted and non-grafted groups, respectively (Table 3.2) in the equicrestal groups. The subcrestal groups, instead, exhibited a loss of 1.95 mm (mean) and 1.28 mm (mean) in the grafted and non-grafted groups, respectively (Table 3.2). This comparison between equicrestal and subcrestal groups achieved statistically significant relevance (Table 3.2). However, this higher crestal bone resorption was compensated by the subcrestal positioning of the implants, which means that despite the crestal bone loss, the peri-implant bone level remained above the implant shoulder in the subcrestal groups.

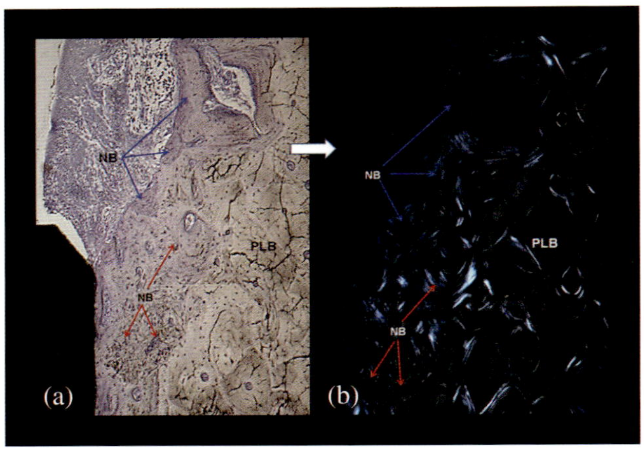

Figure 3.15 (a) The different bone structures. (b) The polarized light: the red arrows showed the new bone (NB) with the lamellar pattern (parallel fibers) (PLB) and, in some areas, a structure with interlaced fibers characterizing the woven bone. The blue arrows showed the new bone (NB) characterized by a parallel-fibered bone (PLB) with residual areas of woven bone (magnification × 10). Toluidine blue stain.

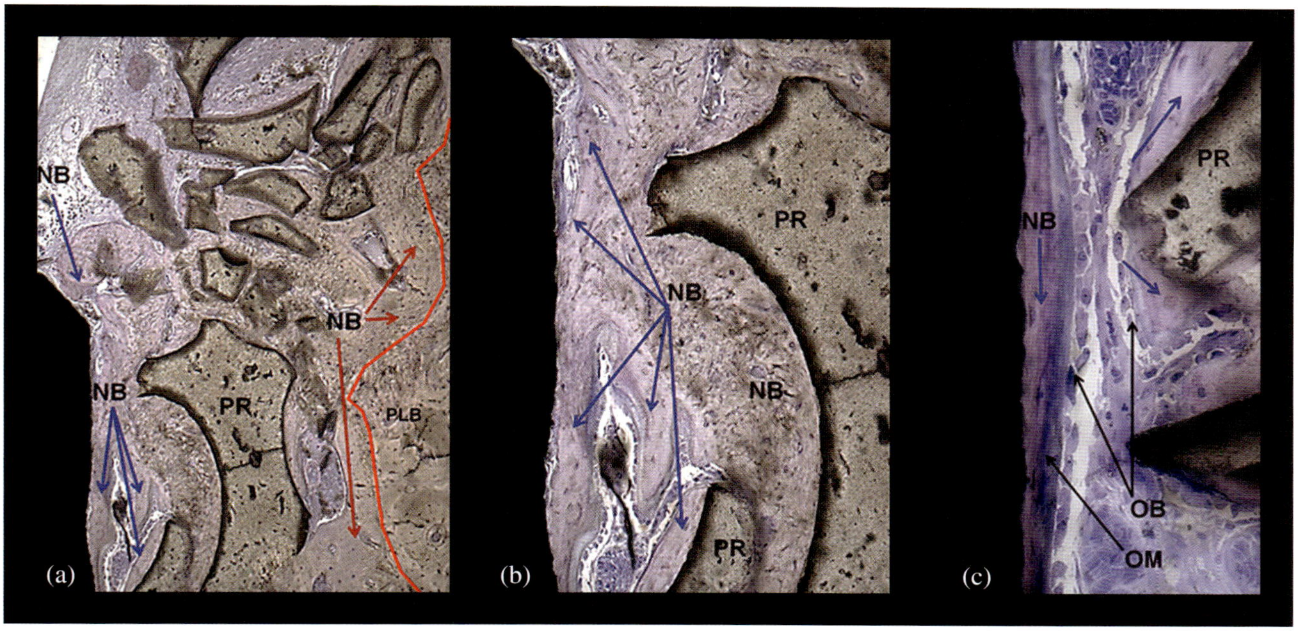

Figure 3.16 Histological images of the control sites. (a) The residual particles of the bone graft (PR) surrounded by new bone (NB; red and blue arrows) (magnification × 10). (b) The implant surface was lined by NB (blue arrows) and its structure established a direct contact with the particles and the new bone forming a bridge between the structures (magnification × 20). (c) The osteoblasts (OB), osteoid matrix (OM), and the NB (blue arrows) in direct contact with the implant surface and residual particles of the bone graft (magnification × 40). Toluidine blue stain.

Table 3.2 Comparisons between equicrestal and subcrestal control and test sites for all histomorphometric parameters: vertical crestal bone resorption (VCBR), vertical bone level (VBL), bone density of new bone total area (NB) (inter- and intragroup analysis of adjacent and distant) and recently formed bone (RFB) (adjacent), and the percentage of residual particles.

							Bone density (%)						
	VCBR(mm)			VBL(mm)			Adjacent (NB–100%)			Distant (NB–100%)			Residual particles (%)
Site	Mean	Med	SD	Mean	Med	SD	Mean	Med	SD	Mean	Med	SD	
ECTG	0.08[a]	0.2	0.7	1.58	1.5	0.95	35.7[b]	35.1	17	16.5	30.3	8	11.16
ECCG	0.20[a]	0.2	0.4	1.67	1.8	0.82	51.4[b,c]	41.8	17	17.3[c]	17.4	9	–
SCTG	1.95[a]	2.0	0.5	1.31	1.2	0.41	45.1[b]	59.1	16	13.7	32.9	4	8.40
SCCG	1.28	1.5	0.6	0.75	0.6	0.33	80[b,c]	86.5	10	18.1[c]	48.6	12	–

Mean; Med: medians; SD: standard deviation.
[a] Intergroup (VCBR parameter) statistically significance difference (Bonferroni post-hoc $p = 0.03$; $n = 8$).
[b] Intergroup (adjacent parameter) statistically significance difference (Bonferroni post-hoc $p = 0.0001$; $n = 8$).
[c] Intragroup statistically significance difference (Wilcoxon test–Bonferroni post-hoc; $p = 0.01$; $n = 8$).

Historically there is no consensus about the better vertical implant positioning in the literature. Negri et al. (2012) also investigated the vertical crestal bone resorption in immediate implants placed equicrestally and 2 mm subcrestally, but without gaps and with flaps performing the surgical approach. Their results demonstrated a mean loss of 1.88 mm in the equicrestal group and 1.26 mm in the subcrestal group, without statistical significant differences. Barros et al. (2009, 2010), who compared the bone remodeling around equicrestally versus 1.5 mm subcrestally contiguous Morse Cone connection implants, found a significantly lower crestal bone resorption in the subcrestal group.

Considering the other histomorphometric parameter evaluated by Suaid et al. (2014), the distance from the implant shoulder to the first bone-to-implant contact, known as vertical bone level, the subcrestal

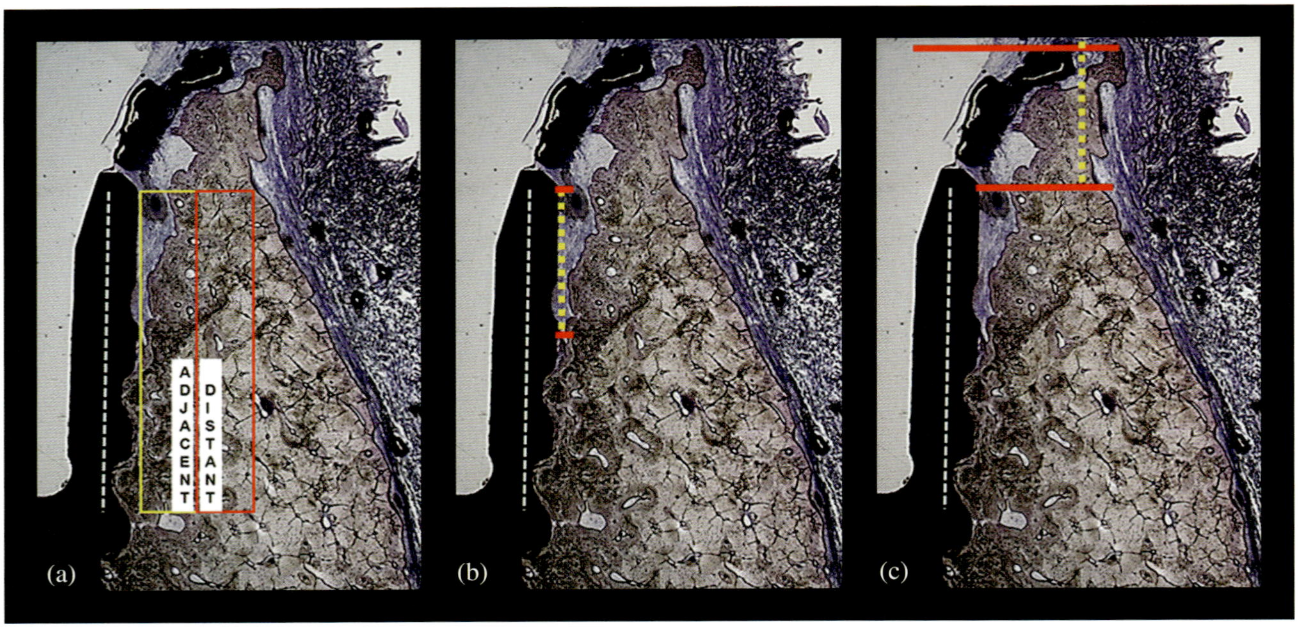

Figure 3.17 Histological images representing the morphometric measurements. (a) Histological "bone density" determined within a rectangle that comprised the region of the defect. The length of 3 mm is always represented by a dashed line on the left of the implant. The adjacent area is the yellow rectangle and the distant area is the red rectangle placed in a mirror image of the first. (b) Vertical bone level (VBL) was calculated on the buccal bone plate of the implants, from the implant shoulder to the first bone-to-implant contact. (c) Vertical crestal bone resorption (VCBR) determined as a linear vertical measurement from an imaginary line from the implant shoulder (second imaginary dotted line) to the highest point of the bone crest (dotted line). Toluidine blue stain. Magnification × 2.5.

Table 3.3 Residual gap (RG) (mm) investigated inside the defects of all the groups equicrestal and subcrestal through linear horizontal measurements: (1) from the implant to the bone at the midpoint of the defect; (2) from the implant to the bone at the most apical point of the defect.

										Mean	Med	SD	Bone fill (BF)
ECTG	1	0	0	0	0.5	0.3	0.2	0.0	0.7	0.24[a]	0.00	0.28	3
	2	0	0	0.0	0.1	0.0	0.0	0	1.1	0.17	0.15	0.37	3
ECCG	1	0.5	0.2	0.0	0.1	0.0	0.0	0.1	0.3	0.19[a]	0.00	0.15	0
	2	0.5	0.2	0.0	0.1	0.0	0.0	0.1	0.3	0.04	0.00	0.07	4
SCTG	1	0	0.1	0	0	0.9	0.2	0	0	0.16	0.16	0.32	5
	2	0.2	0.0	0	0	0	0.4	0	0	0.10	0.00	0.16	4
SCCG	1	0	0	0	0	0	0	0	0.1	0.02[a]	0.13	0.04	6
	2	0.2	0.2	0	0	0	0.2	0	0	0.08	0.04	0.12	4

Mean; Med: median; SD: standard deviation.
[a] Statistically significant (Bonferroni post-hoc $p = 0.04$; $n = 8$).

groups showed an inferior bone loss when compared to the equicrestal groups. Negri et al. (2012) also observed a better vertical bone level for subcrestally positioned implants (2.21 mm) versus 3.39 mm in the equicrestal group. Their bone losses were higher for both groups when compared to those found by Suaid et al. (2014) and can be explained by the flapless approach and the 12-month period of healing provided in the Suaid et al. (2014) study.

Finally, Suaid et al. (2014) revealed a better gap resolution in the subcrestal groups (Figure 3.17a–c and Table 3.3). They used linear horizontal measurements (Figure 3.18a–d) to evaluate the potential of bone fill of the gaps in different circumstances. According to the

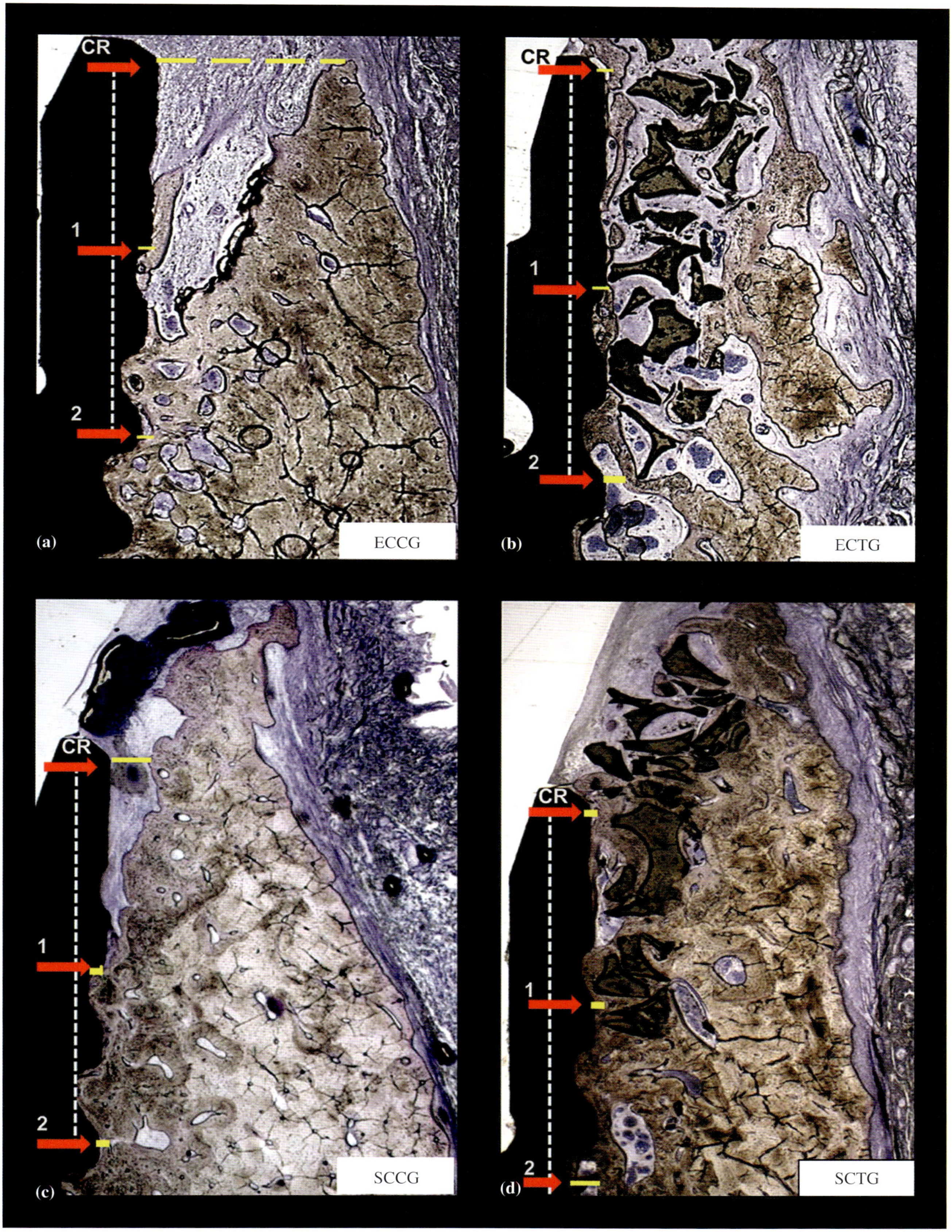

Figure 3.18 Crestal resorption (CR): linear horizontal measurements were made from the most cervical point of the defect to the bone. Residual gap (RG): linear horizontal measurements were made from the midpoint of the defect to the bone (1) and from the most apical point of the defect to the bone (2) to evaluate the bone formation inside the defects. In some specimens, crestal bone resorption was observed, involving the cervical third of the defects and compromising the first horizontal measurement. Toluidine blue stain. Magnification × 2.5.

results, it seems reasonable to suggest that large defects must be considered as a challenge for complete bone fill, but not an impediment. In Table 3.3, a complete bone fill was identified by the number of times in which no distance was found between the new bone and the implant surface (Table 3.3). In accordance with these findings, Araujo et al. (2011), using deproteinized bovine bone mineral in gap defects, demonstrated that the marginal hard tissue of the control sites was markedly different from that of the grafted sites. Thus, while the buccal crestal bone in the grafted sites was comparatively thick and located at or close to the SLA border, the corresponding crest at the control sites was thinner and located a varying distance below the SLA border. According to their conclusion, the placement of Bio-Oss collagen® (Bio-Oss collagen, Geistlich, Switzerland) in the void between the implant and the buccal-approximal bone walls of fresh extraction sockets modified the process of hard tissue healing, provided additional amounts of hard tissue at the entrance to the previous socket, and improved the level of marginal bone-to-implant contact.

Regarding the presence or absence of the gap, de Sanctis et al. (2009) observed a buccal bone loss of 2.5 mm with immediate implants using full-thickness flaps and with gaps of various dimensions. Blanco et al. (2011) placed immediate implants at the bone crest level in flapless surgery with a small gap (<1 mm). The bone crest at the buccal aspect was roughly 0.86 and 1.3 mm apical to the SLA border. In comparison to Suaid et al. (2014) results, analysis shows that wider gaps did not interfere negatively with the maintenance of the buccal bone. Furthermore, it seems that a larger gap promotes better results when compared with its absence, as demonstrated by Negri et al. (2012).

To summarize, Suaid et al. (2014) evidenced little bone loss around immediately placed implants, but their good results were due to the combination of the flapless approach, the grafting of the gap defect, the Morse Cone design of the implants, and also the implant surface treatment. The gap resolution in both test and control groups of Suaid et al. (2014) were compatible, probably again by the careful selection of each surgical step. These advantages on BBP preservation are very important when planning the rehabilitation of esthetic regions.

3.1.5 Presence and Thickness of the Buccal Bone Plate (Tissue Biotype)

The thickness of the BBP in the extraction site seems to have a significant influence on the amount of horizontal and vertical crest resorption in human sockets (Spinato et al. 2014), as well as in implants placed immediately into extraction sockets (Ferrus et al. 2010; Tomasi et al. 2010). This is an important aspect that must be considered in the decision-making process regarding the immediate positioning of the implant into the socket.

Maia et al. (2015) realized a clinical and histomorphometric study to evaluate the influence of gingival thickness and bone grafting on BBP remodeling after immediate implant placement in fresh extraction sockets with thin buccal bone, using a flapless approach. The gingiva of the dogs was thinned at one side of the mandible and all the implants were placed equicrestally with their cervical portion 1.5 mm distant from the BBP (gap). The methodology is similar to that used in Suaid et al. (2014), but the grafting material used was a xenograft (Bio-Oss collagen, Geistlich, Switzerland).

All the animals exhibited a thin buccal bone and the presurgical procedure significantly reduced the gingival thickness in test groups. All the measurements were evaluated on the buccal bone region. The vertical crestal bone resorption (VCBR), vertical bone level (VBL), and the residual gap (RG) were measured according to Suaid et al. (2014). Histologically, all the experimental groups presented the buccal gaps filled with newly formed bone and the buccal bone level was slightly apical to the implant shoulder. There were no statistically significant differences among the groups for the histomorphometric parameters. In general, buccal bone loss (VCBR and VBL) was observed in all the experimental groups, without significant differences between them. Additionally, all groups presented similar histological bone density and RG.

It is important to highlight that the study of Maia et al. (2015) was conducted on small beagle dogs, which were characterized by an inherently thin periodontal biotype. The findings from this study suggest that dimensional changes on the BBP occurred following implant placement into fresh extraction sockets with an initially thin BBP, regardless of the gingival thickness or the association of graft bone filling. The better results observed by Suaid et al. (2014) in terms of buccal bone loss can be explained by the use of large animals (Labradors), which usually have a thicker periodontal type/BBP.

The results of Maia et al. (2015) are in accordance with the scientific literature (Qahash et al. 2008), evidencing that thin BBPs are more likely to resorb, even with flapless implantation and filling the buccal gap with biomaterial.

3.2 Clinical Evidence

Immediate implant placement and provisionalization in the maxillary anterior region must always be treated as a challenging case, although the replacement of a single tooth has been documented with high rates of success and predictability (Mijiritsky et al. 2009).

Nowadays, there is consensus on the participation of the periodontal tissues in the esthetic outcomes involving implants in general. Harmonious esthetic soft tissue contours avoid differences in clinical crown lengths between adjacent teeth and require the presence of papillae and volume of buccal soft tissue (Ahmad 1998). Nevertheless, the achievement of such desired outcomes depends mainly on the preservation of the BBP and proximal bone height, in other words, the underlying hard tissue (Spear 1999). For example, BBP defects detected during or consecutive to immediate implants placement procedures were more frequently associated with the occurrence of gingival recessions, both compromising directly the final esthetic result (Evans and Chen 2008).

As evidenced and supported by our previously described preclinical studies, some strategic factors can influence BBP preservation in immediate implant placement procedures, such as flap-raising techniques, implant positioning, implant surface, periodontal biotype (soft and hard tissue thickness), and also the provisionalization of those implant sites. The understanding of these biological bases is fundamental to the development of a surgical approach that focuses on an optimized esthetic result.

The following clinical case illustrates one treatment strategy based on the compilation of the key-aspects factors elicited in this chapter, which were extensively studied in our scientific research. A 40-year-old female presented the right central incisor with root resorption and an advanced periapical lesion (Figures 3.19–3.21). Considering that there was sufficient apical bone height for primary implant stability and that the periapical lesion cannot be considered as a contraindication (Novaes et al. 2003), an immediate installation was planned. After the restorative crown removal (Figure 3.22), only intrasulcular incisions were performed, as recommended by a flapless intervention. A periotome was used in order to achieve an atraumatic extraction without damaging the buccal and proximal bone (Figure 3.23). A grit-blasted and acid-etched Morse Cone connection implant (ANKYLOS C/X®, DentsplySirona Implants, Mannheim, Germany) was lingually and subcrestally positioned (Figure 3.24), maintaining intact the buccal bone crest. The remaining gap between the implant and the BBP was grafted with a deproteinized bovine bone mineral (Bio-Oss®, Geistlich, Switzerland). As the implant achieved an insertion torque superior to 25 N cm, confirming a good primary stability, the prefabricated prosthetic abutment was connected to the implant (Figure 3.25) and the removed crown was prepared to be used as the provisional crown (Figure 3.26), immediately restoring the lost tooth. Radiographic and tomographic images evidenced the good positioning of the implant, maintaining the bone height, proximally and buccally. The gap left between the BBP and the implant was essential for the preservation of the buccal bone crest thickness (Figures 3.27 and 3.28). Although the periodontal biotype of this patient was not thin, a connective tissue graft was subepithelially positioned using a split-thickness envelope and was maintained in place by absorbable sutures (Figure 3.29).

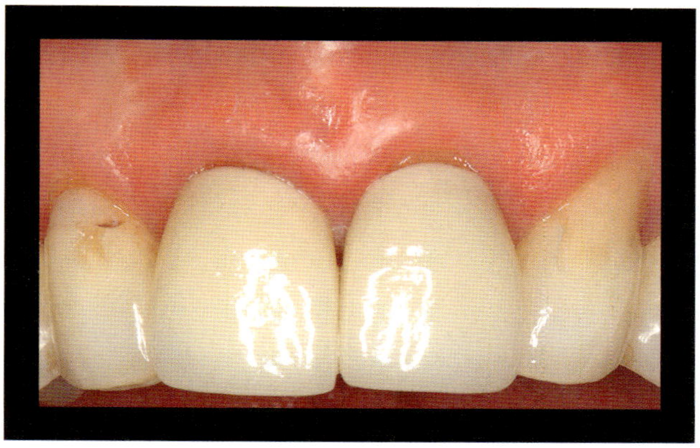

Figure 3.19 Initial presentation of the case with the compromised right central incisor.

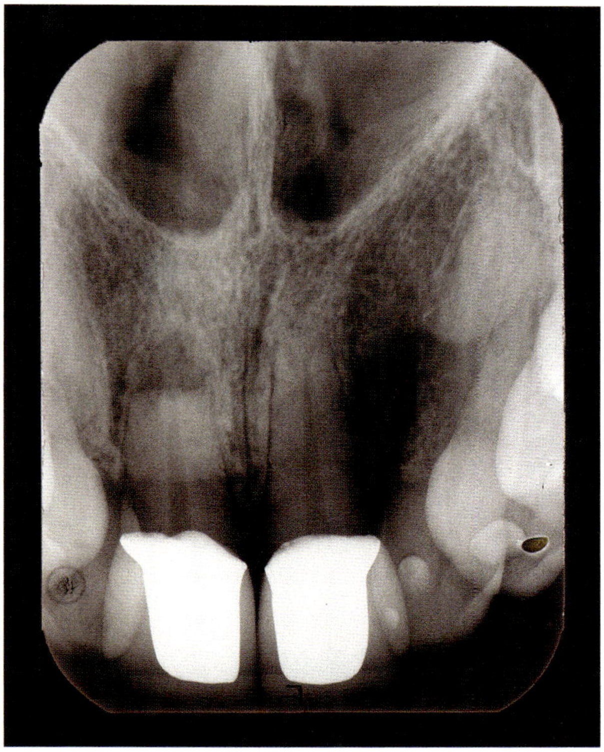

Figure 3.20 Initial radiographic view of the region evidencing periapical lesion on the right central incisor.

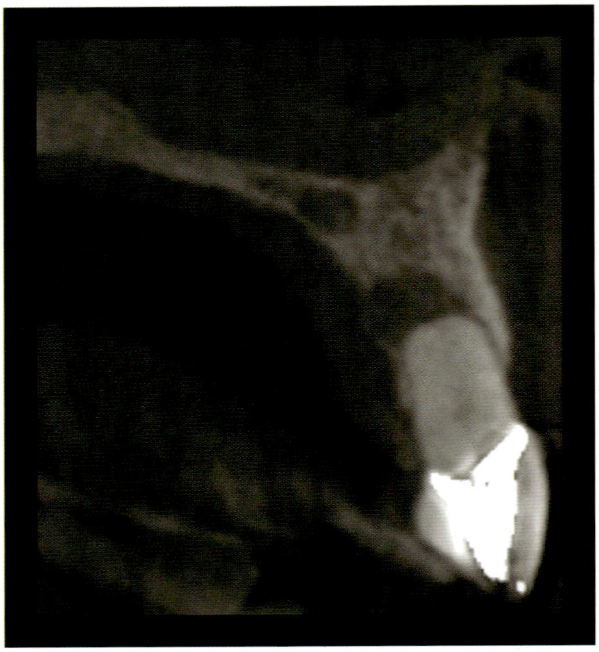

Figure 3.21 A preoperatively cone-beam computed tomographic image slice. Observe the dimension of the periapical lesion and the thickness of the buccal bone plate.

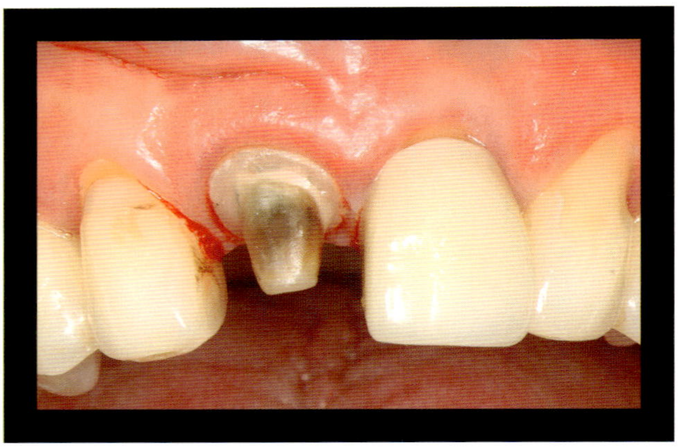

Figure 3.22 After the removal of the restorative crown, only intrasulcular incisions were performed.

Antibiotic and analgesic medications were prescribed, and the patient was instructed to rinse with 0.12% chlorhexidine gluconate solution twice a day for two weeks. A liquid diet was suggested for one week following surgery, and then a soft diet for the next month. After the one-week follow-up, the region appeared edematous, but the soft tissues remained in position without contraction (Figure 3.30). The sutures were totally removed at the one-month follow-up (Figures 3.31 and 3.32). After six months an increased buccal soft tissue was evidenced (Figure 3.33) and the final abutment-level

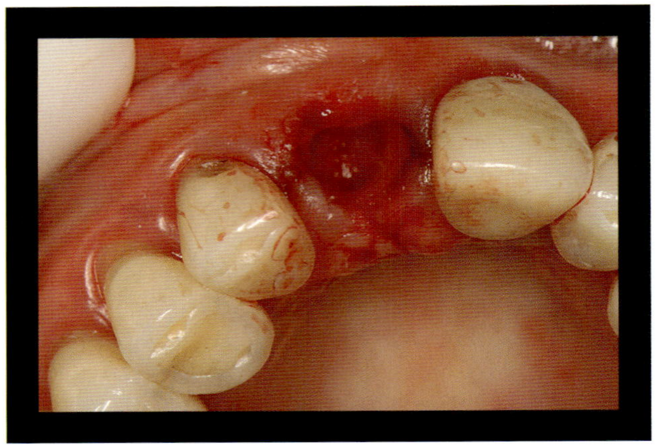

Figure 3.23 Palatal view after the flapless dental extraction. Note the preservation of the tissues.

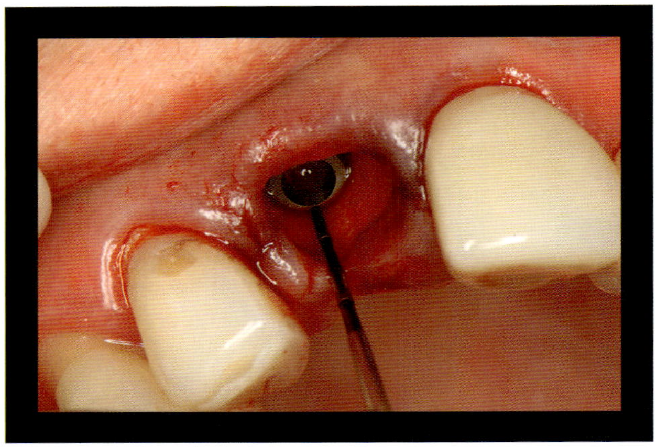

Figure 3.24 The implant was lingually and subcrestally positioned.

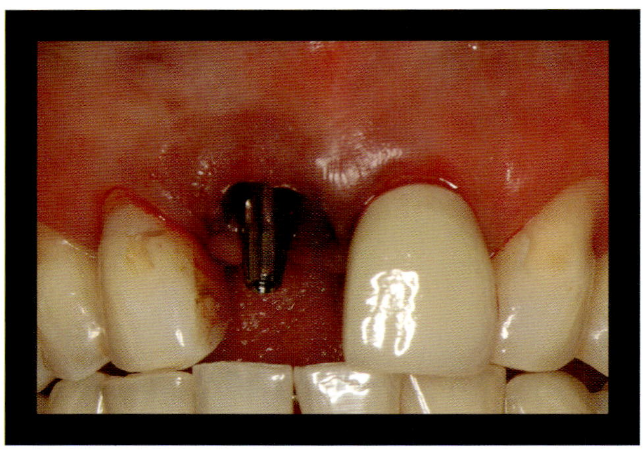

Figure 3.25 A prosthetic abutment was connected to the implant.

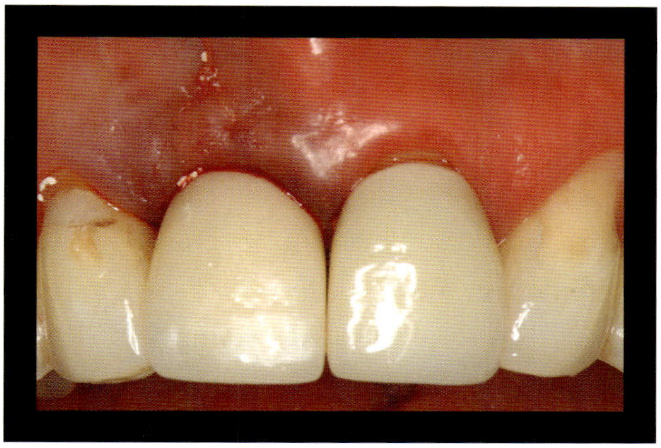

Figure 3.26 The removed crown was prepared to be used as the provisional crown. A connective tissue graft was subepithelially adapted using a split-thickness envelope technique. Absorbable sutures were performed to maintain the graft in place.

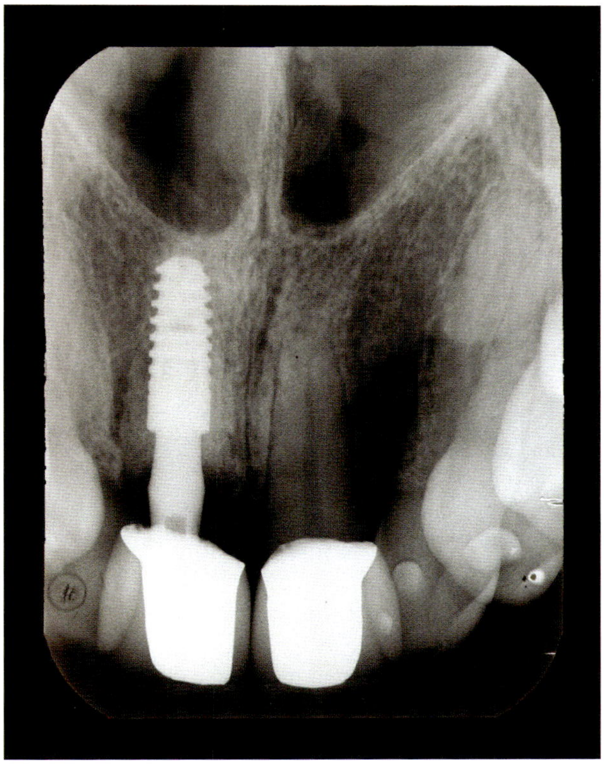

Figure 3.27 Radiographic view of implant subcrestally placed, immediately restored.

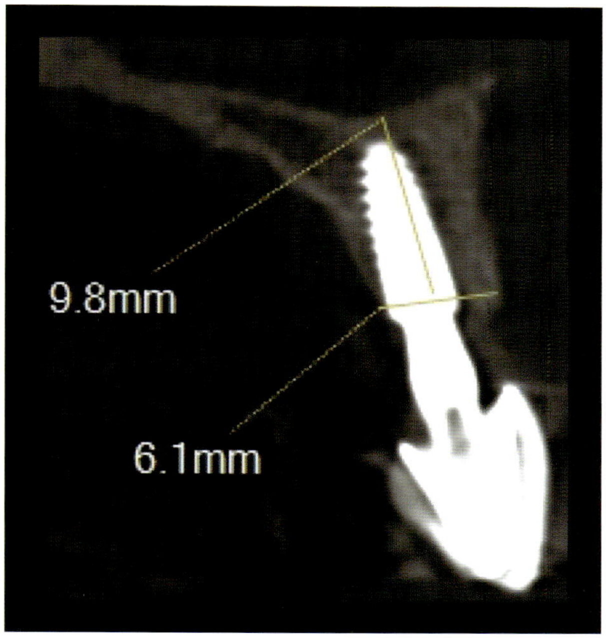

Figure 3.28 The cone beam computed tomographic image was obtained immediately after provisionalization. Observe the lingual positioning of the implant, totally preserving the thickness of the buccal bone crest. The remaining gap between this plate and the implant was filled with a xenograft.

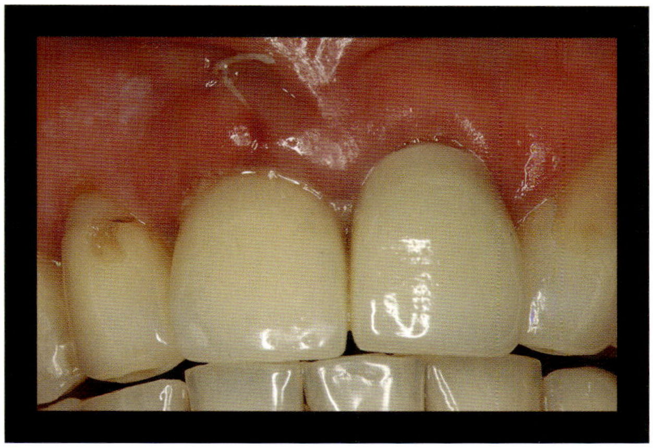

Figure 3.29 Buccal view of the anterior zone, one week after loading. Note the suture keeping in position the connective tissue graft.

impression was made. The zirconia coping was positioned in the gingival sulcus (Figure 3.34). The volume and height of the peri-implant soft tissues were decisive for the natural profile achieved after cementation of the final all-ceramic restoration (Figure 3.35). Radiographically, a perfect integration of the parts of the platform-switching implant–abutment connection was confirmed (Figure 3.36). The two-year postoperative cone-beam computed tomography evidence showed that the bone level was stable (Figure 3.37). It seems reasonable to suggest that the surgical procedures associated with the platform-switched implant with a treated surface were fundamental in the achievement of this success.

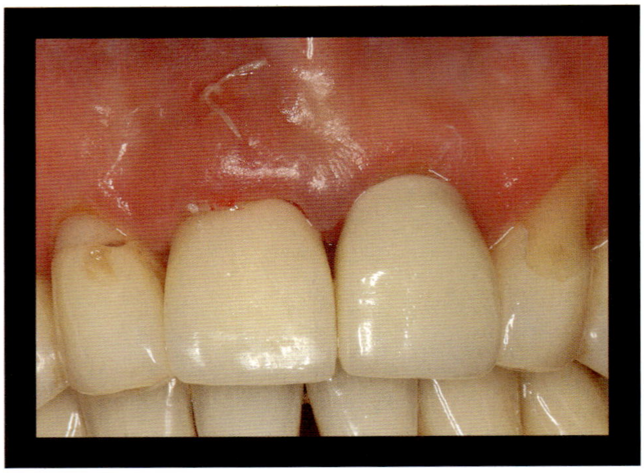

Figure 3.30 After one week, the region appeared edematous. The sutures were maintained in position.

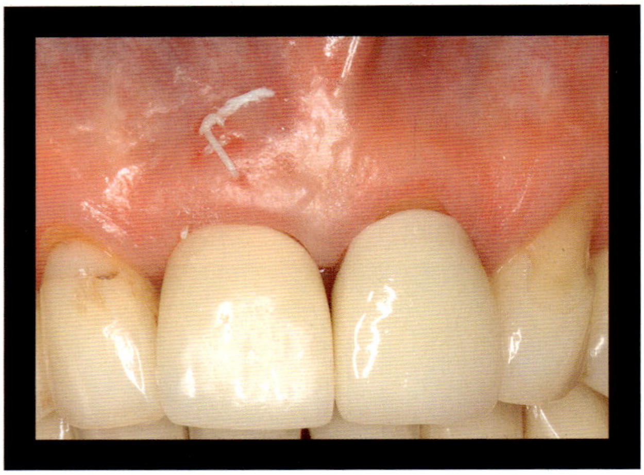

Figure 3.31 At the one-month follow-up, the sutures were totally removed.

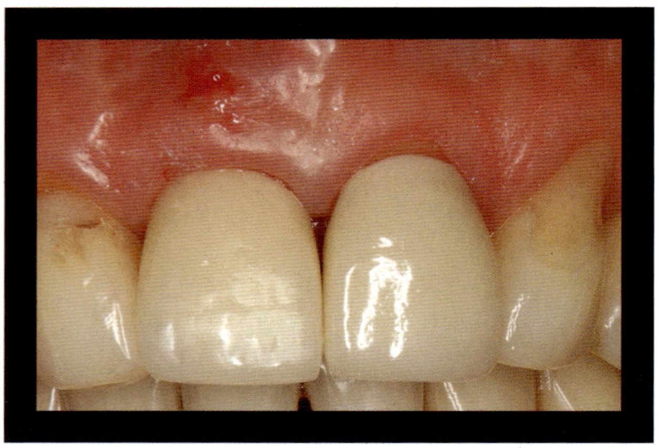

Figure 3.32 Buccal view of the anterior zone, four weeks after loading. Note the suture was removed.

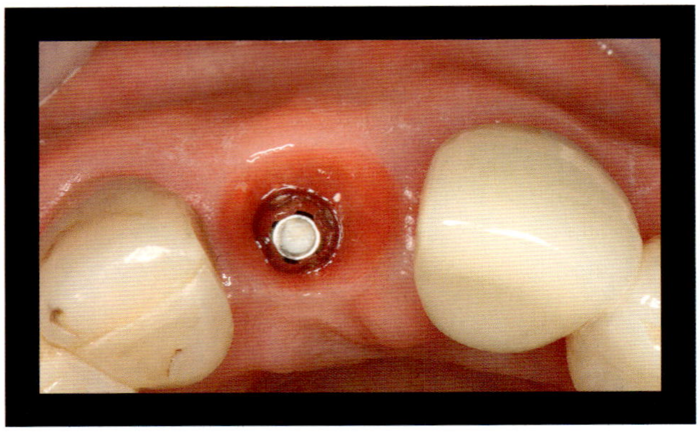

Figure 3.33 After six months, note the appearance and volume of soft tissues in this occlusal view of the implanted region. An excellent profile of the buccal and proximal peri-implant soft tissues can be observed, favoring the final restorative phase and esthetic outcomes.

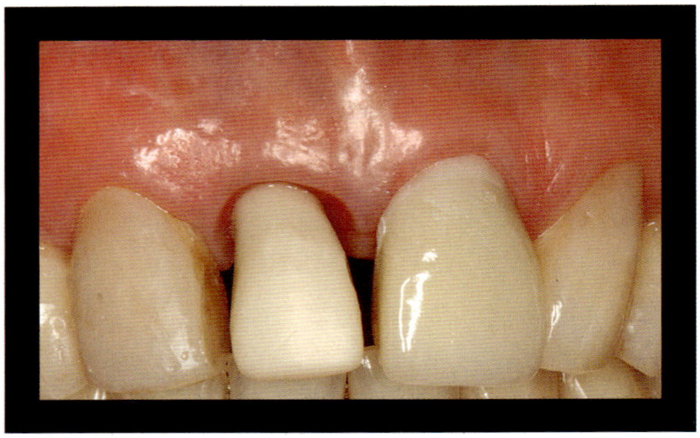

Figure 3.34 The zirconia coping was positioned.

Clinically, it is important that the peri-implant soft tissue thickness and color be considered, in conjunction with the selection of abutment type, and implant–abutment connections have to be in harmony to achieve predictable esthetic and restorative outcomes. Several authors have researched the correlation between peri-implant soft tissue thickness and its color-masking ability (Bressan et al. 2011).

Although there is no consensus on how much peri-implant soft tissue thickness is required, there is agreement that it has an important effect on the esthetic results. The presence and volume of the peri-implant soft tissue affect the implant–abutment selection from the standpoint of restorative material strength. Furthermore, it is known that the soft tissue thickness is critical for the stability of the peri-implant soft tissue and may also help the preservation of the levels of the underlying crestal bone. In other words, it seems that the increase of the peri-implant soft tissue thickness can provide, more successfully, the substrate for color-masking ability and bone stability (Puisys and Linkevicius 2015).

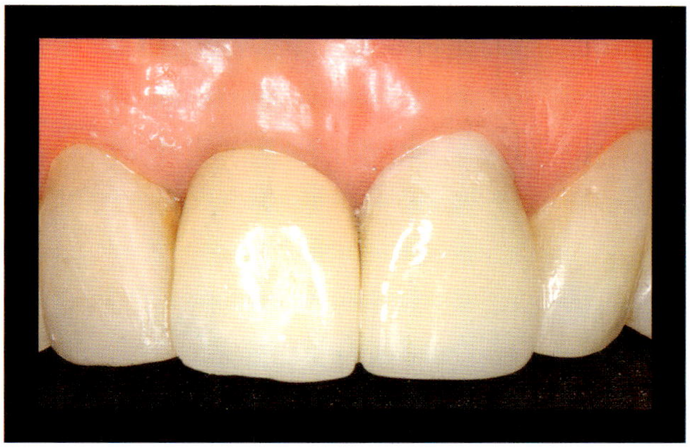

Figure 3.35 After the cementation of the final restoration, the esthetic outcome. The gingival contour favored the natural-looking implant restoration.

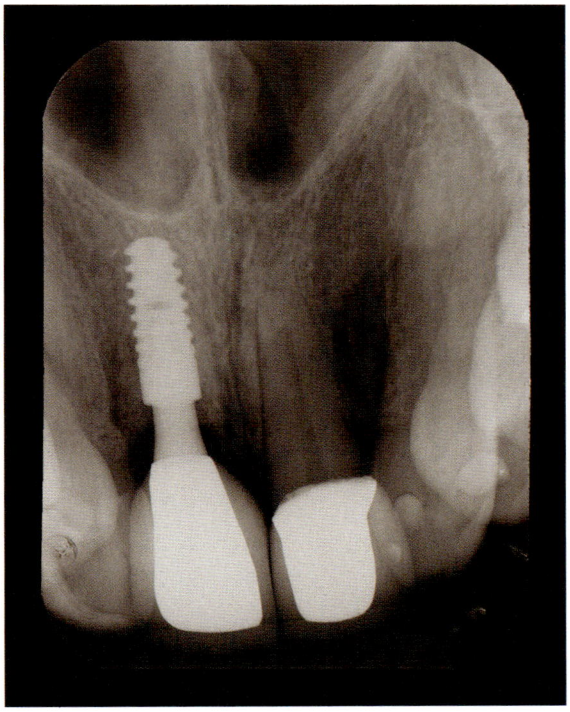

Figure 3.36 The radiograph taken after the final restoration shows a perfect integration of the parts of the switch platform implant-abutment connection.

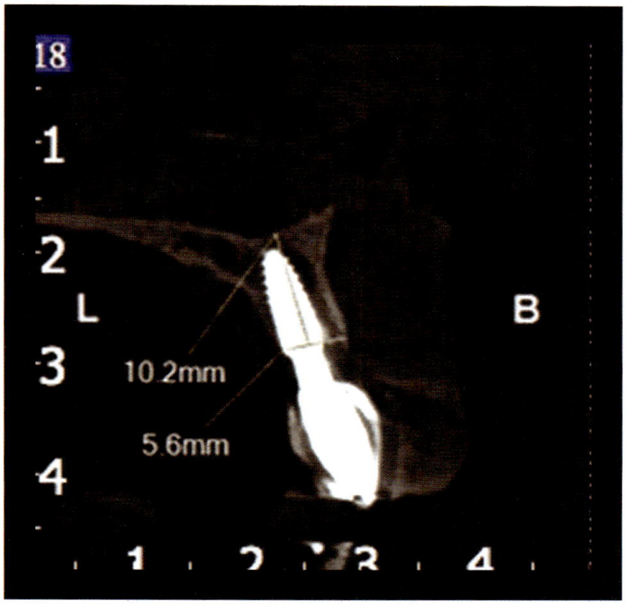

Figure 3.37 The two-year postoperative cone beam computed tomography evidences a stable bone level.

In view of this, subepithelial connective tissue grafts have been associated with the immediate implant placement and provisionalization procedures, exhibiting good esthetic outcomes. The periodontal plastic surgery reported as the gold standard procedure for gingival recessions coverage involving natural teeth has recently been advocated to be used around implants to convert thin gingival biotype regions in those more resistant to recession, thus increasing the dimensions of the peri-implant soft tissue (Waki and Kan 2016).

A previous study evaluated the effect of the association of an autogenous connective tissue graft in immediate implant placement and provisionalization procedures (Rungcharassaeng et al. 2012). The outcomes demonstrated that this approach results in greater peri-implant soft tissue height and thickness. The contours provided by the provisional restorations were conformed in order to support the peri-implant soft tissues, favoring blood clot protection as well as bone graft particles when associated. Another randomized controlled prospective study (Yoshino et al. 2014) using a similar approach showed that subjects who underwent immediate implant placement and provisionalization with a subepithelial connective tissue graft experienced less buccal gingival level change than those who did not receive the connective tissue graft.

To sum up, after careful patient selection, investigating the medical history and risk factors such as smoking habits, a deliberate treatment plan for implant placement and restoration must fulfill the key aspects aforementioned for promising results in the reconstruction of the dentoalveolar complex in a one-stage approach. Undoubtedly, the immediately placed and loaded implants protocols reduce the surgical procedures and the healing period, reduce the toothless period, and increase the patient acceptance of dental rehabilitation following tooth extraction. However, the patients must be precisely selected to achieve excellence in the final esthetic outcomes.

References

Ahmad, I. (1998). Geometric considerations in anterior dental aesthetics: restorative principles. *Pract. Periodontics Aesthet. Dent.* 10: 813–822.

Akimoto, K., Becker, W., Persson, R. et al. (1999). Evaluation of titanium implants placed into simulated extraction sockets: a study in dogs. *Int. J. Oral Maxillofac. Implants.* 14: 351–360.

Araujo, M.G., Sukekava, F., Wennstrom, J.L., and Lindhe, J. (2005). Ridge alterations following implant placement in fresh extraction sockets: an experimental study in the dog. *J. Clin. Periodontol.* 32: 645–652.

Araujo, M.G., Sukekava, F., Wennström, J.L., and Lindhe, J. (2006a). Tissue modeling following implant placement in fresh extraction sockets. *Clin. Oral Implants Res.* 17: 615–624.

Araujo, M.G., Wennström, J.L., and Lindhe, J. (2006b). Modeling of the buccal and lingual bone walls of fresh extraction sites following implant installation. *Clin. Oral Implants Res.* 17: 606–614.

Araujo, M.G., Linder, E., and Lindhe, J. (2011). Bio-Oss collagen in the buccal gap at immediate implants: a 6-month study in the dog. *Clin. Oral Implants Res.* 22: 1–8.

Barros, R.R.M., Novaes, A.B. Jr., Muglia, V.A. et al. (2009). Influence of interimplant distances and placement depth on periimplant bone remodeling of adjacent and immediately loaded Morse cone connection implants: a clinical and radiographic study in dogs. *J. Oral Implantol.* 35: 18–27.

Barros, R.R.M., Novaes, A.B. Jr., Muglia, V.A. et al. (2010). Influence of interimplant distances and placement depth on peri-implant bone remodeling of adjacent and immediately loaded Morse cone connection implants: a histomorphometric study in dogs. *Clin. Oral Implants Res.* 4: 371–378.

Barros, R.R.M., Novaes, A.B. Jr., Queiroz, A., and De Almeida, A.L. (2012). Early peri-implant endosseous healing of two implant surfaces placed in surgically created circumferential defects. A histomorphometric and fluorescence study in dogs. *Clin. Oral Implants Res.* 23: 1340–1351.

Blanco, J., Linares, A., Perez, J., and Munoz, F. (2011). Ridge alterations following flapless immediate implant placement with or without immediate loading. Part II: a histometric study in the Beagle dog. *J. Clin. Periodontol.* 38: 762–770.

Blanco, J., Nunez, V., Aracil, L. et al. (2008). Ridge alterations following immediate implant placement in the dog: flap versus flapless surgery. *J. Clin. Periodontol.* 35: 640–648.

Botticelli, D., Berglundh, T., Buser, D., and Lindhe, J. (2003). The jumping distance revisited: an experimental study in the dog. *Clin. Oral Implants Res.* 14: 35–42.

Bressan, E., Paniz, G., Lops, D. et al. (2011). Influence of abutment material on the gingival color of implant-supported all-ceramic restorations: a prospective multicenter study. *Clin. Oral Implants Res.* 22: 631–637.

Buser, D., Martin, W., and Belser, U.C. (2004). Optimizing esthetics for implant restorations in the anterior maxilla: anatomic and surgical considerations. *Int. J. Oral Maxillofac. Implants* 19: 43–61.

Carlsson, L., Rostlund, T., Albrektsson, B., and Albrektsson, T. (1988). Implant fixation improved by close fit. Cylindrical implant–bone interface studied in rabbits. *Acta Orthop. Scand.* 59: 272–275.

Caudill, R.F. and Meffert, R.M. (1991). Histologic analysis of the osseointegration of endosseous implants in simulated extraction sockets with and without e-ptfe barriers. 1. Preliminary findings. *Int. J. Periodontics Restorative Dent.* 11: 207–215.

Chen, S.T., Darby, I.B., Reynolds, E.C., and Clement, J.G. (2009). Immediate implant placement post-extraction without flap elevation. *J. Periodontol.* 80: 163–172.

de Sanctis, M., Vignoletti, F., Discepoli, N. et al. (2009). Immediate implants at fresh extraction sockets: bone healing in four different implant systems. *J. Clin. Periodontol.* 36: 705–771.

Doring, K., Eisenmann, E., and Stiller, M. (2004). Functional and esthetic considerations for single-tooth Ankylos implant-crowns: 8 years of clinical performance. *J. Oral Implantol.* 30: 198–209.

Evans, C.D. and Chen, S.T. (2008). Esthetic outcomes of immediate implant placements. *Clin. Oral Implants Res.* 19: 73–80.

Ferrus, J., Cecchinato, D., Pjetursson, E.B. et al. (2010). Factors influencing ridge alterations following immediate implant placement into extraction sockets. *Clin. Oral Implants Res.* 21: 22–28.

Fickl, S., Zuhr, O., Wachtel, H. et al. (2008). Tissue alterations after tooth extraction with and without surgical trauma: a volumetric study in the beagle dog. *J. Clin. Periodontol.* 35: 356–363.

Gher, M.E., Quintero, G., Assad, D. et al. (1994). Bone grafting and guided bone regeneration for immediate dental implants in humans. *J. Periodontol.* 65: 881–891.

Hsu, K.M., Choi, B.H., Ko, C.Y. et al. (2012). Ridge alterations following immediate implant placement and the treatment of bone defects with Bio-Oss in an animal model. *Clin. Implant. Dent. Relat. Res.* 14: 690–695.

Karring, T., Thorkild, J., Lindhe, J., and Pierpaolo, C. (2005). Terapia periodontal regenerativa. In: *Tratado de Periodontia e Implantologia Oral*, 4e (ed. J. Lindhe, J.

Thorkild, T. Karring and N.P. Lang), 641–646. Rio de Janeiro, Brazil: Guanabara Koogan.

Knox, R., Caudill, R., and Meffert, R. (1991). Histologic evaluation of dental endosseous implants placed in surgically created extraction defects. *Int. J. Periodontics Restorative Dent.* 11: 364–375.

Maia, L.P., Reino, D.M., Muglia, V.A. et al. (2015). Influence of periodontal tissue thickness on buccal plate remodelling on immediate implants with xenograft. *J. Clin. Periodontol.* 42: 590–598.

Matsuo, M.S.C., Saito, M., Kishi, Y., and Takahashi, K. (2000). Vascularization an unsuccessful case following guided bone regeneration. *Jpn. J. Oral Biol.* 42: 573–579.

Mijiritsky, E., Mardinger, O., Mazor, Z., and Chaushu, G. (2009). Immediate provisionalization of single-tooth implants in fresh-extraction sites at the maxillary esthetic zone: up to 6 years of follow-up. *Implant. Dent.* 18: 326–333.

Molly, L., Vandromme, H., Quirynen, M. et al. (2008). Bone formation following implantation of bone biomaterials into extraction sites. *J. Periodontol.* 79: 1108–1115.

Negri, B., Calvo-Guirado, J.L., Pardo-Zamora, G. et al. (2012). Peri-implant bone reactions to immediate implants placed at different levels in relation to crestal bone. Part I: a pilot study in dogs. *Clin. Oral Implants Res.* 23: 228–235.

Nemcovsky, C.E., Artzi, Z., Moses, O., and Gelernter, I. (2002). Healing of marginal defects at implants placed in fresh extraction sockets or after 4–6 weeks of healing. A comparative study. *Clin. Oral Implants Res.* 13: 410–419.

Nobuto, T., Suwa, F., Kono, T. et al. (2005). Microvascular response in the periosteum following mucoperiosteal flap surgery in dogs: angiogenesis and bone resorption and formation. *J. Periodontol.* 76: 1346–1353.

Novaes, A.B. Jr., Barros, R.R.M., Papalexiou, V., and Almeida, A.L.G. (2011a). Buccal bone loss after immediate implantation can be reduced by the flapless approach. *J. Osseointegration* 3: 45–55.

Novaes, A.B. Jr., Macedo, G.O., Suaid, F.A. et al. (2011b). Histologic evaluation of the buccal and lingual bone plates in anterior dog teeth: possible influence on implant dentistry. *J. Periodontol.* 82: 872–877.

Novaes, A.B. Jr., Marcaccini, A.M., Souza, S.L. et al. (2003). Immediate placement of implants into periodontally infected sites in dogs: a histomorphometric study of bone–implant contact. *Int. J. Oral Maxillofac. Implants* 18: 391–398.

Oh, T.J., Yoon, J., Misch, C.E., and Wang, H.L. (2002). The causes of early implant bone loss: myth or science. *J. Periodontol.* 73: 322–333.

Pietrokovski, J. and Massler, M. (1967). Alveolar ridge resorption following tooth extraction. *J. Prosthet. Dent.* 17: 21–27.

Polimeni, G., Koo, K.T., Qahash, M. et al. (2004). Prognostic factors for alveolar regeneration: bone formation at teeth and titanium implants. *J. Clin. Periodontol.* 31: 927–932.

Puisys, A. and Linkevicius, T. (2015). The influence of mucosal tissue thickening on crestal bone stability around bone-level implants. A prospective controlled clinical trial. *Clin. Oral Implants Res* 26: 123–129.

Qahash, M., Susin, C., Polimeni, G. et al. (2008). Bone healing dynamics at buccal peri-implant sites. *Clin. Oral Implants Res.* 19: 166–172.

Rocci, A., Martignoni, M., and Gottlow, J. (2003). Immediate loading in the maxilla using flapless surgery, implants placed in predetermined positions, and prefabricated provisional restorations: a retrospective 3-year clinical study. *Clin. Implant. Dent. Relat. Res.* 5: 29–36.

Rungcharassaeng, K., Kan, J.Y., Yoshino, S. et al. (2012). Immediate implant placement and provisionalization with and without a connective tissue graft: an analysis of facial gingival tissue thickness. *Int. J. Periodontics Restorative Dent.* 32: 657–663.

Schopper, C., Ziya-Ghazvini, F., Goriwoda, W. et al. (2005). HA/TCP compounding of a porous CaP biomaterial improves bone formation and scaffold degradation – a long-term histological study. *J. Biomed. Mater. Res. B Appl. Biomater.* 74: 458–467.

Schropp, L., Wenzel, A., Kostopoulos, L., and Karring, T. (2003). Bone healing and soft tissue contour changes following single-tooth extraction: a clinical and radiographic 12-month prospective study. *Int. J. Periodontics Restorative Dent.* 23: 313–323.

Schwartz-Arad, D. and Chaushu, G. (1997). The ways and wherefores of immediate placement of implants into fresh extraction sites: a literature review. *J. Periodontol.* 68: 915–923.

Spear, F.M. (1999). Maintenance of the interdental papilla following anterior tooth removal. *Pract. Periodontics Aesthet. Dent.* 11: 21–28.

Spinato, S., Galindo-Moreno, P., Zaffe, D. et al. (2014). Is socket healing conditioned by buccal plate thickness? A clinical and histologic study 4 months after mineralized human bone allografting. *Clin. Oral Implants Res.* 25: e120–e126.

Suaid, F.A., Novaes, A.B. Jr., Queiroz, A.C. et al. (2014). Buccal bone plate remodeling after immediate implants with or without synthetic bone grafting and flapless surgery: a histomorphometric and fluorescence study in dogs. *Clin. Oral Implants Res.* 25: e10–e21.

Tomasi, C., Sanz, M., Cecchinato, D. et al. (2010). Bone dimensional variations at implants placed in fresh extraction sockets: a multilevel multivariate analysis. *Clin. Oral Implants Res.* 21: 30–36.

Waki, T. and Kan, J.Y. (2016). Immediate placement and provisionalization of maxillary anterior single implant with guided bone regeneration, connective tissue graft, and coronally positioned flap procedures. *Int. J. Esthet Dent.* 11: 174–185.

Wikesjo, U.M., Susin, C., Qahash, M. et al. (2006). The critical-size supra-alveolar peri-implant defect model: characteristics and use. *J. Clin. Periodontol.* 33: 846–854.

Wilderman, M.N., Wentz, F., and Orban, B.J. (1960). Histogenesis of repair after mucogingival surgery. *J. Periodontol.* 31: 283–299.

Yoshino, S., Kan, J.Y., Rungcharassaeng, K. et al. (2014). Effects of connective tissue grafting on the facial gingival level following single immediate implant placement and provisionalization in the esthetic zone: a 1-year randomized controlled prospective study. *Int. J. Oral Maxillofac. Implants* 29: 432–440.

Zeren, K.J. (2006). Minimally invasive extraction and immediate implant placement: the preservation of esthetics. *Int. J. Periodontics Restorative Dent.* 26: 171–181.

4

Novel Concepts in Restoring Defective Labial Plate of Bone in Immediate Implant Therapy

4.1 Introduction

The concept of oral implant integration that was introduced by Branemark has definitely changed the face of dentistry, as well as the basic knowledge of dental surgery and prosthetics (Branemark et al. 1977). Since then, oral implantology has become one of the most investigated topics in dental medicine. Data shows that the number of implants used for oral rehabilitation in the United States increased 10-fold between 1983 and 2002 and 10-fold from 2000 to 2010 (Misch 2014). Investigators are now placing the focus on shortening treatment time, simplifying surgical techniques, and esthetic improvement (Prakash 2015; Turkyilmaz, Company and McGlumphy 2010). Dental implants opened doors for global research: in a MEDLINE electronic literature search conducted recently, the PubMed search initially identified 15 695 publications and 5048 additional results were identified from a hand search. Among the most covered surgical topics in the literature were immediate loading (14.3%), bone substitutes (11.6%), immediate implant placement (7.5%), simultaneous implant placement with bone augmentation (6.4%), onlay grafting (4.3%), medically compromised patients (4.0%), healing modality (3.7%), transcrestal sinus floor elevation (3.0%), flapless surgery (2.7%), socket grafting (2.6%), and guided surgery (2.4%). Immediate loading (14.3%), cross-arch implant bridges (8.0%), early loading (4.5%), and platform switching (1.7%) were ranked as the most prevalent prosthodontic issues in current oral implant research (Pommer et al. 2015). Immediate implant placement offers success rates that are strongly evidenced in the literature; results are considered to be equivalent to that of the delayed implant placement modes (Becker 2005; Meredith, Alleyne and Cawley 1996) (see Figure 4.1a and b).

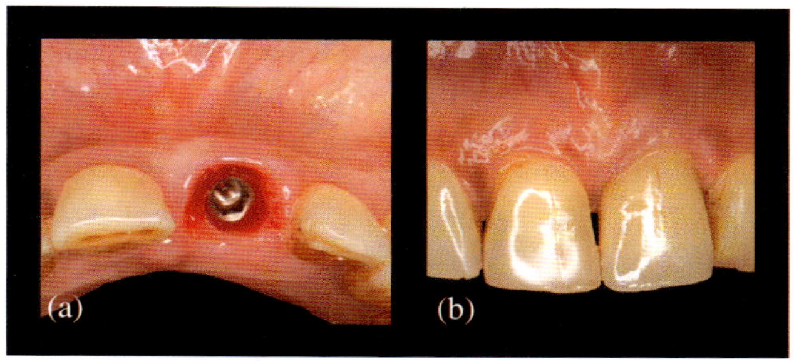

Figure 4.1 (a) and (b) Successful result of immediate implant placement and loading.

4.1.1 Treatment Benefits of Immediate Implant Placement in the Esthetic Zone

The high demand by patients to attain high esthetic results with implant-supported restorations has led to optimizing the outcome with implants placed in fresh extraction sites (Paolantonio et al. 2001). This has encouraged clinicians to improve esthetic outcome, especially for implants that are placed in more demanding esthetic situations. Although the first clinical procedures for the placement of implant fixtures immediately following tooth removal were described long ago (Hammerle et al. 2004), it is only recently that the details of such clinical approaches have been studied thoroughly. Initial observations on placing dental implants in fresh extraction sites indicated that the procedure itself helps retain osseous heights around the implant fixture, thus preventing post-extraction bone resorption and hence maintaining the original shape of the ridge (Paolantonio et al. 2001); however, findings reported from a clinical study by Botticelli et al. (2003) failed to support this hypothesis.

There are some clinical factors that should be taken into consideration prior to selecting an immediate implant placement protocol versus the other clinical approaches, such as: (1) bone topography, (2) level of crestal and interproximal bone from the adjacent contact point of the natural tooth, (3) smile line, (4) condition of the gingival tissues, (5) pathological and morphological condition of the alveolar socket, (6) soft tissue biotype, (7) the need for preservation of interdental papilla, (8) the need to prevent alveolar ridge resorption, and (9) patient demands (Elaskary 2008).

4.1.1.1 Reduced Treatment Time

Nowadays advances in clinical techniques and biomaterials have facilitated a great expansion in the indications for dental implant treatment options. Not only are the total time of the treatment and number of operations reduced but there are also improved implant survival rates, better esthetics, and higher patient satisfaction compared with delayed implants (Norton 2011). Reductions in the number of surgical interventions, a shorter treatment time, an ideal three-dimensional implant positioning, and soft tissue esthetics have been claimed as the potential benefits of this treatment approach.

Different placement and loading protocols have evolved over time to provide fast delivery of implant supported restorations. Immediate placement of a dental implant in an extraction socket was initially described by Schulte and Heimke (1976). The intention was to try to preserve tissue contour, dimension, and also to decrease treatment time (Capelli et al. 2013). Immediate implant placement in fresh extraction sites has provided an outstanding reduction in the overall treatment time (Covani et al. 2004; Lazzara 1989; Schwartz-Arad and Chausu 1997) via the reduction in the number of surgical treatments and reduction of the time between tooth extraction and the placement of the definitive prosthesis. However, there are still some situations that could jeopardize the success of the aforesaid therapy, such as the presence of an infection caused by periodontal disease or periapical lesions (Marconcini et al. 2013).

4.1.1.2 Improved Patient Acceptance

Long-term survival of osseointegrated implants in the absence of symptoms and minimal progression of peri-implant bone loss were considered the primary end-points to determine the success of dental implant therapy (Albrektsson et al. 1986); however, some of these original parameters have changed over time (Misch et al. 2008; Albrektsson et al. 2012). Maintenance of functionally loaded, osseointegrated implants in an adequate state of health and esthetics has emerged as the new therapeutic goal. The importance of patient satisfaction, the absence of peri-implant inflammation, the stability of marginal bone levels, and the optimal restoration and peri-implant soft tissue esthetics has been widely recognized (Annibali et al. 2012; Furhauser et al. 2005; Papaspyridakos et al. 2012; Sohrabi et al. 2012).

4.1.1.3 Better Esthetics

In general in the esthetic anterior regions, the labial cortical plates are thinner than the lingual plate and are the first to be lost after tooth extraction or trauma. The labial alveolar bone often undergoes rapid resorption after natural tooth loss, with an approximately 25% decrease in volume during the first year, followed by a 40–60% decrease in width in the next three years, leading to the labial cortex of bone more medial than its original position. This sequel of resorption after tooth loss jeopardizes the functional and esthetic outcome of treatment. Many authors (Barzilay 1993; Hammerle et al. 2004; Werbitt and Goldberg 1992) proposed that simultaneous implant placement along with bone grafting of the deficient site offers several advantages; these include a more accurate implant position; preservation of bone at the site of implantation; optimal soft tissue esthetics; fewer surgeries; and reduced treatment time of up to six months, so minimizing the overall treatment time and incidences of morbidity, and lower costs to the patients. The importance of a sound and intact labial bone after tooth extraction is the main prerequisite for fresh socket implants to enjoy long-term stability and success, as shown in Figure 4.2.

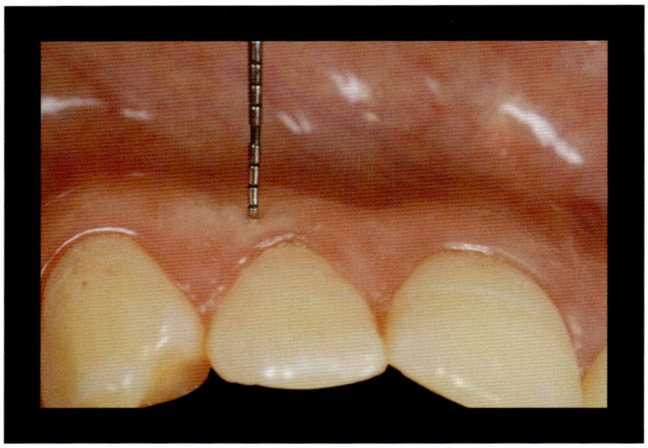

Figure 4.2 Effect of thickness of soft tissue and thickness of the labial plate of bone.

Future resorption of a thin labial plate after prosthesis connection may result in gingival recession, with exposure of the unsightly implant abutment or fixture. Therefore the proper maintenance of the crestal anatomy tends to maintain those parameters that are recognized as essential for esthetic treatment.

According to Camargo et al. (2002) and Covani et al. (2004), reflecting a mucoperiosteal flap might induce gingival recession, papilla destruction, and crestal bone resorption. Hence, the immediate implant placement procedure without reflecting a mucoperiosteal flap was proposed by Al-Ansari and Morris in 1998. They noticed reduced bleeding, maintenance of tissue contour, and reduced postoperative patient discomfort with a flapless immediate implant placement. Moreover, maintenance of the available anatomical structure is much easier than reconstruction of the new one.

4.1.2 Treatment Complications with Immediate Implant Placement

4.1.2.1 Facial Recession

The recession of the facial mucosa around dental implant fixtures placed immediately in fresh extraction sites is the main esthetic complication observed (Becker 2005; Blanes et al. 2007; Botticelli et al. 2006; Buser et al. 2004; Ferrus et al. 2010; Grunder, Gracis and Capelli 2005). However, it has been reported that flapless immediate placement did not prevent marginal mucosal recession from occurring. In a recent systematic review, Chen and Buser (2014) concluded that immediate implant placement is associated with a greater variability in clinical outcome and attains a higher frequency of recession of >1 mm of the mid-facial mucosa. In a retrospective study of immediate implant placement with bone graft, the facial bone wall was not detectable on cone-beam computed tomography (CBCT) in 36 and 57% of sites. These sites had more recession of the mid-facial mucosa compared to sites with detectable facial bone (Chen and Buser 2014), which is the reason for suggesting that increasing the thickness of the facial mucosa with the addition of a connective tissue graft beneath the facial flap at the time of implant placement may reduce this risk of recession (Kan et al. 2005). However, Chen, Wilson and Hämmerle (2004) failed to show that the addition of a connective tissue graft at the time of surgery had any influence on the incidence or extent of mucosal recession.

4.1.2.2 Dropped Facial Contours

Immediate implant placement therapy has proved its reliability and clinical efficacy (Blanes et al. 2007; Chen, Darby and Reynolds 2007; Evans and Chen 2008; Kan, Rungcharassaeng and Lozada 2003; Lazzara 1989; Tolstunov 2007; Wheeler, Vogel and Casellini 2000). However, some recent studies in animals have shown pronounced resorption of the buccal bone plate and the lingual bone plate occurred after immediate implant therapy (Araujo and Lindhe 2005; Becker et al. 1998; Paolantonio et al. 2001).

It has been also reported that bone to implant contact established during the early phase of socket healing following implant installation was partly lost when the buccal bone wall underwent continued resorption (Araujo and Lindhe 2005). In some cases where tissue phenotype is thin, once the labial plate of bone is resorbed, the overlying soft tissue starts to drop facially, and marginal bone loss ultimately led to a poor esthetic outcome. To overcome these problems, several researchers have recommended placing the implant into the extraction sockets with minimal flap elevation (Becker 2005) or without elevation of surgical flaps (Schwartz et al. 1998). In animal studies, flap exposure during periodontal mucoperiosteal procedures resulted in 2–4 mm of crestal bone loss (Pennel et al. 1967; Wildermann and Wentz 1970) (see Figure 4.3).

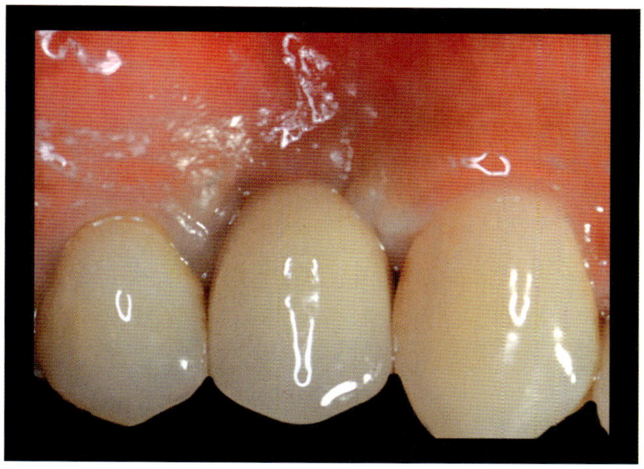

Figure 4.3 Poor esthetics as a result of missing the labial plate of bone.

Animal studies proved that implant placement in a fresh extraction socket might result in an early hard tissue fill of the marginal socket gap, but at a later phase, tissue remodeling starts followed by crestal bone loss (Araujo and Lindhe 2005, 2009). In the same study, the buccal bone wall was shown to be more susceptible to resorption than the lingual plate (probably due to its thickness) (Araujo and Lindhe 2005; Botticelli, Berglundh and Lindh 2004). However, in this study, roots were hemisectioned which would have induced more bone resorption, mucoperiosteal flaps were elevated which induces surgical trauma and would involve bone loss, the gap size was not stabilized in the work done, and no tissue phenotype was mentioned. On the other hand, a human study evaluating the dimensional alveolar ridge alterations following tooth extraction, noted that the marginal gaps in buccal and palatal/lingual locations were filled with new bone formation from inside the defects and substantial bone resorption occurred on the outer side of the ridge, and the implant fixture was surrounded with bone throughout the study (Botticelli et al. 2004). The hypothesis that claims that the esthetic success of dental implants depends more on an ideal three-dimensional implant position, adequate buccal bone over the implant surface, and tissue biotype probably makes better sense and gives a wider view (Chiapasco et al. 2004).

A retrospective review on the esthetic outcomes of immediate implant placement was reported a high degree of predictability to integrate in the surrounding bone, thus suggesting that careful case selection and high surgical skills are required to achieve a good esthetic outcome (Evans and Chen 2008).

4.1.2.3 Poor Esthetics and Tissue Discoloration

The outstanding esthetic outcome of the immediate implant placement in fresh sockets might not be sustained in cases of labial plate of bone resorption, or in cases of implant-related gingival recession, and further consequences would be shrinkage of the adjacent interdental papillae.

When buccal plate bone thickness is lost over time, which may be followed by soft tissue recession, the metallic hue of the implant fixture or the abutment base starts to show, giving a metallic gray tinge to the gum overlying the substructure (see Figure 4.4).

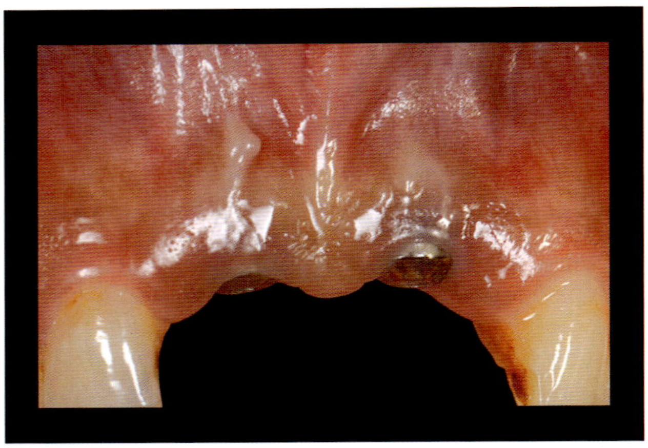

Figure 4.4 Clinical example of implant-related soft tissue discoloration as a result of labial plate of bone resorption.

4.2 Reasons for Inconsistent Outcome with Immediate Implant Placement

4.2.1 Lack of Diagnostic Tools

Diagnosis and proper case investigations are the key factors for a successful treatment outcome for implant placements in fresh extraction sockets. Careful diagnosis and treatment planning with proper evaluation of the dimensions of the available alveolar bone is an important prerequisite for a favorable outcome. The investigations that are usually done include visual examination, intraoral periapical radiographs, CBCT (see Figures 4.5, 4.6 and 4.7 a–c) and three-dimensional implant virtual planning software (Becker and Goldstein 2000).

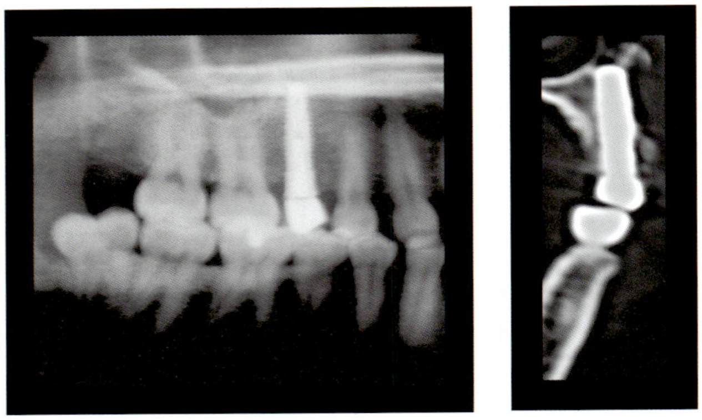

Figures 4.5 and 4.6 Panoramic view showing excellent implant positioning; CT view showing the same implant position violating the labial plate of bone.

Poor diagnostic skills or poor diagnostic aids may be detrimental to the success and esthetic outcome of the proposed treatment. Among the diagnostics to run is the check for the presence of periapical infections (Andersson et al. 2003). The accurate assessment of the buccolingual dimension of the osseous ridge is also needed and should be obtained from the CBCT scan. The use of computerized tomography is paramount in the execution of immediate implant placement for evaluation of the buccolingual ridge width (Ziegler et al. 2002) (see Figure 4.8a–q).

The conventional panoramic radiograph belongs to history as it gives only a general idea on the patient condition, but it attains a degree of distortion and magnification can be misleading in many instances. Whereas the CBCT scans give the clinician the exact details of the hard and soft tissue structures necessary for proper diagnosis and accurate treatment planning. CBCT creates real-time images in axial, coronal, sagittal, and oblique planes, which provide accurate 3D information (Hatcher, Dial and Mayorga 2003). It generates 3D images of oral structures, soft tissues, nerve pathways, and bone in the craniofacial region in a single scan. CBCT helps the clinician to access all the required measurements during implant placement (Van Assche et al. 2007). It provides highly accurate 3D images of the area concerned from a single low-radiation scan, and thus delivers comprehensive details of the patient's jaw and

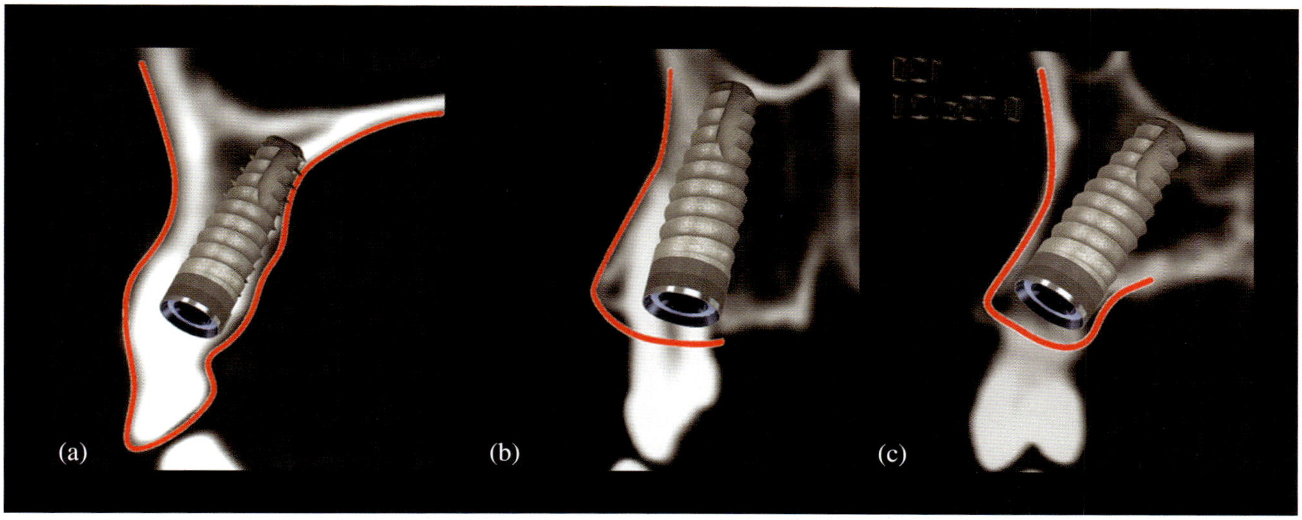

Figure 4.7 (a–c) CT is a valuable diagnostic tool in flapless implant placements.

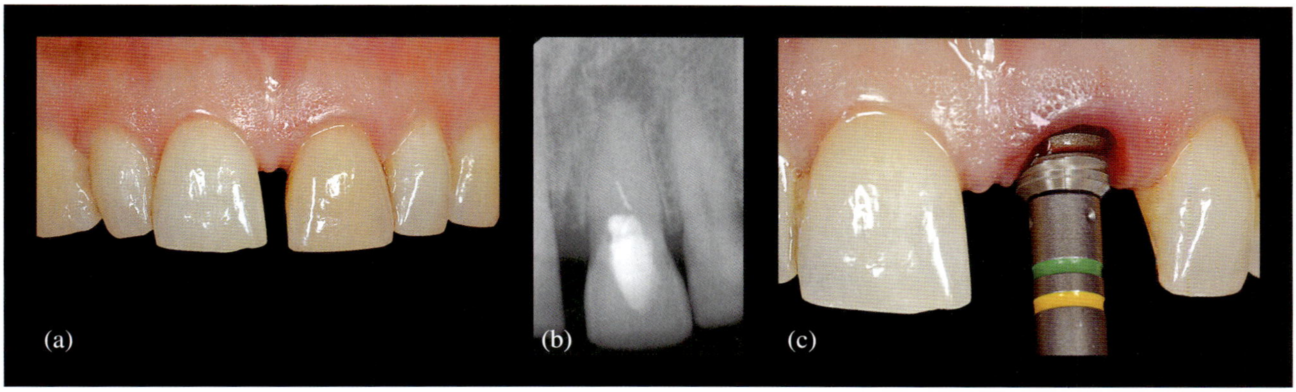

Figure 4.8 (a) Preoperative view showing a failed maxillary left central incisor. (b) Periapical radiographic view showing the failed tooth due to a broken file with periapical infection and blocked nerve canal. (c) An implant (platform switched) is inserted in the socket after tooth extraction and is placed without making a CBCT scan in the flapless mode.

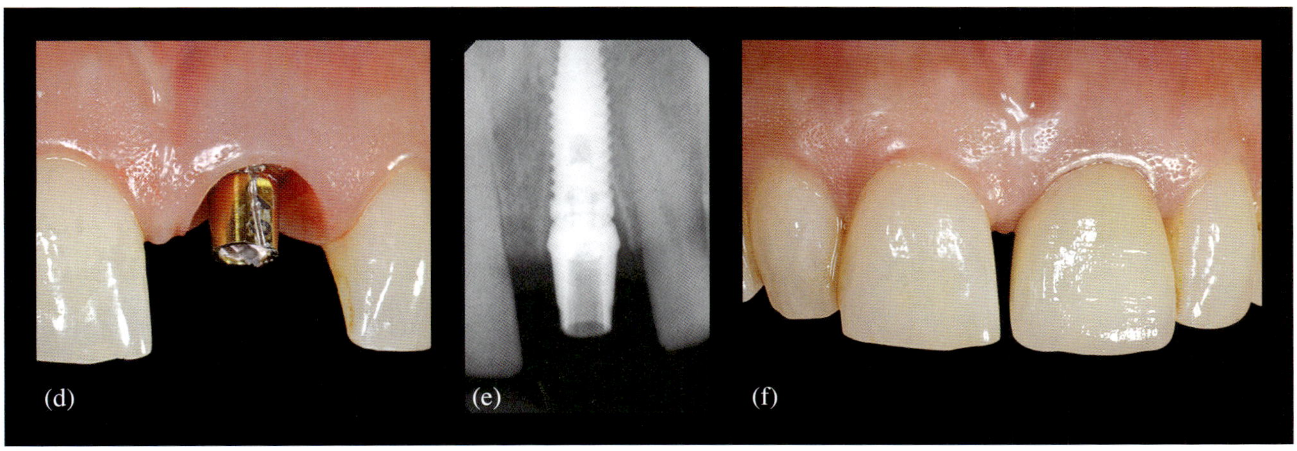

Figure 4.8 (d) Abutment is connected and soft tissue maturation allowed. (e) Periapical radiographic view showing the implant in position without a CBCT scan. (f) Final case restored.

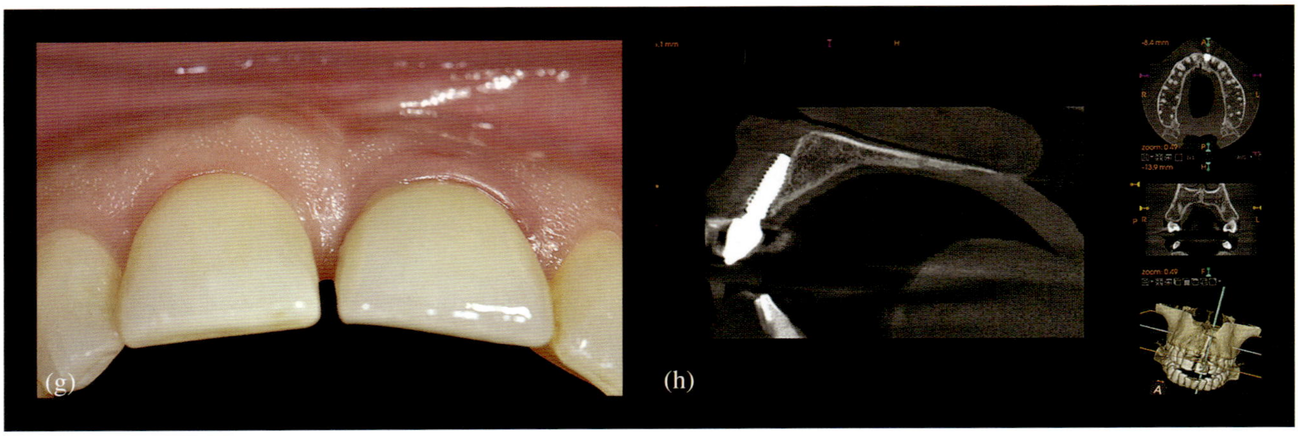

Figure 4.8 (g) One year later, the patient showed up with a missing labial profile. (h) CBCT view showing the complete resorption of the labial plate of bone as a result of blind placement, and the placement of the implant closer to the labial plate of bone.

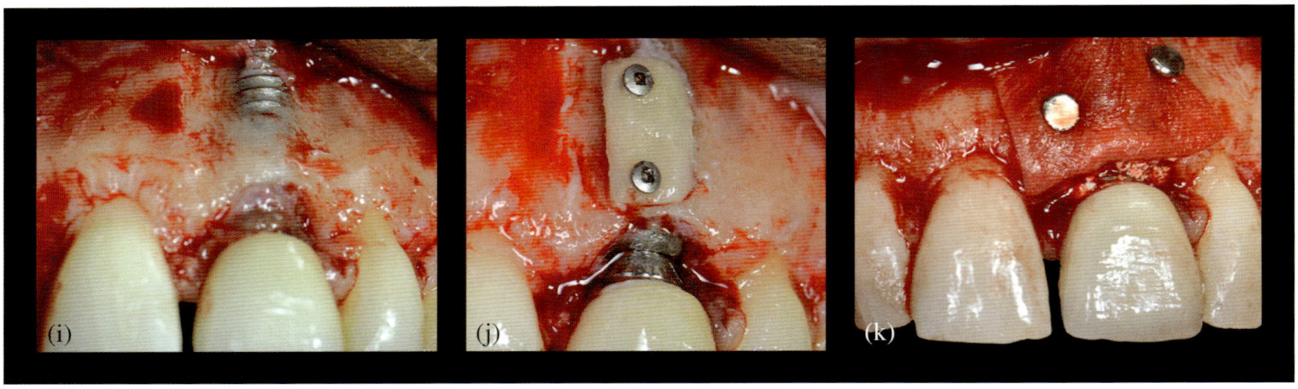

Figure 4.8 (i) Intraoperative view showing labial plate of bone resorption. (j) Corticocancillus block harvested from the chin is stabilized over the defect. (k) Collagen membrane stabilized over the block with two membrane tacs.

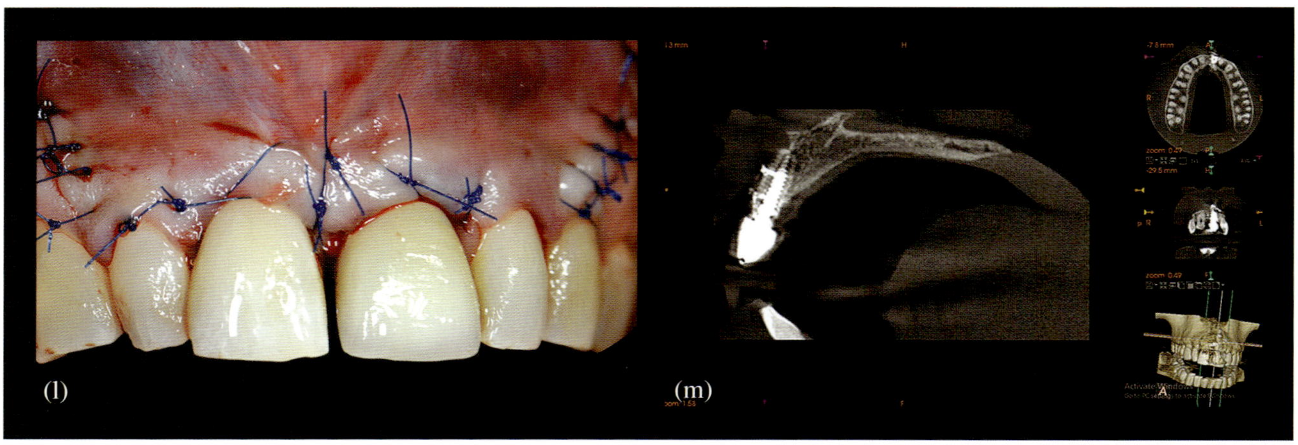

Figure 4.8 (l) Flap sutured. (m) CBCT view showing the complete restoration of the labial plate of bone.

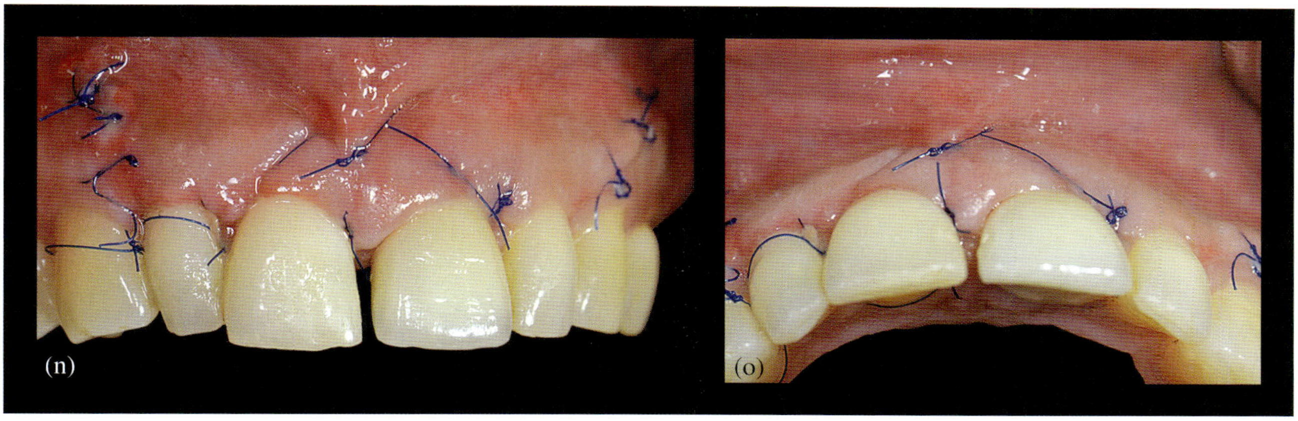

Figure 4.8 (n) and (o) One week post-operative view showing favorable tissue healing and restoring labial contour.

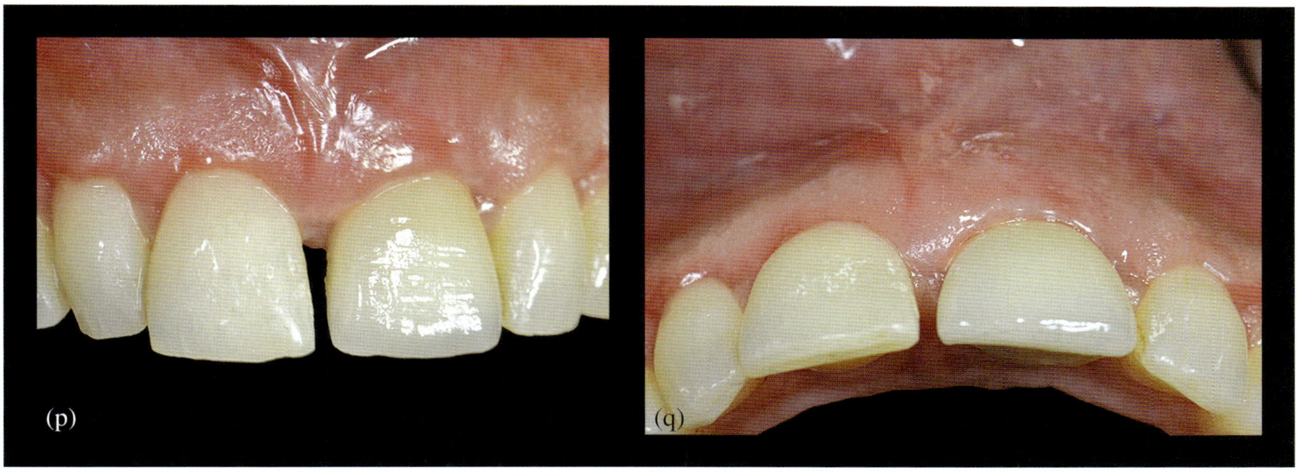

Figure 4.8 (p) and (q) Final case healing after three weeks showing an excellent healing condition.

the anatomical landmarks necessary to properly plan and provide treatment, ensuring a better prognosis and outcome for implant placement. The evaluation of alveolar bone with CBCT helps the clinician to assess the quality and quantity of cortical and cancellous bone (Jung et al. 2009) and (Sonick 1994; Sukovic 2003) (see Figure 4.9a–f).

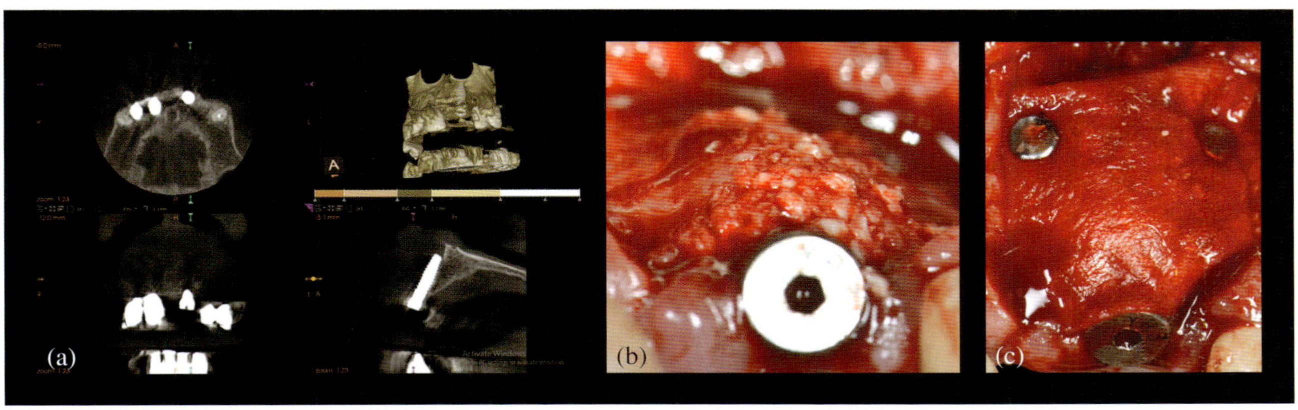

Figure 4.9 (a) CBCT scan showing the violation of the labial plate of bone as a result of not using a surgical guide (arbitrary placement). (b) and (c) A new implant fixture is inserted in the in the correct position. The osseous defect is grafted with particulated bone graft and a collagen membrane stabilized with two auto tacs.

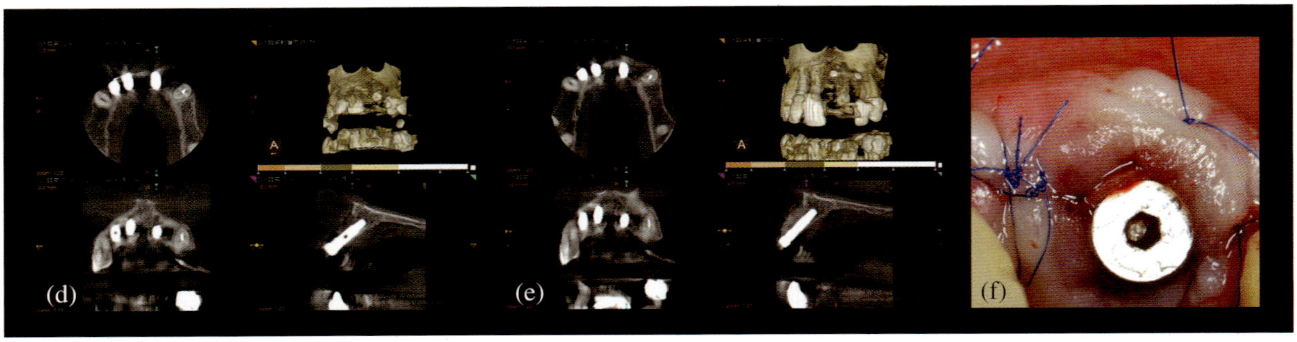

Figure 4.9 (d) CBCT scan showing the new position of the implant and the grafted site. (e) Post grafting CBCT showing the amount of bone built to restore the labial bone defect. (f) Flap sutured.

4.2.2 Reduced Levels of Technical Skills

Predictable implant-based esthetic treatment requires meticulous attention to detail in all phases of the treatment. Therefore, for clinicians to thrive they must develop their surgical and prosthetic skills, because reports have shown that clinical success in regenerating peri-implant defects is strongly dependent on the technical skills of the surgeon (see Figure 4.10a–k).

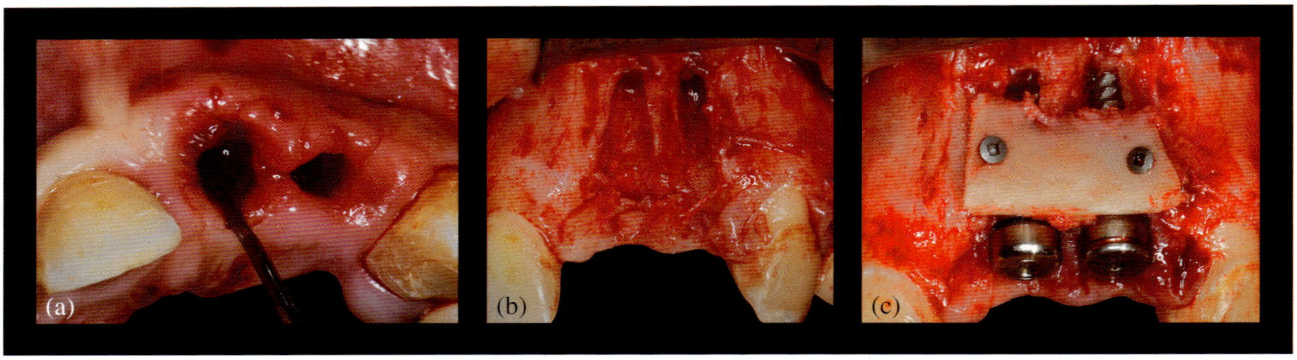

Figure 4.10 (a) Two implants failed and removed leaving two sockets. (b) Complete absence of the labial plate of bone due to faulty placement. (c) The case planned for non-staged implant placement (Laser-Lock, BioHorizons, Birmingham, AL, USA) along with monocortical bone graft stabilized with two titanium screws (KLS Martin, GmbH, Tuttilngen, Germany).

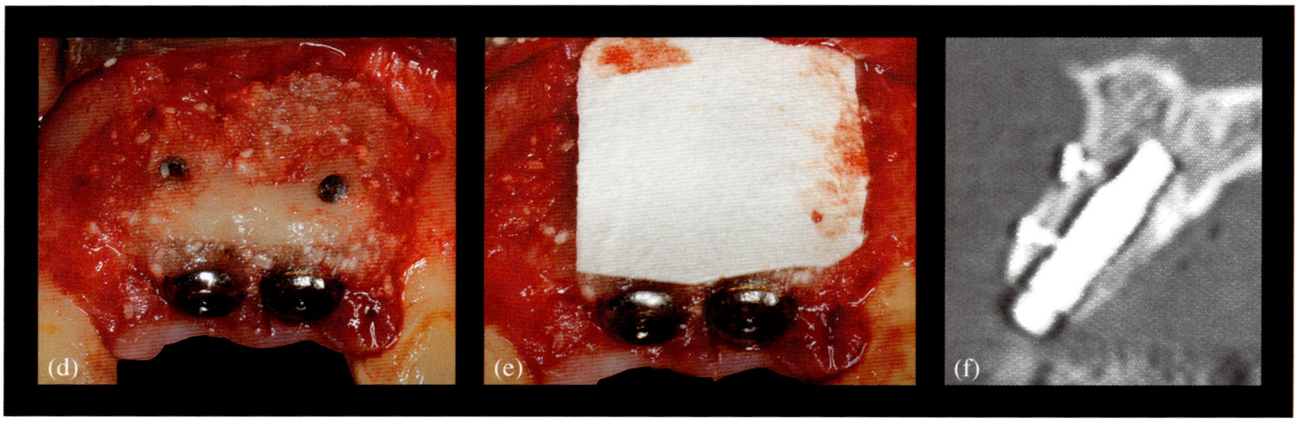

Figure 4.10 (d) Voids filled with allograft (Mineross, BioHorizons, Birmingham, AL, USA). (e) Collagen membrane is placed (Mem-Lock, BioHorizons, Birmingham, AL,USA). (f) CBCT showing complete restoration of the labial plate of bone.

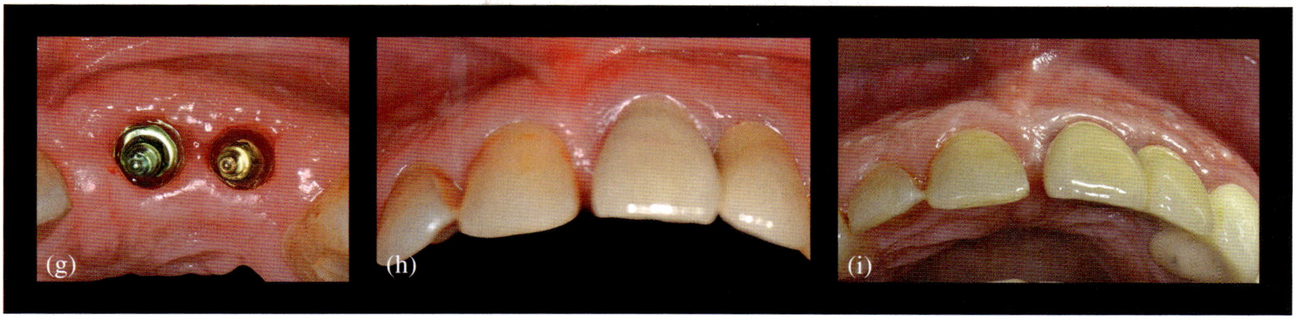

Figure 4.10 (g) Three months postoperative view showing the complete restoration of labial contour. (h) Final case restored with two PFM crowns. (i) Five years follow-up showing excellent stable tissue profile.

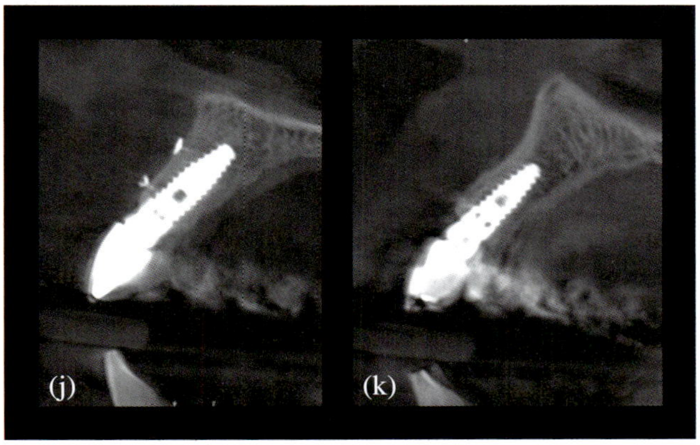

Figure 4.10 (j) and (k) CBCT showing a highly predictable osseous regenerative outcome.

Recently, many techniques have been introduced to optimize the clinical outcome of the immediate implant placement procedure in the esthetic zone, some authors claimed that the root retention may be able to avoid tissue alterations after tooth extraction. Filippi, Pohl and von Arx (2001) noted in a case report that decoronating of an ankylosed tooth preserved the alveolar bone before implant placement. The technique of retaining roots to avoid alveolar bone remodeling was adopted from dental traumatology. Multiple experimental and clinical studies have shown that the decoronation of teeth predictably preserves the alveolar ridge contour (Cohenca and Stabholz 2007; Filippi et al. 2001; Sapir and Shapira 2008). The retained root portion appears to preserve its characteristics with respect to its attachment to the periodontal ligament and the supraperiosteal fibers. O'Neal et al. (1978) reported on a study of 16 submerged endodontically treated mandibular premolar roots in four dogs. Results after one to four months depicted coronal overgrowth of bone, with no periapical and limited pericoronal inflammation. The major findings of the histological analysis were that the internal aspect of the root was covered with new cementum and new periodontal attachment. In addition, in areas where the implant was placed into the root fragment, cementum could be detected on the implant surface. In a study conducted by Buser et al. (1990), when the implant fixtures were placed in close relationship to the root fragment, examination of the undecalcified sections revealed a cementum layer on the implant surface with intervening collagen fibers. The socket shield approach bone (Hurzeler et al. 2010) is yet another modality for leaving the natural tooth root in its place to prevent further labial plate bone resorption. At the time of tooth extraction, the root fragment is reduced only along its vertical axis to the level of the height of the alveolar ridge to prevent perforation of the buccal mucosa during the healing period, the buccal shield should be thinned in its horizontal dimension to a height of less than 1 mm to ensure that the former tooth socket is filled with a maximum amount of bone and only minimal dentin at the time of reopening. Preserving the periodontal ligament and the supracrestal attachment of the tooth on the buccal aspect in conjunction with immediate implant placement appears to have a great potential.

However, in the world of reality these techniques are considered to be highly technique sensitive, the average clinician might not be able to perform these techniques with adequate perfection, these methods involve certain risks, such as the formation of a peri-implant periodontal membrane (Parlar et al. 2005) or the development of peri-implant infections, as well as alveolar bone resorption, and the exposure of the natural root throughout the gingiva. Several errors have been recorded using these methods, which include leaving a significant amount of tooth structure in situ (see Figure 4.11a–c).

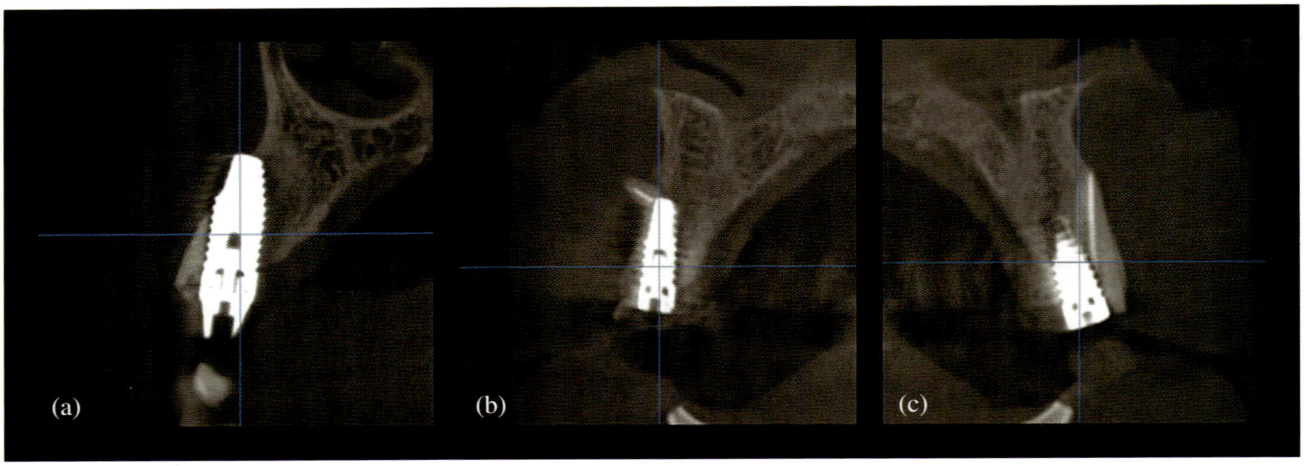

Figure 4.11 (a–c) Different faulty applications of the socket shield technique that complicates the treatment outcome, leading to failure of the immediate implant placement procedure.

4.2.3 Accuracy of Positioning of the Implant

The concept of reverse planning (Neves et al. 2004) allows for virtual planning and determination of an accurate implant position and its associated prosthetic components, which insures a successful treatment plan. The emergence of computerized tomography has revolutionized image examinations by obtaining much clearer images of the anatomical structures and three-dimensional reconstructions. Associating the concept of stereolithography and CAD/CAM technology, it becomes possible to generate prototyped surgical guides with high precision (Geng et al. 2015; Malo, de Araujo Nobre and Mangano 2007; Patel 2010; Sarment, Sukovic and Clinthorne 2003). This technology is based on real images of the bone anatomy obtained through CT scans and the design of a computerized prototyped surgical guide to implant placement based on mathematical 3D models.

The CT scan images are manipulated on a specific software, enabling virtual surgery that simulates the implant placement of the future prosthesis to be used (Geng et al. 2015; Malo et al. 2007; Patel 2010; Sarment et al. 2003). Guided surgeries are suitable for the most varying types of rehabilitation with implants, including edentulous patients, and partial or single unit restorations. This technology has been widely used with scientifically proven success (Schnitman and Hayashi 2015; Tallarico et al. 2015; Van de Wiele et al. 2015). Guided surgery may be considered as a viable alternative for the rehabilitation of edentulous spaces within the correct indications. The highlight of this technique is the detailed planning necessarily performed prior to the surgery. Therefore the optimal implant position can be obtained either by a highly skillful surgeon, or via using the surgical guides that provide an even a better clinical outcome when there is no room for error. One should anticipate using a surgical guide and avoid arbitrary implant positioning so that serous treatment complications do not arise.

4.2.4 Nature of the Labial Plate of Bone

When using dental implants in the esthetic zone to rehabilitate lost dental esthetics, there are numerous factors that contribute to the success of the overall procedure, because the main focus of any oral rehabilitation procedure is to focus on its long-term success. One of the main factors that influences the success of immediate implants placed in fresh extraction sites is the condition of the labial plate of bone, as this unique part of the oral anatomy constitutes the most valuable element of the treatment. It is only a few years ago that the behavior and influence of its physiology and response to the implantation procedure has been completely understood. This chapter is dedicated to the preservation, management, protection, and repair of the labial plate of bone.

The labial alveolar bone often undergoes a rapid remodeling physiologic process after natural tooth loss with an approximately 25% decrease in volume during the first year, followed by a 40–60% decrease in width in the next three years, leading to a labial cortex of bone that is more medial than its original position (Mechery, Thiruvalluvan and Sreehari 2015) (see Figure 4.12a and b).

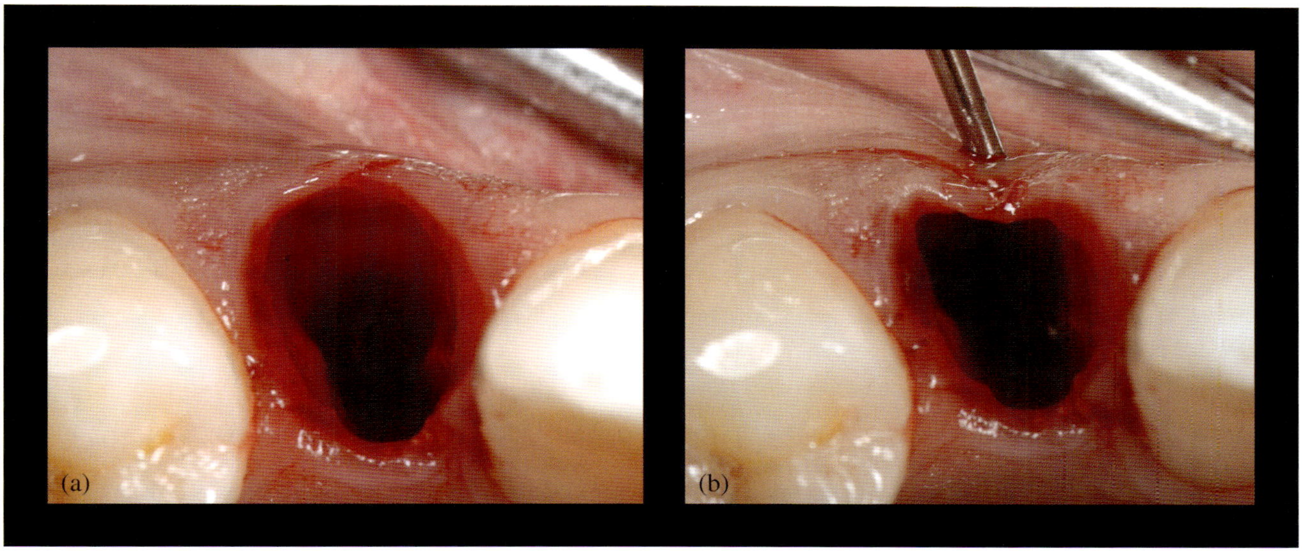

Figure 4.12 (a) and (b) The absence of the labial plate of bone at the time of tooth extraction could be a common clinical event.

Misch, Dietsh-Misch and Misch (1999) proposed that the loss of crestal bone height and width of the buccal plate after tooth extraction is partially due to the reduction of the blood supply the alveolus followed by the remodeling of the labial cortical plates in response to an inadequate blood supply after the extraction. Ashman (2000) reported that tooth extraction creates sequelae, resulting in approximately 40–60% loss of bone height and width, respectively, within two to three years (see Figure 4.13a–d).

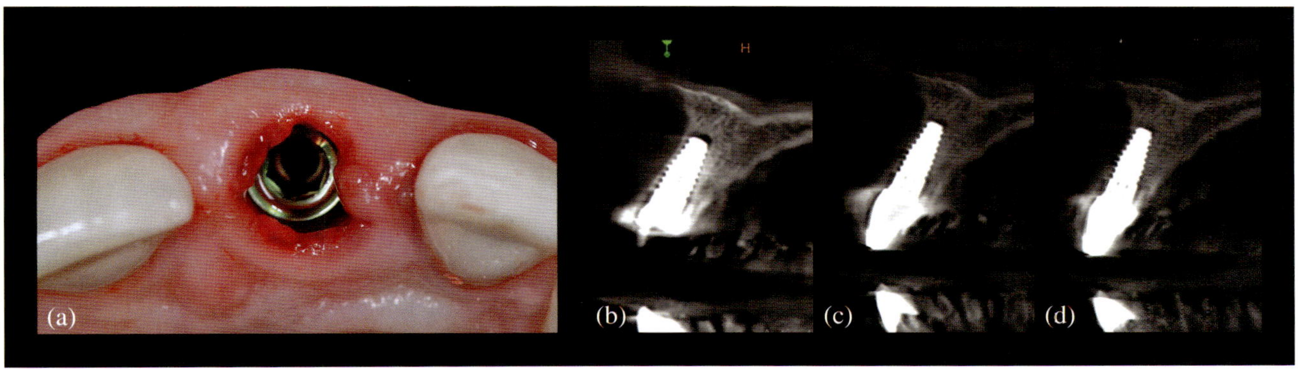

Figure 4.13 (a) Clinical view of a fresh extraction socket with abundant keratinized mucosa that received an immediate implant. (b) Immediate postoperative CT scan showing the proximity of the implant to the inner surface of the labial plate of bone on 13 December 2016. (c) CT scan approximately two months postoperative on 5 February 2017 showing complete resorption of the labial plate of bone. (d) Further bone resorption occurred on 14 March 2017.

4.2.5 Influence of Implant Fixture Diameter

Wide implants in the esthetic zone are no longer used. Clinical observations have lead to the recommendation of a wider gap distance that increases the discrepancy between the implant diameter and the tooth to be replaced, as wide implants violate the integrity of the labial plate of bone and may obstruct the blood supply to the labial plate, leading to postoperative gingival recession. There is no formula to use to decide on the right diameter to be used in the esthetic zone, but the choice should be based on the diameter of the tooth to be replaced, the osseous architecture, and the available implant fixture diameter. Attempts should be made to place dental implant collars away from the crest of the labial plate of bone to avoid poor post-operative consequences (See Figure 4.14).

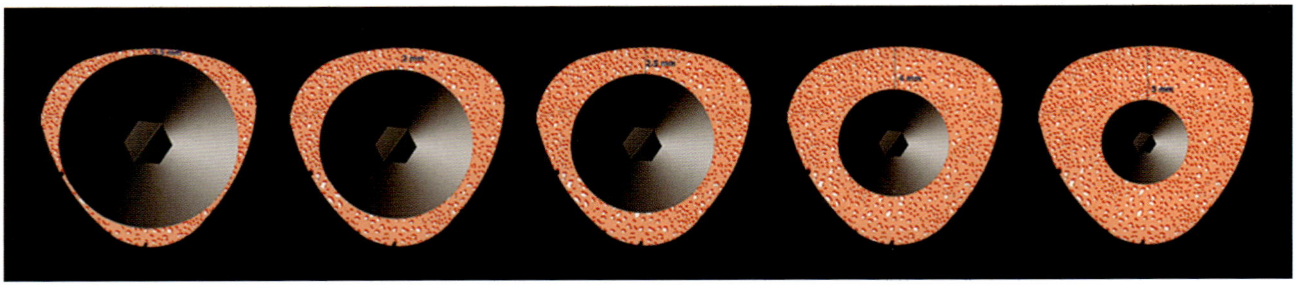

Figure 4.14 The different implants width in relation to the socket size, warrants the accurate selection of the smallest implant diameter that provides the optimal prosthetic result.

It has been reported that mucosal recession of 0.5 mm or more occurs in more than 33% of immediately placed implants, with one-fifth of the sites having 1–2 mm of recession (Beagle 2013; Buser, Martin and Belser 2004; Chen et al. 2007). Wide-diameter implants were often used in the past immediately in extraction sockets because it was thought to increase stability by reaching the socket wall (Jiansheng et al. 2012; Vandeweghe and De Bruyn 2012). In addition, they may improve bone-to-implant contact due to the increased implant surface area (Khayat et al. 2001; Krennmair et al. 2010; Olate et al. 2010), which could enhance the osseointegration of implant to bone and establish better implant stability (Jiansheng et al. 2012), and might compensate for the lack of bone height or density (Brink, Meraw and Sarment 2007) (see Figure 4.15a–m).

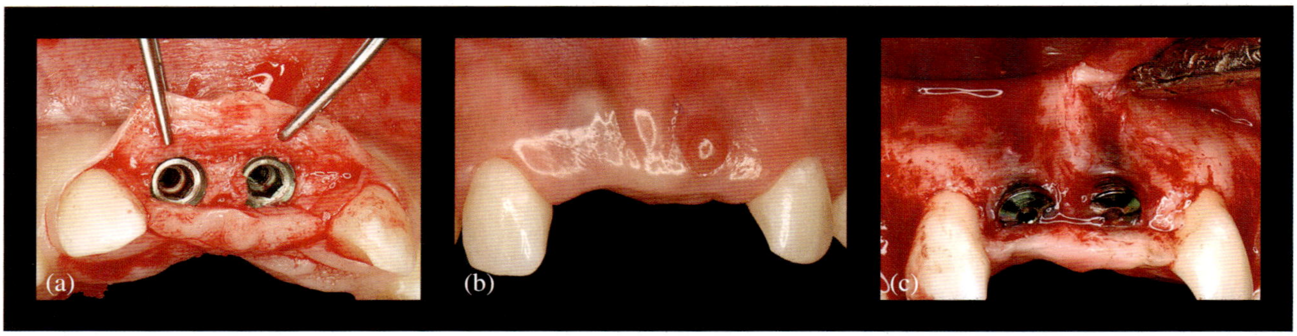

Figure 4.15 (a) Two wide implants; note the labial edge of the implant has a very thin labial plate of bone. (b) One month post implant placement showing related soft tissue thinning as a result of labial plate of bone resorption. (c) Mucoperiosteal flap reflected showing labial plate of bone resorption related to both implants due to the placement of a wide diameter implant body in a pre-existing narrow socket.

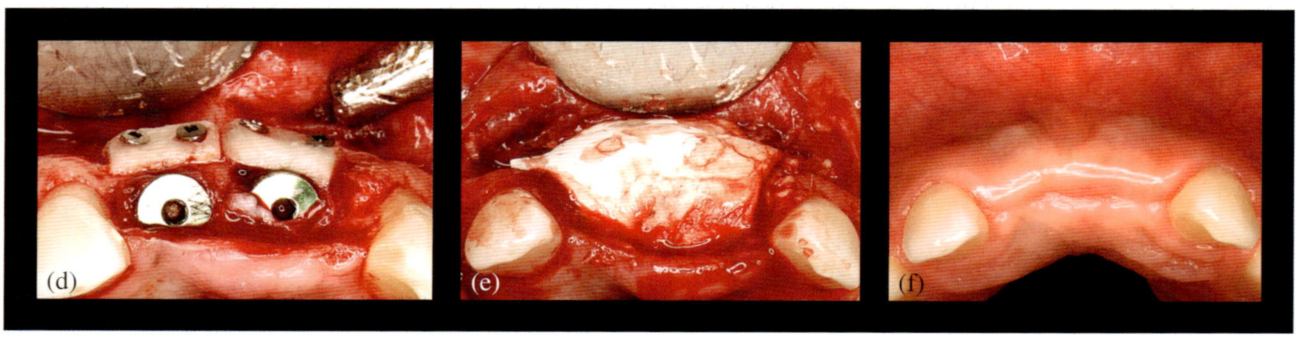

Figure 4.15 (d) Facial and incisal view of two chin block grafts stabilized with two microtitanium screws (KLS Martin, GmbH, Tuttilngen, Germany). (e) Collagen membrane (Mem-Lock, BioHorizons, Birmingham, AL, USA) is used to cover the graft and is stabilized by two membrane tacs (Auto Tac, BioHorizons, Birmingham, AL, USA). (f) One month post-surgery.

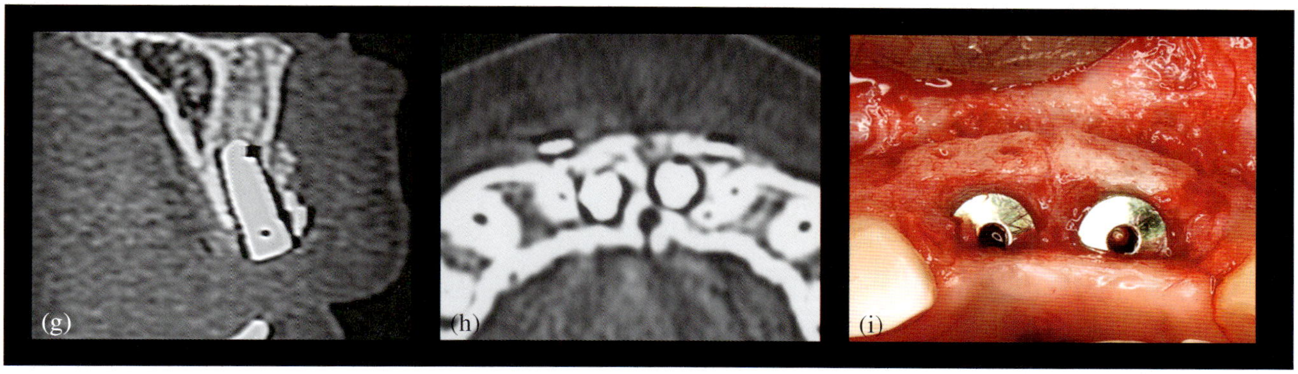

Figure 4.15 (g) and (h) CT scan showing complete integration of the graft. (i) Four months after grafting showing complete integration of the graft.

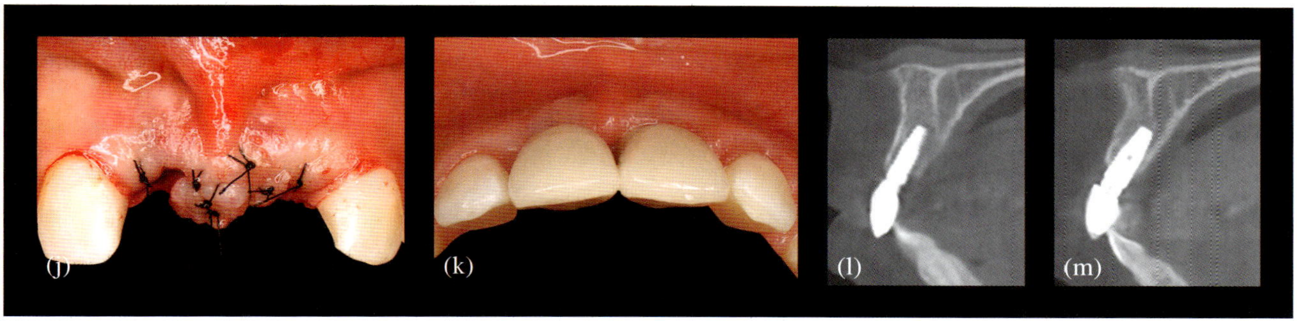

Figure 4.15 (j) Second-stage surgery with palatal rotational flap to improve the papilla height. (k) Case finally restored. (l) and (m) Three years follow-up.

On the other hand, a low survival rate (82%) had been described by Ivanoff and associates: reporting on the influence of variations in the Branemark implant diameter in a three- to five-year retrospective clinical study, the authors found the highest implant failure rate (18%) for 5 mm diameter implants, compared with 3% for 4 mm wide implants and 5% for the 3.75 mm diameter implants (Ivanoff et al. 1999). Eckert and colleagues also found statistically higher failure rates for wide-diameter implants in both maxilla (29%) and mandible (19%); according to the authors, a critical bone volume was needed for osseointegration, which was sometimes hampered by wide-diameter implants (Eckert et al. 2001). Similar results were reported in a retrospective study by Shin and colleagues, with survival rates of 80.41 and 96.8% for wide- and regular-body implants, respectively (Shin et al. 2009), while Hultin-Mordenfeld and co-workers reported a higher implant failure rate with wide-diameter implants, with better results in the mandible (94.5%) than the maxilla (78.3%) (Hultin-Mordenfeld et al. 2004) (see Figure 4.16a–j).

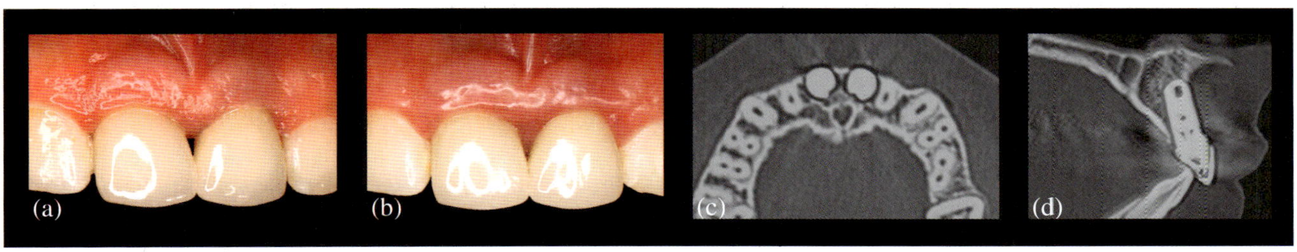

Figure 4.16 (a) Case restored two months after implant placement. (b) One year post restorative showing gingival discoloration. (c) and (d) CT view showing absence of the labial plate of bone related to the use of wide diameter implants.

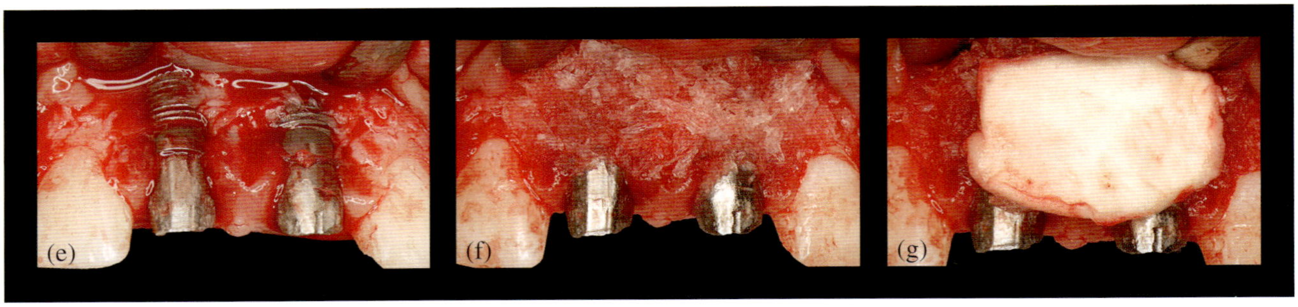

Figure 4.16 (e) Mucoperiosteal flap showing complete loss of the labial plate of bone due to resorption. (f) The labial defect is grafted with allograft (Grafton, BioHorizons, Birmingham, AL, USA). (g) The bone graft is covered with a cellular dermal graft (Alloderm, BioHorizons, Birmingham, AL, USA) to improve soft tissue quality.

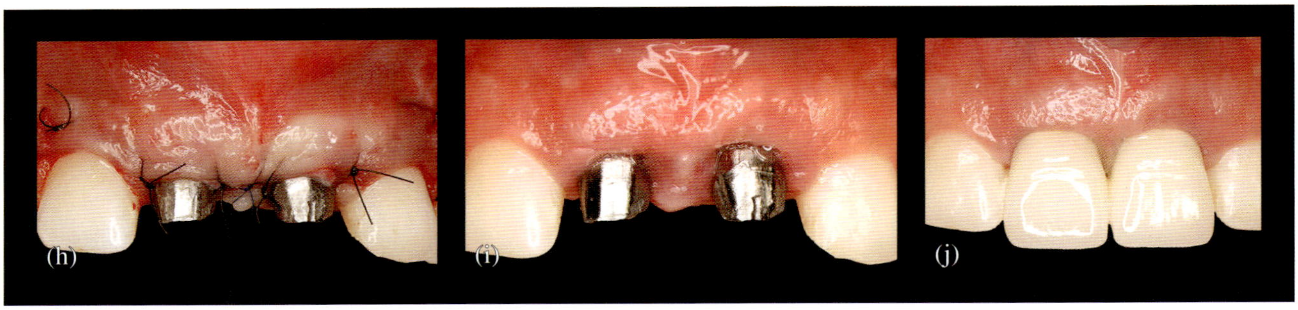

Figure 4.16 (h) Flap sutured. (i) Three weeks post-surgery showing remarkable improvement in both labial profile and soft tissue quality. (j) Case restored.

4.2.6 Risk Factors

4.2.6.1 Socket Trauma

Maxillofacial trauma results in significant loss of teeth and associated soft and hard tissues. Often the teeth that remain after trauma show signs of significant damage and may not be restorable. Others may have been luxated or avulsed and subsequently re-implanted, which might result in a questionable long-term prognosis. Specifically oral traumas often lead to esthetic, functional, and healing problems. According to Andreasen, Andreasen and Andersson (2007), recovery of root fractures is divided into four different types: (1) recovery with hard tissue, (2) recovery with conjunctive tissue interposition, (3) recovery with bone and conjunctive interposition between the fragments, and (4) recovery with granulation tissue between the fragments (see Figure 4.17a–f).

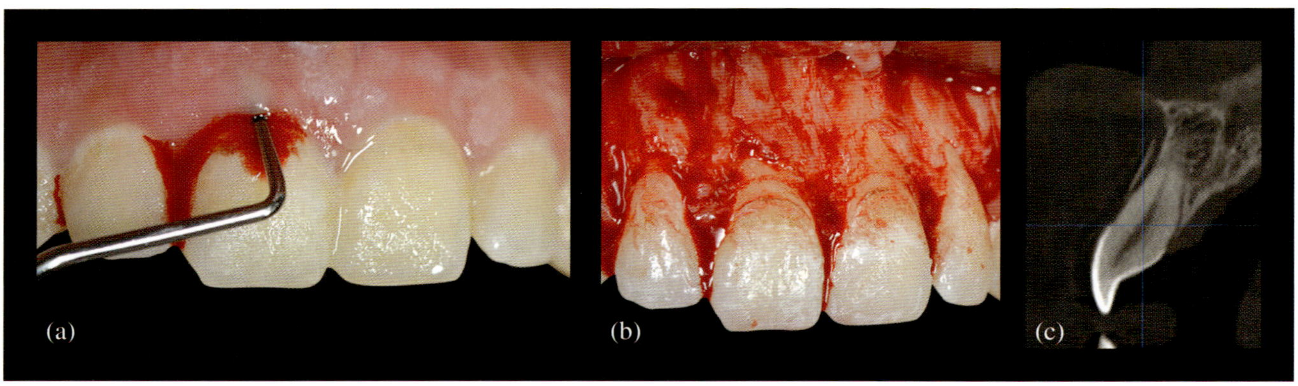

Figure 4.17 (a) and (b) Tooth trauma leads to pocketing and fracture of labial plate of bone. (c) CBCT showing the fracture of the labial plate of bone.

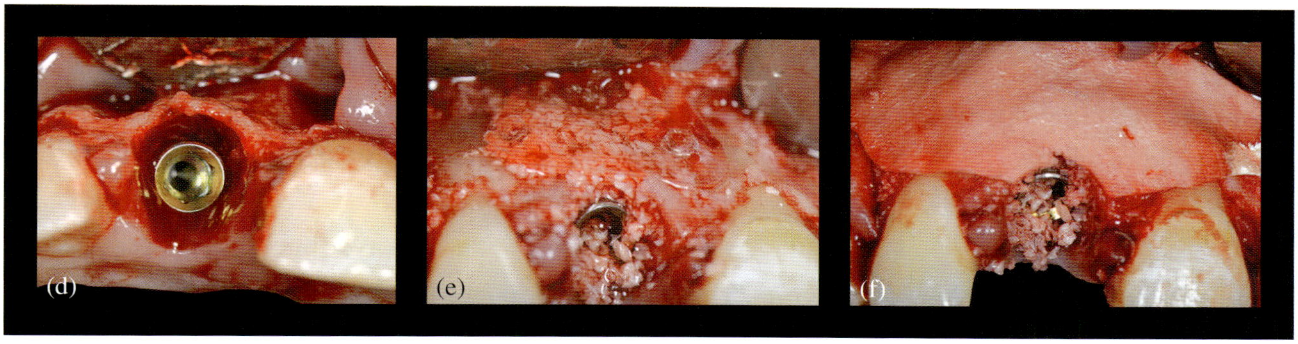

Figure 4.17 (d) Tooth extracted and replaced with an implant. (e) Labial plate of bone is grafted. (f) Collagen membrane is placed and stabilized.

According to the aforementioned literature, if the volume of the alveolar ridge can be maintained after extraction of the damaged tooth, dental implant insertion would be a straightforward procedure; however, most traumas involve labial plate of bone avulsion. Loss of alveolar bone associated with tooth avulsion would require that ridge augmentation, perhaps using guided bone regeneration or other regenerative techniques, is incorporated into the reconstruction treatment plan. In addition, the deleterious effects of soft tissue scarring on the final esthetic outcome would be anticipated. A post-traumatic malocclusion may necessitate a combined orthodontic, prosthodontic, and oral surgical approach to rehabilitation.

Rehabilitating patients who have had severe dentofacial trauma can be challenging. Careful planning is required to assess the prognosis of the remaining teeth, the bone volume available, the amount of keratinized soft tissue present, and occlusal relationships. In some cases, rehabilitation of the alveolar ridge and the use of the bone around the extraction site for implant placement is needed. In other cases, bone grafting is required and when a large bone defect, many grafting procedures can be implemented that can result in a predictable outcome. Barone et al. (2013) reported that the use of corticocancellous porcine substitute and resorbable membrane succeeded in reducing alveolar contour from remodeling when compared to non-preserved extraction sockets. Kim et al. (2014) reported in a series of their cases that autogenous tooth bone graft material can be a preferable bone substitute for extraction socket graft because of its good bone remodeling and osteoconductivity. Cheah et al. (2014) demonstrated that both calcium sulfate–platelet rich plasma and calcium sulfate were effective GTR in socket preservation applications and the amount of mineralized bone component was significantly higher in the calcium sulfate–platelet rich plasma group in comparison to the calcium sulfate group. The design of the final prosthesis plays a vital role in the overall esthetic appearance after surgical intervention; however, good oral hygiene should be maintained daily by the patient during the course of treatment. Ultimately, this will determine the long-term success and survival of the rehabilitation (see Figure 4.18a–i).

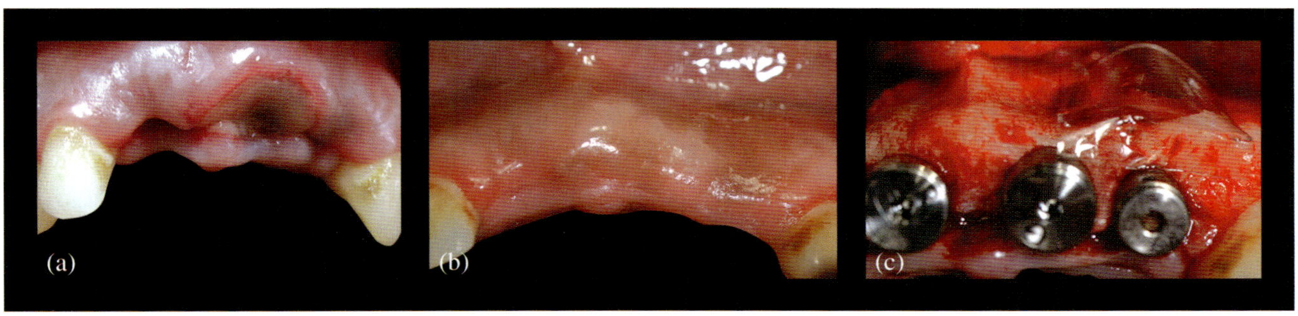

Figure 4.18 (a) Preoperative view showing root avulsion as a result of trauma. (b) Staged approach elected. (c) Implants were placed and PDLLA membrane is tried in; note the space making for the bone graft.

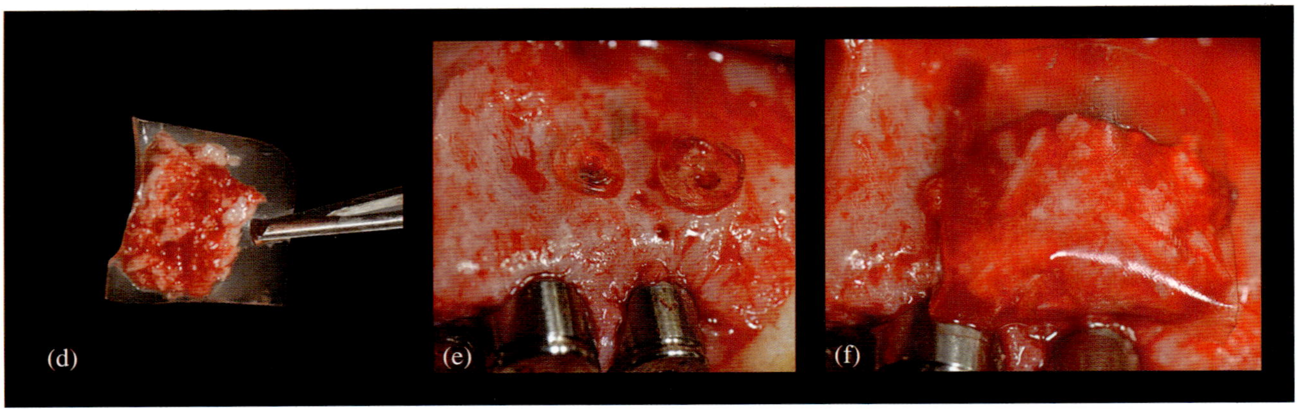

Figure 4.18 (d) Particulated bone graft was placed inside the carrier. (e) and (f) The carrier is stabilized.

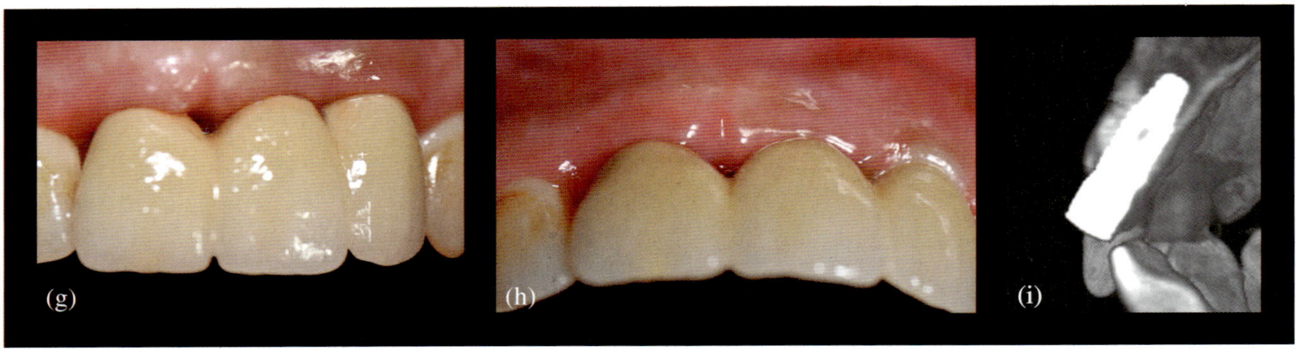

Figure 4.18 (g) and (h) Finally case restored. (i) CBCT scan showing the enhancement of thin labial plate of bone.

4.3 Arbitrary Flapless Implant Fixture Installation

Flapless implant placement technique has increasingly been used recently to offer several clinical advantages, but the technique requires strict meticulous clinical handling to achieve an optimal treatment outcome. There are some factors that are considered to be detrimental to this treatment modality, including: 1) a lack of direct visibility as it is considered to be a blind surgical technique when used without a surgical guide, 2) the innaccurate duplication of the CT scan preoperative planning to the socket with manual implant placement, 3) the increased risk of this modality might add more cost to the treatment, 4) and the limited ability to augment any ridge deficiencies (see Figure 4.19a–u).

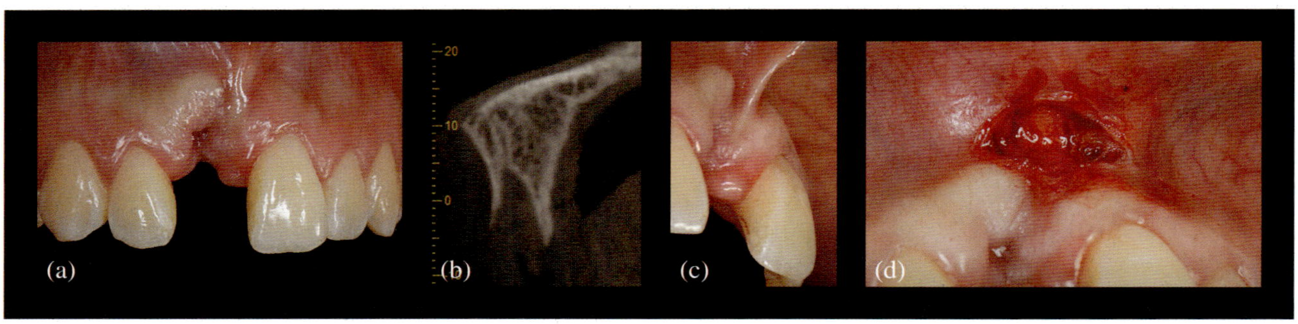

Figure 4.19 (a) Preoperative view of two weeks old socket trauma reveals soft and hard tissues deficiencies. (b) CBCT scan showing partial loss and thinning of labial plate. (c) and (d) The presence of high attached frenum, frectenomy performed with classic surgery.

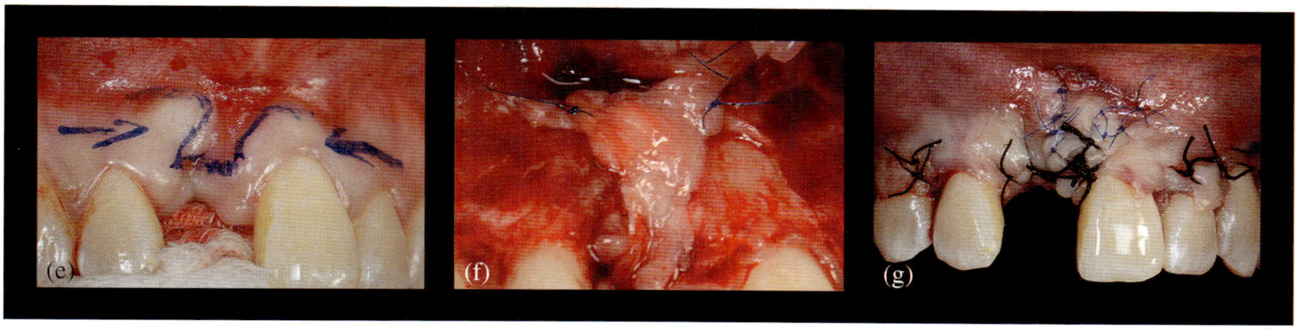

Figure 4.19 (e) Preoperative view of soft tissue deficiency and loss of criticized tissue band (double papillary approximation and vestibular tissue excision is planned). (f) Rotated palatal pedicel flap (partial thickness) is stabilized to the labial tissue with two sutures. (g) flap sutured.

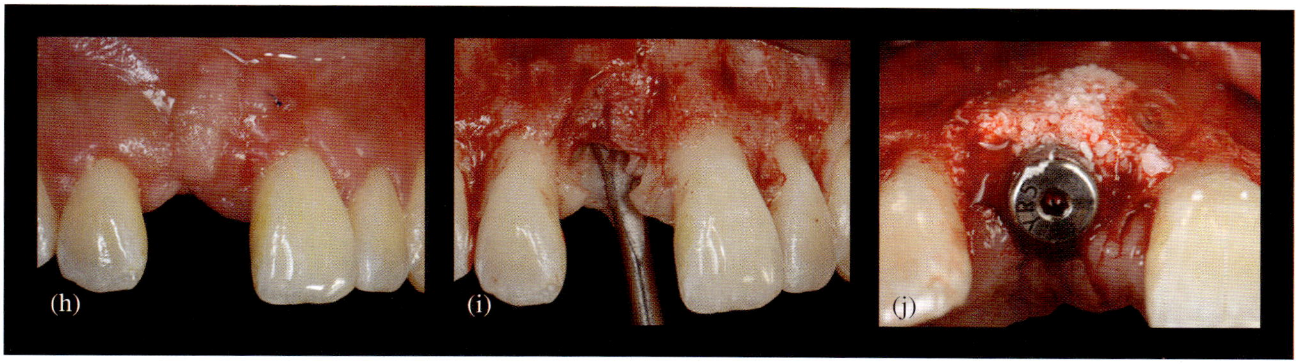

Figure 4.19 (h) Two weeks postoperative healing showing the regain of keratinized tissue band. (i) Four weeks post soft tissue surgery, intraoperative view showing labial plate of bone loss. (j) Particulate bone graft is placed along with PDLLA membrane and an implant is stabilized.

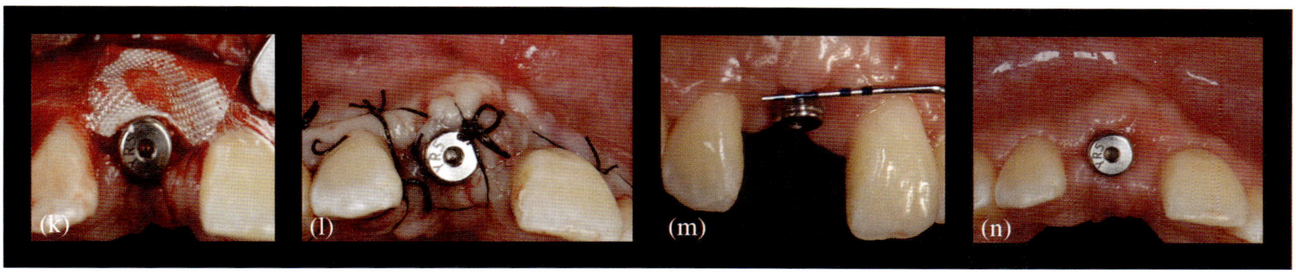

Figure 4.19 (k) Cellulose membrane is placed on top to facilitate soft tissue adherence. (l) Flap sutured. (m) and (n) Ten days postoperative view showing excellent healing.

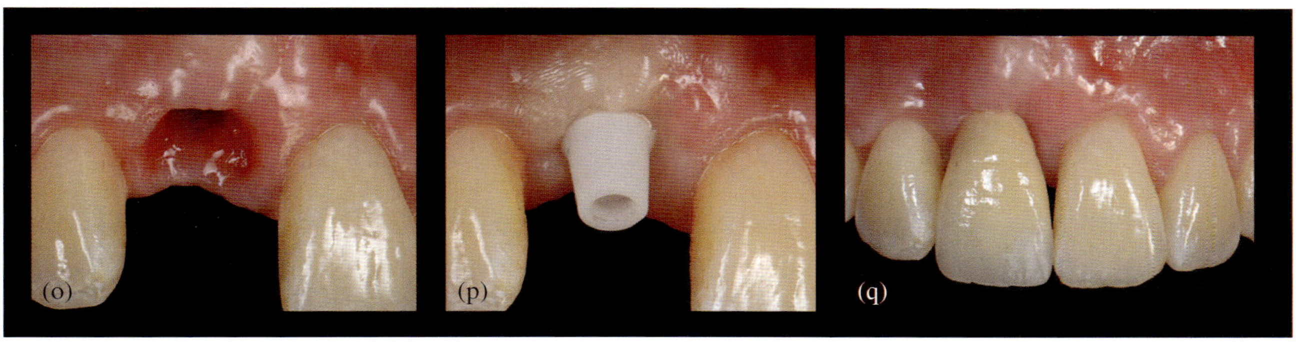

Figure 4.19 (o) and (p) Final soft tissue maturation and zirconia abutment is connected. (q) Case finally restored.

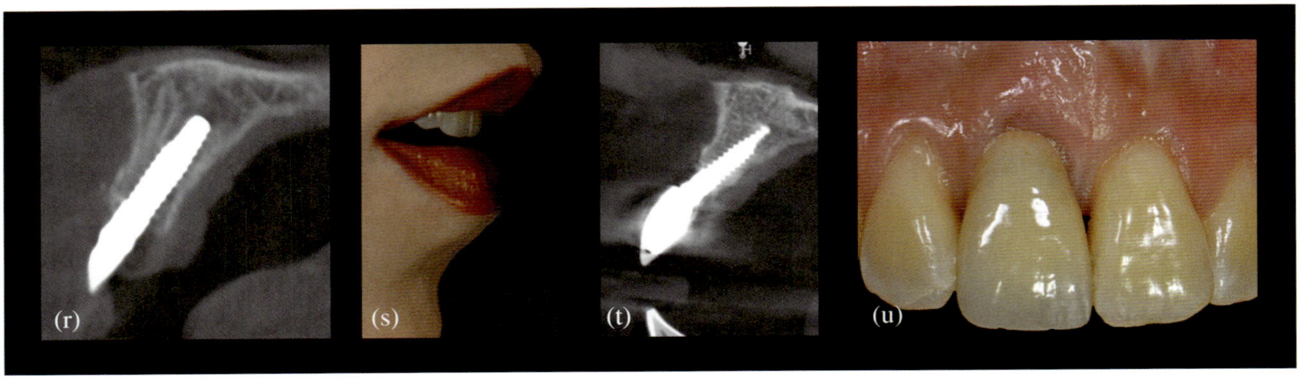

Figure 4.19 (r) CBCT of three months post-surgery. (s) Extra oral side view showing enhanced esthetic result. (t) Two years postoperative view showing stable bone thickness. (u) Three years postoperative assessment showing excellent tissue stability.

The technique of placing dental implants in delayed protocol or in healed sites via the flapless approach was presented by Campelo and Camara (2002), who placed dental implants in 359 patients to restore both completely edentulous and partially edentulous arches with fixed prostheses or removable complete dentures. Each patient was examined after three months, six months, one year, and then once every year. The cumulative success rate for implants placed using a flapless single-stage surgical technique after a 10-year period varied from 74.1% for implants placed in the year of 1990 to 100% in the year of 2000. However, flapless implant placement is considered a generally "blind" surgical technique, so extra care must be taken when placing implants. Angulation of the implants affected by drilling is critical to avoid perforation of the cortical plates, either lingual or buccal, especially on the lingual in the mandibular molar areas and the anterior maxilla. This technique has showed several disadvantages, which include the possible perforation of the labial plate of bone without notice; therefore installing dental implants via the flapless method in delayed healed sites should not be used except in very limited surgical situations and must include the patient's acceptance to share the responsibility for the high unexpected increased failure rate. In conclusion, the flapless approach is still a blind surgical procedure that should be approached with caution even when performed by skillful experienced clinicians (see Figures 4.20a–d and 4.21a, b).

Becker (2006) observed that the implants were stable upon insertion and demonstrated increased stability at three months without significant differences between surgical protocols. The histologic evaluation showed high bone–implant contact (flapless surgery: 54.7% ± 8.4%; control: 52.2% ± 13.0%; $P > 0.05$) without evidence of gingival tissue or foreign body inclusions. There were no significant differences in marginal bone levels between the surgical protocols. Postinsertion and at three months, Implant Stability Quotient (ISQ) values depend on the torque delivered to the implant at placement. Immediately postinsertion, for every one unit increase in torque value, the ISQ increased by 0.3 (95% confidence interval: 0.1–0.4;

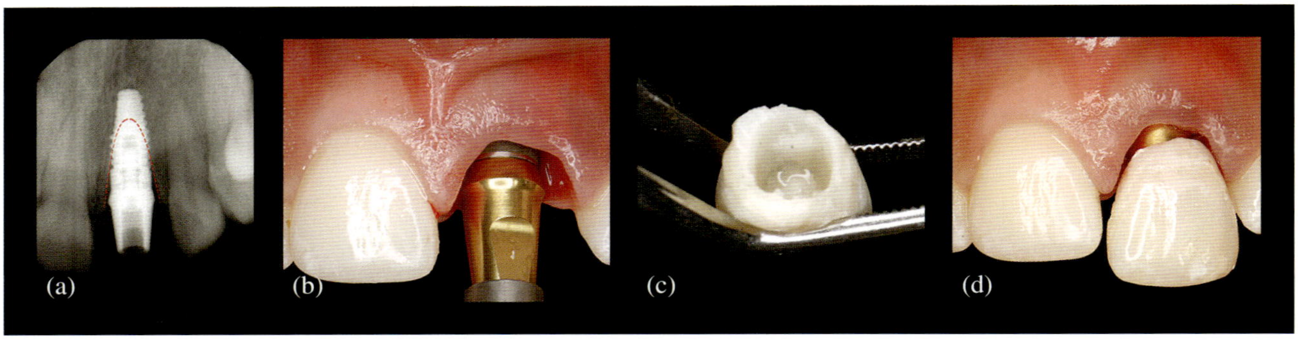

Figure 4.20 (a) Implant primary stability is obtained via extending the implant fixture 3 mm or more above the root apex; the dotted red line indicates the socket outline, this can minimize the treatment time. (b) The optimal implant size and position will lead to the optimal esthetic and functional outcome. (c) Immediate support to the gingival margin with the provisional restoration will help minimize soft tissue shrinkage postoperatively. (d) Using accurate esthetic contours will impact the final soft tissue outcome when placing an immediate implant in a fresh extraction site.

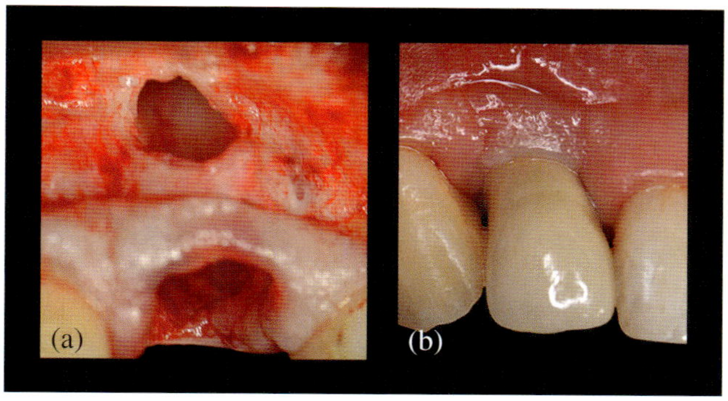

Figure 4.21 (a) and (b) Esthetic buccal flap might not be a predictable solution for providing tissue stability.

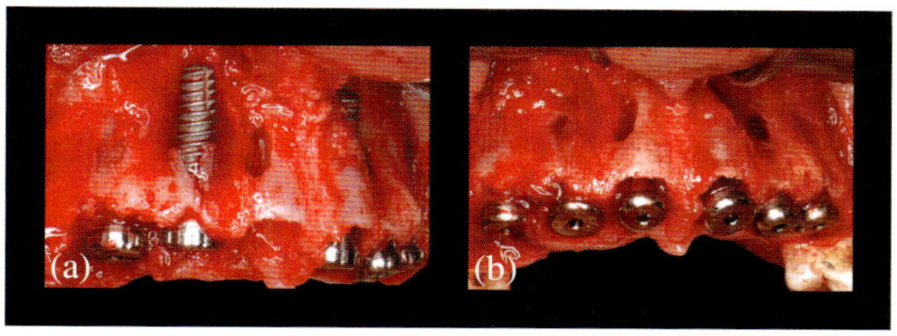

Figure 4.22 (a) and (b) Violating the labial plate of bone with faulty implant angulation as a result of blind placement of the flapless implant positioning.

$P = 0.0043$). Three months postoperatively, for every one unit increase in torque the ISQ value decreased by 0.2 (9556 confidence interval: −0.4 to −0.1; $P = 0.0012$). The effect of torque on ISQ values was independent of treatment effects and remained significant after adjustment for treatment. The results suggest that implants placed without flap reflection remain stable and exhibit clinically relevant osseointegration similar to when implants are placed with flapped procedures. Greater torque at implant placement resulted in less implant stability at three months (see Figure 4.22a and b).

From another perspective, the literature reported the use of a flapless approach for immediate and delayed dental implant placement in the alveolar ridge in order to maintain the natural soft tissue contours, reduce intraoperative bleeding, reduce postoperative patient discomfort, preserve alveolar ridge integrity, and avoid additional soft tissue trauma by raising a mucoperiosteal flap. The preservation of the delicate vascular network adjacent to implant receptor sites may be an important factor in maintaining facial bone height and esthetics. In edentulous regions where the vascular network is compromised by tooth loss, the associated periosteum and soft tissues may serve as primary blood sources for the area (Al-Ansari and Morris 1998; Landsberg 2008) (see Figure 4.23a–e).

A study by Covani et al. (2004), however, evaluated 15 patients (9 men and 6 women) aged 31–54 years old, and each had at least 4 mm of bone beyond the root apex. They calculated flapless implant placement and its related soft tissue response. Teeth with multiple roots were excluded from this study. The second-stage surgical procedure was performed six months after the first procedure. The following clinical parameters were evaluated at the time of implant placement and at second stage surgery: levels of mesial and distal papillae, width of keratinized mucosa, position of the muco gingival junction relating to the surrounding tissues, peri-implant radiolucency, and marginal bone loss, which were evaluated radiographically. The postsurgical healing period was uneventful for all patients. Soft tissue closure over the implant sites was achieved in one to three weeks after surgery at all sites. At second-stage surgery, no peri-implant bone defects were observed or detected by probing around all the experimental implants. The soft tissue anatomy was considered clinically acceptable in all patients.

Another study by Schwartz et al. (1998) evaluated the clinical success of osseointegration achieved with nine

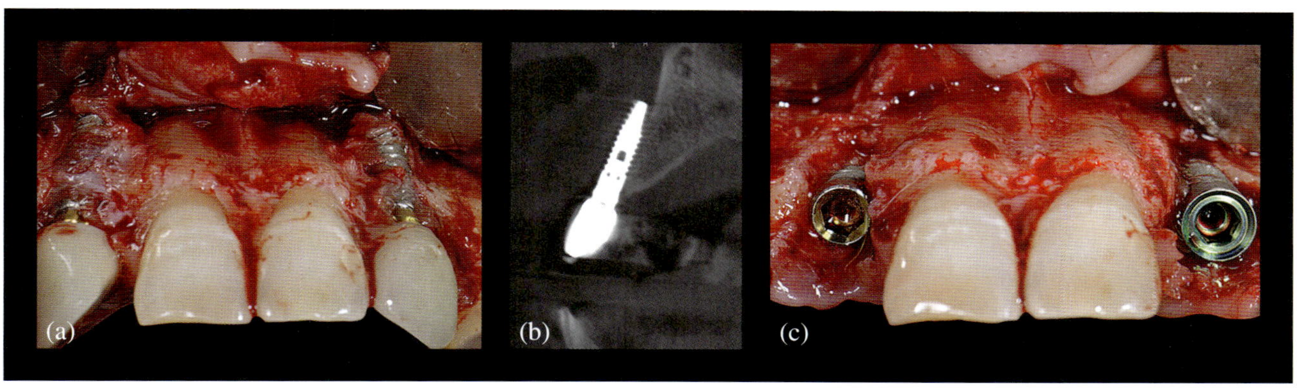

Figure 4.23 (a) and (b) Another example of labial plate of bone violation as a result of arbitrary positioning. (c) Two new implants placed with excellent primary stability.

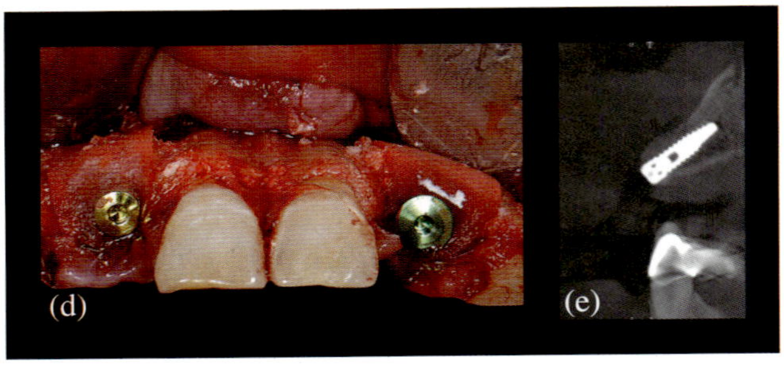

Figure 4.23 (d) The alveolar ridge defect is grafted using particulated bone graft. (e) CBCT scan showing the restoration of the labial plate of bone.

immediate implants placed without incisions in fresh extraction sites, and without any guided bone regenerative membranes being used; the only allowed grafting material to fill the socket gaps was autogenous bone chips harvested from the drilling procedure. It starts with atraumatic extraction of the unsalvageable teeth. Drilling is then performed through a surgical template using a buccally placed guiding finger to avoid perforating the labial plate of bone. Autogenous bone chips are collected from the drill flutes and packed back into the surgical site around the implant fixture to fill any existing gaps, though the drilling should be based on the CBCT profile of the available ridge. Finally, the wound edges are approximated and may be sutured; the results showed high clinical success without soft tissue primary closure.

Another example of the arbitrary implant placement in delayed implant placement protocol where soft tissue punching is used to expose the bone for the drilling procedure and implant placement, involved a higher risk of morbidity and many treatment errors were recorded as a result of using an arbitrary placement of the dental implants in the healed sites without using a surgical guide. A conservative palatal flap may be reflected during implant placement, which can reveal the condition of the labial plate of bone; it can be viewed through the palatal side at a 45° angle to the occlusal plane. This modified palatal approach adds more predictability by helping to detect any labial osseous defect before implant placement.

On another hand, successful immediate implants in debrided infected alveoli depends on the complete removal of all contaminated tissue and the controlled regeneration of the alveolar defect. Experienced clinicians consider immediate implants as a viable treatment option in patients with dentoalveolar infections (Casap et al. 2007).

4.3.1 The Effect of Loading Protocol

When it comes to loading dental implants, many factors are to be considered, such as the number of implants used, bone quality, quantity, the position of the implants placed, the type of future prostheses, the physical design of the implant used, type of occlusion, nature of the opposing arch, the decision of the clinician, and detection of the risk factors involved in each case individually. Some authors (Branemark et al. 1977) applied the immediate loading of dental implants with certain criteria with a high degree of success (see Figure 4.24a–c).

Immediate functional loading of dental implants involved patients receiving prostheses with occlusal function on the day of implant placement, whereas nonfunctional immediate loading (termed immediate restoration by this consensus group (Degidi and Piattelli 2003) involved the provision of a prosthesis 1–2 mm away from the occlusal contact. Early loading of dental implants has been defined as restoration of implants in or out of

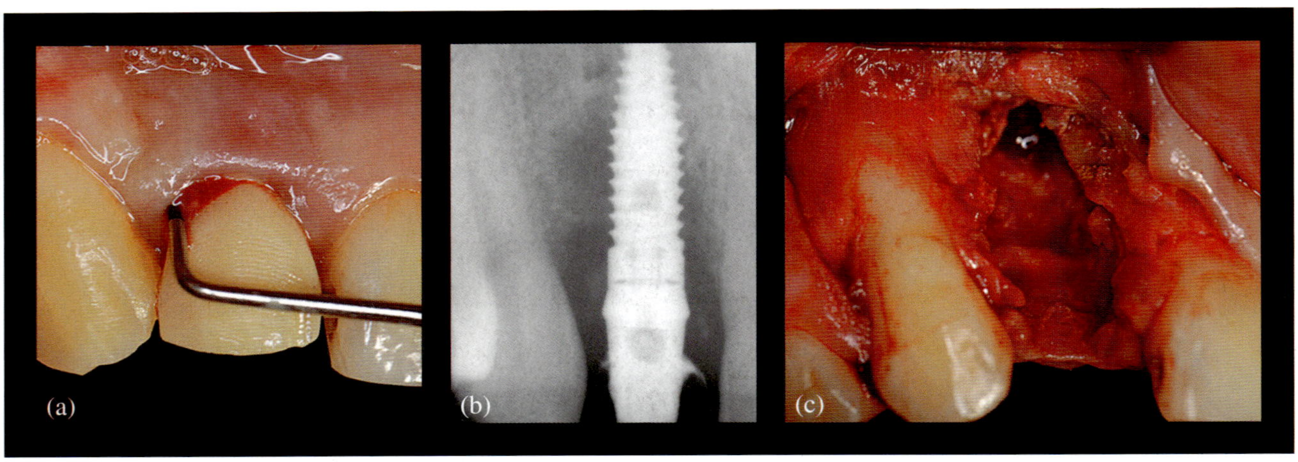

Figure 4.24 (a) Severe pocketing and bone loss due to improper application of immediate load concept. (b) Periapical radiographic view showing a classic picture of bone breakdown related to the implant surface. (c) Resultant osseous defect.

occlusion at least 48 hours after implant placement (Ganeles and Wismeijer 2004), but at a shorter time interval than conventional healing. Different implant surface characteristics, in particular surface properties (e.g. roughness, bioactive coatings, extent of the surface in direct contact with the bone), seem to be of major importance for successful early loading results. Several authors (Aparicio, Rangert and Sennerby 2003; Ganeles and Wismeijer 2004) have detailed clinical factors to be considered when assessing the applicability of immediate restoration or loading, such as: (1) primary clinical stability of the implants, (2) adequate implant splinting where appropriate, (3) provisional restorations that promote splinting and reduce or control the mechanical load applied to the implants, (4) prevention of provisional restoration removal during the recommended period of implant healing, and (5) incorporation of the team approach and the use of surgical templates. In addition, some authors (Ganeles and Wismeijer 2004) have identified risk factors associated with immediate restoration or loading of dental implants. These include: (1) the presence of high masticatory or parafunctional forces, (2) poor bone quality or volume, and (3) the presence of infection.

A consensus stated that most publications that cover immediate and early loading indicated that implant survival rate with immediate restoration was comparable to the results with conventional and early loading protocols (Ganeles and Wismeijer 2004). However, they stated that these conclusions may be misleading statistical phenomena and limited data suggest that immediate restoration of implants in the esthetic zone might facilitate and stabilize gingival architecture more than a delayed approach. They also stated that there is no evidence suggesting that deleterious gingival complications can be directly attributed to immediate restoration or loading protocols.

Chiapasco et al. (2004) stated that limited histological data supporting the reliability of immediate loading or widespread use of immediate or early loading of implants in all clinical situations; he indicated that only when torque applied to the implant insertion was more than 35 N cm in immediately loaded implants offered a higher degree of bone formation and remodeling in comparison to unloaded implants.

De Wijs, Cune and De Putter (1995) also demonstrated the formation of transversely oriented collagen fibers in the peri-implant bone. The study used four to six immediately loaded and unloaded dental implants with a microstructured surface, which were placed in the mandible and the maxilla in seven minipigs. A total of 85 implants were placed. After a four month healing period, all implants were retrieved. Histomorphometry was performed. The study aimed to prove that when the insertion torque on the dental implants was more than 35 N cm, secondary osteons were present, while a higher quantity of collagen fibers with a more parallel orientation were also present. This was a logical explanation for the benefits of the immediate loading concept on the bone remodeling and formation rate.

4.3.2 The Influence of Socket Related Pathology

The immediate implant placement in extraction site offers the higher esthetics and a reduction in surgery time and the overall treatment (Lindeboom, Tjiook and Kroon 2006). However, the concept of immediate implant placement after extraction of a tooth with The immediate implant placement in the extraction site offers better esthetics and a reduction in surgery time (Lindeboom, Tjiook and Kroon 2006). However, the concept of immediate implant placement after extraction of a tooth with periapical disease raises many questions, with few scientific studies reported (see Figure 4.25). Some authors suggest that the immediate implant placement in an infected socket has a questionable prognosis , because the implant surface becomes contaminated with bacteria (Becker and Becker 1990). Others recommended meticulous debridement of the infected socket combined with an antibiotic curettage. Liljenqvist et al. (2003) claimed that osseointegration between the titanium surface and the bone occur, despite the presence of infection. In addition, Novaes and Novaes (1995) have shown that proper debridement and prophylactic use of antibiotics would not jeopardize implant placement in an infected socket (see Figure 4.27a and b).

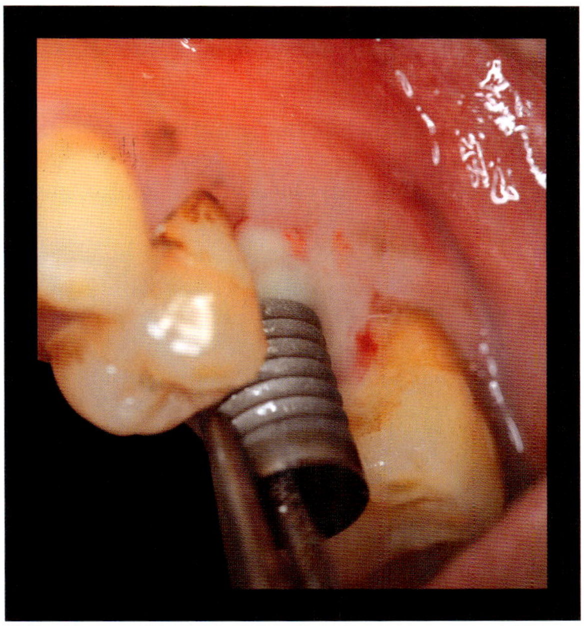

Figure 4.25 Implant related infection.

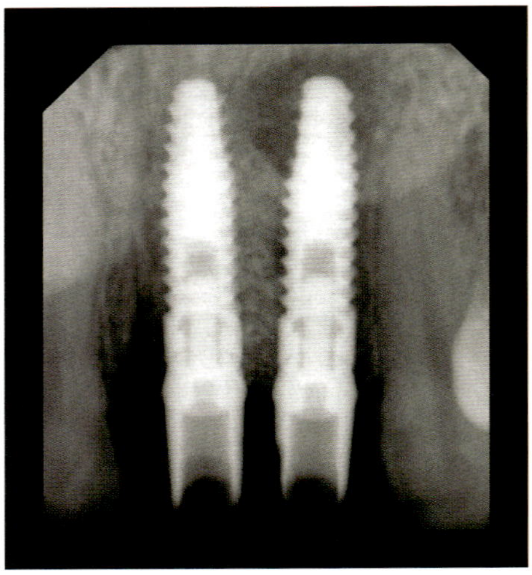

Figure 4.26 Peri-apical implant related infection.

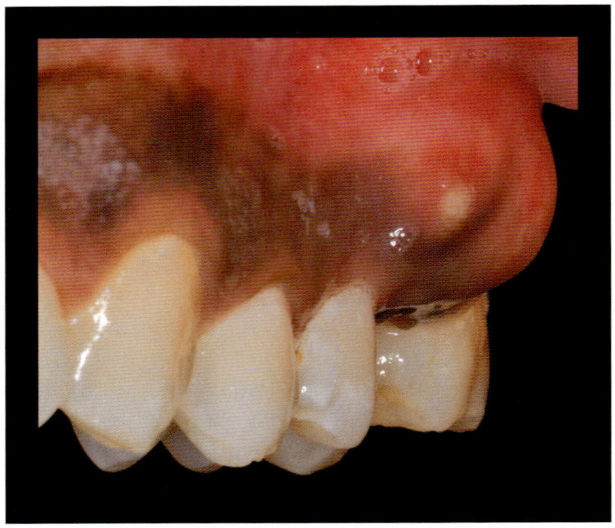

Figure 4.28 Acute periapical infection related to the maxillary molar which contraindicates immediate implant placement.

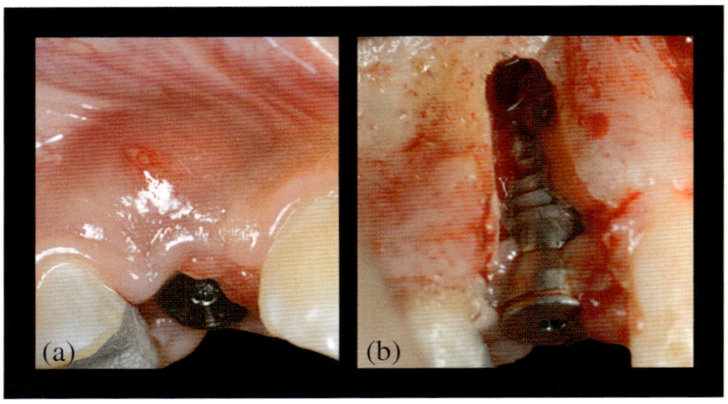

Figure 4.27 (a) and (b) Clinical views showing peri-implant infection manifested by swelling and redness. Lost labial plate of bone as a result of infection.

Alsaadi et al. (2007), in a case–control study, reported a greater loss of implants in those sockets with periapical lesions, especially when machined surface implants were placed. An increased loss of endosseous implants has also been associated with periodontal disease (Alsaadi et al. 2007; Cardaropoli et al. 2005; Evian et al. 2004). However, there are few clinical data regarding the immediate implant placement in sockets associated with chronic periapical infectious processes. Some clinical studies have suggested that a history of periodontal disease and periapical infection could be used as a predictive marker for the onset of the peri-implant disease, as well as predicting implant failure (Ayangco and Sheridan 2001; Karoussis et al. 2003); therefore the placement of implants in the presence of periapical and periodontal pathology is discouraged. It was related to the potential contamination of the implant fixture during the initial phase of wound healing (Karoussis et al. 2003) (see Figure 4.28).

Implant survival rates were significantly reduced after immediate implantation in post-extraction sockets associated with chronic periapical disease (90.8%) than in healthy post extraction sockets (98.1%) (Hita-Iglesias and Sanchez-Sanchez 2016). On the other hand Casap et al. (2007) showed satisfactory results in the immediate implant placement in sockets with chronic periapical disease. The sites must be thoroughly debrided prior to placement (Waasdrop, Evian and Mandracchia 2010). Researchers, such as Siegenthaler et al. (2007) and others, concluded that immediate implant placement performed at extraction sockets exhibiting periapical pathology did not lead to an increased rate of complications and rendered an equally favorable type of tissue integration of the implants where primary stability was achieved (Crespi, Capparè and Gherlone 2010; Del Fabbro, Boggian and Taschieri 2009; Lindeboom et al. 2006).

Novaes and Novaes recommended postoperative antibiotic coverage for the placement of immediate implants in sites associated with chronic periapical infection. In a histomorphometric study in dogs, Novaes et al. (1998) demonstrated that the osseointegration levels in those immediate implants in fresh extraction sockets associated with infection (study group) did not differ significantly from those implants in healthy sockets. Yet another study by Crespi et al. (2010) reported that the marginal bone level in those immediate implants in sockets with a history of infection remained at levels similar to those with healthy socket implants. Similar results were obtained by Villa and Rangert (2005, 2007), who evaluated the survival rates of immediate implants after extraction of teeth with periodontal and endodontic lesions followed by a thorough socket curettage of the apical socket and irrigation with an antibiotic solution. No signs of implant-associated local infection were detected after one year (see Figure 4.29a–i).

Siegenthaler et al. (2007) investigated immediate implant placement with signs of chronic periapical periodontitis (periapical images, and presence of fistula and purulent discharge); a mucoperiosteal flap was

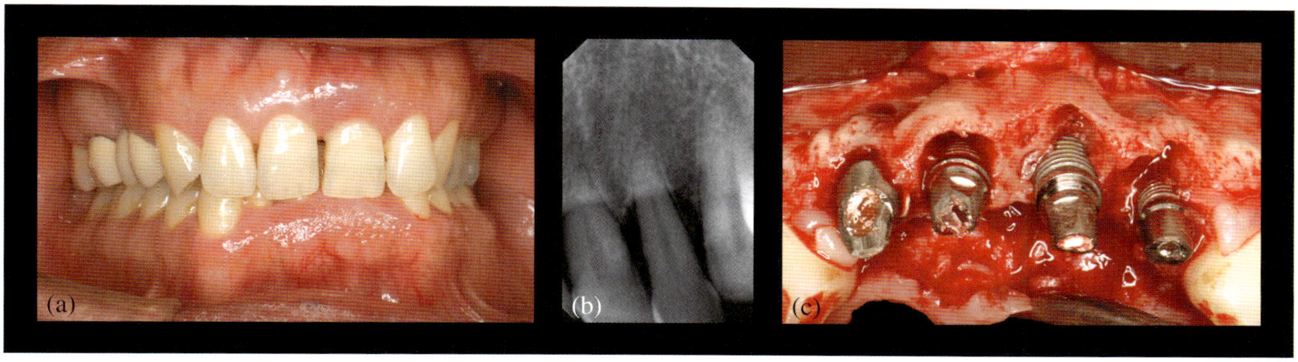

Figure 4.29 (a) Preoperative view of four periodontally involved maxillary and mandibular teeth. (b) Radiographic view showing bone resorption pattern. (c) Four implants are placed in the maxilla and two implants placed in the mandible, revealing an osseous defect that is to be augmented.

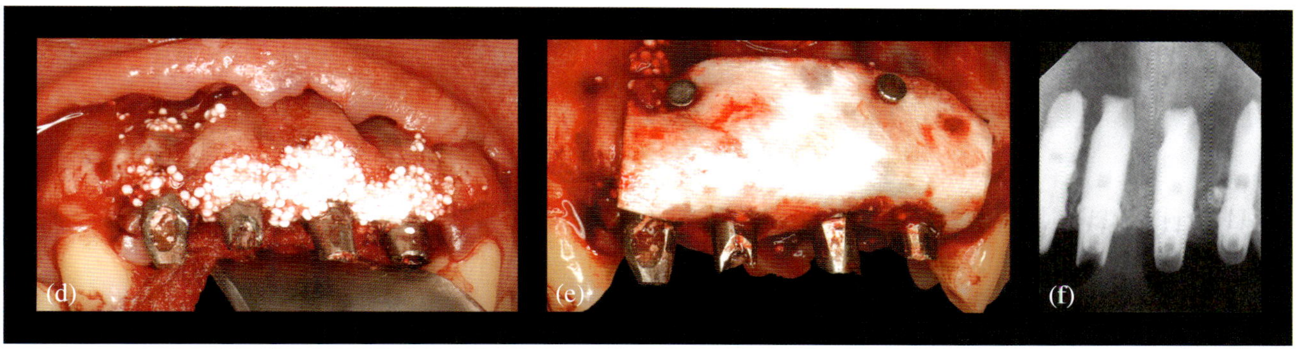

Figure 4.29 (d) The osseous defect is grafted with an osseoconductive grafting material. (e) Collagen membrane (Mem-Lock, BioHorizons, Birmingham, AL, USA) is used and stabilized with membrane tacs (Auto Tac, BioHorizons, Birmingham, AL, USA). (f) Post-grafting radiographic view.

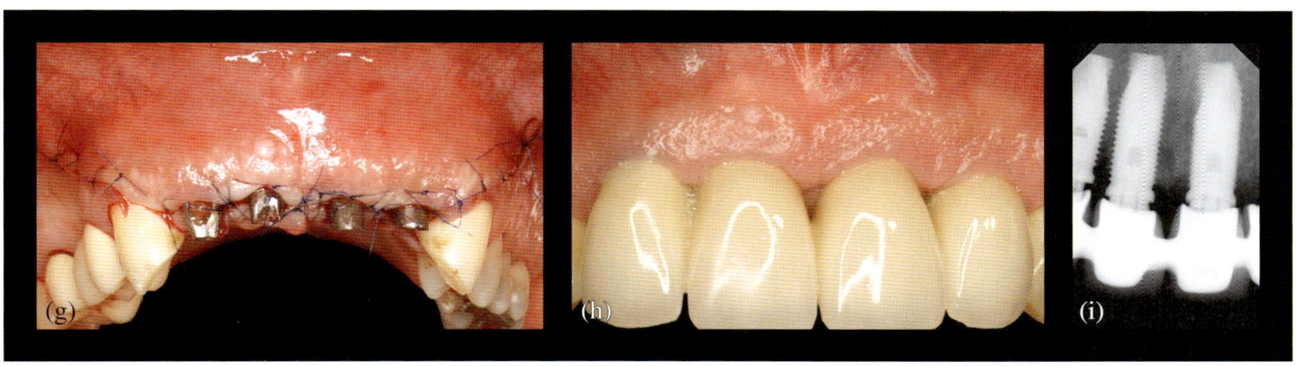

Figure 4.29 (g) Flap sutured. (h) Three months after the final restoration showing reduced pocket width and normal soft tissue architecture. (i) Ten years follow-up periapical view showing intact bone crest level.

raised, the apical granulation tissue was thoroughly cleaned out, and irrigated with sterile saline. Crespi et al. (2010) explained the high success rate of immediate implants in sockets with the presence of acute infections associated with anaerobic bacteria (*Fusobacterium, Prevotella, Porphyromonas, Actinomyces, Streptococcus, Peptostreptococcus*); they claimed that accurate socket debridement and lavage eradicated the associated endo-periodontal microbiota.

Both Lindeboom et al. (2006) and Siegenthaler et al. (2007) used preoperative antibiotics (clindamycin 600 mg, one hour before surgery), and Casap et al. (2007) recommended the preoperative use of a daily dose of 1.5 g of amoxicillin four days prior to surgery, maintaining the same dose for 10 days during the postoperative course.

Another study has indicated that the presence of periodontal pockets may serve as reservoirs for bacterial colonization around adjacent implants (Quirynen et al. 2005). The similarity in microbial flora responsible for aggressive periodontitis and peri-implantitis supports the concept that periodontal pathogens may be associated with peri-implant infections and failing implants (Valente and Andreana 2016) (see Figure 4.30a–c).

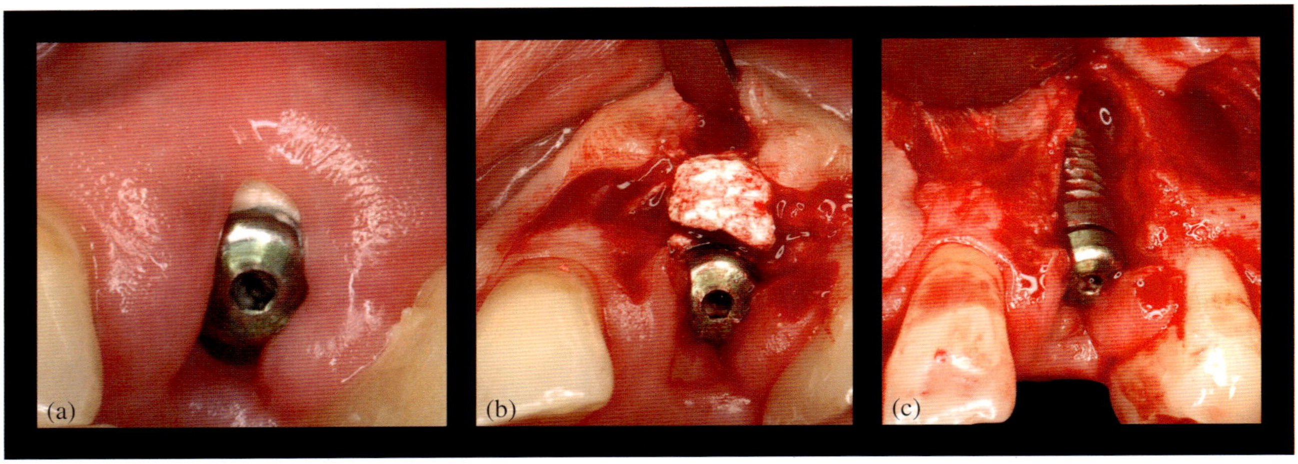

Figure 4.30 (a) Sign of soft tissue infection (marginal redness and swelling) three weeks after immediate implant placement. (b) Complete separation and deterioration of the grafting material (sequestration). (c) Socket lavage and implant surface decontamination revealing a labial osseous defect.

In a study by Crespi et al. (2010), 37 patients were included in which a total of 275 implants were placed and immediately loaded in extraction sockets, 197 implants in periodontally infected sites (infected sites group) and 78 implants in non-infected sites (non-infected sites group). Marginal bone levels and clinical parameters (plaque accumulation and bleeding index) were evaluated at baseline and 12, 24, and 48 months after implant placement. It was observed that at 48 months follow-up, the infected group presented a survival rate of 98.9%; the non-infected group reported a survival rate of 100%. The marginal bone level was 0.79 ± 0.38 mm for the infected group and 0.78 ± 0.38 mm for the non-infected group, plaque accumulation was 0.72 ± 0.41 for the infected group and 0.71 ± 0.38 for the non-infected group, and the bleeding index was 0.78 ± 0.23 for the infected group and 0.75 ± 0.39 for the non-infected group. No statistically significant differences were reported between the infected group and non-infected group over time and between time points. Therefore it was concluded that at 48 months follow-up, dental implants that were placed and immediately loaded in periodontally infected sockets showed no significant differences compared to implants placed in uninfected sites (see Figure 4.31a–c).

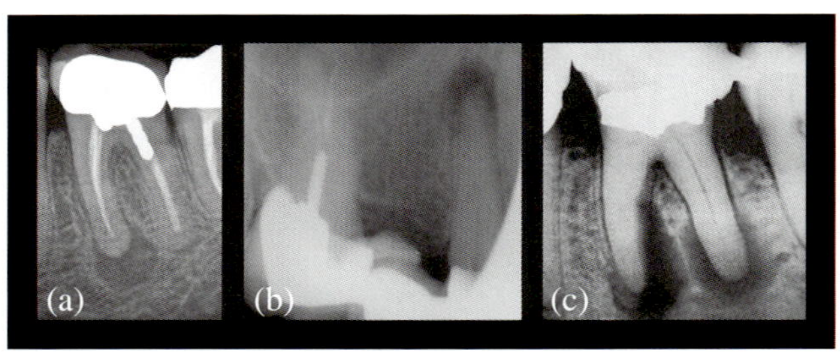

Figure 4.31 (a) Asymptomatic chronic lesion that is considered a low risk for implant placement. (b) Moderate risk pathological lesion for implant placement. (c) High risk pathological lesion that would jeopardize immediate implant placement.

Novaes et al. (2003) showed in a histomorphometric analysis, a mean bone–implant contact of 62.4% in the control group and 66.0% in the experimental group (induced periodontitis) in dogs, a difference that was not statistically significant. It was concluded that periodontally infected sites may not be a contraindication for immediate implantation in this animal model system, if adequate pre- and postoperative care is taken.

In contrast, Deng et al. (2010) evaluated the clinical performance of implant fixtures placed immediately after tooth extraction in patients with severe periodontitis. They concluded that there was a heightened risk of failure for immediate implants placed in a periodontally compromised site.

Marginal bone loss around implants in patients with generalized aggressive periodontitis as compared with implants in healthy patients or chronic periodontitis patients was not significantly greater in short-term studies but was significantly greater in long-term studies. In short-term studies, the success rates of implants were between 97.4 and 100% in patients with generalized aggressive periodontitis, and there were no significant differences for the implant success between the three groups except in one study that involved smokers and patients with systemic diseases (Mengel and Flores-de-Jacoby 2005). The survival rates of implants were between 83.3 and 96% in patients with generalized aggressive periodontitis in long-term studies (Kim and Hun-Mo Sung 2012). In conclusion immediate implant placement in patients with generalized aggressive periodontitis is not contraindicated provided that adequate preoperative infection control and an individualized maintenance program are assured (see Figure 4.32a–c).

An infection that compromises the labial plate of bone is infection of the bone graft material used for socket gap filling, whether composed of human or animal origin. As the use of bone graft material may induce microbial colonization that result in a biofilm, which may prove hard to eliminate (Costerton et al. 1999, 2005). Del Fabbro et al. (2009) reported an infection associated with a mineralized bone allograft, while Crespi et al. (2007) reported an infection of autogenous bone chips. A prospective study evaluating the healing of marginal defects in immediate transmucosal implants grafted with bovine bone matrix was performed. Thirty implants in the esthetic zone were analyzed for 30 patients who had randomly received Bio-Oss (n = 10), Bio-Oss and resorbable collagen membrane (n = 10), or no graft as a control group (n = 10). No significant differences were found for vertical defects, although horizontal resorption was significantly greater in the control group (Chen et al. 2007).

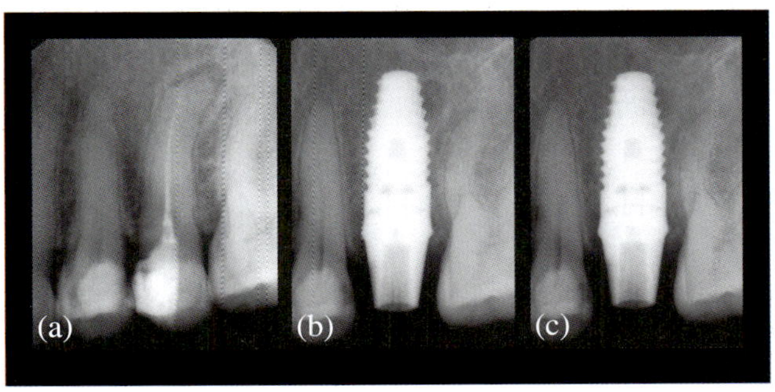

Figure 4.32 (a) Localized periapical infection (apical granuloma) with no intraoral symptoms. (b) An implant is placed after preoperative antibiotics are administered and intraoperative local curettage and debridement were made. (c) Three months after implant placement radiographic view showing complete healing of the osseous defect and resolution of infection.

4.3.3 Discussion

Further studies are needed to evaluate the clinical and histologic outcome of placing dental implants in periodontal or periapical infected sites. Further research should be directed toward the indication of antibiotic therapy prior to surgery (Álvarez-Camino, Valmaseda-Castellón and Gay-Escoda 2013). Most publications ignored the extent of the socket infection and did not supply information about the patient's current systemic condition. The degree/severity/type of infection, that is, acute, chronic diffuse, localized granulomatous, etc., has also not been accurately described. Further long-term studies specific to various other risk factors and other systemic or patient-related factors is needed to yield a definite protocol and its efficacy.

According to the author's suggestion, a risk assessment protocol has been formulated as a clinical guideline sets a level of risk for each category of socket related infection, which guides the clinician to verify any risks involved prior to the start of treatment (see Figure 4.33a–c) or to make a general view on the risk involved.

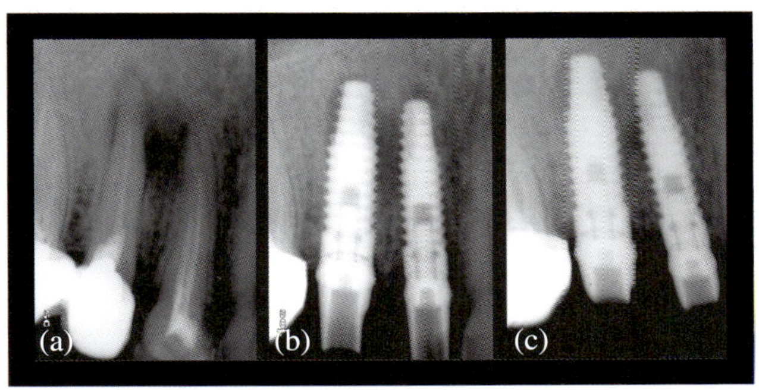

Figure 4.33 (a–c) *Medium* risk pathological lesions.

Class 1: All forms of asymptomatic apical pathology, asymptomatic apical periodontitis, granulomas and or apical cyst, pose no risk. A thorough debridement followed by an immediate implant placement under postoperative antibiotic coverage suffices for such situations (see Figure 4.34a–e).

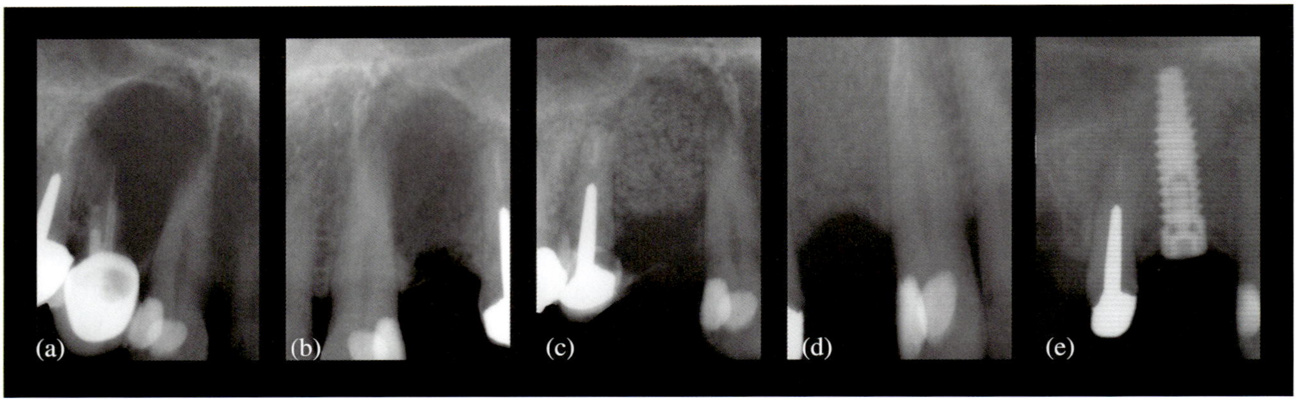

Figure 4.34 (a) Preoperative radiographic view of a huge radiolucent periapical lesion related to the first maxillary premolar. (b) Preoperative radiographic view after tooth extraction. (c) Pre-operative radiographic view of the grafted socket four weeks post extraction. (d) Preoperative radiographic view four months after grafting showing improved osseous architecture. (e) Preoperative radiographic view showing an implant fixture installed (Tapered Internal, BioHorizons, Birmingham, AL, USA).

Class 2: Non-suppurative periodontal pathology and symptomatic chronic disuse lesions presented with pain on percussion (see Figure 4.35a–c) present a moderate risk to placing immediate implants (see Figure 4.36a–f).

Treatment for such cases includes immediate implant placement under pre-and postoperative systemic antibiotics, accurate, and thorough socket debridement and lavage is mandatory.

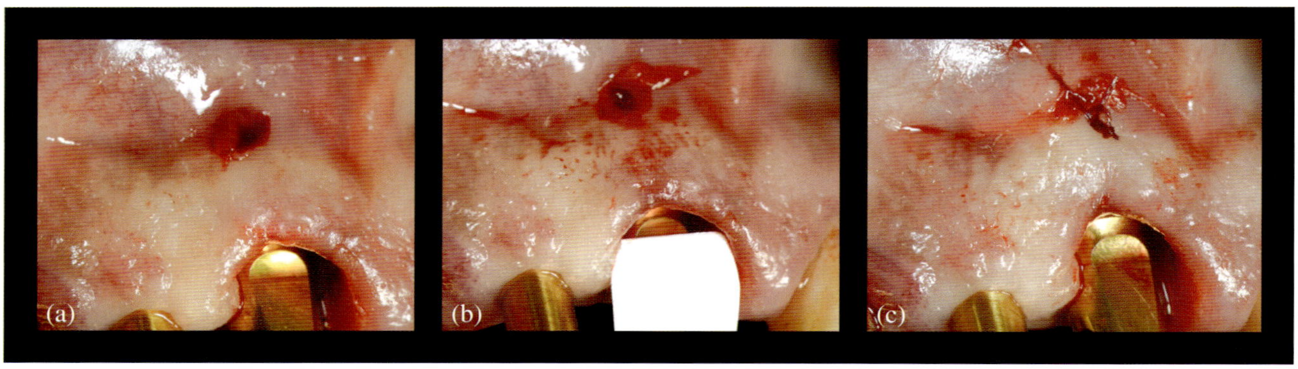

Figure 4.35 (a) De-epithialization of the fistulas tract. (b) Introduction of collagen membrane to isolate the fistula orifice from the socket environment. (c) *Fistula* orifice closure.

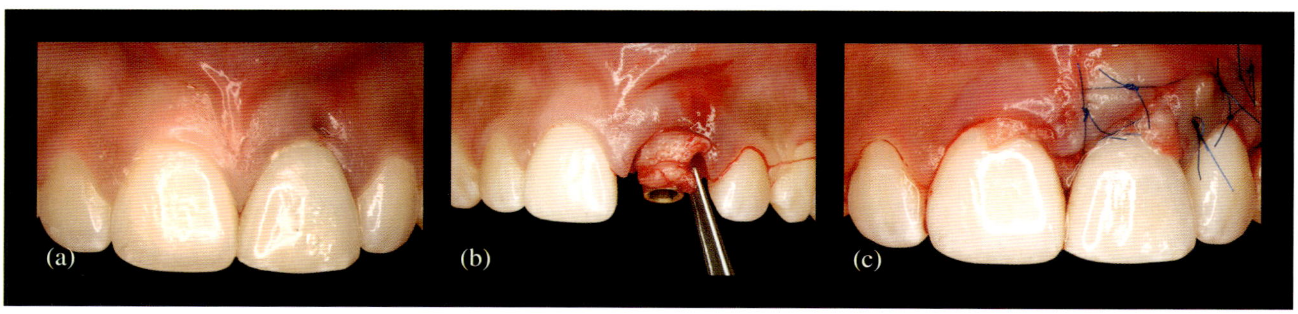

Figure 4.36 (a) Two weeks after implant insertion showing soft tissue defect in the place of the previous sinus tract. (b) Connective tissue graft is introduced underneath the flap. (c) Flap sutured and connective tissue graft stabilized.

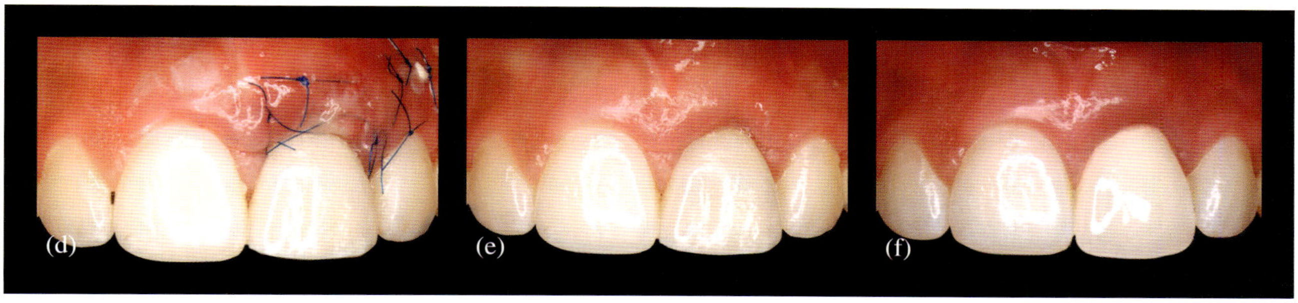

Figure 4.36 (d) One week post-surgery showing excellent healing condition and revascularization. (e) Clinical view four weeks post-surgery. (f) One year post-surgery.

Class 3: All forms of symptomatic apical periodontitis, presented with sinus tract and/or tenderness, or an acute periapical abscess with suppuration, swelling, and pain, fall under the high-risk category. A delayed implant placement protocol might be undertaken; it involves tooth extraction, thorough debridement, antibiotic regimen, a sufficient healing period, and an implant installation. Although this staged approach took more time and an additional surgical procedure, it allowed for a more predictable functional and esthetic reconstruction (Moghadam 2009; Rabelo et al. 2010).

4.4 Socket Preservation Therapy

Socket preservation is an intervention completed at the time of dental extraction that is claimed to preserve socket walls and osseous anatomy of the extraction site, and the future implant site (Iasella et al. 2003; Lekovic et al. 1998). Tan-Chu et al. (2014) described the application of socket preservation therapy, which entails using collagen membrane contoured into a modified V-shape. The membrane should be strong so that it can be sutured and maintain a long absorption time to allow for guided bone regeneration. The membrane must also be firm enough to allow insertion into the socket without collapsing. An absorbable collagen membrane that can be sutured without tearing may be used. The narrow part of the trimmed membrane (i.e. a V-shaped cone) is placed into the socket and should be wide enough to extend laterally past the defect in the buccal wall, while keeping in mind that placing the membrane on the external aspect of the buccal wall may compromise its blood supply and cause an increased chance of resorption. The wider part of the membrane should be trimmed to cover the opening of the socket following graft placement. Following final shaping, the membrane is positioned into the socket lining the buccal tissues. The socket is then filled with a bone graft; pressure from the graft against the membrane will help keep it in place and push out the contour of the buccal tissue. Ideally, the graft material should be compressed into the socket and remain in place. The graft material recommended for this technique is a small-particle, mineralized cancellous freeze-dried bone allograft (FDBA) (i.e. 0.25–1 mm). This graft material should be hydrated for five minutes and retain enough moisture for the particles to aggregate when inserted. An allograft material compresses well and, because it is mineralized, slowly resorbs. After the graft is compressed, the top part of the membrane is extended over the opening of the socket. The membrane is then sutured with absorbable sutures to the palatal tissue. No sutures are needed on the buccal aspect because the membrane is kept in place by the pressure from the graft against the buccal tissue (see Figure 4.37a–d).

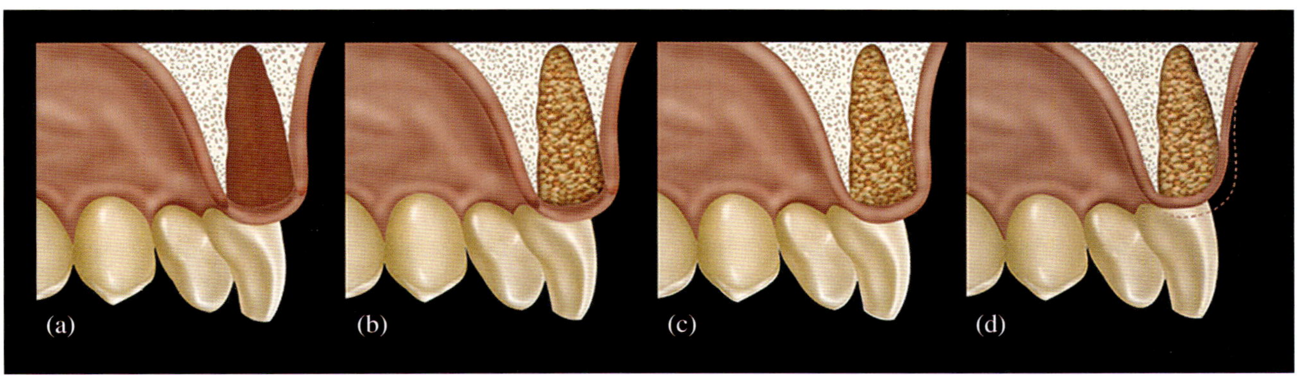

Figure 4.37 (a–d) Resorption of the alveolar plate of bone continues immediately after tooth extraction regardless of the socket filler placement, which makes the socket preservation therapy limited to only filling a socket gap not preventing the labial plate of bone remodeling.

Buser et al. (1990) reported successful ridge augmentation with GBR in humans using an e-PTFE membrane and tenting pins. He described 12 patients who received alveolar ridge augmentation prior to dental implant placement. Surgical protocol involved reflection of a mucoperiosteal flap, and perforations of the cortical plate within the defect using a round bur to increase blood supply to the graft. Titanium mini screws placed within the defect helped to provide tenting support to the overlying e-PTFE membrane. Following 6–10 months of healing, the authors demonstrated an increase in bone volume sufficient to allow placement of dental implants in 9 of the 12 sites. The gain in new bone formation ranged from 1.5 to 5.5 mm. The authors concluded that the biologic principle of osteopromotion by exclusion was highly predictable for ridge enlargement or defect regeneration.

Lekovic et al. (1998) compared the outcome of ridge augmentation with or without absorbable barrier membranes. They observed lesser crestal bone loss (−0.38 versus −1.50 mm) in the membrane group and more internal socket fill (−5.81 versus. −3.94 mm) and less horizontal ridge resorption (−1.31 versus −4.56 mm). Iasella et al. (2003) combined the use of tetracycline hydrated FDBA and a collagen membrane. After a six month healing period they reported an average of a 1.3 mm ridge height gain in the preserved group, against a 1 mm crestal loss in the control group.

Shapoff et al. (1980) studied the particle size of FDBA for hard tissue grafting around teeth and reported that 100–300 μm was the ideal particle size that would allow the bone particles to remain at the grafted site for a sufficient length of time while optimizing vascularization. Particles that are too small (<125 μm) provoke a macrophage reaction and are resorbed too quickly, with little to no bone formation. Particles that are too large may restrict interparticle space for vascularization and may be sequestered.

Zaner and Yukna (1984) also studied the particle sizes of autogenous bone obtained by different collection methods and FDBA. They found that the bone blend had the smallest and most uniform particle size (21 μm × 105 μm), osseous coagulum and FDBA had particle sizes of 300–500 μm, and chiseled bone chips had the largest and least uniform particle size (789 μm × 1559 μm). In addition, they suggested that the most appropriate graft particles size was 380 μm.

Wood and Mealey (2012) conducted a study of 40 extraction sockets divided into two groups. Either DFDBA or FDBA was randomly selected and grafted in the extraction sockets. Histologic samples were obtained at four–five months post-grafting during implant placement. There were no significant differences when comparing changes in alveolar ridge dimensions of the two groups. DFDBA had a significantly greater percentage of vital bone at 38.42% versus FDBA at 24.63%. The DFDBA group also had a significantly lower mean percentage of residual graft particles at 8.88% compared to FDBA at 25.42%.

Hoang and Mealey (2012) evaluated the use of DFDBA bone putty with different particle sizes. Particle sizes ranging from 125 to 710 μm had a mean of 49% vital bone, 8% residual graft, and 43% CT. The other group (particle sizes ranging from 125 to 710 μm in addition to 2–4 mm particles in putty) had 53%, 5%, and 42%, respectively. Patients in both groups lost a mean of <1 mm alveolar height on the buccal and lingual aspects and <1.5 mm of total ridge width. There were no statistically significant differences between the two groups for any clinical or histologic parameters.

Authors concluded that the placement of a biomaterial in an extraction socket may modify bone remodeling rate following tooth removal (Araujo and Lindhe 2009). A human study using 25 patients compared placing Bio-Oss collagen® (Geistlich Pharma AG, Wolhusen, Switzerland) into intact extraction sockets versus controls (clot only) in 39 sites. Their results after 12 weeks showed that new bone formation in augmented sites (test) was only 25% compared to non-augmented sites (control) of 44% (Eskow 2013).

A study was conducted that evaluated extraction sockets grafted with decalcified bovine bone mineral (DBBM) at nine months. The authors noted that it was present uniformly throughout the socket and averaged an overall 30% residual graft (Artzi, Tal and Dayan 2000). One year later, while DBBM still remained in the socket at nine months, no connective tissue was in contact with the graft, thus allowing the authors to claim that DBBM is a biocompatible socket filler that can be used in ridge preservation procedures (Artzi et al. 2000). Another study found that DBBM was a favorable graft for ridge preservation, compared DBBM to irradiated cancellous allograft (ICA), and to solvent-dehydrated allograft (SDA) when used to preserve extraction sockets (Lee et al. 2009). Very few particles were in contact with stromal connective tissue, suggesting no evidence of fibrous encapsulation (Lee et al. 2009).

Froum et al. (2002) evaluated extraction sockets that had buccal defects and there was no attempt to gain primary closure when grafted with hydroxyapatite (HA) and noted approximately 31% vital bone present at six to eight months. In that same study, bovine bone yielded an average of 29.75% vital bone.

An alternate material may be sponges made of collagen or polylactic/polyglycolic acid. Serino et al. (2003) conducted studies with Fisiograft® (GHIMAS S.p. A, Bologna, Italy), a synthetic co-polymer composed of polylactic and polyglycolic acids, used as a space filler during ridge preservation. At six months, the implants were placed and core biopsies obtained for histological analysis. Ridge dimensions were not significantly different between any of the groups. Histologically the test sites revealed new bone that was mineralized and well structured. No residual graft material was detected in the extraction sites. Five years later, the same clinical trial was repeated with the exception of not waiting six months to place the implant. In this study they re-entered the grafted sites and controls at three months. Histological analysis revealed that the grafted sites had healed with mineralized, well-organized bone with no residual graft particles (Serino et al. 2003).

Then comes a technique described by Sclar (1999), called the Bio-Col technique, involving the placement of DBBM particles in the extraction socket which is then covered with a collagen plug or a membrane sutured into place. Results yielded an adequate ridge preservation that allowed implant placement (Sclar 1999). On average a reduction of 0.15 ± 1.76 mm in height and 1.31 ± 0.96 mm in width was seen for the test sites and for controls a 0.56 ± 1.04 mm reduction in height and a 1.43 ± 1.05 mm reduction in width were observed, though the difference in height was significant. Histology revealed that mean bone density was significantly superior in the test group (TG) (2.08 ± 0.65 versus 3.33 ± 0.65). Histomorphometric analyses revealed similar percentages of bone vitality (test: 29.92% ± 8.46%; control: 36.54% ± 7.73%). Comparable percentages of bone marrow and fibrous tissue were also were observed (test: 65.25% ± 6.41%; control: 62.67% ± 7.41%). Only 6.25% of the Putty P15 particles remained at four months in the analyzed biopsies (Neiva et al. 2008).

Iasella et al. (2003) performed a six-month randomized, controlled, blinded clinical study to establish whether ridge preservation would prevent post extraction alveolar ridge resorption changes, assessed by clinical and histologic parameters. The width of the FDBA and collagen membrane group decreased from 9.2 to 8.0 mm, while the width of the control group decreased from 9.1 to 6.4 mm, a difference of 1.6 mm.

Lindeboom et al. (2006) carried out a prospective randomized trial on 50 patient with 50 implants followed up for one year. Patients with a tooth demonstrating radiographic signs of chronic apical periodontitis were randomized into two groups (n = 25 each): (1) Immediate placement (IP) and (2) delayed placement (DP), three months post extraction. Primary stability at the time of implant placement was an inclusion criterion for the study. In the IP group, implants were placed following thorough degranulation of the socket, and bone augmentation utilizing ground corticocancellous bone harvested from the trigonum retro molar or chin regions was performed to cover the buccal surface and implant. A bioresorbable collagen membrane (Bio-Gide) was placed to cover the graft and implant. In the DP group, implant placement was carried out after 12 weeks of healing. All implants were submerged and allowed to heal without loading for six months. Implant success criteria included: no clinical implant mobility at second-stage surgical procedures or follow-up evaluations, no radiographic evidence of peri-implant radiolucency, no signs or symptoms of infection, and no bone loss in excess of the bone loss criteria reported by Albrektsson et al. (2012). Thirty-two implants were placed in the anterior maxilla and 18 implants in the premolar region. Every patient required augmentation of the buccal bone (autograft) at the time of implant placement. Cumulative implant success rates after six months were 92% in the IP group and 100% in the DP group. At the one-year follow-up, all implants remained in function.

A study by Eskow (2013) compared the use of cortical versus cancellous FDBA from a single donor in ridge preservation; 38 patients were enrolled in the study and histologic analysis was performed on 33 cores obtained at 18 weeks following extraction. The histology showed more residual graft material present in the cortical samples and only 13–16% new bone formation, respectively, for cancellous and cortical FDBA at 18 weeks. The dimensional ridge changes for both materials were similar and both showed a loss of ridge height and width, with the cortical FDBA preserving more lingual/palatal ridge height than the cancellous FDBA. In 11 of 35 patients, the residual ridge at implant placement required additional bone grafting on the buccal aspect due to thin remaining bone or dehiscence, thus confirming other studies showing that ridge preservation techniques will improve the outcome for site preparation for implants with some loss of bone still expected (Ten Heggeler et al. 2011).

Attempting to graft fresh extraction sites with any grafting material will not preserve the labial plate of bone. While grafting materials usually take 3-6 months to mature and form viable bone, the labial plate of bone undergoes a fast resorption process that may take as little as 40 days in thin plates. Thus, socket preservation therapy should be only used to fill an empty socket until the socket environment is ready for implant placement, as often socket preservation therapy may be an additional surgical procedure that provides no great clinical benefit and adds cost to the patient, and increase the duration of the overall treatment plan. The artificial bone, irrespective of the origin, fails to support the buccal plates of bone from the physiologic resorption perspective. It is the author's recommendation that whenever there is a opportunity for implant fixture primary stability in damaged sockets (minimum of 3 mm apically), a non-staged approach is advised, along with the preferred method of bone grafting, which would help minimize alveolar bone remodeling and support the surrounding soft tissues. The non-staged approach stabilizes the interproximal papillae and adjacent labial soft tissues. The only indication for implementing socket preservation therapy would be when implant installation is not achievable for any valid clinical reason.

4.5 Novel Concepts to Treat Defective Labial Plate of Bone

A number of classifications have been proposed in the literature to classify socket types, including a simplified popular classification proposed by Elian et al. (2007). This classification allows easier documentation and better communication between clinicians, researchers, and authors. The classification is divided into three socket types: (1) type I socket: the facial soft tissue and buccal plate of bone are at normal levels in relation to the cementoenamel junction of the pre-extracted tooth and remain intact post extraction; (2) type II socket: the facial soft tissue is present but the buccal plate is partially missing following extraction of the tooth; and (3) type III socket: the facial soft tissue and the buccal plate of bone are both markedly reduced after tooth extraction (see Figures 4.38, 4.39, 4.40 and 4.41a–c).

Type I sockets offers the easiest and most predictable treatment outcome, when tissue phenotype is favorable (Kan et al. 2003). Type III sockets, are very difficult to treat and require a combined sophisticated soft tissue and hard tissue augmentation. As shown in Figure 4.42a–c type II sockets are oftentimes the most difficult to diagnose. These sockets can be very deceptive, and can be confused with type I sockets and as a result post-treatment soft tissue recession may occur. Managing type III sockets conditions requires a high level of experience, skills, and patient compliance.

There are versatile socket defects which involve several osseous defects that are different in nature, as well different soft tissue conditions related to the alveolar socket; on another hand, there are numerous available bone grafting materials, techniques each has it regenerative capacity and terms of use. The clinician should choose the best possible technique that offers the fastest recovery, less trauma, and minimal tissue morbidity along with the best treatment predictability. Selecting the technique will depend on the operators skills, the availability of the regenerative material, the type of the bone defect, the need for soft tissue grafting, the patient's compliance, the condition of the adjacent teeth, the level of the patient's oral hygiene, the patient's habits (e.g. smoking and alcohol intake), and any pre-existing socket pathology. Several methods are described later to treat defective soft tissue conditions (see Figure 4.43a and b).

4.5.1 Block Autografts

Intramembranous autogenous osseous grafts, including the mandibular ramus, mandibular symphysis, angle of mandible, maxillary tuberosity, and intraoral exostoses, are called the "gold standard" for improving intraoral osseous volume to facilitate the placement of implants (Chiapasco et al. 1999). Alveolar defects can be restored by many forms of autologous grafts including cortico-cancellous blocks, compressed particulate cancellous bone and marrow chips, cancellous chips, and mono-cortical grafts; each form has its indication. For example, cortico-cancellous blocks can be used to treat large osseous defects; however micro-titanium screws are required for fixation, the patient must accept having a donor site surgery, and the clinician must have the skills required to perform such procedures, and the cortico-cancellous graft has a higher resorption rate that can reach up to 40% of its size, which explains that it should be oversized (Bahat and Handelsman 1996). A mono-cortical graft can be used as a scaffold because it lacks a blood supply, and

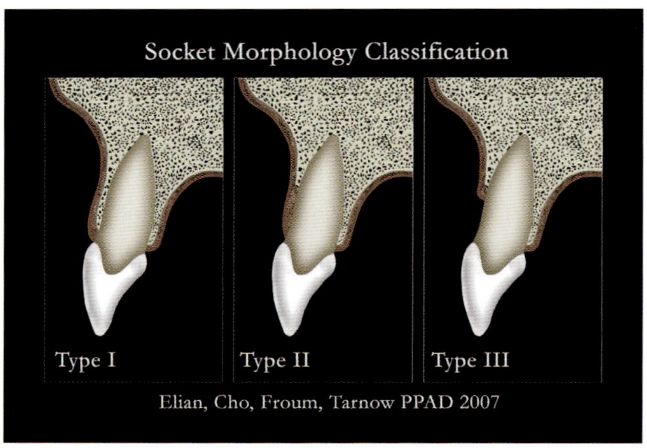

Figure 4.38 Socket morphology classification.

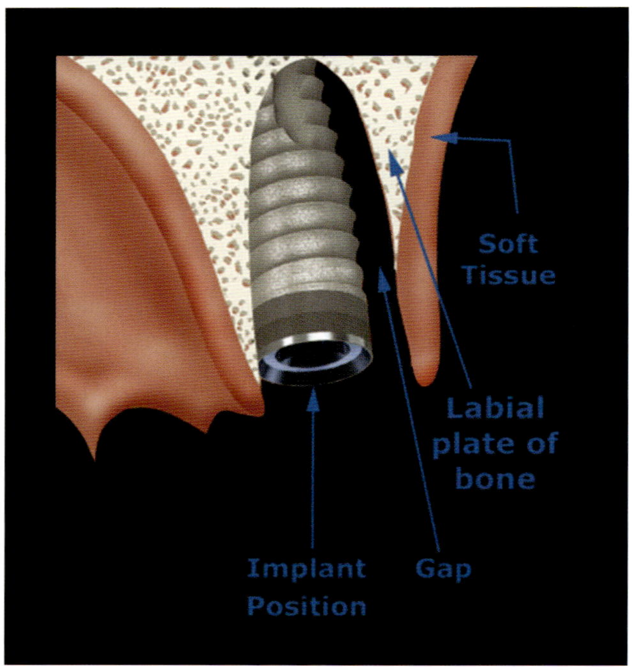

Figure 4.39 Influential elements affecting immediate implant placement therapy.

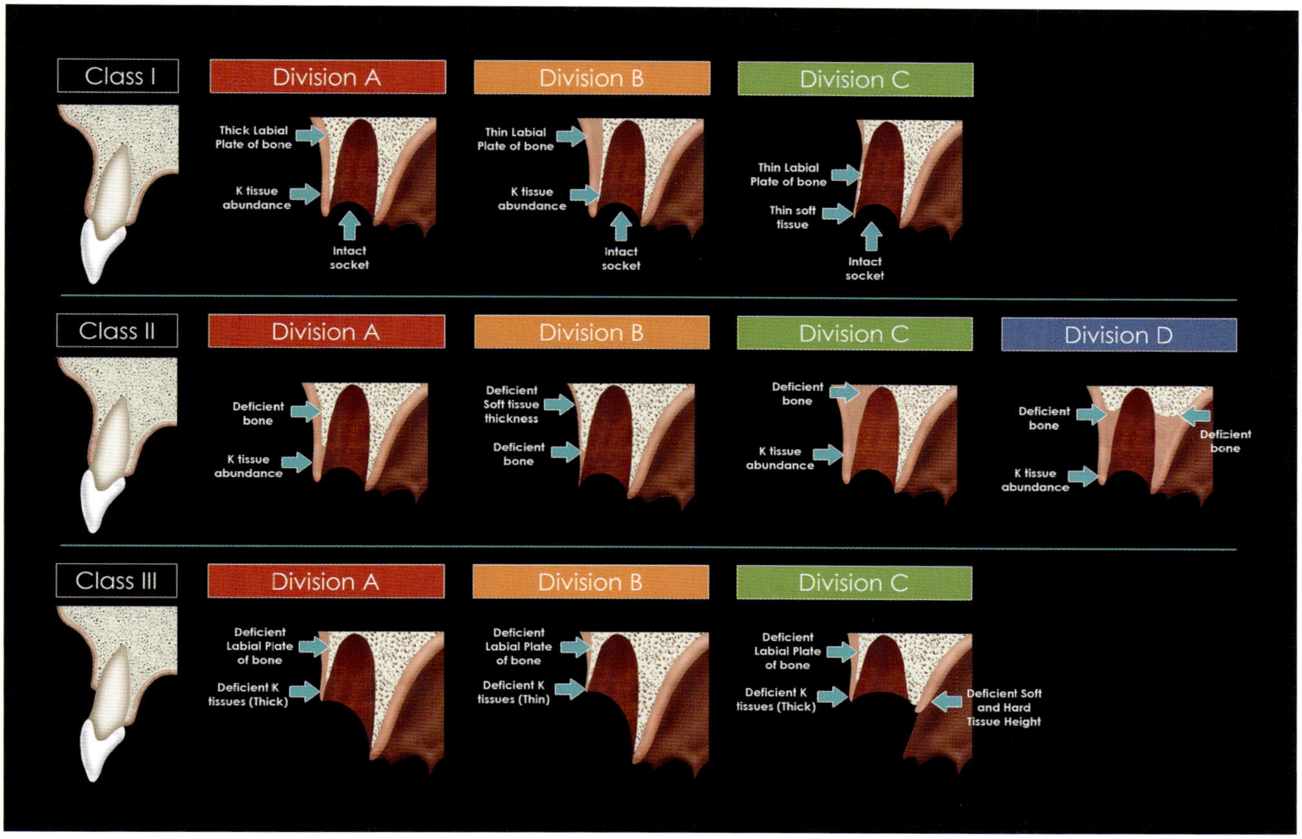

Figure 4.40 A new classification system developed by the author that details the different clinical situations of the labial plate of bone (soft and hard tissue conditions), Class I intact labial plate of bone, Class II thin labial plate of bone with intact soft tissue (thick), Class III fenestrated labial plate of bone with intact soft tissue, Class IV thin fenestrated labial plate of bone with thin soft tissue, Class V mild labial plate of bone resorption (vertical 2 mm) with intact soft tissue, Class VI moderate labial plate of bone deficiency (2–4 mm vertically) with intact soft tissue, Class VII completely lost labial plate of bone, Class VIII Completely lost labial and palatal labial plate of bone, this novel classification system gives more details on the different clinical situation of the condition of the fresh extracted sites (that is confirmed by both clinical and radiographic assessment).

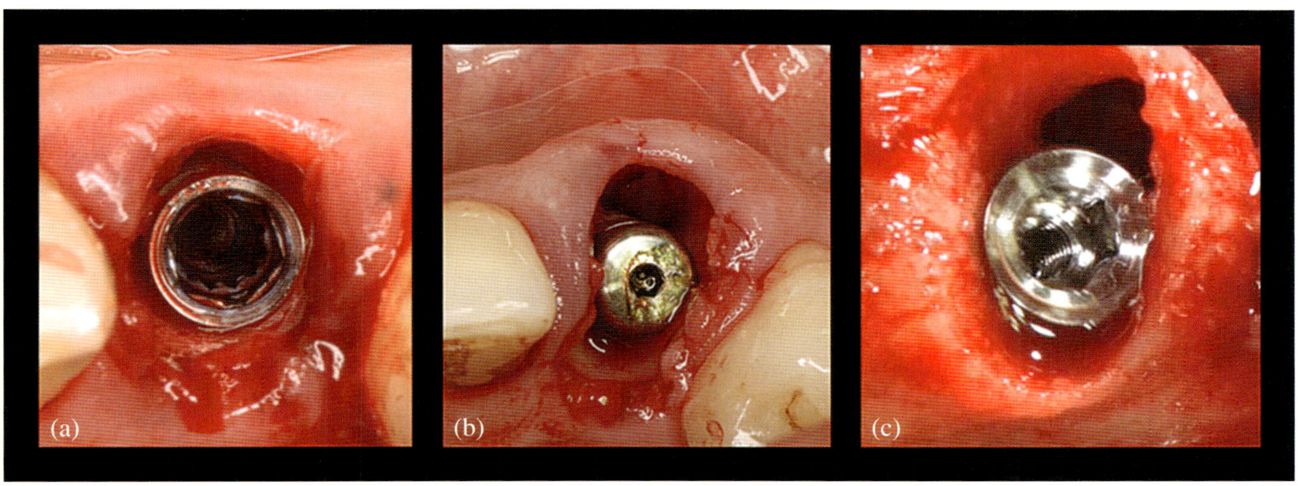

Figure 4.41 (a) Class I socket gap. (b) Class II socket gap. (c) Class III socket gap.

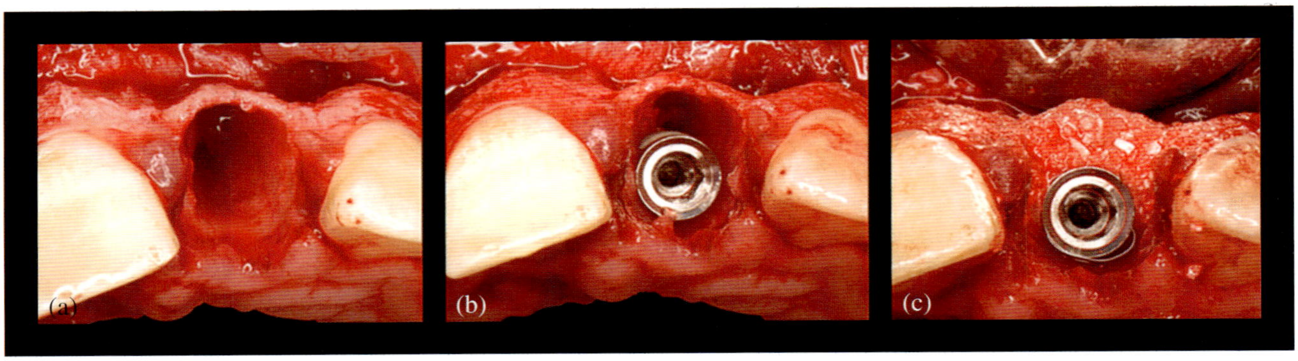

Figure 4.42 (a) Fresh extraction socket with thin labial wall. (b) Class III socket gap. (c) The gap is filled with particulated bone graft.

it can be placed to protect another autogenous graft underneath it to provide a viable bone. It is also easily broken when manipulated. However, the use of autogenous graft chips alone will not offer many advantages, because it should be mixed with synthetic or allograft bone supplement (Elaskary 2008) to minimize its resorption rate while adding an osteogenic boost to the particulate graft.

However, cortico-cancellous grafts do not usually require the use of an overlying membrane unless the dimensions of the graft are inadequate, but they take longer time to integrate.

4.5.2 Fitted Autogenous Bone Veneers

The need for an intact and sound labial bone plate is of paramount value, especially in the maxillary anterior region. In practice, the labial bone may not always be intact after tooth extraction. In such instances, the clinician has to decide if it is more appropriate to carry out ridge preservation and delay the implant placement.

When a there is a defective labial plate of bone, the classic surgical correction might entail the use of a block autograft to repair the missing labial plate of bone. However, block fixation of grafts requires more operating time spent in preparing the screw access holes, while the placement of the graft and securing it with the screws can be time consuming and requires high surgical skills. Furthermore, after the healing phase, some fixation screws may penetrate through the soft tissue, which mandates their removal later.

The author introduced a friction-fitted autograft veneer, using leverages on friction fitting the graft into the socket walls to secure the graft, and hence eliminating the need for fixation screws. This technique not only reduces the time needed to stabilize the block graft after healing but also avoids an additional step to remove the fixation screws. The method is indicated specially for class 2 socket type.

This technique is illustrated on Styrofoam™ models to show the steps involved in preparing the host bed and the block bone graft preparation (see Figure 4.43a–d).

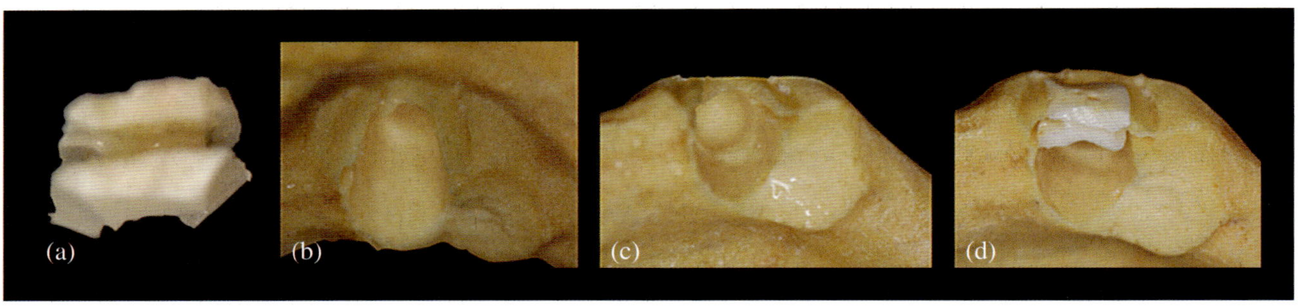

Figure 4.43 (a–d) The steps of autograft bone veneer preparationand placement on a Styrofoam model.

The labial proximal walls of the extraction socket (the recipient site) were indented from both sides to form two projections along the defect with a long shank fissure bur to receive the block graft. Then an autogenous cortico-cancellous graft of an average size is harvested from either the chin or the external oblique ridge that is similar to the defect size or a bit larger, then engraved from both sides with two slots on the sides to engage the lateral walls of the previously prepared socket wall projections. A CBCT evaluation was carried out at four and eight months after implant restorations. Eight partially edentulous patients, having a class 2 socket type or a moderate defect of the alveolar ridge were selected.

The criteria precluded patients with bad oral hygiene, patients who smoked, patients previously treated for chronic periodontitis, and patients systemically contraindicated to implant surgery. After a thorough preoperative examination, comprising a complete medical history, and clinical and radiographic examinations, a preoperative CBCT scan was carried out to assess the defect size. Each surgery was performed under local anesthesia (Articaine hydrochloride, Ubistesin™ forte, 3 M ESPE) of 40 mg mL^{-1}, with adrenaline, 1:80 000). After a sulcular incision, full mucoperiosteal flaps were raised on the facial aspect and the alveolar bone crest was curetted to remove all related soft tissues. The defect dimensions were measured to determine the approximate size of the block graft to be harvested (see Figure 4.44a–k). The donor sites for the block graft were from the chin area.

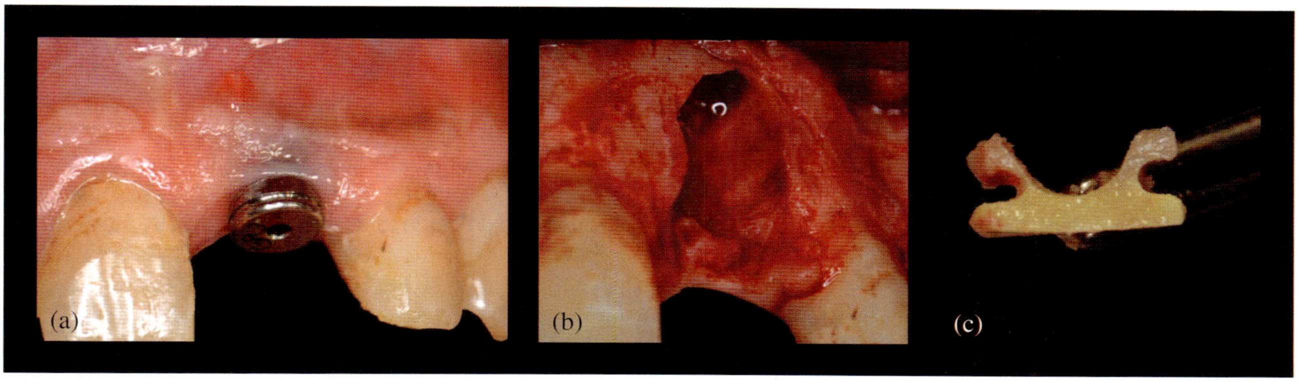

Figure 4.44 (a) Failed implant features fistulous tract with thinning of related soft tissue. (b) Implant removed, socket degranulated. (c) Autograft bone veneer is harvested and prepared.

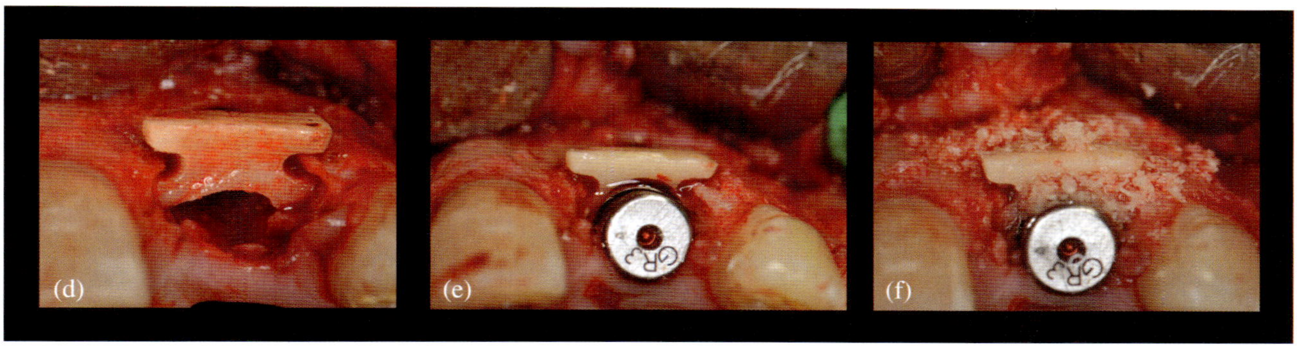

Figure 4.44 (d) Bone veneer is fitted in place. (e) Implant fixture (Laser-Lock, BioHorizons, Birmingham, AL, USA) is placed. (f) Voids are filled with allograft (Mineross, BioHorizons, Birmingham, AL, USA).

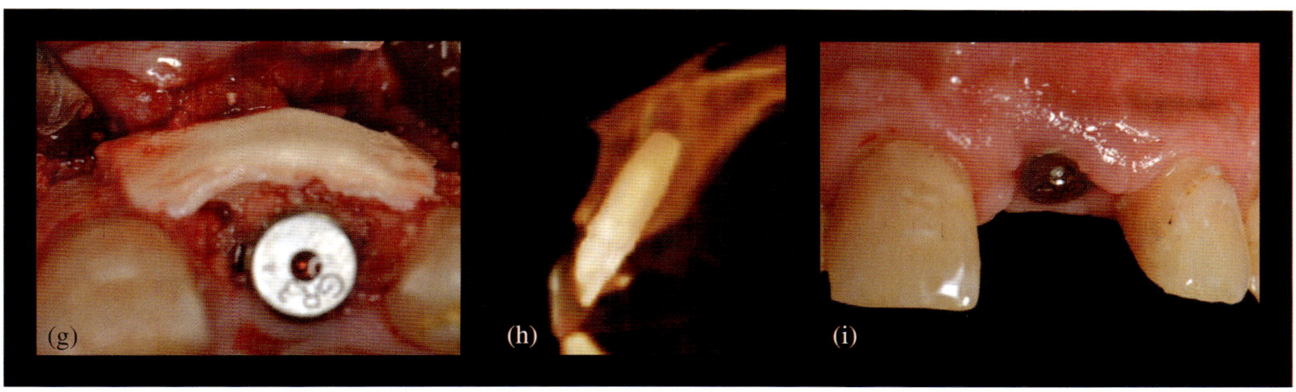

Figure 4.44 (g) A cellular dermal graft is placed to seal the graft from the overlying soft tissue pre-existingsinus tract (Alloderm, BioHorizons, Birmingham, AL, USA). (h) Four months postoperative CT scan showing complete maturation of the labial plate of bone. (i) Final healing occurred showing remarkable improvement of the keratinized tissue.

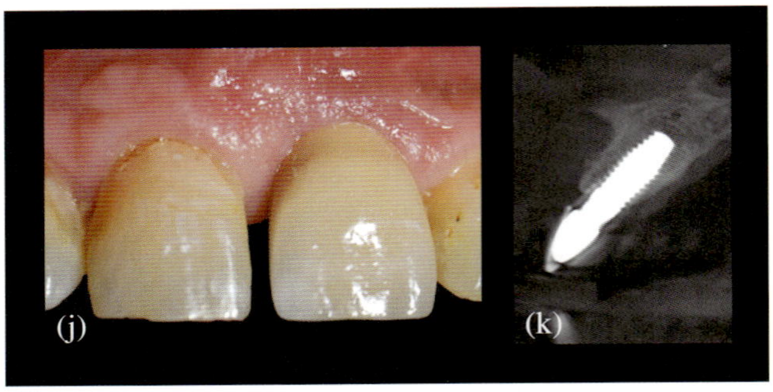

Figure 4.44 (j) Final case restored. (k) Six years follow up radiographic view showing an excellent bone formation and intact labial plate of bone.

The graft block is then harvested using piezoelectric surgery. The block is then sculpted along the sides of the graft using a 170-carbide bur (Mani, Inc., Japan) to acquire two proximal slots to engage and fit the lateral walls of the socket, thus stabilizing the graft in its place via snuggling friction, eliminating the use fixation screws (see Figure 4.45a–e).

Particulate bone graft (MinerOSS, BioHorizons, USA) mixed with autogenous bone chips were used to fill the voids between the grafts and the host bed. Acellular dermal grafts (AlloDerm, BioHorizons, USA) may be used to enhance soft tissue quality whenever needed (see Figure 4.46a–g).

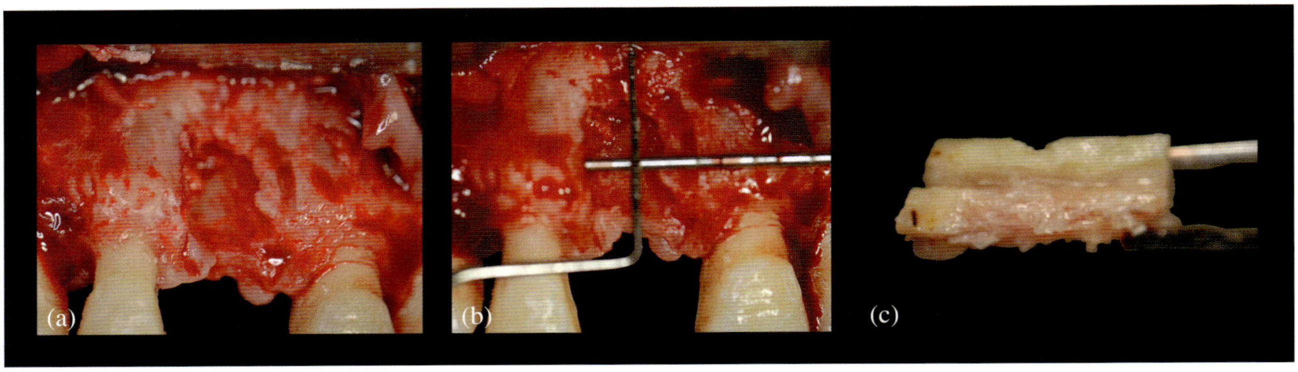

Figure 4.45 (a) Osseous bed is prepared. (b) Graft size is calculated. (c) Bone veneer is prepared.

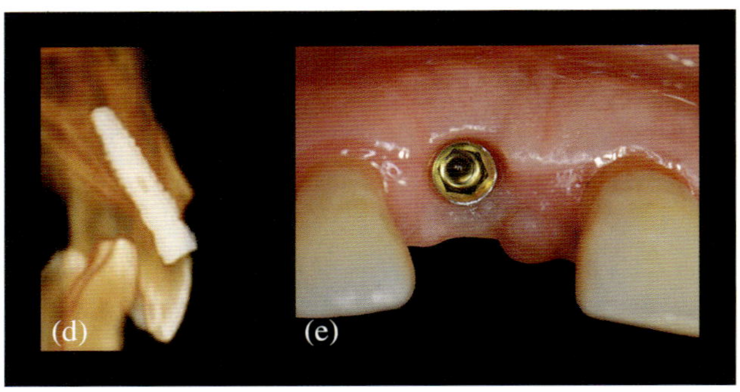

Figure 4.45 (d) Implant is positioned (Laser-Lock, BioHorizons, Birmingham, AL, USA), the bone veneer fitted in place showing in postoperative CBCT scan. (e) Three months after grafting showing complete integration of the graft and healed soft tissues ready for restorative phase.

The implants (Laser-Lok implants, BioHorizons, USA) were placed using a series of drills with increasing diameters under abundant irrigation using a sterile saline solution. Primary implant stability was achieved for all cases. Deep periosteal incisions were made to allow flap mobilization and tension-free primary wound closure. Flaps were closed with horizontal mattress sutures until the incisions were perfectly sealed.

Antibiotics were prescribed (Tavanic, Sanofi Aventis; 500 mg once daily for five days), together with Ibuprofen (Catafast, Novartis; 500 mg three times a day for three days) and antiseptic mouthwash (Listerine, Johnson & Johnson; 0.064% thymol, 0.092% eucalyptol, 0.060% methyl salicylate, 0.042% menthol) three times a day for seven days post-surgery. Sutures were removed seven days post-surgery. Clinical and radiographic follow-up examinations were performed at baseline and at four and eight months after rehabilitation. The success criteria were accepted as: (1) postoperative absence of bone graft exposure and infection; (2) incorporation of the graft into the receptor bed and increased bone volume of the labial plate of bone; (3) enhanced gingival contour with no recession; (4) absence of clinically detectable implant mobility, and (5) absence of exudate, persistent inflammation, patient discomfort, or radiolucency. After

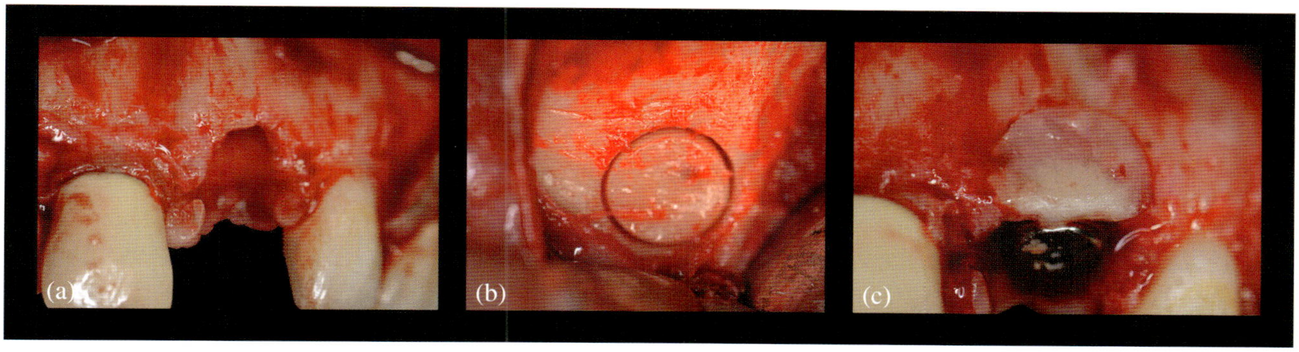

Figure 4.46 (a) Moderate labial plate of bone resorption related to the labial plate of bone. (b) Cortico-cancellous trephine core harvested from the chin. (c) Implant (Laser-Lock, BioHorizons, Birmingham, AL, USA) is placed.

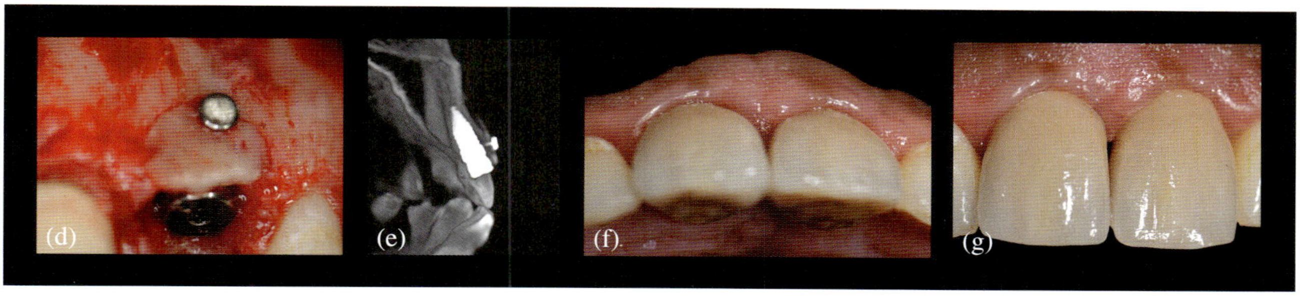

Figure 4.46 (d) Membrane tac is used to achieve further security of stabilization of the veneer graft (Auto Tac, BioHorizons, Birmingham, AL, USA). (e) CT view showing the restoration of the labial profile. (f) and (g) Final case restored showing complete restoration of the labial profile.

restoration of the implants, CBCT was used to measure the thickness of the labial bone at four and eight months postoperatively (see Figure 4.47a–p).

A dedicated software was used for all statistical analyses of the results. For clinical parameters and radiographic bone levels (mesial, distal, and mean bone loss), data were calculated for each implant and reported as the mean standard deviation (SD) at baseline and at four and eight months. To compare the differences between the test group and control group (CG) data at every time point, Student's two-tailed t test was adopted. $P < 0.05$ was considered the threshold for statistical significance. After eight months follow-up, a survival rate of 100% was reported for all implants. Integration of the graft into the receptor bed and increased bone volume were reported. More than half of the total cases were observed to have moderate to excellent bone gain. No clinically detectable implant mobility was detected, and no pain, mucositis, or flap dehiscences with suppuration were found.

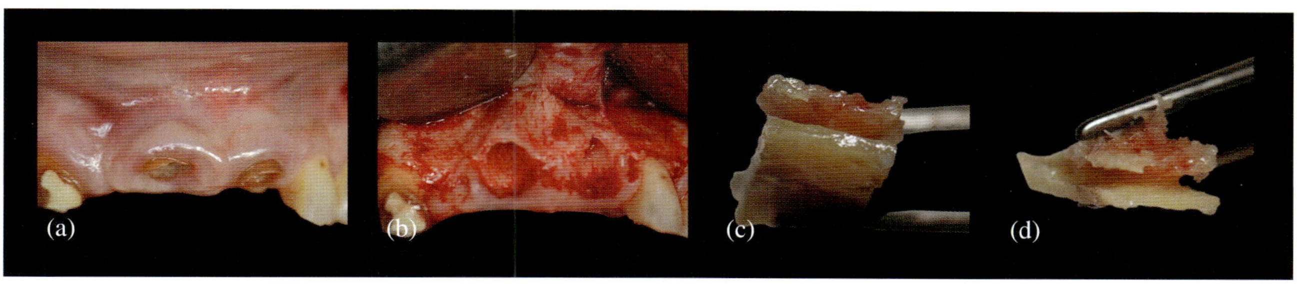

Figure 4.47 (a) Preoperative view of missing multiple anterior maxillary teeth. (b) Intra-operative view showing the thin fenestrated labial plate of bone. (c) and (d) Autogenous bone veneer is ready for use.

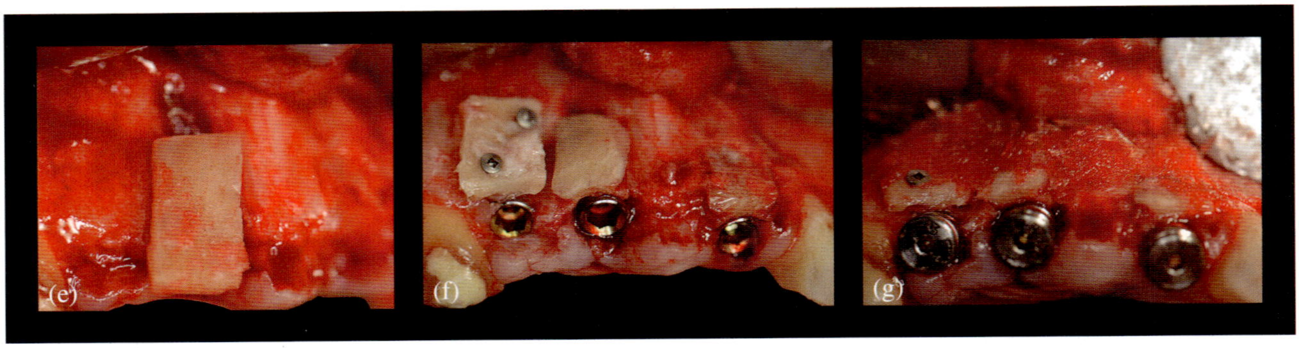

Figure 4.47 (e) Fraction fit of the lumineers in position. (f) Onlay monocortical graft is secured with two titanium screws (KLS Martin, GmbH, Tuttilngen, Germany) to autofitted blocks and placed in voids filled with bone allograft (Grfton, BioHorizons, Birmingham, AL, USA). (g) Incisal view showing the complete rehabilitation of the labial profile.

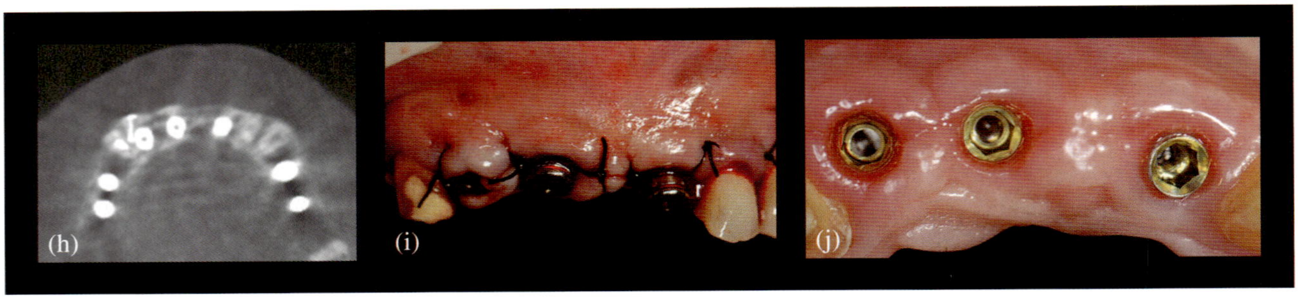

Figure 4.47 (h) CBCT view showing the complete restoration of the labial plate of bone. (i) Flap sutured. (j) Three months after healing abutment removal.

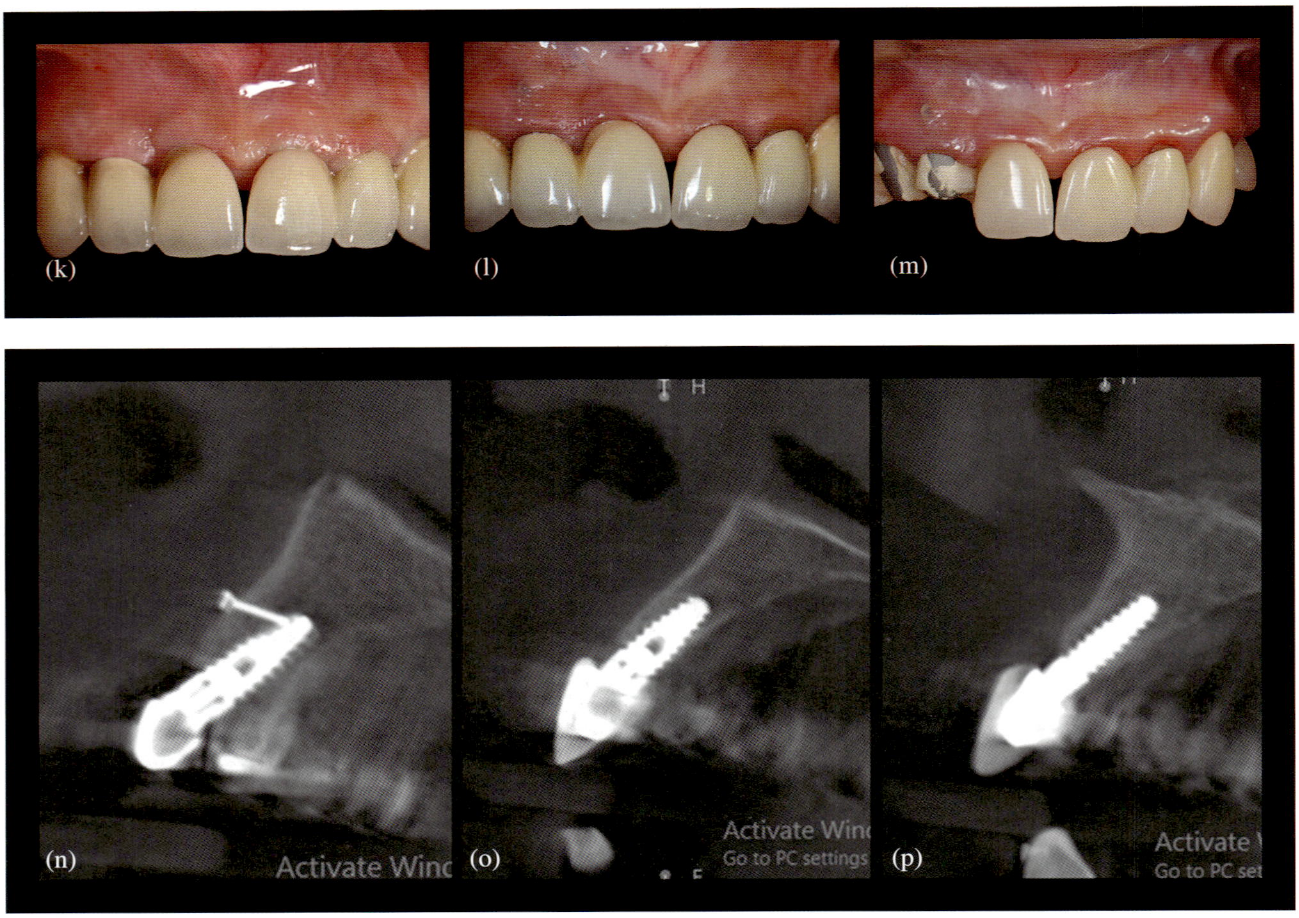

Figure 4.47 (k) Case finally restored. (l) Two years follow-up showing excellent tissue stability. (m–p) Six years follow-up, the patient showed up for fractured prosthesis; the clinical picture and CBCT images revealed excellent tissue stability and osseous architecture.

The CBCT follow-up concludes that the use of friction-fitted autogenous veneers offers practitioners an alternative way of graft fixation that is predictable, easy to carry out, and devoid of the woes contributed by fixation screws. The main benefit of this modality is that it restores exactly the defect size. Other cases with fitted autogenous bone veneers are depicted in series (see Figure 4.48a–j).

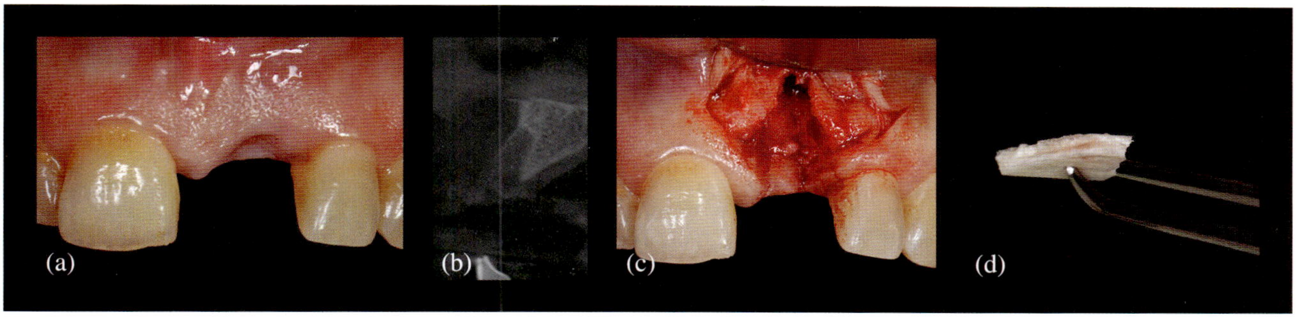

Figure 4.48 (a) Clinical picture of missing maxillary left central incisor. (b) CBCT showing lost and very thin remaining labial plate of bone that indicates doubling its thickness. (c) Intra-operative view showing the lost labial plate of bone. (d) The use of xenograft cortical sheet (2 mm thick) modified to act as a bone veneer, with two slots on the sides.

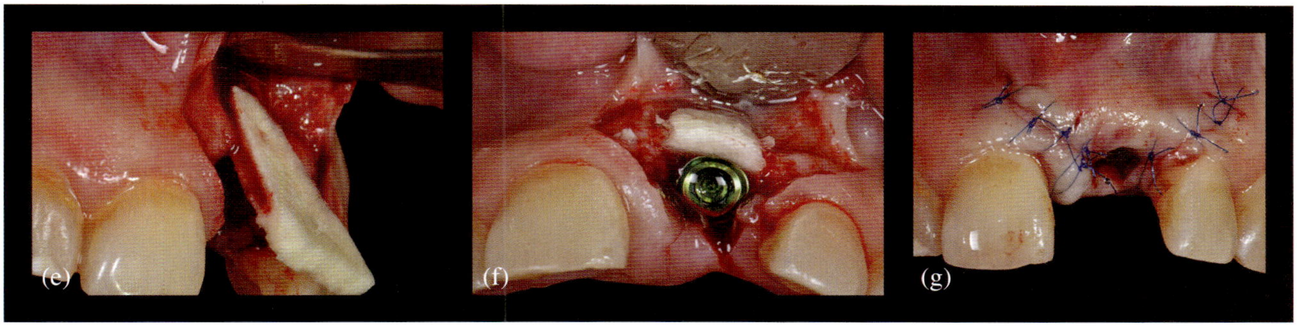

Figure 4.48 (e) The attempting positioning of the graft veneer. (f) The graft finally stabilized in place. (g) Flap closure.

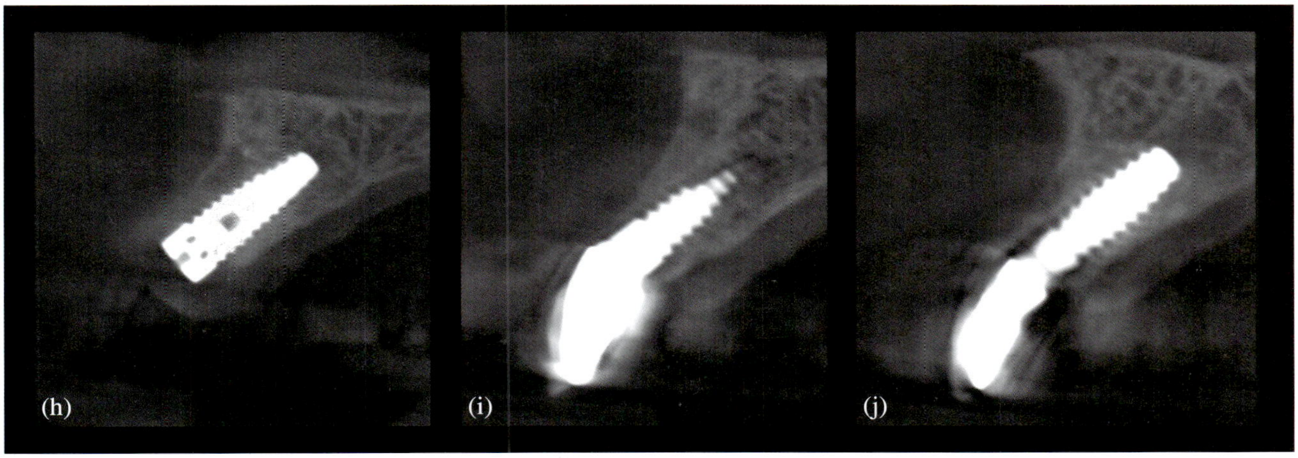

Figure 4.48 (h–j) CBCT of the patient at immediate postoperative, at two months and at four months time consecutively, showing the regenerated labial plate of bone.

4.5.3 Using Monocortical Allografts

Monocortical allografts can serve as a satisfactory allografting material alternative to autografts as it can be used in many clinical applications. However, it requires more attention to detail and meticulous handling to prevent the progression of complications to graft failures. In Acocella et al.'s (2012) study, 18 blocks were placed, and each patient received either 1 or 2 blocks. During the sampling procedures, all the grafts were found to be firm in consistency, well-incorporated, and vascularized. A total of 34 implants were placed into the grafts with a minimum of 40-N cm torque in all cases. The follow-up period ranged from 18 to 30 months. No implants were lost. The histological analysis revealed vital bone with mature and compact osseous tissue surrounded by marrow spaces. They have concluded that it can be used safely in areas of implant placement as a suitable alternative to autogenous grafts. The advantage of using allograft sheets is to avoid harvesting from the donor site, thus reducing the possibility of donor site morbidity (see Figures 4.49a–z and 4.50a–u).

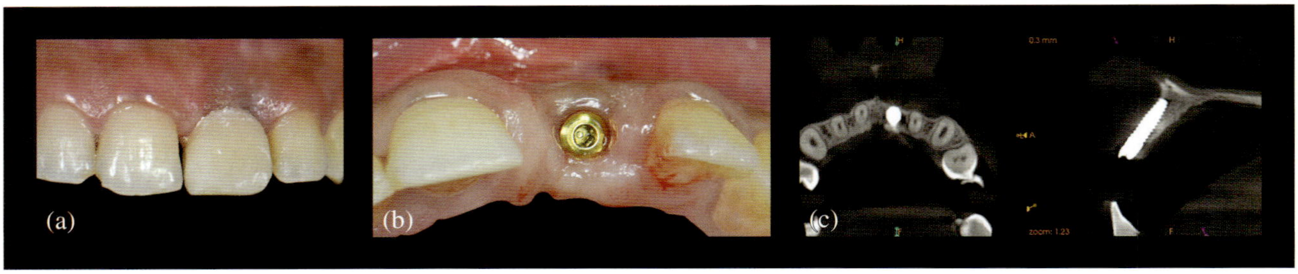

Figure 4.49 (a) and (b) Frontal and incisal clinical views showing poorly made provisional restoration that reveals the implant fixture grayish shade beneath the gingiva, along with dropped facial contour. (c) CBCT view showing complete loss of the labial plate of bone.

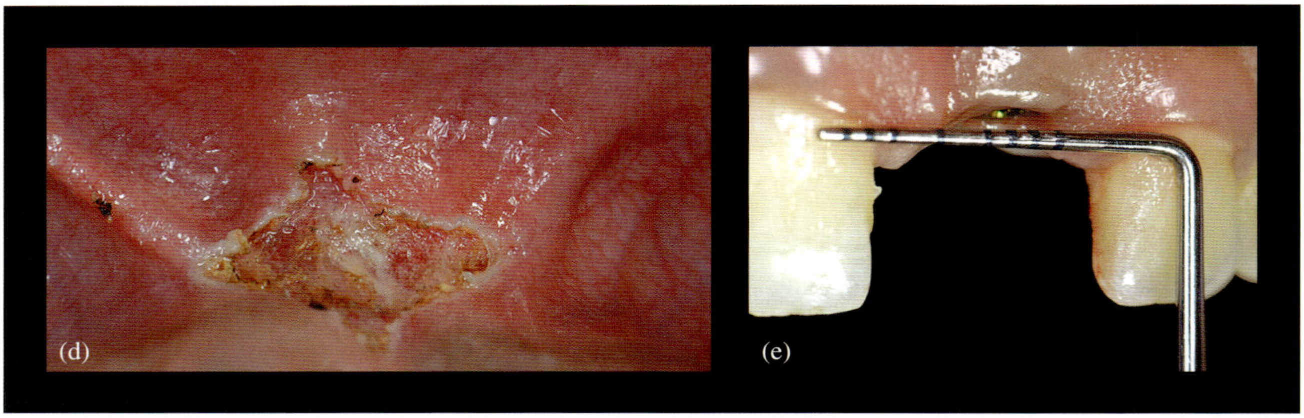

Figure 4.49 (d) Frenectomy is made to release muscular activity at the site. (e) Preoperative view showing the too far incisal position implant fixture.

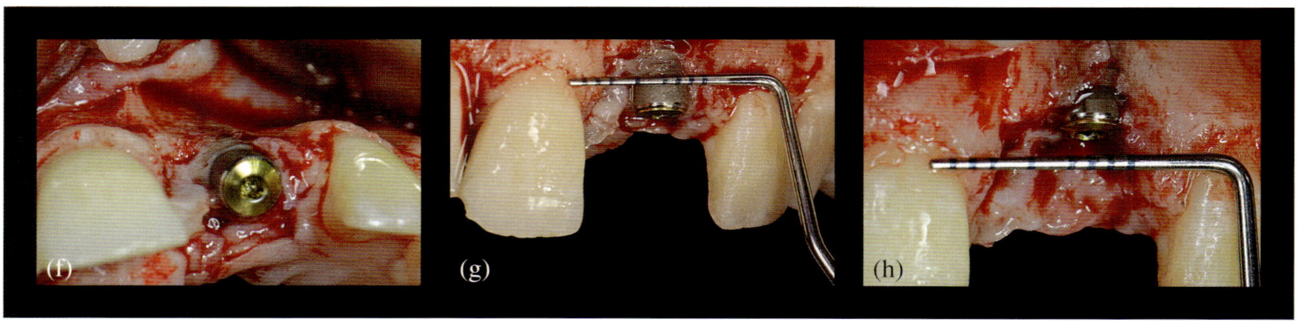

Figure 4.49 (f) and (g) Intra-operative view showing the complete loss of the labial plate of bone, and the faulty implant position. (h) A new implant is placed according to the 3D esthetic protocol.

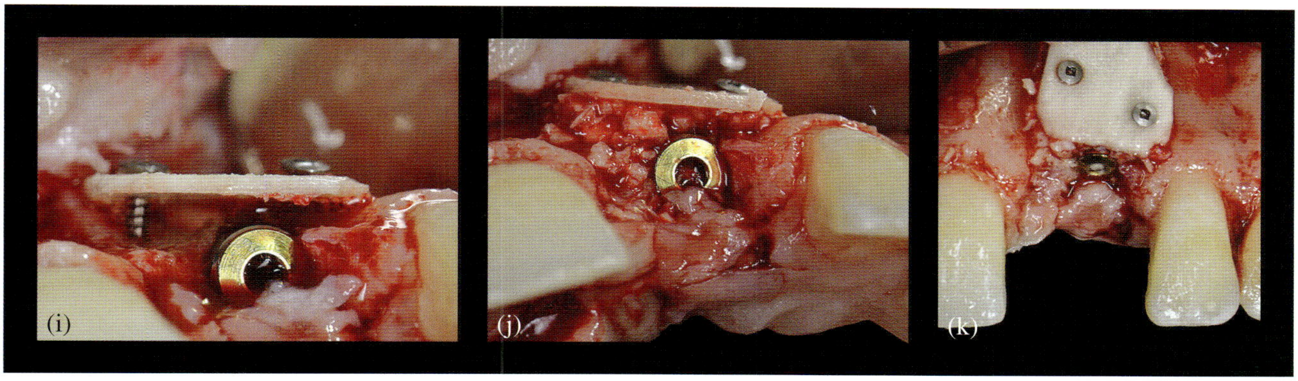

Figure 4.49 (i) An allograft bone monocortical sheet is positioned, leaving grafting space underneath. (j) and (k) Allograft cortical sheet is stabilized suing two micro titanium screws and the space is grafted with particulate bone graft.

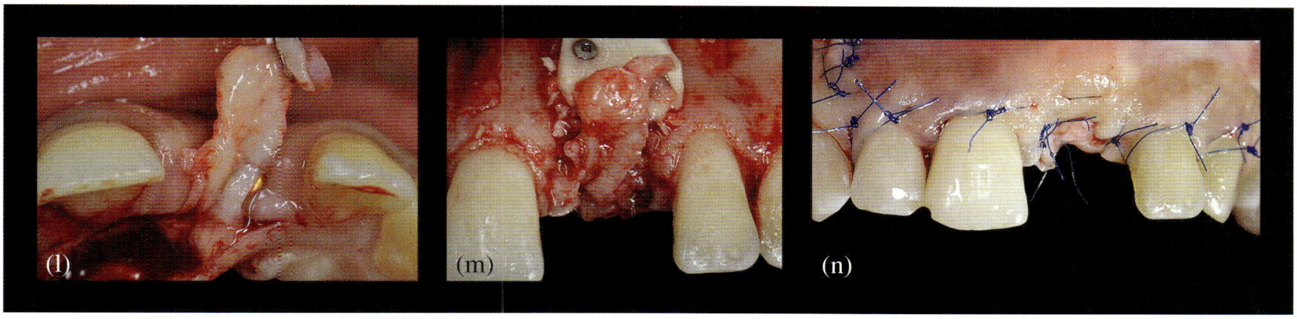

Figure 4.49 (l) and (m) Subepithelial pedicle connective tissue graft is harvested and rotated. (n) Flap sutured.

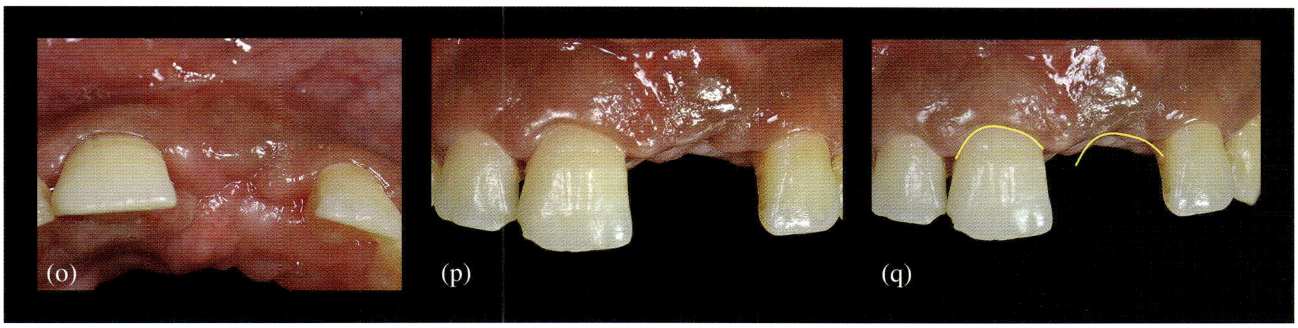

Figure 4.49 (o) and (p) One week post-operative view. (q) One month post-surgery showing the regain of the keratinized tissue band and the regain of the missing labial contour.

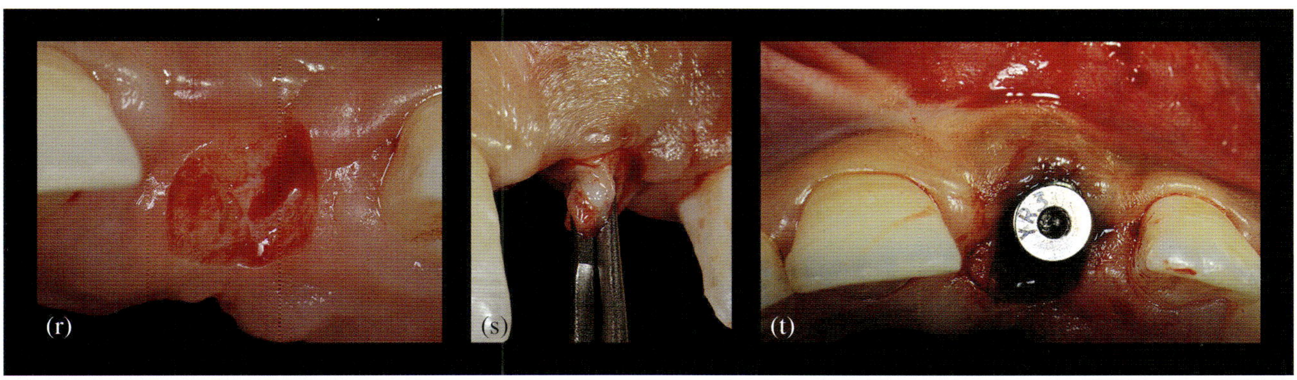

Figure 4.49 (r–t) Second stage surgery and healing abutment connection.

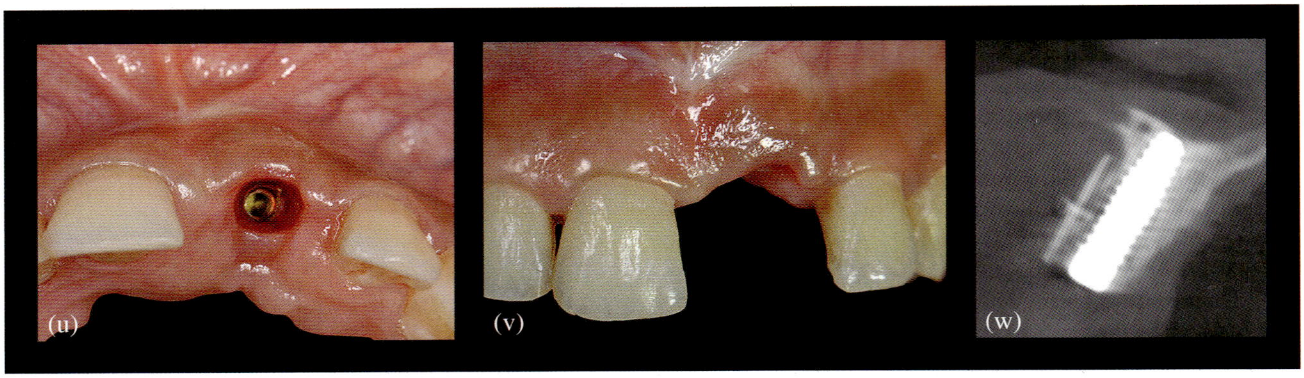

Figure 4.49 (u) and (v) Final tissue maturation. (w) CBCT scan showing the new implant and the grafted bone.

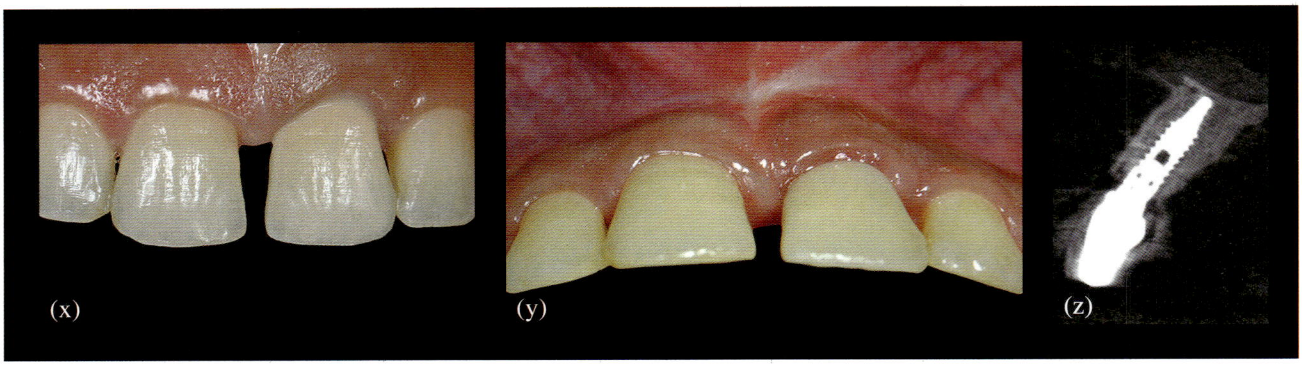

Figure 4.49 (x) and (y) Frontal and incisal views showing the restorative outcome. (z) Two years postoperative CBCT scan showing the final bone graft maturation.

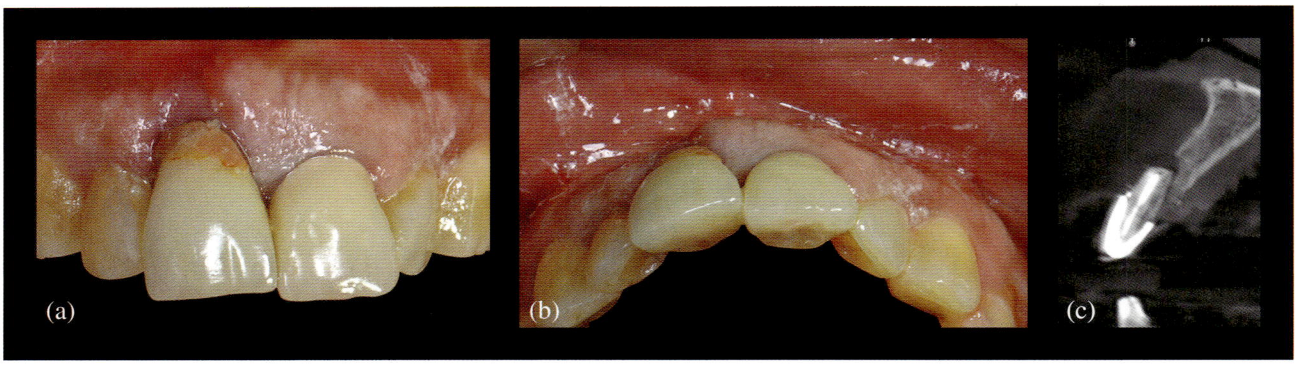

Figure 4.50 (a) and (b) Frontal and incisal views of two hopeless central incisors rotated showing severe tissue deficiency. (c) CBCT scan showing the labial plate of bone status.

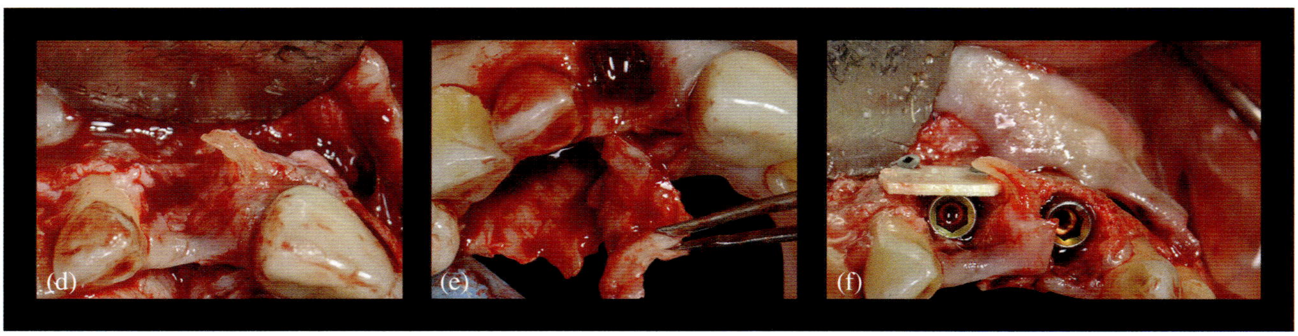

Figure 4.50 (d) Intra-operative view showing the loss of labial plate of bone. (e) Rotated subepethelial connective tissue graft is prepared. (f) Monocortical allograft sheet is stabilized along with two implant fixtures.

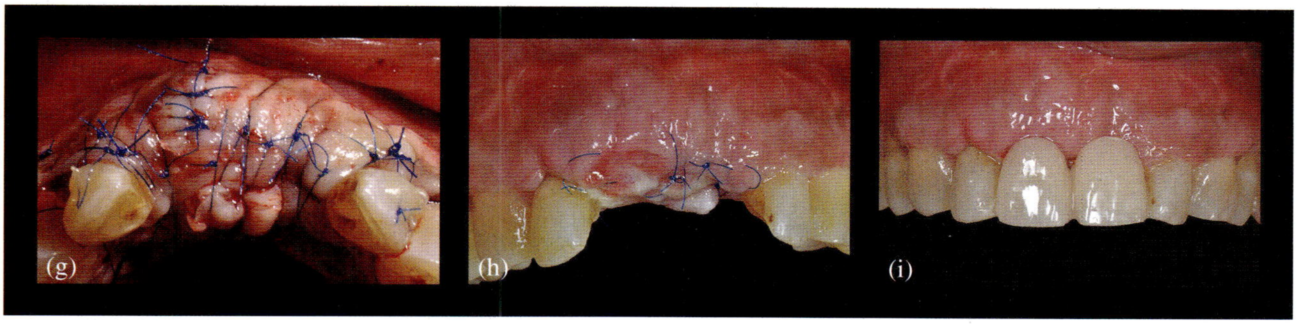

Figure 4.50 (g) Flap sutures. (h) and (i) Two weeks post-surgery showing the uneventful healing with a resin bonded bridge attached to the adjacent teeth, also reveals abundant keratinized mucosa.

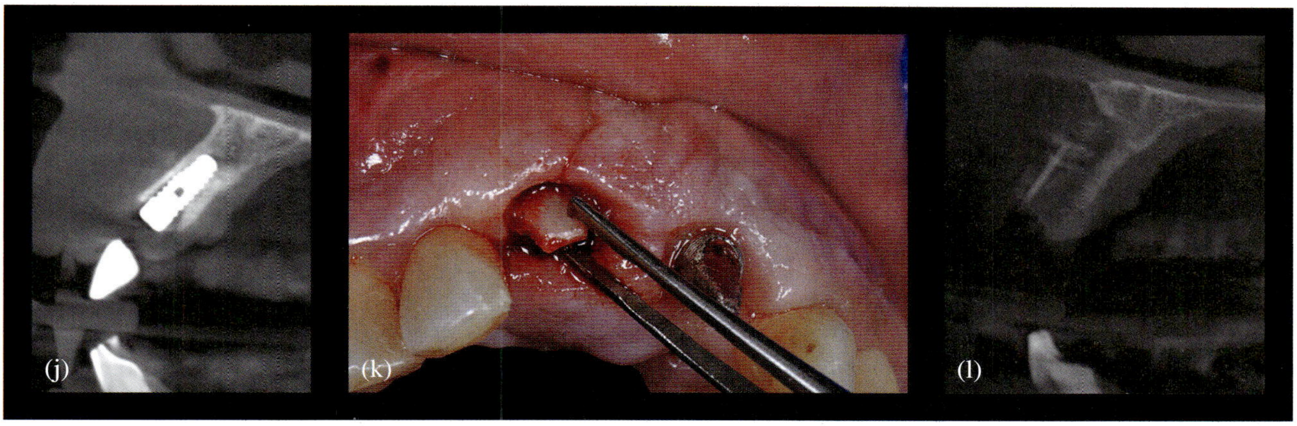

Figure 4.50 (j) Two months post-surgery CBCT view showing the implant fixture in place. (k) Three months post-surgery showing the implant fixture is lost along with the failed allograft cortical sheet as a result of infection. (l) CBCT view showing the lost implant and the Brocken allograft sheet.

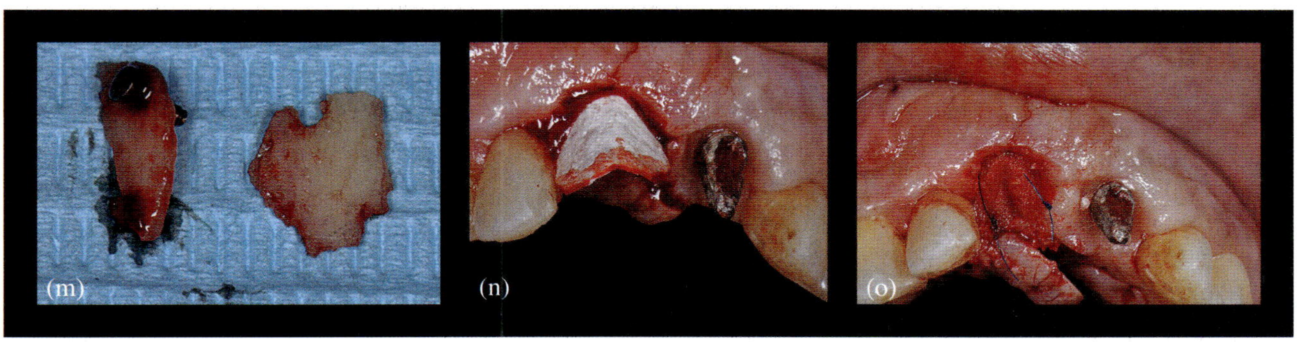

Figure 4.50 (m) The removed cortical allograft sheet. (n) and (o) Ice-cream cone technique is used to augment the socket that will be filled with particulated bone graft.

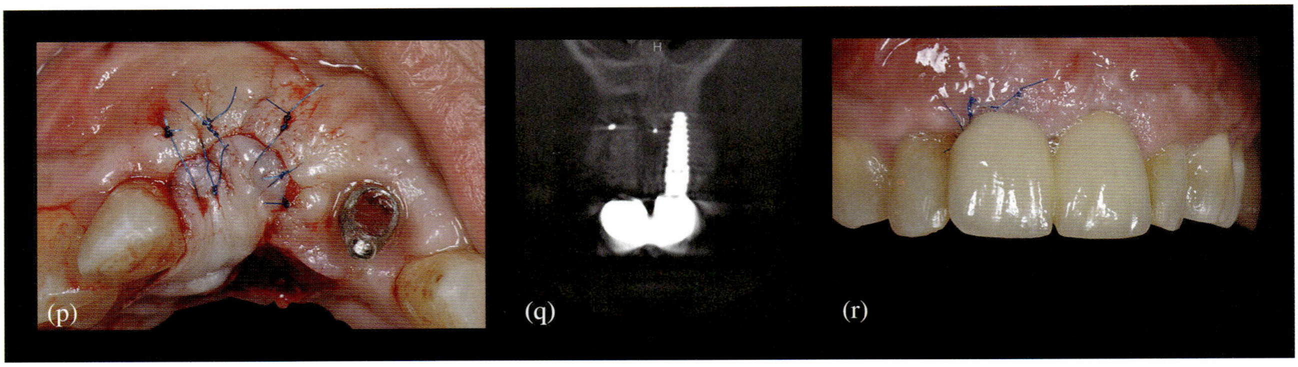

Figure 4.50 (p) Full thickness rotated palatal flap is used to close the socket orifice to protect the bone graft. (q) CBCT showing the bone graft in place. (r) Uneventful healing one week postoperative.

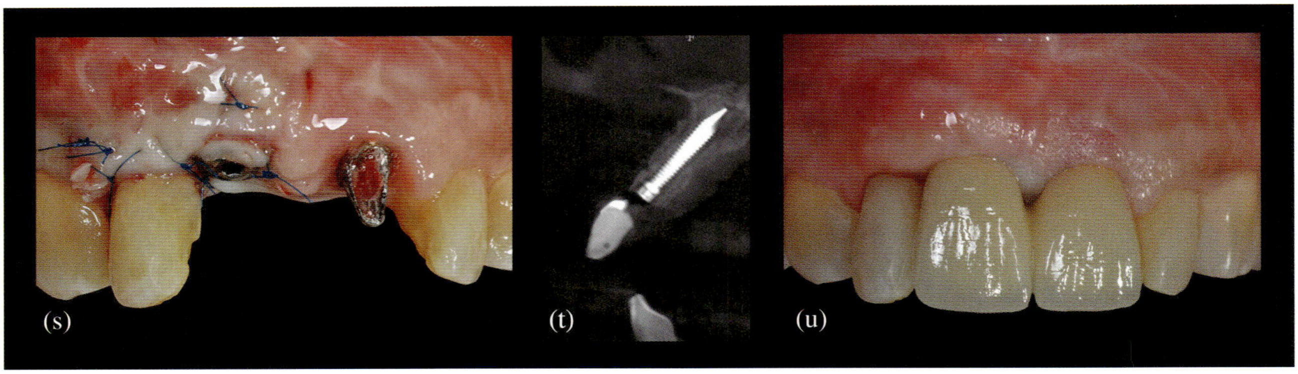

Figure 4.50 (s) Another connective tissue graft is used to improve the marginal tissue levels. (t) CBCT scan showing the new placed implant in place. (u) Final restoration in place.

4.5.4 Using Guided Tissue Regeneration

Guided tissue regenerative membranes were applied in the maxillofacial region to regenerate periodontal and osseous defects (Garg 2004; Ikada 2006; Kinoshita and Amagasa 2002; Villar and Cochran 2010); they were also used to secure the grafting material (Barrows 1986). The two broad categories of bioresorbable membranes include natural and synthetic membranes. Natural membranes are made of collagen or chitosan, whereas synthetic products are made of six aliphatic polyesters, primarily poly-L-lactic acid (PLLA) and poly-L-lactic-co-glycolide acid (PLGA) copolymers (Pontoriero, Wennström and Lindhe 1999) (see Figure 4.51a–j).

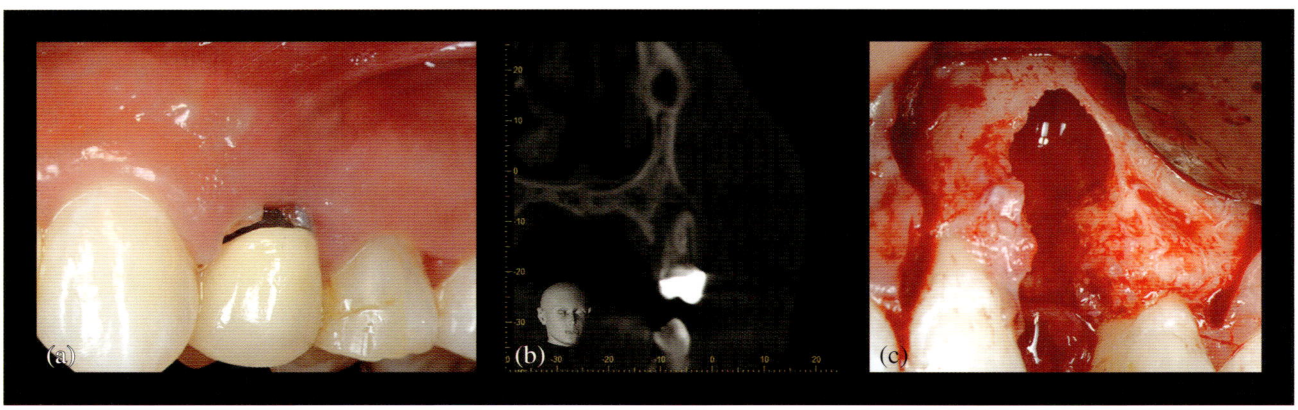

Figure 4.51 (a) Preoperative view of failed maxillary first pre molar. (b) CBCT view showing sever bone loss, complete loss of the labial plate of bone that requires definitive repair. (c) Intra- operative view showing the labial plate of bone condition.

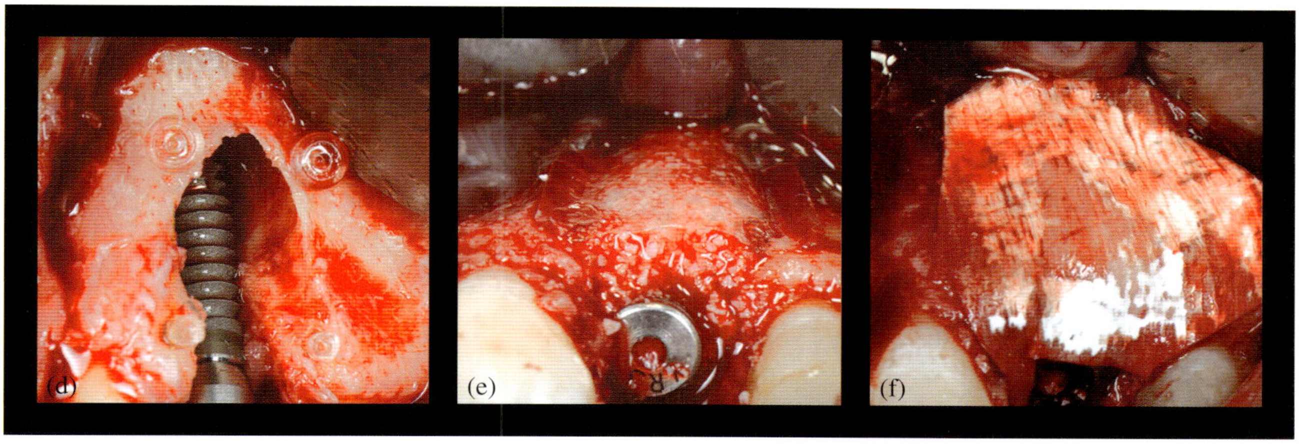

Figure 4.51 (d) Stabilization of an implant within the bone housing (primary stable). (e) PDLLA membrane was stabilized to cover particulate bone graft. (f) Collagen membrane was used to cover the grafting mix.

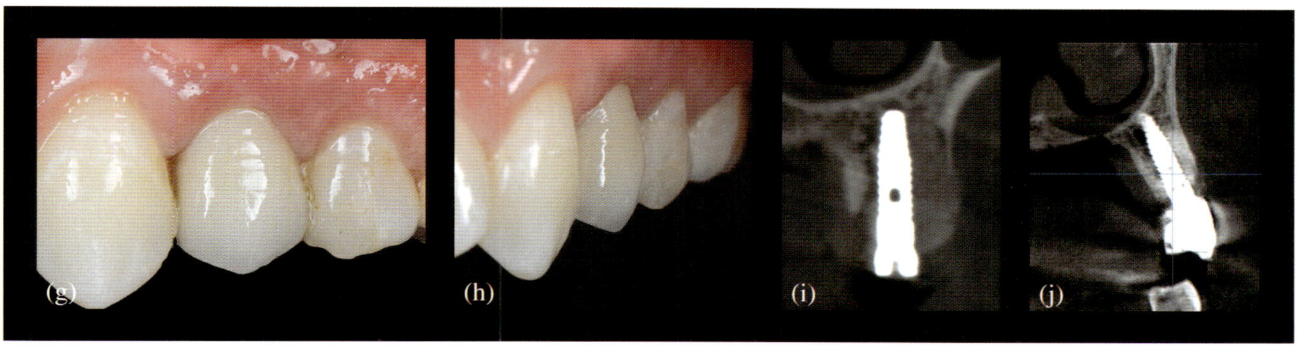

Figure 4.51 (g) and (h) Final case restored showing enhanced labial contour. (i) CBCT showing complete restoration of labial plate of bone. (j) Six years CBCT view showing abundance of labial plate of bone thickness and maintained crestal height.

D-lactide, L-lactide (each 50%) membrane (PDLLA) is a thermoplastic and biodegradable polymer. It is degraded by simple hydrolysis in the body to finally generate non-toxic water and carbon dioxide. PDLLA has been clinically applied in various surgical applications due to its biocompatibility, thermoplasticity, and mechanical strength (Buser et al. 1990) (see Figure 4.52a–g).

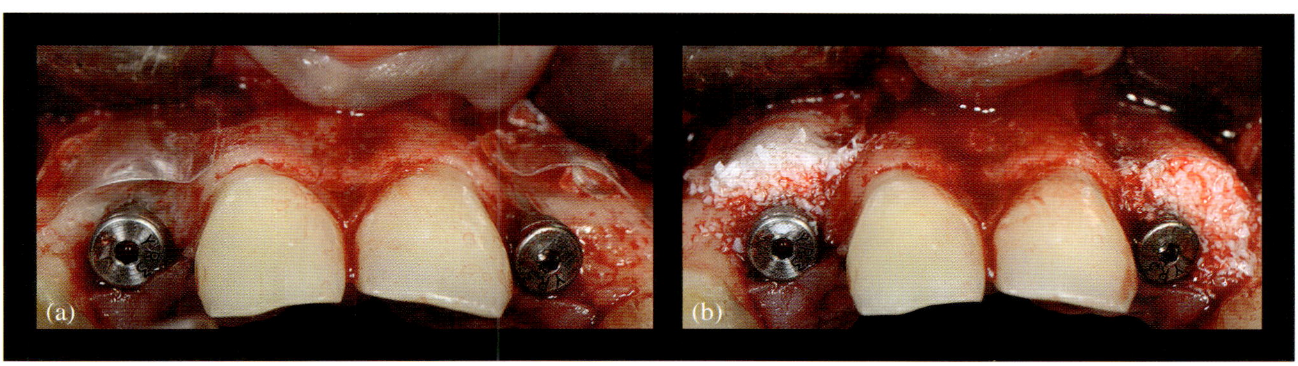

Figure 4.52 (a) Lost labial plate of bone being corrected using PDLLA membrane that is stabilized and positioned leaving space underneath for the particulate bone graft. (b) The particulate bone graft was filled underneath the membrane.

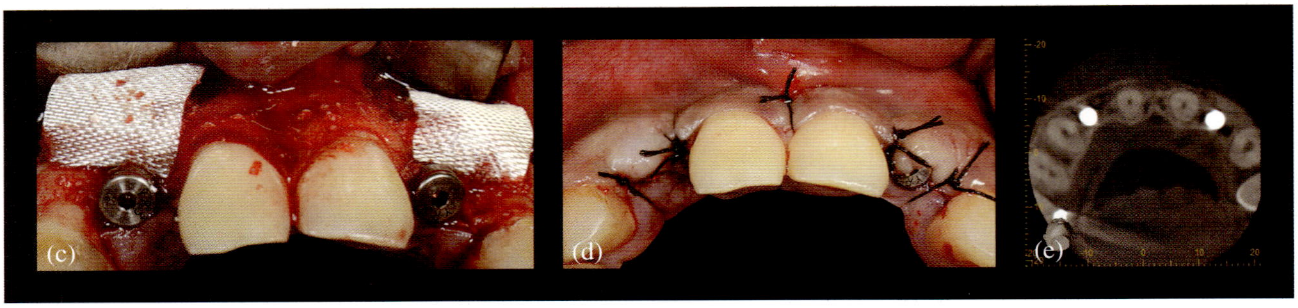

Figure 4.52 (c) Cellulose membrane was used to cover the grafting complex. (d) Flap sutured. (e) CBCT view showing complete regeneration of the missing labial contour.

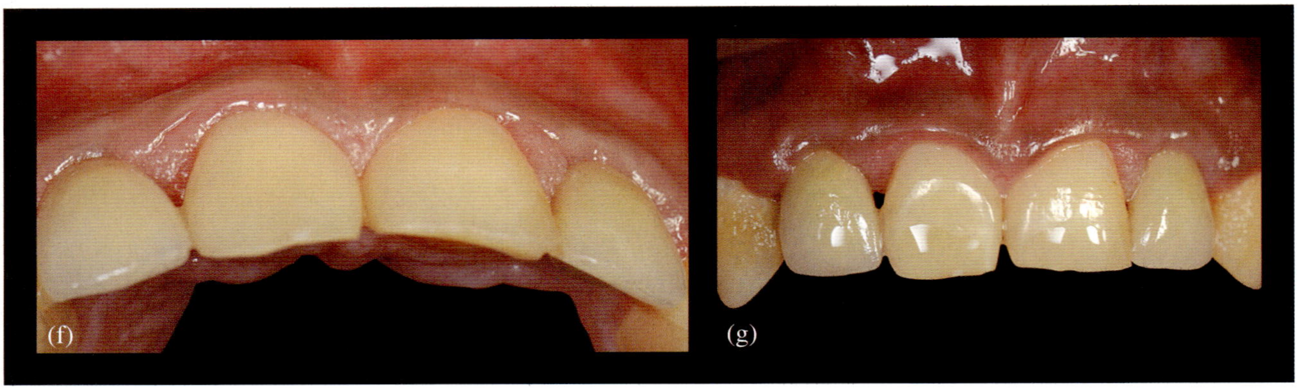

Figure 4.52 (f) and (g) Case finally restored showing complete restoration of the labial tissue bulk.

Cell adhesion to PDLLA materials is low and the proliferative activity is poor because of surface hydrophobicity. Low cell adhesion to PDLLA membrane prevents soft tissue invasion. In the histologic analysis, a close contact between PDLLA devices and the surrounding bone was always found, without traces of inflammatory tissue or signs of infection (Nuss and Rechenberg 2008) (see Figure 4.53a–f).

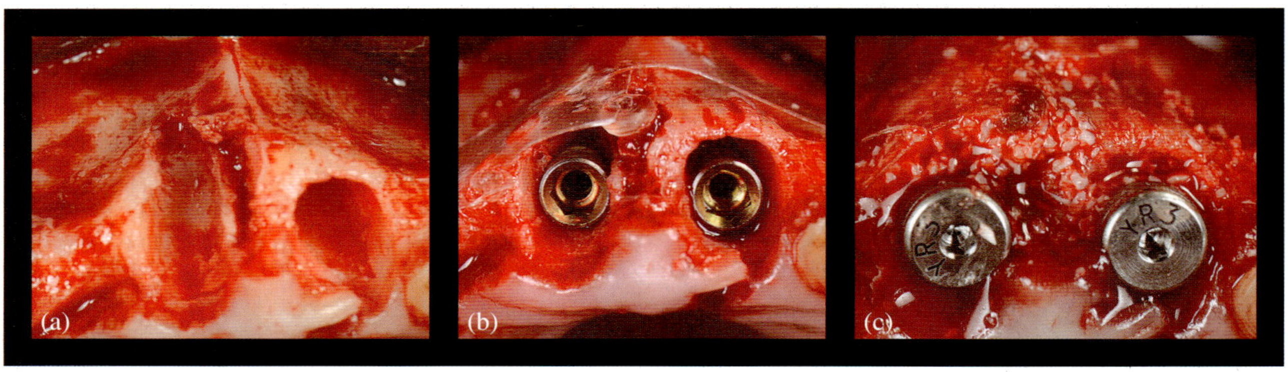

Figure 4.53 (a) Intraoperative view showing completely lost labial plate of bone. (b) Two implants were placed to restore the missing teeth. (c) Gap filled with particulated bone graft material.

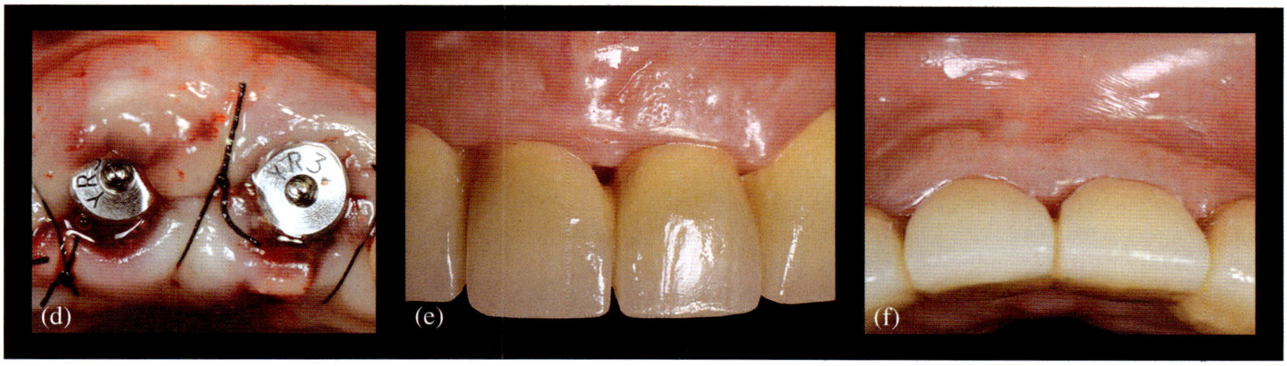

Figure 4.53 (d) Flap sutured. (e) and (f) Postrestorative view showing restored labial contour.

Poly-L-lactic acid membrane (PLLA) is used for the preparation of different bioabsorbable membranes, characterized by thermal plasticity, suitable mechanical properties, and biocompatibility (Garg 2004; Ikada 2006). PLLA has the disadvantage of being slowly resorbed for up to four years (Kinoshita and Amagasa 2002; Matsusue et al. 1995). To overcome this problem, copolymers of lactide and e-caprolactone, glycolide, trimethylene carbonate, etc., have been formulated to reduce the resorption time (see Figure 4.54a–e).

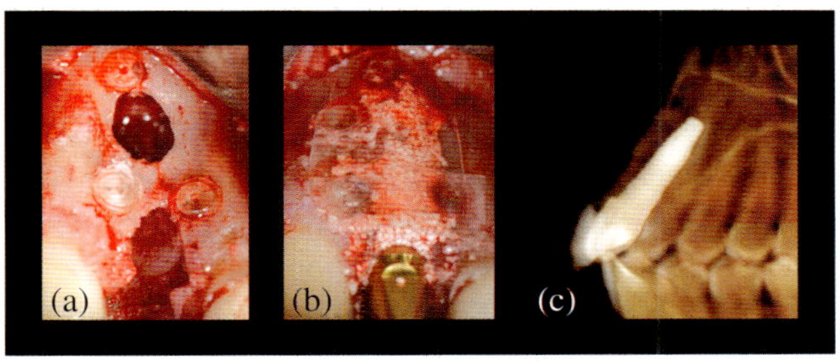

Figure 4.54 (a) Thin, fenestrated labial plate of bone. (b) Bone graft material placed underneath a PDLLA membrane. (c) CBCT showing enhanced restored labial profile.

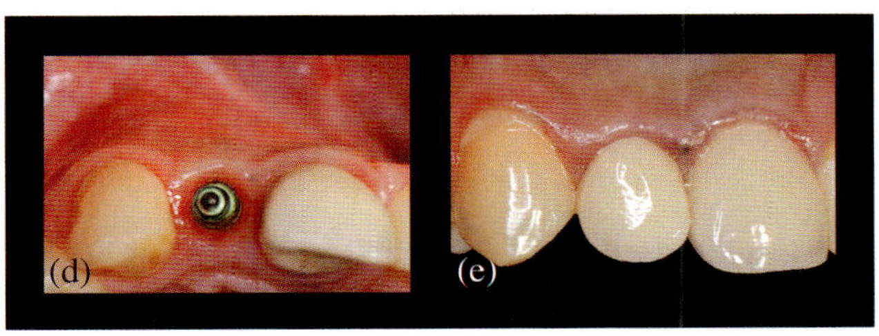

Figure 4.54 (d) Soft tissue profiling using provisional restoration. (e) Case finally restored.

There are several studies in humans where bioabsorbable membranes have been used for reconstruction of segmental or large mandibular bone defects using a bioresorbable PLLA barrier membrane (mesh) in combination with an autologous bone graft (Carini et al. 2014). The bioresorbable PLLA synthetic membrane was particulated in combination with autologous cancellous bone graft or bone marrow. Preliminary results showed healing of the defects and a satisfactory function in all cases (Barrows 1986). Synthetic resorbable materials, such as poly-lactic acid (PLA), poly-glycolic acid (PGA), poly-ε-ca-prolactone (PCL), poly-hydroxyl valeric acid, poly-hydroxyl butyric acid, and their copolymers have been widely considered for orthopedic applications due to their low rigidity, tuned biodegradation (Haidar 2010).

The Guidor® (Sunstar, Inc., Schaumburg, IL, USA) Matrix Barrier is a biodegradable membrane, first used for the regeneration of tissues in periodontology, consisting of polylactic acid treated with acetyltributylcitrate to achieve flexibility to guarantee close barrier adaptation to the bone defect. Guidor Matrix Barrier has a matrix with two differently perforated layers. The external layer, allowing integration of the overlying gingival flap, has large rectangular pores to promote tissue integration and to enable gingival connective tissue to penetrate quickly into the matrix. The inner layer has small circular pores able to retard tissue penetration but allowing nutrient permeation. The two layers are separated by many inner spacers forming an interspace into which tissue can grow (Araujo, Berglundh, Lindhe 1998; Gottlow 1993).

Resolut® (Gore & Associates, Inc., Flagstaff, Arizona, USA) is another commercially available product consisting of two layers: a PLGA compact layer that prevents epithelial cell penetration and a porous network of polyglycolide fibers, promoting tissue integration. Histological studies showed a similar effectiveness to non-resorbable membranes and complete resorption five to six months after placement (Pontoriero et al. 1999). Fibers of polyglactin 910, a copolymer of glycolide and L-lactide (9:1 wt/wt) were used to produce a woven mesh (Vicryl Periodontal Mesh®). The polyglactin 910 is inert (no reactions in the surrounding tissue during its adsorption were observed), preserves its physicomechanical properties during the first three to four weeks (De Sanctis and Zucchelli 1996).

Atrisorb® (Evaluate Ltd. London, United Kingdom) membrane is the first liquid product applied directly at the surgical site: it consists of poly-DL-lactic acid dissolved in *N*-methyl-2-pyrrolidone. Membrane thickness is 600–750 μm, and it is positioned into the defect site by applying a moderate finger pressure. A histological complete resorption was observed 6–12 months after implantation (Coonts et al. 1998; Hou et al. 2004). Clinical studies reported its efficacy in the treatment of periodontal defects (Camargo et al. 2002).

The Epi-Guide® (Curasan, NC, USA) Bioresorbable Barrier Matrix is a porous membrane consisting of poly-DL-lactic acid with a unique three-layer technology, used as an adjunct to periodontal restorative surgery. The Epi-Guide maintains its structure and functions for five months after implantation with a complete bioresorption after one year (Takata, Wang and Miyauchi 2001). The layer in contact with the gingiva is porous to promote fibroblast infiltration and attachment. In contrast, the layer in contact with the bone defect has a limited porosity that supports fluid uptake, helps adherence to the tooth surface, and inhibits fibroblast movement (Bilir et al. 2007; Takata et al. 2001).

Membranes based on copolymers of lactic acid and e-caprolactone have been produced, showing a lower degradation time as compared to pure PLA membranes. PCL is characterized by higher hydrophobicity and lower water solubility than PLA, PGA, and their copolymers. A commercial product, called Vivosorb® (Polyganics, Groningen, The Netherlands), consisting of poly-DL-lactide-e-caprolactone, was found to be biocompatible, non-cytotoxic, occlusive, and space maintaining (Meek et al. 2004). However, different studies have shown its potential for GBR applications (Gielkens et al. 2008; Hoogeveen et al. 2009). The most important commercial collagen membrane are Bio-Gide® (Geistlichpharma, wolhusen, Switzerland), Mem-Lock (BioHorizons, Birmingham, AL, USA), and BioMend® (Zimmer-Dental, Carlsbad, California, USA) which is based on xenogenic collagen type I made from porcine skin and is characterized by a bilayered structure with a dense and a porous layer. The dense layer has a smooth surface able to avoid epithelial cell infiltration into bone defects, while the porous layer allows tissue integration (Taguchi et al. 2005).

A type I collagen membrane is manufactured from bovine Achilles tendon (BioMend®, Zimmer-Dental, Carlsbad, California). The membrane is semi-occlusive with nano-sized pores and is resorbable within eight weeks. Clinical studies revealed a partial effectiveness, (Maksoud 2001; Sela et al. 2003).

Hydroxyapatite (HA), β-tricalcium phosphate (β-TCP), bioactive glass, and glass–ceramic are synthetic materials that have been formulated to provide adequate properties for applications in the field of GBR (Balasundaram, Sato and Webster 2006; Schwarz et al. 2007). However, in reality and with more understanding of the optional osteogenic power of the graft materials, alloplasts showed very minimal or no osteoinductive properties. Kikuchi et al. (2004) reported a complete integration of the composite membranes in beagles' mandible defects (10 mm × 10 mm × 10 mm). Moreover, in several works, the addition of bioactive glass into PGA or PLA membranes has been shown to stimulate different biological processes, such as the enhancement of osteoblastic activity and new collagen production (Lu et al. 2003).

4.5.5 Socket Repair Kit

An innovative method for the repair of the defective labial plate of bone in fresh extraction sockets (type 2) has been proposed by the author, using PDLLA (KLS Martin Group, Tuttlingen, Germany) barrier membrane and an ultrasound-aided biodegradable pin fixation system (see Figure 4.55a and b).

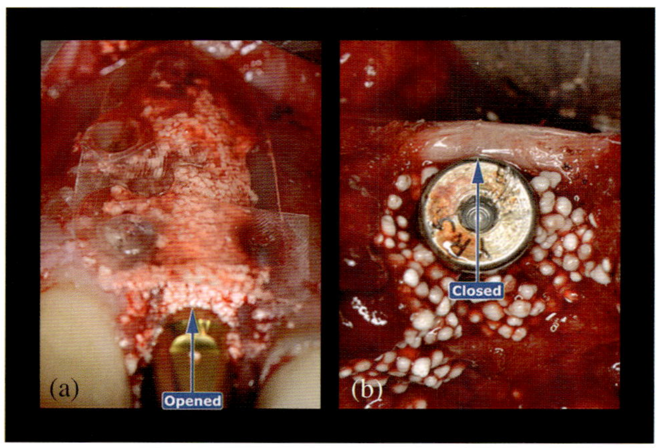

Figure 4.55 (a) and (b) The difference between using ordinary grafting techniques when the socket orifice is opened while on the other hand using the socket template when the orifice is closed (protected from bacterial invasion and prevented from epithelial down growth).

The basic idea of the socket repair kit is to mold the membrane to exactly restore the defective plate of bone, which is then filled with an autograft chips to induce and regenerate bone at the defective site. The technique entails measuring the osseous defect of the socket wall clinically and then tailoring the PDLLA membrane to cover the defective area of the socket (see Figure 4.56a–c).

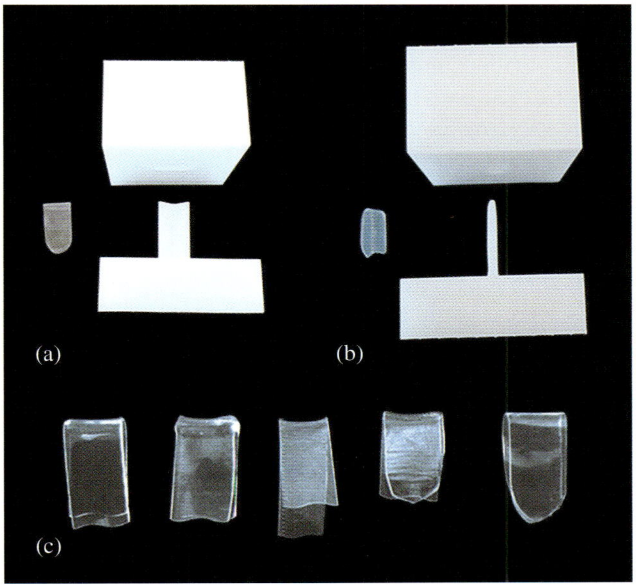

Figure 4.56 (a–c) The Preliminary lab model of fabricating the PDLLA socket repair template.

Once this is done, the PDLLA membrane is folded into a U-shape and filled with the particulate autogenous bone graft chips. The U-shaped PDLLA membrane is then filled with the bone graft and stabilized to the defective socket wall, using PDLLA biodegradable pins through the membrane into a predrilled hole apical to the defective labial bone site. As ultrasound energy is applied to the biodegradable pins, they will melt and cause biodegradable polymers to flow into the bone. Once the energy source is removed, the pin solidifies, locks into the bone, and secures the membrane. Implant site preparation may then be carried out for a regular immediate implant placement procedure.

The Socket Repair Kit (International Patent Number: PCT/EG2012/000005), is planned to consist of pre-U-shaped PDLLA membrane made of assorted sizes, usually three sizes that are commonly used to treat other minor, moderate, or major labial plate bone defects (thickness about 1.5 mm, height ranging from 3 to 7 mm, widths of 3–6 mm), and assorted PDLLA membrane shields to fit different socket defect sizes, along with specially designed clamp forceps to hold the U-shaped membrane to stabilize it in to the defective socket, making it easy to use and minimizing treatment time, as shown in Figure 4.57a–c.

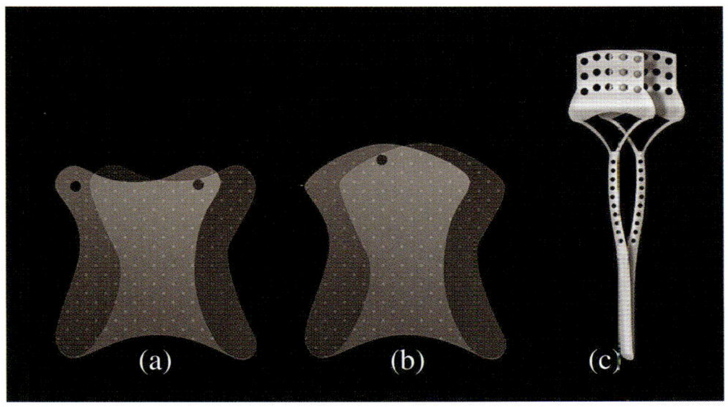

Figure 4.57 (a–c) Final design of the socket repair template with the clip holder.

The socket repair kit is an easy and efficient method to treat minor to severe labial plate bone defects in freshly extracted sockets (class II). It acts like a carrier to carry and protect any grafting material, preferably autogenous bone chips harvested with any type of bone shaver (see Figure 4.58a–c).

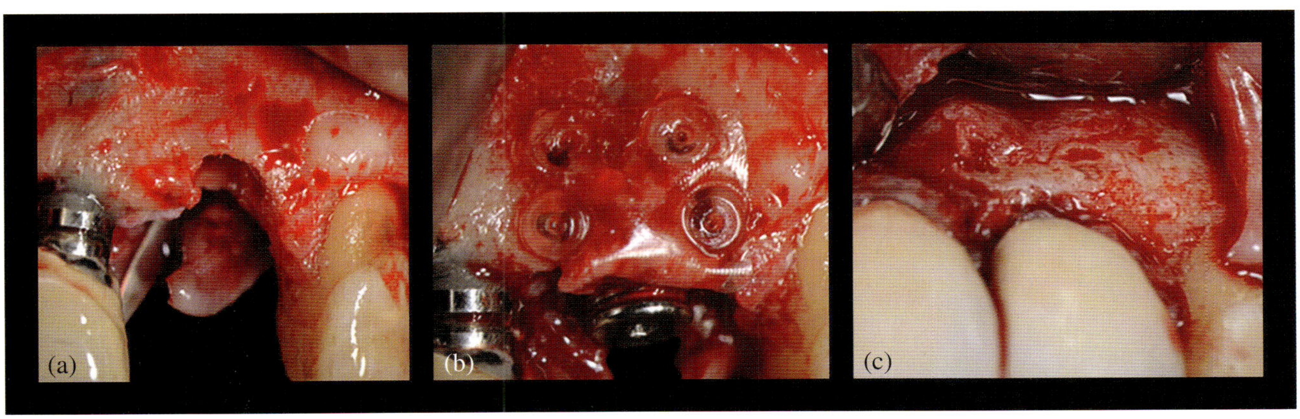

Figure 4.58 (a–c) Clinical pictures showing the fate of the PDLLA socket template showing the complete replacement of the defect with natural bone over a seven months period.

The advantage of the carrier is that it totally eliminates the hassle of harvesting the autoblock from the ramus or the chin. It is very predictable for regenerating the defective socket wall, because it isolates the graft material completely and restores the original socket dimensions, is easy to handle, and does not require any extra surgical skills to perform.

The author studied 10 patients presenting anterior single-tooth type II sockets after extraction. All eight patients received a preoperative screening including a complete medical history, as well as clinical and radiographic examinations. All patients were free of any untreated systemic disease. Each surgery was performed under local anesthesia (Articaine hydrochloride, Ubistesin forte, 3M ESPE) of 40 mg mL^{-1}, with adrenaline, 1:80 000. After the anesthesia had taken effect, initial incisions were made using sharp surgical 15-C surgical blades (B Braun, Tuttlingen, Baden-Württemberg, Germany) circumferentially around the teeth to be extracted then extended vertically. A full periosteal flap was raised beyond the mucogingival junction with relieving incisions made to include one tooth mesial to and one tooth distal to the extracted tooth. Scoring of the periosteumat the base of the flap was carried out where additional flap mobility was needed to facilitate tension-free closure. Traumatic teeth extractions were then carried out with the additional use of periotomes and root elevators. The local socket area is first cleaned with hand curettes to eliminate any existing residual granulation tissues then debrided and irrigated with normal saline. The socket defect size is then measured with a periodontal probe moving in both apical and coronal directions (see Figure 4.59a–i).

The PDLLA membrane was first cut to the right size to fit the defect site, then soaked for 30 seconds in a warm sterile water bath (60–70 °C) and thermoplastically molded to the desired U-shape. Autogenous bone chips were carefully packed into the U-shape PDLLA membrane. A 1.6-mm twist drill was first used to prepare the sites for pin placement. The PDLLA pins with diameters of 2.1 mm were then welded into the funnel-shaped predrilled holes approximately 2–3 mm into the bone to secure the U-shaped membrane filled with bone chips. Immediate implant placements were then carried out. Implant fixture (Laser-Lok implants, BioHorizons, Birmingham, USA) is placed using a series of drills with increasing diameters under copious saline irrigation.

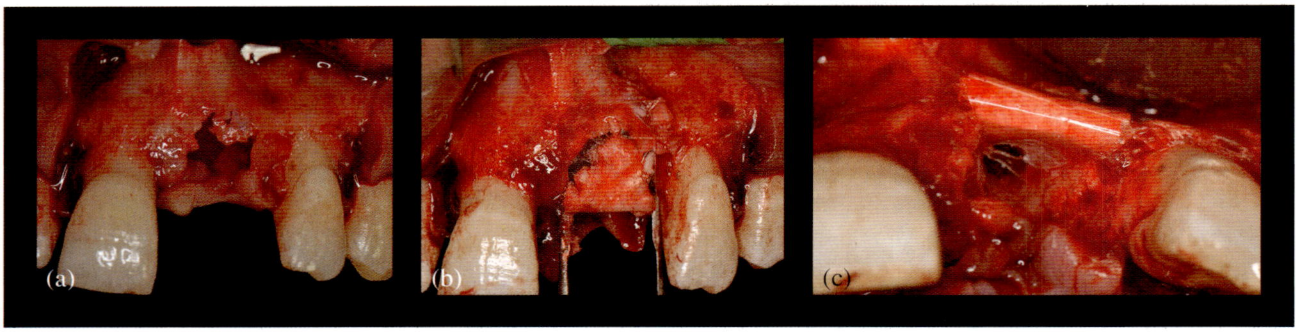

Figure 4.59 (a) Intra-operative picture showing a thin and resorbed labial plate of bone. (b) Socket template tried in place. (c) Socket carrier stabilized with two PDDLA screws.

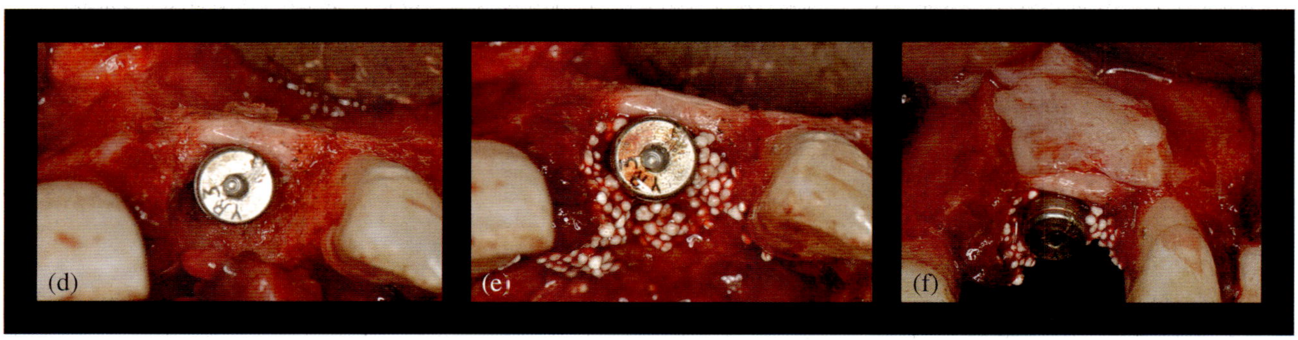

Figure 4.59 (d) Incisal view showing the implant in position. (e) Gap filled with alloplast. (f) Connective tissue graft is used to enhance the labial grafting.

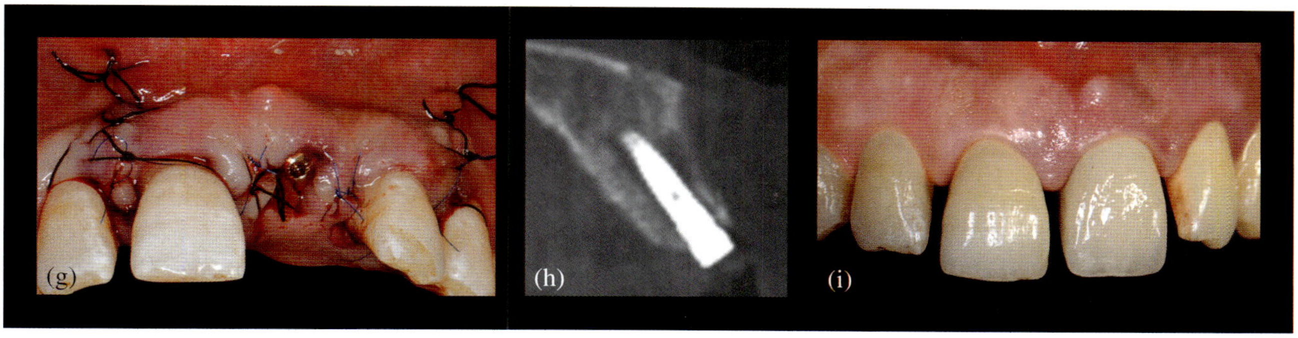

Figure 4.59 (g) Flap sutured. (h) CBCT scan three months post-surgery showing the complete restoration of the labial plate of bone. (i) Case restored.

After placement, an optional socket filler may be used to fill the gap (Mineross, BioHorizons, Birmingham, USA). A connective tissue graft or cellular dermal matrix (AlloDerm, LifeCell Corp., Branchburg, NJ, USA) can be used to cover the PDLLA membrane to increase soft tissue thickness when needed. Tension-free closure was then achieved with Vicryl 5.0 (Ethicon, Johnson & Johnson, USA) and black silk 4.0 sutures (B Braun, Tuttlingen, Baden-Württemberg, Germany) using interrupted sutures. Postoperative instructions given to the patients included gentle brushing near the surgical site and rinsing with 0.12% chlorhexidine mouth rinse twice a day for one week. Amoxicillin (500 mg) three times a day for a five-day duration was prescribed to prevent infection. Clinical and radiographic follow-up examinations were performed at baseline, and at four-, six-, and twelve-month intervals after rehabilitation.

During this study, two implants failed, and were omitted from the study. The remaining eight implants healed uneventfully and were included in the follow-up protocol. During the entire follow-up period, implants showed no evidence of clinical mobility, no pain, and no mucositis nor flap dehiscence. Measurements taken from the CBCT scan postoperatively showed the stability of the bone regenerated. At the end of the follow-up period, all cases showed remarkable improvement of the labial wall thickness. The CBCT scan follow-up revealed successful repair of the defective labial bone in class 2 extraction sockets. It was concluded that this technique is a viable alternative for repairing the defective labial bone in class 2 extraction sockets with ease and with more predictability.

4.5.6 Composite Grafts

Misch et al. (1999) introduced a novel grafting method called the modified composite autograft; the graft was made of a core graft harvested with a trephine drill consisting of epithelial tissue on the top surface of the core, a connective tissue layer, periosteum, cortical bone, and cancellous bone, it is harvested from the tuberosity area then trimmed to be introduced to fill and seal a defective socket. The autogenous bone graft composite core integrates to the socket walls by osteogenesis and osteoinduction. After peeling of the epithelial part, the connective tissue portion of the graft merges and blends with the adjacent keratinized tissues, providing keratinized epithelium on top of the socket with a color and texture similar to that of the surrounding original tissues (Dahlin et al. 1989) (see Figure 4.60a–f).

Misch and Dietsh (1993) have also recommended the use of platelet-derived growth factor (PDGF) to boost overall healing and to enhance bone formation. The procedure entails a thorough curettage and decortication of the defective socket walls. The soft tissue around the rim of the extraction socket is then de-epithelialized with a diamond burr or a sharp scalpel (freshen the socket rim edges). A wide-diameter trephine drill that is larger than the diameter of the socket orifice is used to harvest the composite graft from the tuberosity. A slow-speed, high-torque handpiece with copious internal and external saline irrigation should be used during the harvesting procedure to avoid overheating the graft (see Figure 4.61a–j).

A green stick fracture of the composite graft is performed at its base to separate it from the donor site. A preoperative X-ray film or digital imaging can help determine the extent of drilling needed. The keratinized layer of the graft core is then peeled with a sharp scalpel to remove only the surface epithelium, leaving almost 3 mm of connective tissue attached to the bone core. If the bone core is found to be larger than the socket orifice, it should be trimmed so that it will fit snugly in the socket. The apical third of the extraction socket is subsequently filled with demineralized freeze-dried bone and a puffy coat containing PDGF. The trimmed composite graft is introduced into the socket and tapped gently into place using a mallet and a blunt instrument (see Figure 4.62a–m).

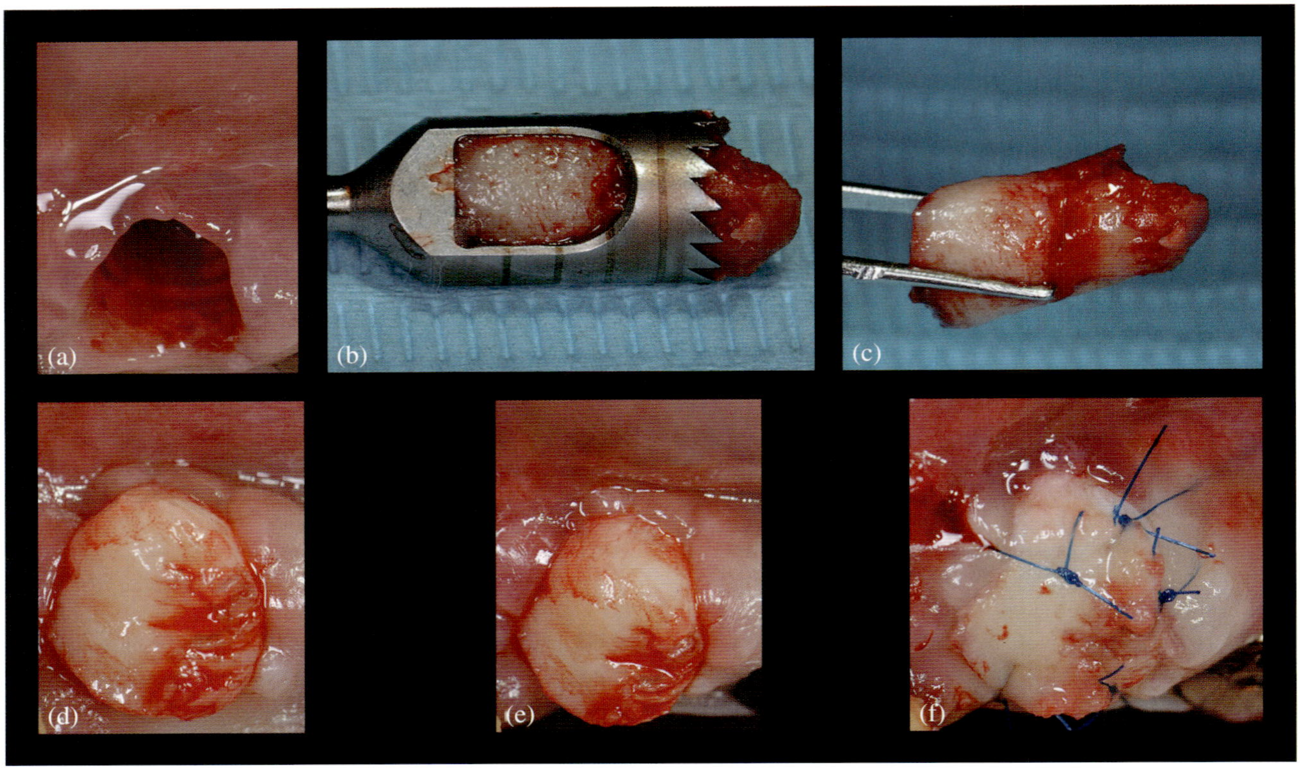

Figure 4.60 (a–f) Steps of harvesting and securing a composite graft from the tuberosity to a fresh extraction socket.

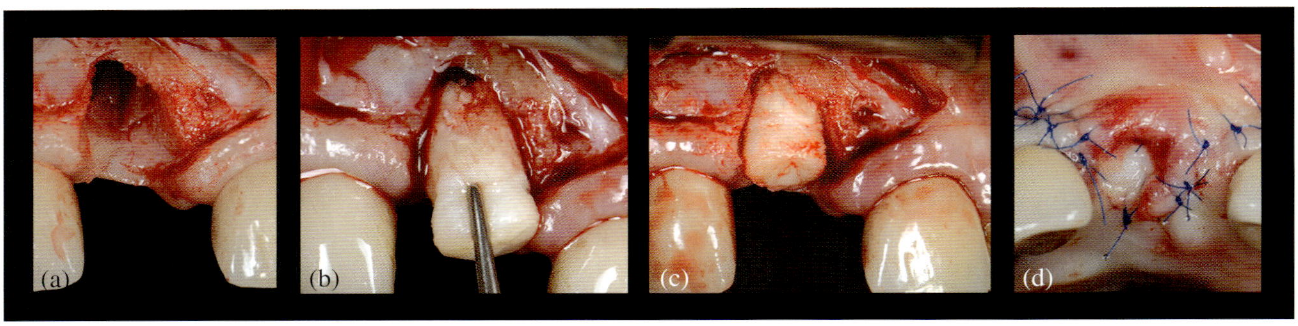

Figure 4.61 (a) Intra-operative view showing missing labial plate of bone with empty socket. (b) The composite core is trimmed to snugly fit the socket. (c) The core fitted inside the socket. (d) Flap sutured.

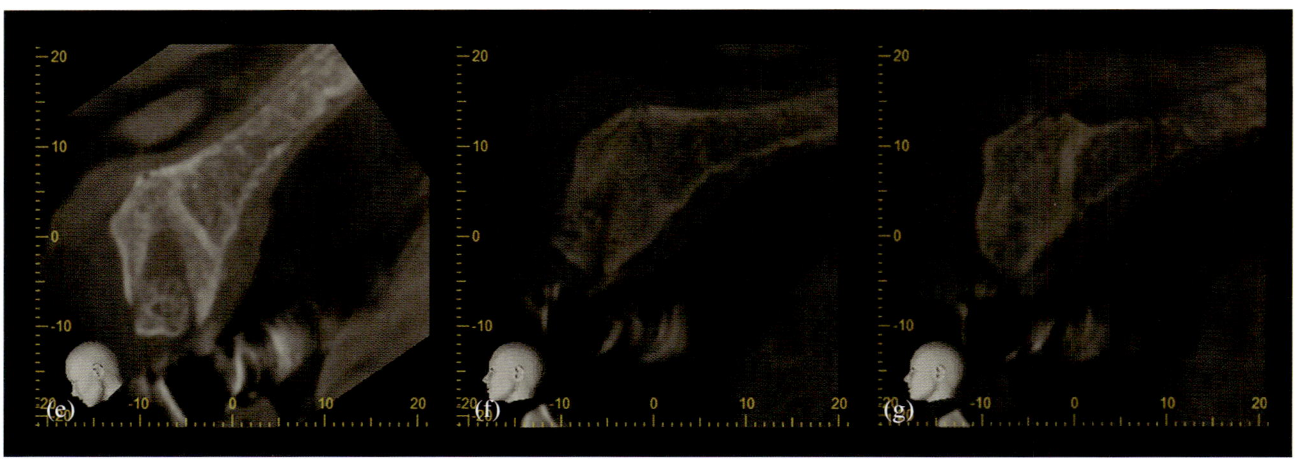

Figure 4.61 (e–g) CBCT scan showing the integration of the composite core restoring the labial plate.

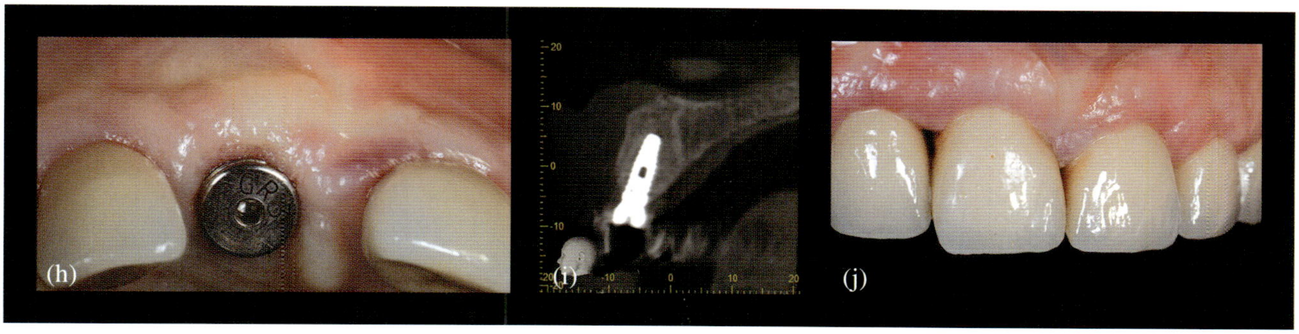

Figure 4.61 (h) Two months postimplant placement with the healing abutment connected. (i) CBCT scan showing implant in place. (j) Final case restored.

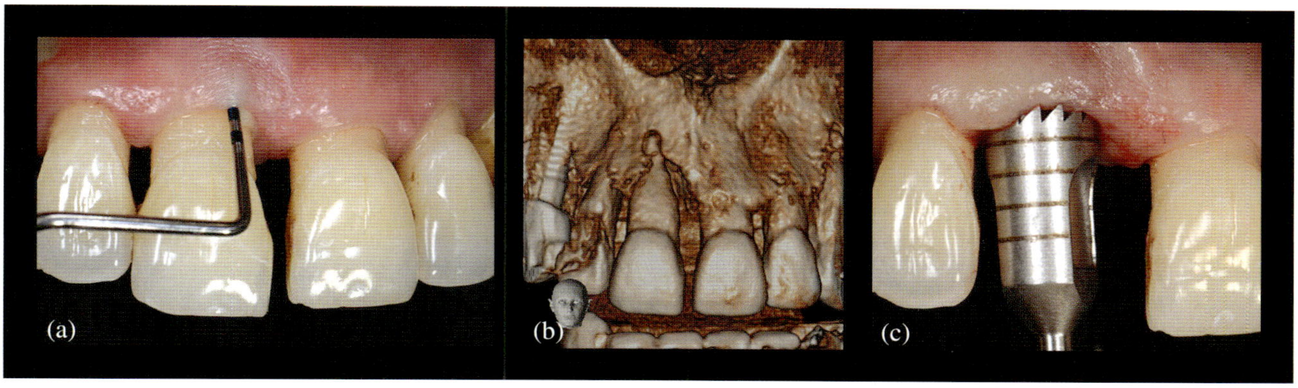

Figure 4.62 (a) and (b) Clinical and radiographical preoperative view showing failed natural tooth as a result of deep pocketing and angular bone resorption. (c) Measuring the socket orifice size by trying the core punch technique.

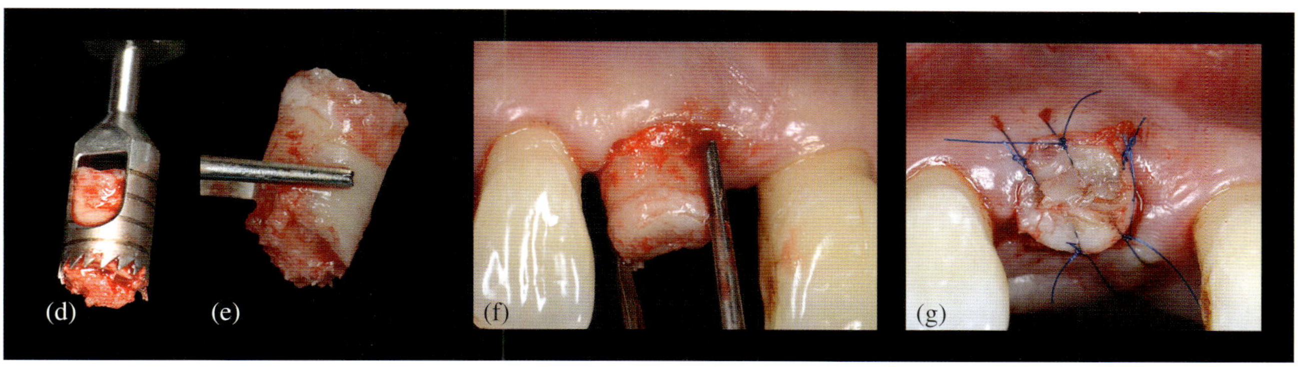

Figure 4.62 (d) and (e) Composite core harvested from the tuberosity. (f) Composite core fitted in. (g) Composite core sutured and stabilized.

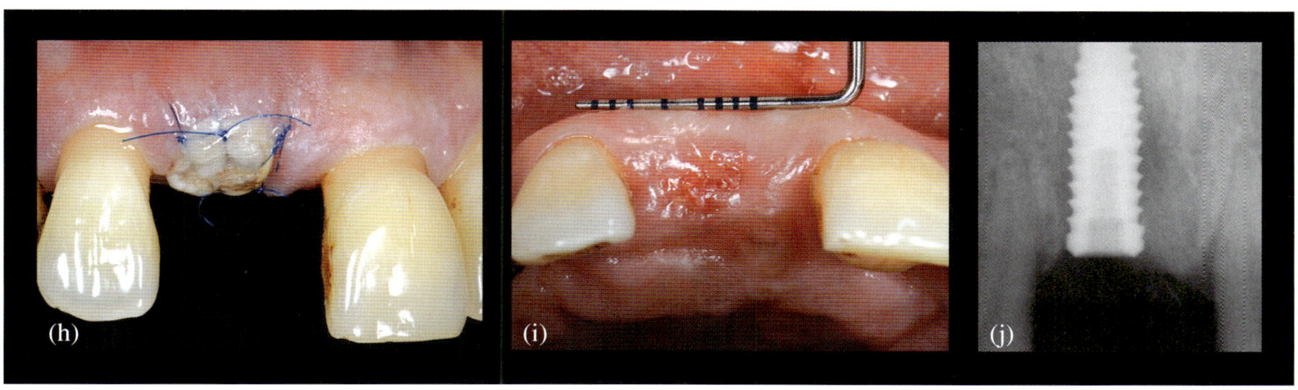

Figure 4.62 (h) Healing at one and two weeks, respectively. (i) Healing at one month after healing showing the complete restoration of the labial plate of bone and abundance of keratinization mucosa. (j) Radiographic view of implant in place.

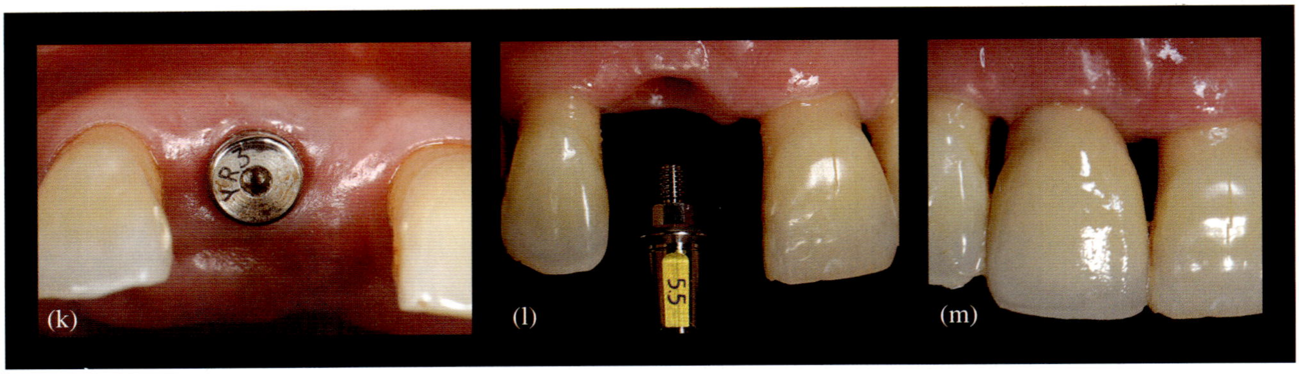

Figure 4.62 (k) Healing abutment connected. (l) Laser etched abutment base (one time abutment) is connected. (m) Final case restoration.

Upon seating, the surface of the composite graft should level up with the crestal contour of the socket; it may be positioned slightly below the surrounding marginal gingival. This is to allow for epithelial migration from the sides of the socket on top of the connective tissue graft. The connective tissue portion of the graft is then sutured to the surrounding gingival tissues. Provisional removable prosthesis should not be allowed during the first few weeks after surgery, because the composite graft may move upon pressure and become sequestrated due to premature loading of the bone that results from fitting the surface of the prosthesis.

The osteotomy hole of the donor site can be filled with any bone-grafting material or heavily packed with collagen sponge, an acrylic template may be used to seal the area of the defect until it heals by secondary intention.

This technique reduces the risk of morbidity, because the quality of the bone harvested from the tuberosity offers the best environment for regeneration and bone formation in its cancellous compartments. It also offers faster and more predictable bone regeneration inside the socket, thus improving the overall prognosis for any future implant placement. There are many defective alveolar ridges that have both soft and hard tissue defects; the use of these grafts would offer a better alternative. When there is a need for a graft that contains a cortico-cancellous component, connective tissue, periosteum, and keratinized tissues, the composite autograft becomes an outstanding solution (Elaskary 2002).

A modified approach introduced by the author to the later technique entails the use of a composite autograft in a that can be used for treating implant-related ridge deficiencies. The author introduced and evaluated the use of the composite autograft technique to treat alveolar ridge combined soft and hard tissue deficiencies around esthetic dental implants. The graft is composed of an autogenous block bone covered with periosteum and connective tissues that is attached at the same time to keratinized gingival tissue at its rim. The keratinized gingival portion of the graft aids in expanding the width of keratinized mucosa as well as the mucosal volume and quality around the dental implant (see Figure 4.63a and b).

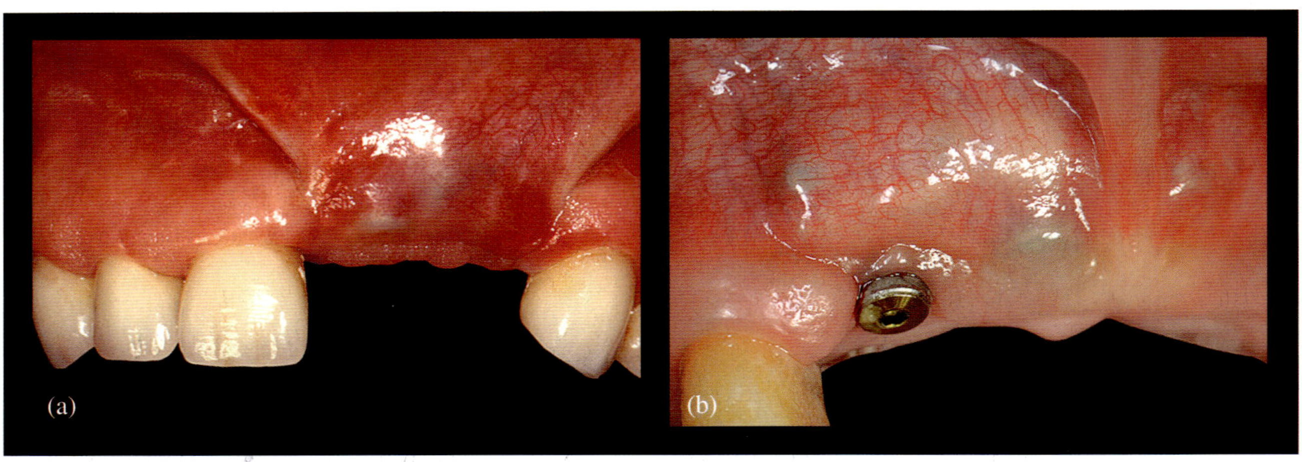

Figure 4.63 (a) and (b) A common clinical picture after autograft treatment, revealing a lack of keratinization tissue band as a result of periosteal stripping and flap advancement.

This eliminates the need to perform a staged grafting approach. The periosteum layer of the graft provides protection for the bone graft. The osseous component of the graft provides a predictable osteogenic potential to increase bone volume (Hislop, Finlay and Moos 1993) (See Figure 4.64a–t).

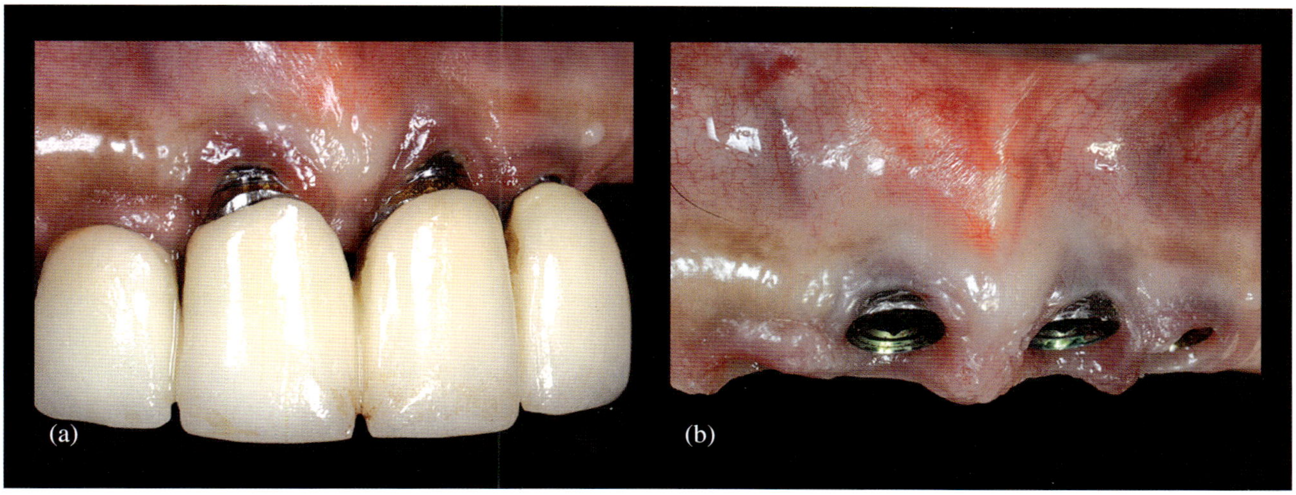

Figure 4.64 (a) Preoperative view showing lack of keratinized tissue and thin tissue phenotype. (b) Restoration removed.

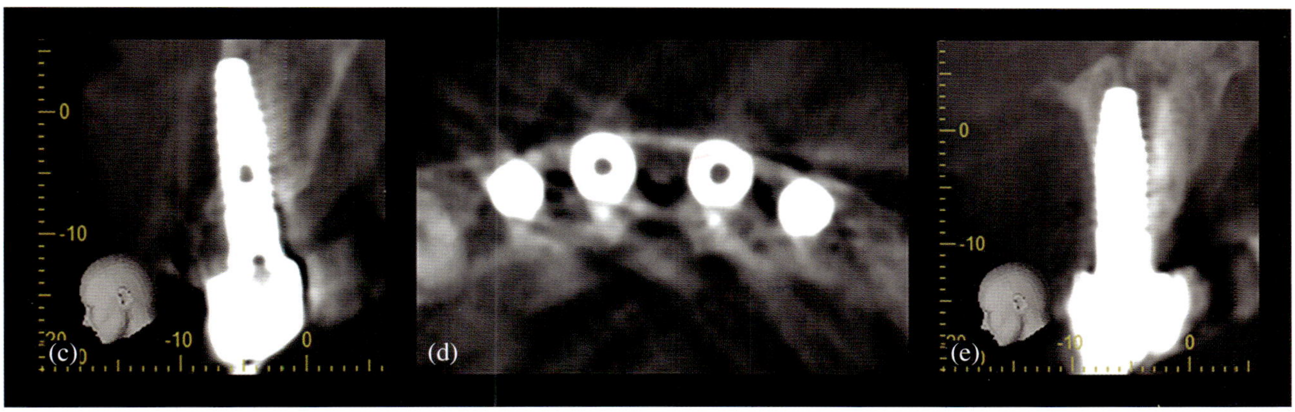

Figure 4.64 (c–e) CBCT scan showing missing labial plate of bone.

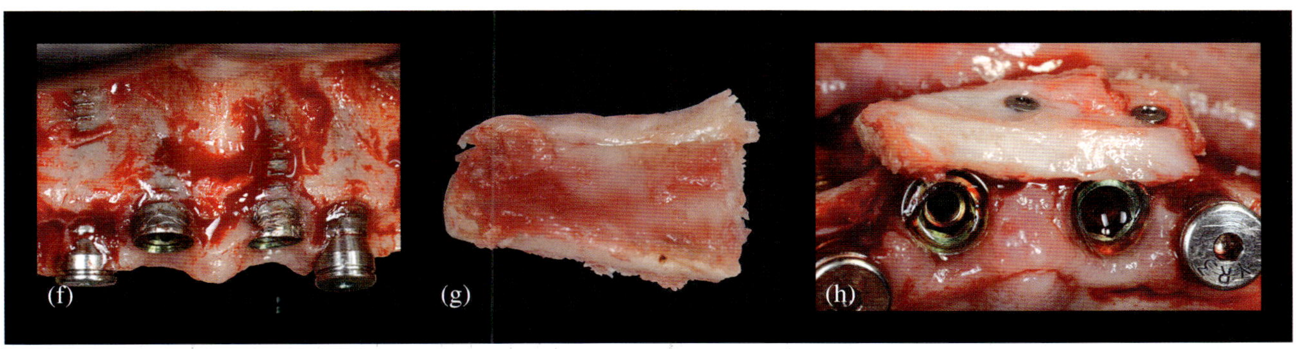

Figure 4.64 (f) Intra-operative view showing missing labial plate of bone. (g) Modified composite autograft composed of epithelial keratinized rim connective tissue with underlying periosteum and cortical bone block. (h) The autograft being fitted and stabilized with two titanium microscrews.

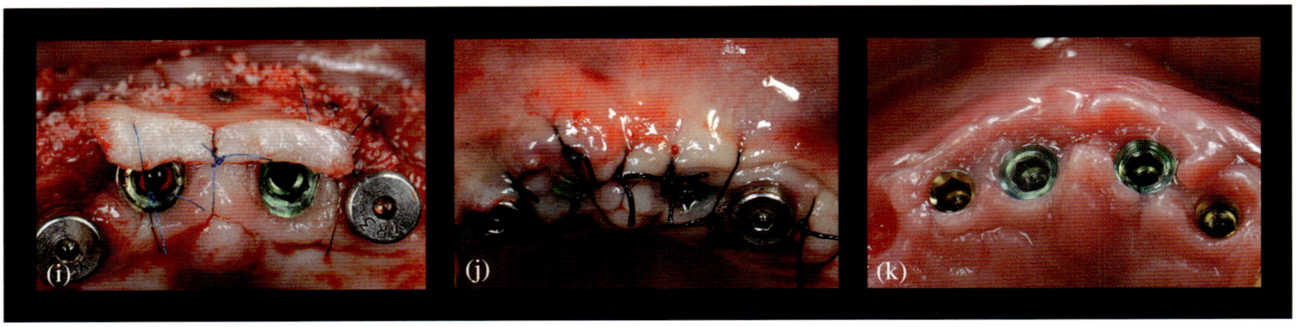

Figure 4.64 (i) Epithelial soft tissue rim is stabilized with suturing to the palatal mucosa. (j) Flap sutured. (k) Two weeks postoperative view showing abundance of keratinization and doubling the thickness of the labial volume.

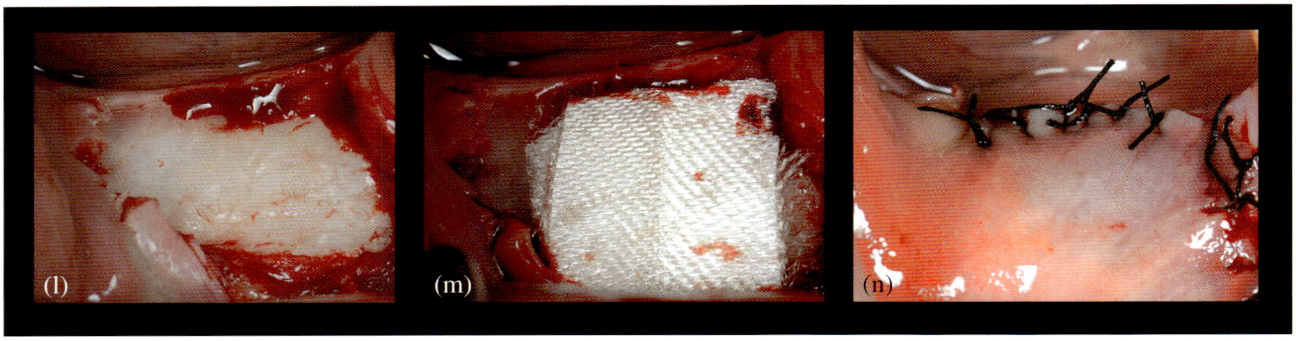

Figure 4.64 (l) Donor site (external oblique ridge) is filled with bone wax. (m) Cellulose sheet is placed on top. (n) Donor site sutured.

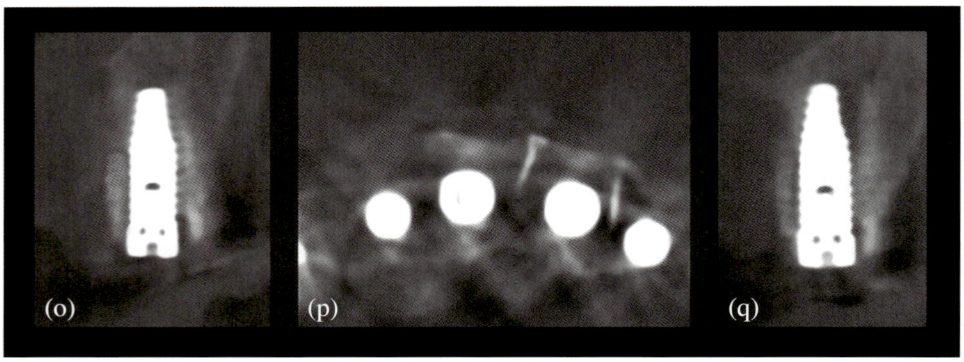

Figure 4.64 (o–q) CBCT scan showing the enhancement of the labial profile with amendment of the labial plate of bone.

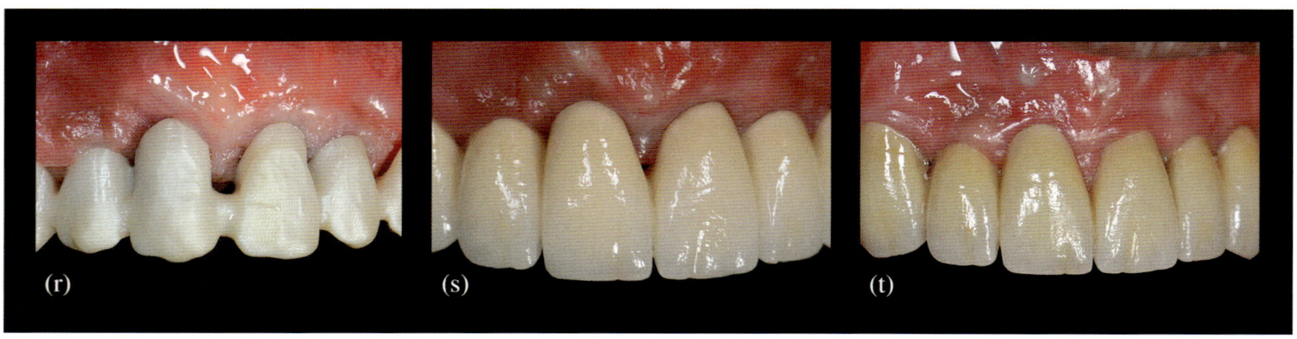

Figure 4.64 (r) Four week postoperative view showing that an excellent amount of labial tissue bulk is regenerated, and zirconia core try-in showing the abundance of tissue keratinization. (s) Final restoration in place. (t) Three years after restorative result showing marginal tissue stability.

This modified autograft has the advantage of augmenting hard and soft tissues concurrently, hence reducing the need for multiple surgical interventions. Thickening of the soft tissue will aid in long-term stabilization of the soft tissue profile. This has the advantage of reducing both the need for additional surgical procedures as well as patient morbidity (see Figure 4.65a–j).

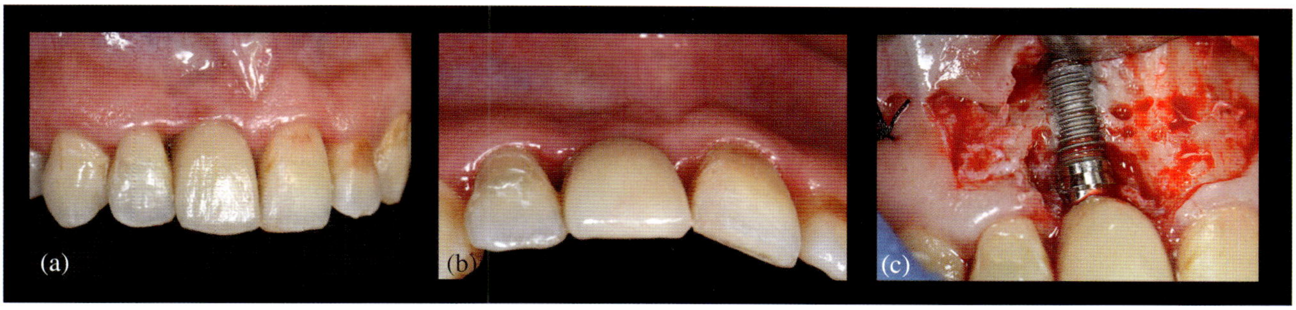

Figure 4.65 (a) and (b) Preoperative view showing loss of keratinized tissues and lost labial plate of bone (lost labial profile). (c) Full thickness periosteal flap elevated showing complete loss of labial plate of bone.

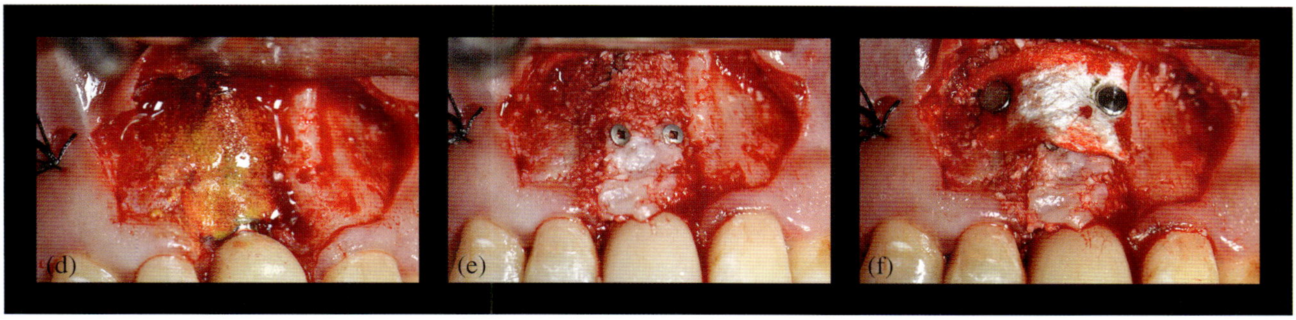

Figure 4.65 (d) Implant surface decontamination using tetracycline slurry for two minutes. (e) Modified composite bone graft stabilized with titanium screws and particulated bone graft filling the remaining gaps. (f) Collagen membrane stabilized.

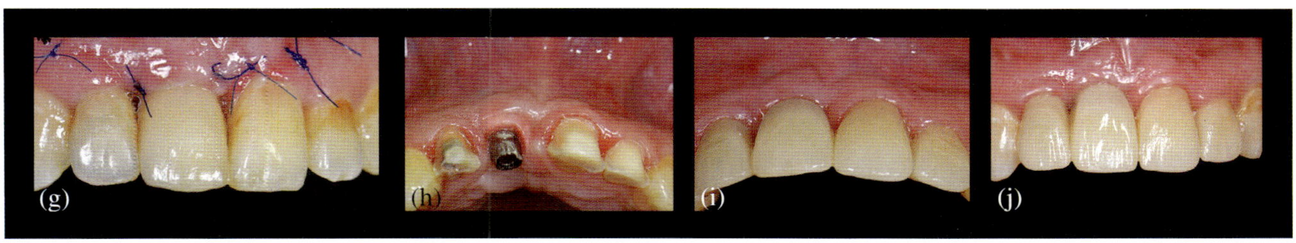

Figure 4.65 (g) One-week postoperative clinical picture. (h) Abutment connected, note the gain in soft tissue thickness well supported by underlying labial plate of bone. (i) Incisal view showing labial volume. (j) Frontal final view of the case restored.

The procedure involves obtaining accurate patient medical history, and carrying out soft and hard tissue examinations. Preoperative CBCT is taken to assess the amount of the osseous defect as well as the potential location of donor site of the graft. A local anesthetic (Articaine hydrochloride, Ubistesin forte, 3M ESPE) of $40\,mg\,mL^{-1}$, with adrenaline (1:80 000) was administered at both the recipient and donor sites, the composite autograft is harvested either from the external oblique ridge or the tuberosity area through the use of a piezotome ultrasonic surgery unit (Satelec, Acteon). At the donor site, an initial buccal-sulcular incision from the retromolar area to the second premolar region was made. An incision up the ramus was made lateral to the retromolar pad at the height of the occlusal plane. A partial thickness flap instead of a full mucoperiosteal flap was raised, exposing the lateral aspect of the ramus, while vertical and horizontal cuts of the graft were made, with the superior horizontal cut of the graft extended beyond the raised partial thickness flap border to include 2–3 mm of gingival tissue. A thin chisel was then used to gently tap the cut sections along their entire length. This was followed by a wider-wedged chisel, which was inserted and levered to pry free the bone block segment, hence completing the greenstick fracture of the graft from the donor area, hemostasis was achieved at the donor site by using bone wax and any hemostatic gauze (Salvin dental, USA). Primary closure of the donor site was completed after removal and fixation of the composite graft to the recipient site.

Any pre-existing implant restorations and abutments should be first removed. At the recipient site, a partial thickness mucoperiosteal flap is reflected until reaching the osseous defect, where it becomes a full thickness flap. All granulation tissues were removed to expose the underlying bone. The modified composite autograft is trimmed and contoured for a better fit into the recipient site and then fixed to the recipient site with two to three fixation micro-titanium screws, positioned so that the keratinized tissue rim of the graft matches the adjacent gingival margins. Bone particulates collected during drilling were mixed with minerOss (BioHorizons, Birmingham, AL, USA) to fill the small discrepancies and spaces around the block graft. Interrupted sutures (5-0 Polyglactin, Ethicon, Johnson & Johnson, and Boston, MA) were further used to secure the gingival tissue of the composite graft to the palatal tissue of the recipient site. The mucoperiosteal flap at the recipient site was then closed without tension using interrupted nylon 6.0 sutures (B Braun, Tuttlingen, Germany). The patient was given postoperative instructions and prescribed 500 mg Amoxicillin to be taken three times a day for five days. Patients were seen for postoperative care at one day, one week, one month, and four months. A post-treatment CBCT was also carried out at the fourth month to check the stability and integration of the graft to the underlying bed. Impressions were then taken to fabricate the final implant crowns (see Figure 4.66a–i).

It is worth noting that tension-free closure of the recipient site is imperative to the success of the treatment as the main risk with onlay bone grafts is wound dehiscence and graft exposure. The CBCT follow-up revealed a thick layer of bone on the buccal aspect of the dental implants. This provides an insight that a modified composite autograft is a predictable alternative procedure for treating implant-related gingival

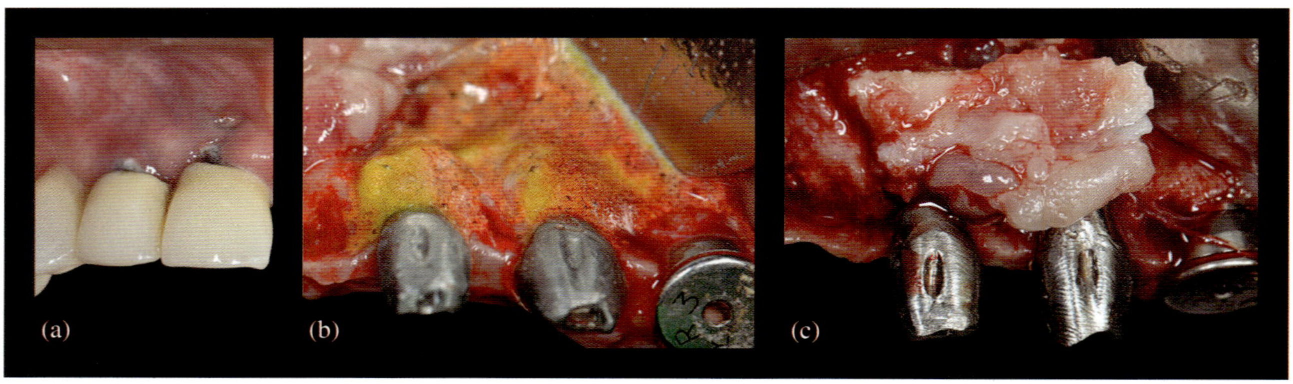

Figure 4.66 (a) Front view of three unites implant supported restoration that reveals soft tissue thinning and fenestrations. (b) Decontamination of the implant surface with tetracycline slurry for two minutes. (c) Modified composite graft being tried in.

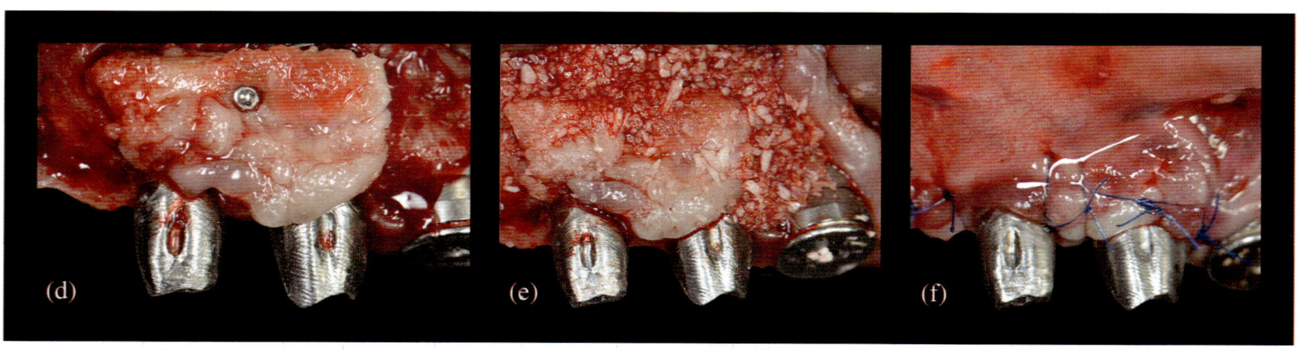

Figure 4.66 (d) Modified composite graft being stabilized with one micro-screw. (e) Particulated bone graft filled adjacent to the modified composite graft. (f) Flap sutured.

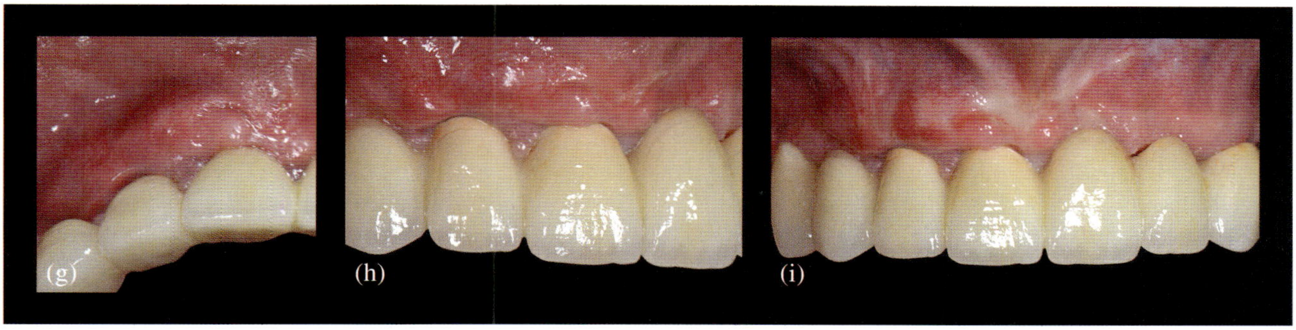

Figure 4.66 (g) Incisal view of the case showing the improved labial profile. (h) and (i) Frontal view of the case finally restored.

deficiencies without having to go through multiple surgical interventions.

As in the case with the free gingival graft, a thick blood clot between the donor's and the host's tissue would disrupt circulation during the initial phase of healing and increase the risk of necrosis. Therefore, the graft must be well fitted to the recipient site. It is thus advisable to maintain a constant pressure over the gingival site of the modified composite autograft against the recipient site with a piece of wet gauze for a few minutes to minimize the possible formation of hematoma. Similarly for any bone grafting procedure to achieve a predictable outcome, principles such as tension-free coverage, space creation, and wound stability must be respected (Buser et al. 1990) (see Figure 4.67a–h).

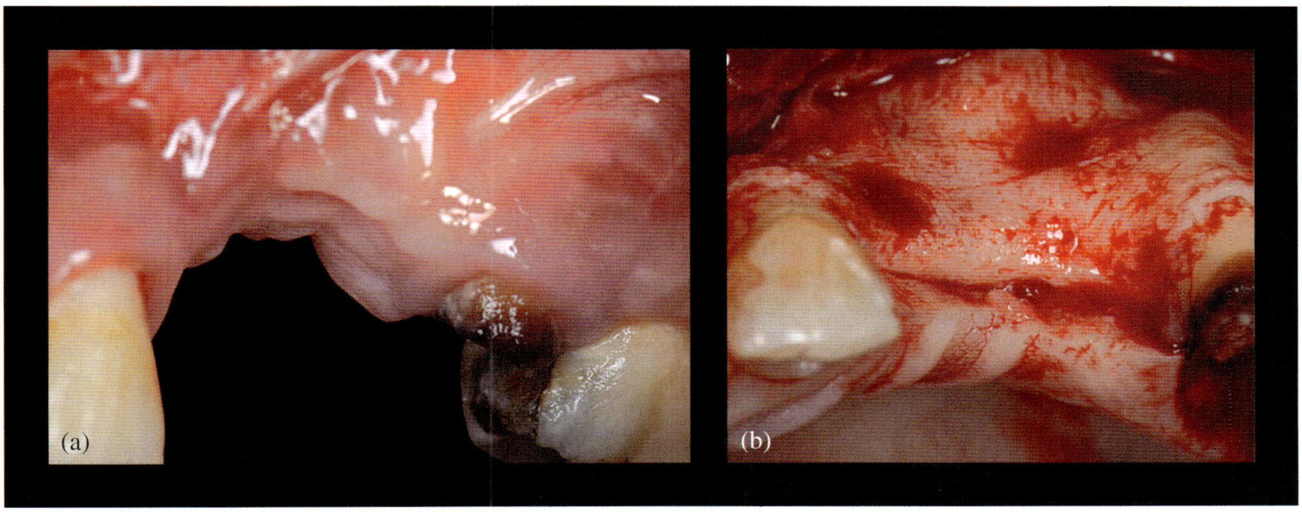

Figure 4.67 (a) Loss of horizontal and vertical bone height along with the deficiency of the keratinized tissue band. (b) Intraoperative view showing lack of labial bone bulk.

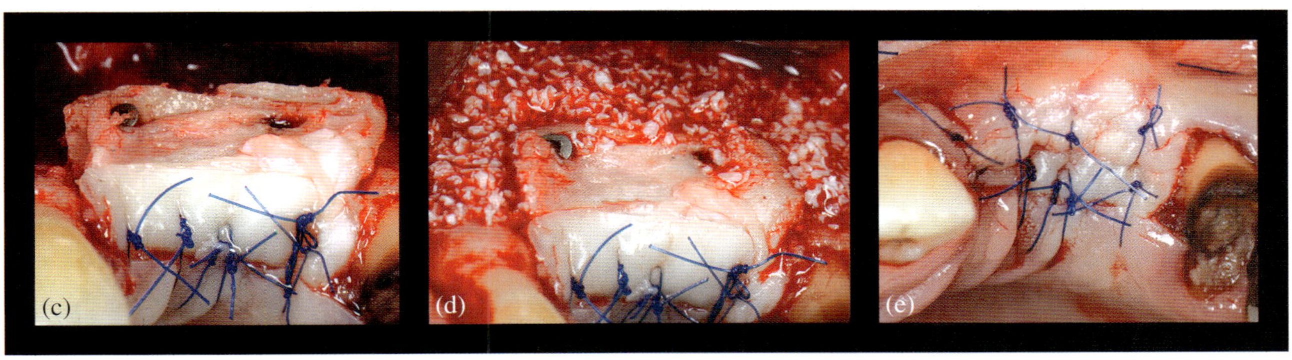

Figure 4.67 (c–d) Modified composite autograft fitted and stabilized. (e) Flap sutured.

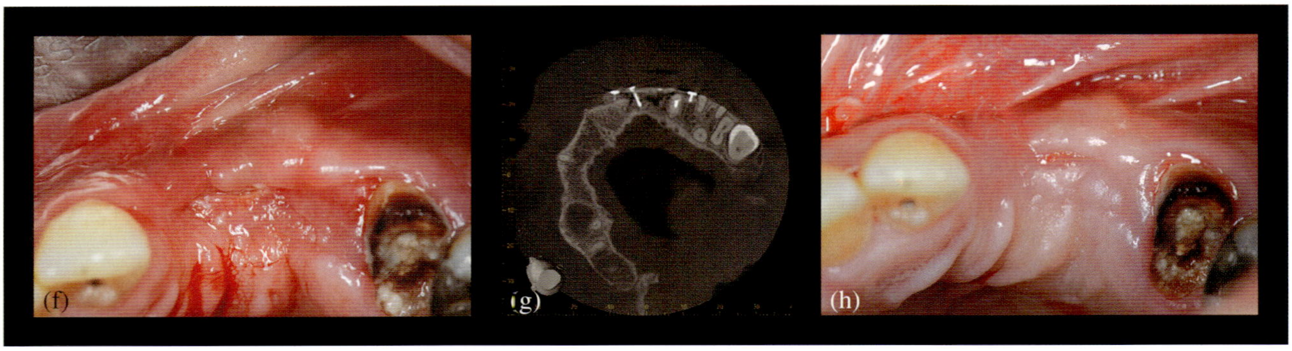

Figure 4.67 (f) Three weeks after healing. (g) CBCT scan showing the restoration of missing labial tissue volume. (h) Two months of healing showing abundance of keratinization tissue and restoration of labial bulk in horizontal direction.

4.6 Conclusion

Dental implantology continues to evolve with new advances in all aspects of dentistry, including the developments of new surgical and prosthodontic techniques and armamentarium. Nuances in esthetic implantology have been followed over decades. Novel concepts have emerged for enhanced treatment planning and diagnosis, guided surgeries, and microsurgery. With the treatment protocols detailed earlier in this chapter, there is no strict indication for the use of each method to treat a particular condition. It is the clinician's decision to select the best, fastest, and easiest method that he or she can master. The purpose of these techniques is to offer a wide variety of treatment options for clinicians to choose from, without any obligation or restriction, which cover most clinical indications (see Figure 4.68a–t).

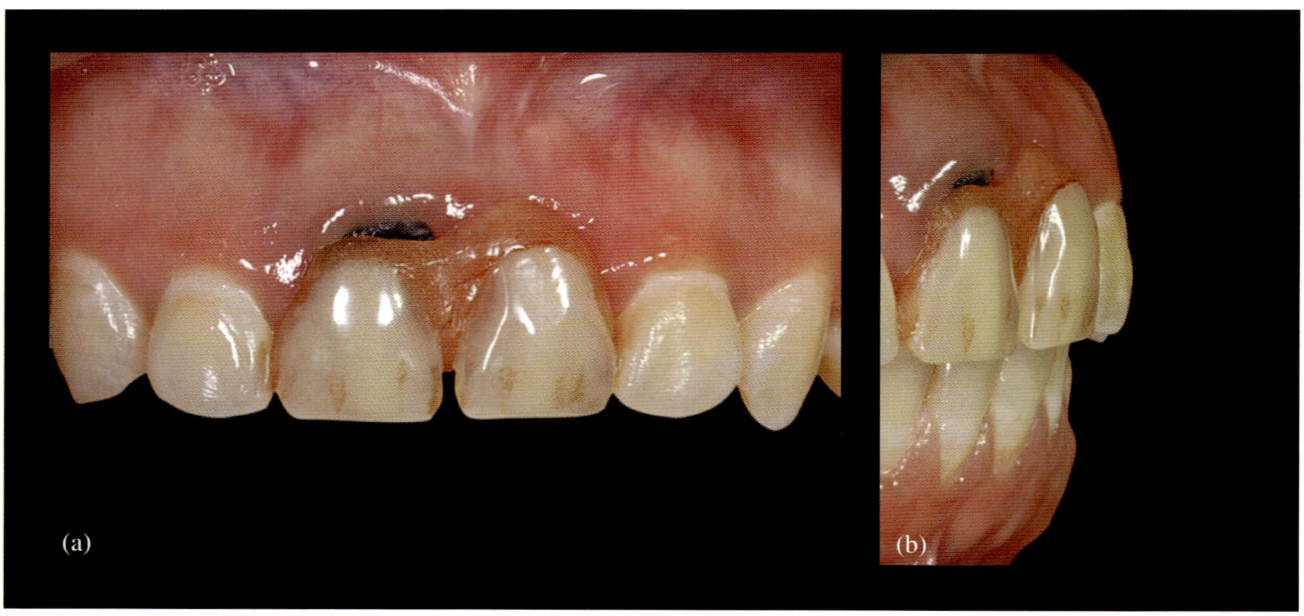

Figure 4.68 (a) and (b) Preoperative clinical frontal and side views of poor prosthetic construction of left missing maxillary central incisors and failed right central maxillary incisor. Note the thin nature of the local tissues.

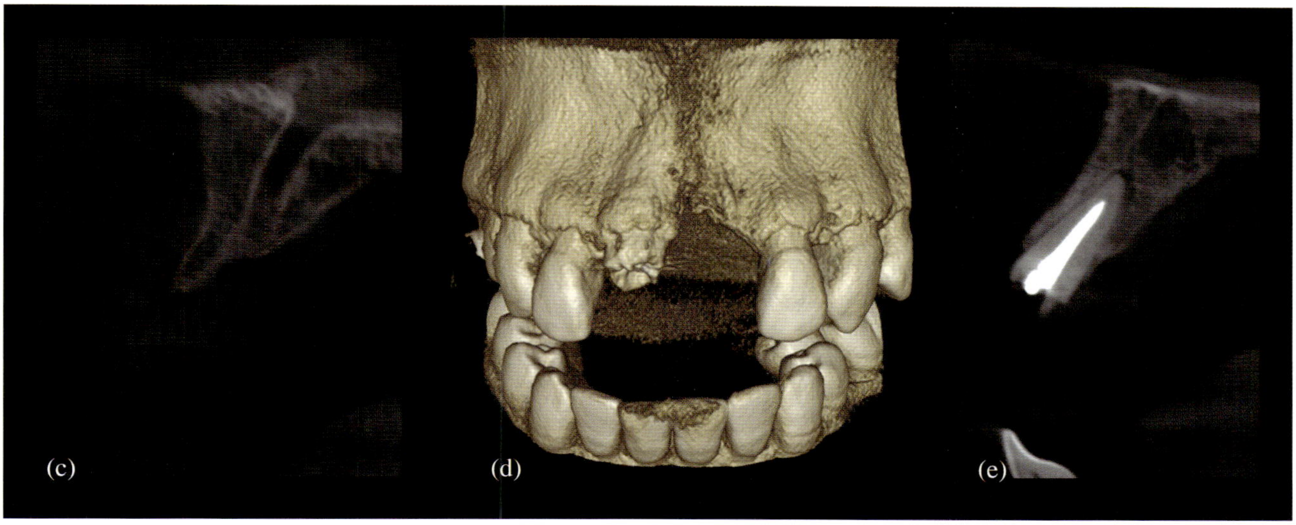

Figure 4.68 (c–e) CBCT scan sections showing the vertical bone deficiency in the place of the left central incisor, and the thin nature of the labial plate of bone.

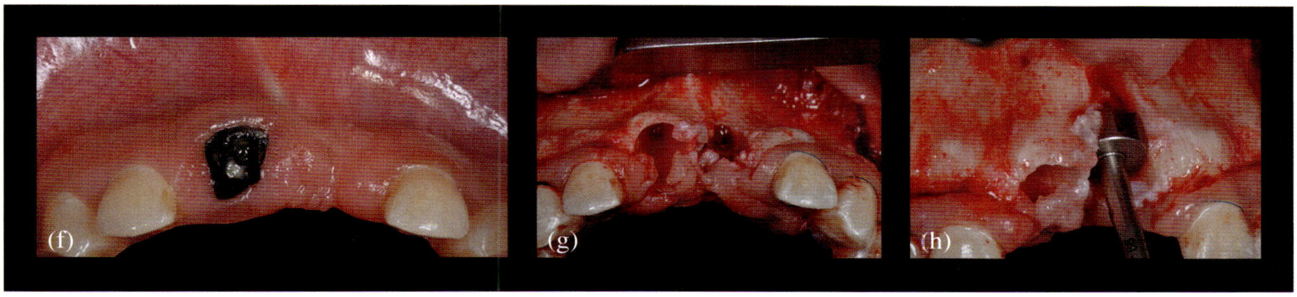

Figure 4.68 (f) Prosthetics removed. (g) Intra-operative view at the surgery time. (h) Preparing the osseous bed for the allograft bone ring.

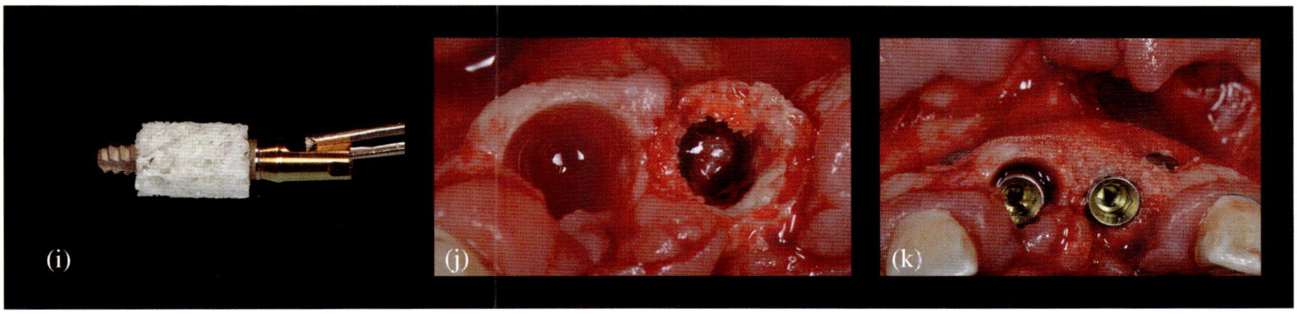

Figure 4.68 (i) The bone ring is manipulated and trimmed to fit the implant fixture size. (j) The bone ring is fitted in place showing the restoration of the labial plate of bone continuity and the vertical defect. (k) Two implants placed in the location and a collagen membrane on top is stabilized with two membrane tacs.

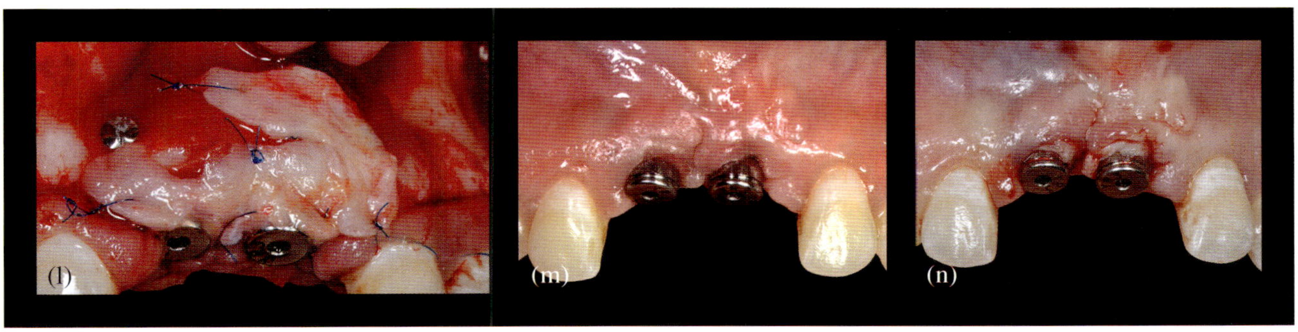

Figure 4.68 (l) Connective tissue graft is secured on top of the grafted complex. (m) Two weeks postoperative healing. (n) One month post-surgery showing another connective tissue graft is used to add more marginal stability and reform he gingival margins.

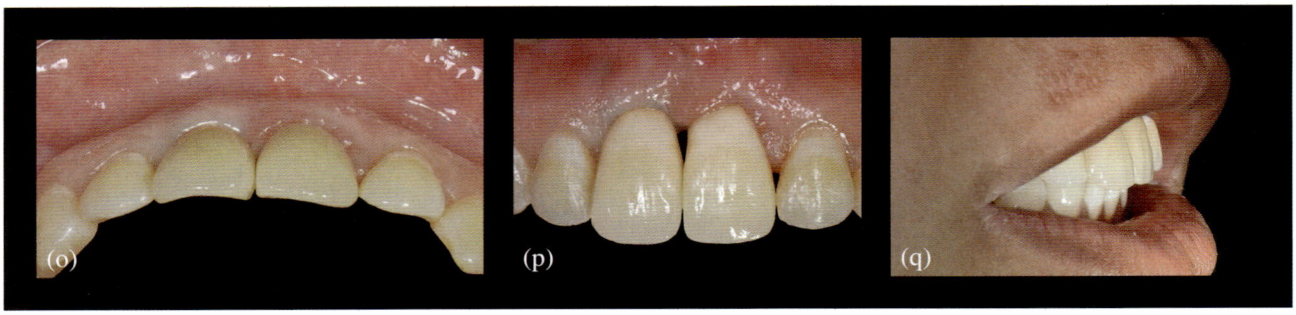

Figure 4.68 (o) and (p) Incisal and facial views showing the final prosthetics in place. (q) Profile extra-oral view of the patient post restorative.

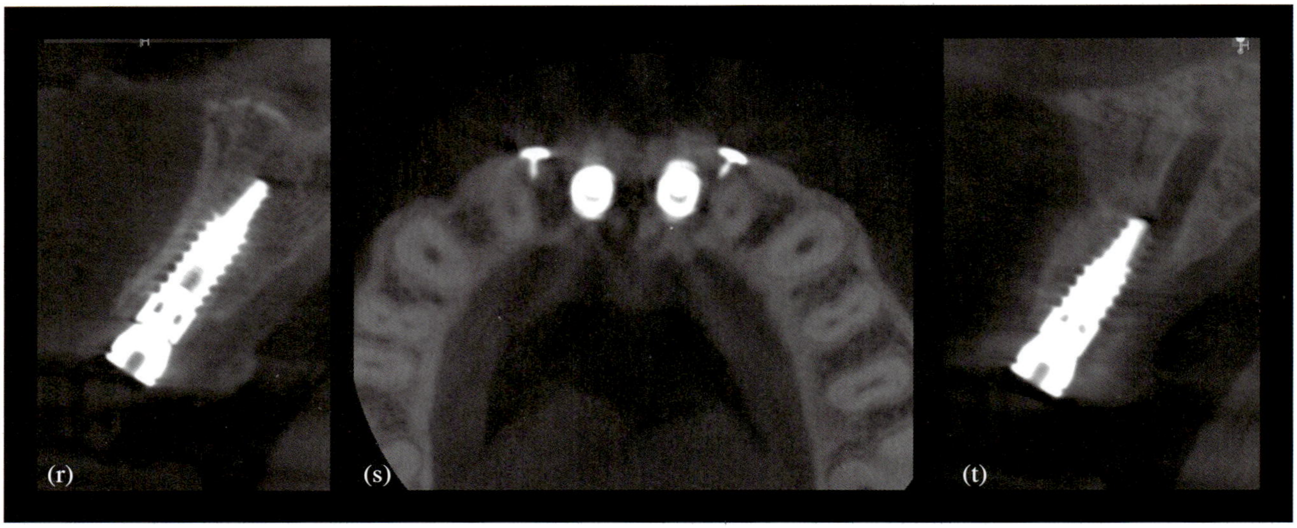

Figure 4.68 (r–t) CBCT scans showing the labial plate of bone restored.

References

Acocella, A., Bertolai, R., Ellis, E. 3rd et al. (2012). Maxillary alveolar ridge reconstruction with monocortical fresh-frozen bone blocks: a clinical, histological and histomorphometric study. *J. Craniomaxillofac. Surg.* 40 (6): 525–533.

Al-Ansari, B.H. and Morris, R.R. (1998). Placement of dental implants without flap surger: a clinical report. *Int. J. Oral Maxillofac. Implants* 13 (6): 861–865.

Albrektsson, T., Buser, D., and Sennerby, L. (2012). Crestal bone loss and oral implants. *Clin. Implant Dent. Relat. Res.* 14 (6): 783–791.

Albrektsson, T., Zarb, G., Worthington, P., and Eriksson, A.R. (1986). The long-term efficacy of currently used dental implants: a review and proposed criteria of success. *Int. J. Oral Maxillofac. Implants* 1: 11–25.

Alsaadi, G., Quiynen, M., Komärek, A., and van Steenberghe, D. (2007). Impact of local systematic factors on the incidence of oral implant failures, up to abutment connection. *J. Clin. Periodontol.* 34: 610–617.

Álvarez-Camino, J.-C., Valmaseda-Castellón, E., and Gay-Escoda, C. (2013). Implants placed in fresh sockets associated to periapical infections. *Med. Oral Patol. Oral Cir. Bucal.* 18 (5): September 1): e780–e785.

Andersson, B., Glauser, R., Maglione, M., and Taylor, A. (2003). Ceramic implant abutments for short-span FPDs: a prospective 5 year multicenter study. *Int. J. Prosthodont.* 16 (6): 640–646.

Andreasen, F.M., Andreasen, J.O., and Andersson, M.C. (2007). *Textbook and Color Atlas of Traumatic Injuries to the Teeth*, 4e. Oxford: Blackwell.

Annibali, S., Bignozzi, I., Cristalli, M.P. et al. (2012). Peri-implant marginal bone level: a systematic review and meta-analysis of studies comparing platform switching versus conventionally restored implants. *J. Clin. Periodontol.* 39 (11): 1097–1113.

Aparicio, C., Rangert, B., and Sennerby, L. (2003). Immediate/early loading of dental implants: a report from the Sociedad Espanola de Implants World Congress consensus meeting in Barcelona, Spain 2002. *Clin. Implant Dent. Relat. Res.* 5 (1): 57–60.

Araujo, M.G., Berglundh, H., and Lindhe, J. (1998). GTR treatment of degree III furcation defects with 2 different resorbable barriers. An experiemental study in dogs. *J. Clin. Periodontol.* 25 (3): 253–259.

Araujo, M.G. and Lindhe, J. (2005). Dimensional ridge alterations following tooth extraction. An experimental study in the dog. *J. Clin. Periodontol.* 32: 212–218.

Araujo, M.G. and Lindhe, J. (2009). Ridge preservation with the use of Bio-Oss collagen: a 6-month study in the dog. *Clin. Oral Implants Res.* 20 (5): 433–440.

Artzi, Z., Tal, H., and Dayan, D. (2000). Porous bovine bone mineral in healing of human extraction sockets. Part 1: Histomorphometric evaluations at 9 months. *J. Periodontol.* 71 (6): 1015–1023.

Ashman, A. (2000). Ridge preservation: important buzzwords in dentistry. *Gen. Dent.* 48 (3): 304–312.

Ayangco, L. and Sheridan, P.J. (2001). Development and treatment of retrograde peri-implantitis involving a site with a history of failed endodontic and apicoectomy procedures: a series of reports. *Int. J. Oral Maxillofac. Implants* 16: 412–417.

Bahat, O. and Handelsman, M. (1996). Use of wide implants and double implants in the posterior jaw: a clinical report. *Int. J. Oral Maxillofac. Implants* 11: 379–386.

Balasundaram, G., Sato, M., and Webster, T.J. (2006). Using hydroxyapatite nanoparticles and decreased crystallinity to promote osteoblast adhesion similar to functionalizing with RGD. *Biomaterials* 27: 2798–2805.

Barone, A., Ricci, M., Tonelli, P. et al. (2013). Tissue changes of extraction sockets in humans: a comparison of spontaneous healing vs. ridge preservation with secondary soft tissue healing. *Clin. Oral Implants Res.* 24: 1231–1237.

Barrows, T.H. (1986). Degradable implant materials: a review of synthetic absorbable polymers and their applications. *Clin. Mater.* 1: 233–257.

Barzilay, I. (1993). Immediate implants: their current status. *Int. J. Prosthodont.* 6 (2): 169–175.

Beagle, J.R. (2013). *Surgical Essentials of Immediate Implant Dentistry*, 32. Oxford, UK: Wiley-Blackwell.

Becker, B.E., Becker, W., Ricci, A., and Geurs, N. (1998). A prospective clinical trial of endosseous screw-shaped implants placed at the time of tooth extraction without augmentation. *J. Periodontol.* 69 (8): 920–926.

Becker, S. (2006). Osteopromotion by beta-tricalcium phosphate/bone marrow hybrid implant for use in spine surgery. *Spine* 31 (1): 11–17.

Becker, W. (2005). Immediate implant placement: diagnosis, treatment planning and treatment steps/or successful outomes. *J. Calif. Dent. Assoc.* 33 (4): 303–310.

Becker, W. and Becker, B.E. (1990). Guided tissue regeneration for implants placed into extraction sockets and for implant dehiscences: surgical techniques and case report. *Int. J. Periodontics Restorative Dent.* 10: 376–391.

Becker, W. and Goldstein, M. (2000). Immediate implant placement: treatment planning and surgical steps for successful outcome. *Periodontol. 2000* 47: 79–89.

Bilir, A., Aybar, B., Tanrikulu, S.H. et al. (2007). Biocompatibility of different barrier membranes in cultures of human CRL 11372 osteoblast-like cells: an immunohistochemical study. *Clin. Oral Implants Res.* 18: 46–52.

Blanes, R.J., Bernard, J.P., Blanes, Z.M., and Belser, U.C. (2007). A 10-year prospective study of ITI dental implants placed in the posterior region. II: influence of the crown to implant ratio and different prosthetic treatment modalities on crestal bone loss. *Clin. Oral Implants Res.* 18 (6): 707–714.

Botticelli, D., Berglundh, T., and Lindhe, J. (2004). Hard tissue alterations following immediate implant placement in extraction sites. *J. Clin. Periodontol.* 31: 820–828.

Botticelli, D., Berglundh, T., Buser, D., and Lindhe, J. (2003). The jumping distance revisited. An experimental study in the dog. *Clin. Oral Implants Res.* 14 (1): 35–42.

Botticelli, D., Persson, L.G., Lindhe, J., and Berglundh, T. (2006). Bone tissue formation adjacent to implants placed in fresh extraction socket: an experimental study in dogs. *Clin. Oral Implants Res.* 17 (4): 351–358.

Branemark, P.I., Hansson, B.O., Adell, R. et al. (1977). Osseointegrated implants in the treatment of the edentulous jaw. Experience from a 10-year period. *Scand. J. Plast. Reconstr. Surg. Suppl.* 16: 1–132.

Brink, J., Meraw, S.J., and Sarment, D.P. (2007). Influence of implant diameter on surrounding bone. *Clin. Oral Implants Res.* 18: 563–568.

Buser, D., Bragger, U., Lang, N.P., and Nyman, S. (1990). Regeneration and enlargement of jaw bone using guided tissue regeneration. *Clin. Oral Implants Res.* 1 (1): 22–32.

Buser, D., Martin, W., and Belser, U.C. (2004). Optimizing esthetics for implant restorations in the anterior maxilla: anatomic and surgical considerations. *Int. J. Oral Maxillofac. Implants* 19 (Suppl): 43–61.

Camargo, P.M., Lekovic, V., Weinlaender, M. et al. (2002). Platelet-rich plasma and bovine porous bone mineral combined with guided tissue regeneration in the treatment of intrabony defects in humans. *J. Periodontal Res.* 37: 300–306.

Campelo, L.D. and Camara, J.R. (2002). Flapless implant surgery: a 10 year clinical retrospective analysis. *Int. J. Oral Maxillofac. Implants* 17 (2): 271–276.

Capelli, M., Testori, T., Galli, F. et al. (2013). Implant–buccal plate distance as diagnostic parameter: a prospective cohort study on implant placement in fresh extraction sockets. *J. Periodontol.* 84 (12): 1768–1774.

Cardaropoli, G., Araújo, M., Hayacibara, R. et al. (2005). Healing of extraction sockets and surgically produced – augmented and non-augmented – defects in the alveolar ridge. An experimental study in the dog. *J. Clin. Periodontol.* 32: 435–440.

Carini, F., Longoni, S., Amosso, E. et al. (2014). Bone augmentation with TiMesh. Autologous bone versus autologous bone and bone substitutes. A systematic review. *Ann Stomatol (Roma)* 5 (Suppl 2 to No. 2): 27–36.

Casap, N., Zeltser, C., Wexler, A. et al. (2007). Immediate placement of dental implants into debrided infected dentoalveolar sockets. *J. Oral Maxillofac. Surg.* 65: 384–392.

Cheah, C.W., Vaithilingam, R.D., Siar, C.H. et al. (2014). Histologic, histomorphometric, and cone-beam computerized tomography analyses of calcium sulfate and platelet-rich plasma in socket preservation: a pilot study. *Implant Dent.* 23 (5): 593–601.

Chen, S.T. and Buser, D. (2014). Esthetic outcomes following immediate and early implant placement in the anterior maxilla – a systematic review. *Int. J. Oral Maxillofac. Implants* 29 (Suppl): 186–215.

Chen, S.T., Darby, I.B., and Reynolds, E.C. (2007). A prospective clinical study of non-submerged immediate implants: clinical outcomes and esthetic results. *Clin. Oral Implants Res.* 18 (5): 552–562.

Chen, S.T., Wilson, T.G. Jr., and Hämmerle, C.H. (2004). Immediate or early placement of implants following tooth extraction: review of biologic basis, clinical procedures, and outcomes. *Int. J. Oral Maxillofac. Implants* 19 (Suppl): 12–25.

Chiapasco, M., Abati, S., Romeo, E., and Vogel, G. (1999). Clinical outcomes of autogenous bone blocks or guided bone regeneration with e-PTFE membranes for the reconstruction of narrow edentulous ridges. *Clin. Oral Implants Res.* 10 (4): 278–288.

Chiapasco, M., Romeo, E., Casentini, P., and Rimondini, L. (2004). Alveolar distraction osteogenesis vs. vertical guided bone regeneration for the correction of vertically deficient edentulous ridges: a 1–3 year prospective study on humans. *Clin. Oral Implants Res.* 15 (1): 82–95.

Cohenca, N. and Stabholz, A. (2007). Decoronation – a conservative method to treat ankylosed teeth for preservation of alveolar ridge prior to permanent prosthetic reconstruction: literature review and case presentation. *Dent. Traumatol.* 23 (2): 87–94.

Coonts, B.A., Whitman, S.L., O'Donnell, M. et al. (1998). Biodegradation and biocompatibility of a guided tissue regeneration barrier membrane formed from a liquid polymer material. *J. Biomed. Mater. Res.* 42: 303–311.

Costerton, J.W., Montanaro, L., and Arciola, C.R. (2005). Biofilm in implant infections: its production and regulation. *Int. J. Artif. Organs* 28 (1): 1062–1068.

Costerton, J.W., Stewart, P.S., and Greenberg, E.P. (1999). Bacterial biofilms: a common cause of persistent infections. *Science* 284: 1318–1322.

Covani, U., Barone, A., Cornelini, R., and Crespi, R. (2004). Soft tissue healing around implants placed immediately after tooth extraction without incision: a clinical report. *Int. J. Oral Maxillofac. Implants* 19: 549–553.

Crespi, R., Capparè, P., and Gherlone, E. (2010). Fresh-socket implants in periapical infected sites in humans. *J. Periodontol.* 81: 378–383.

Crespi, R., Vinci, R., Capparè, P. et al. (2007). Calvarial versus iliac crest for autologous bone graft material for a sinus lift procedure: a histomorphometric study. *Int. J. Oral Maxillofac. Implants* 22 (4): 527–532.

Dahlin, C., Sennerby, L., Lekholm, U. et al. (1989). Generation of new bone around titanium implants using a membrane technique: an experimental study in rabbits. *Int. J. Oral Maxillofac. Implants* 4: 19–25.

De Sanctis, M. and Zucchelli, G. (1996). Guided tissue regeneration with a resorbable barrier membrane (Vicryl) for the management of buccal recession: a case report. *Int. J. Periodontics Restorative Dent.* 16: 435–441.

De Wijs, F.L., Cune, M.S., and De Putter, C. (1995). Delayed implants in the anterior maxilla with the IMZ-implant system. *J. Oral Rehabil.* 22 (5): 319–326.

Degidi, M. and Piattelli, A. (2003). Immediate functional and non-functional loading of dental implants: a 2 to 60 month follow-up study of 646 titanium implants. *J. Periodontol.* 74 (2): 225–241.

Degidi, M., Piattelli, A., Iezzi, G., and Carinci, F. (2007). Wide-diameter implants: analysis of clinical outcome of 304 fixtures. *J. Periodontol.* 78: 52–58.

Del Fabbro, M., Boggian, C., and Taschieri, S. (2009). Immediate implant placement into fresh extraction sites with chronic periapical pathologic features combined with plasma rich in growth factors: preliminary results of single-cohort study. *J. Oral Maxillofac. Surg.* 67: 2476–2484.

Deng, F., Zhang, H., Zhang, H. et al. (2010). A comparison of clinical outcomes for implants placed in fresh extraction sockets versus healed sites in periodontally compromised patients: a 1-year follow-up report. *Int. J. Oral Maxillofac. Implants* 25: 1036–1040.

Eckert, S.E., Meraw, S.J., Weaver, A.L., and Lohse, C.M. (2001). Early experience with wide platform MKII implants. Part I: implant survival. Part II: evaluation of risk factors involving implant survival. *Int. J. Oral Maxillofac. Implants* 16: 208–216.

Elaskary, A.S. (2002). The use of connective tissue grafts to enhance the esthetic outcome of implant treatment. *J. Prosthet. Dent.* 87: 129–132.

Elaskary, A.S. (2008). *Fundamentals of Esthetic Implant Dentistry*. Blackwell publishing –John Wiley.

Elian, N., Cho, S.C., Froum, S. et al. (2007). A simplified socket classification and repair technique. *Pract. Proced. Aesthet. Dent.* 19 (2): 99–104.

Eskow, A.J. (2013). Evaluation of healing following tooth extraction with ridge preservation using cortical versus cancellous freeze-dried bone allograft. *J. Periodontol.* 85 (4): 1–10.

Evans, C.D. and Chen, S.T. (2008). Esthetic outcomes of immediate implant placements. *Clin. Oral Implants Res.* 19 (1): 73–80.

Evian, C.I., Emling, R., Rosenberg, E.S. et al. (2004). Retrospective analysis of implant survival and the influence of periodontal disease and immediate placement on long-term results. *Int. J. Oral Maxillofac. Implants* 19: 393–398.

Ferrus, J., Cecchinato, D., Pjetursson, E.B. et al. (2010). Factors influencing ridge alterations following immediate implant placement into extraction sockets. *Clin. Oral Implants Res.* 21 (1): 22–29.

Filippi, A., Pohl, Y., and von Arx, T. (2001). Decoronation of an ankylosed tooth for preservation of alveolar bone prior to implant placement. *Dent. Traumatol.* 17 (2): 93–95.

Friberg, B., Ekestubbe, A., and Sennerby, L. (2002). Clinical outcome of Brånemark System implants of various diameters: A retrospective study. *Int. J. Oral Max. Fac. Implants* 17 (5): 671–677.

Froum, S., Cho, S.C., Rosenberg, E. et al. (2002). Histological comparison of healing extraction sockets implanted with bioactive glass or demineralized freeze-dried bone allograft: a pilot study. *J. Periodontol.* 73: 94–102.

Furhauser, R., Florescu, D., Benesch, T. et al. (2005). Evaluation of soft tissue around single-tooth implant crowns: the pink esthetic score. *Clin. Oral Implants Res.* 16 (6): 639–644.

Ganeles, J. and Wismeijer, D. (2004). Early and immediately restored and loaded dental implants for single-tooth and partial arch applications. *Int. J. Oral Maxillofac. Implants* 19: 92–102.

Garg, A.K. (2004). Augmentation and grafting of the maxillary anterior alveolar ridge. In: *Bone Biology, Harvesting and Grafting for Dental Implants: Rational and Clinical Application* (ed. A.K. Garg), 213–240. Quintessence Publishing Co. Inc.

Geng, W., Liu, C., Su, Y. et al. (2015). Accuracy of different types of computer-aided design/computer-aided manufacturing surgical guides for dental implant placement. *Int. J. Clin. Exp. Med.* 8: 8442–8449.

Gielkens, P.F., Schortinghuis, J., de Jong, J.R. et al. (2008). Vivosorb, Bio-Gide, and Gore-Tex as barrier membranes in rat mandibular defects: an evaluation by microradiography and micro-CT. *Clin. Oral Implants Res.* 19: 516–521.

Gottlow, J. (1993). GTR using resorbable and nonresorbable devices: initial healing and long term results. *J. Periodontol.* 64: 1157–1165.

Grunder, U., Gracis, S., and Capelli, M. (2005). Influence of the 3 D bone to implant relationship on esthetics. *Int. J. Periodontics Restorative Dent.* 25 (2): 113–119.

Haidar, Z.S. (2010). Bio-inspired-functional colloidal core-shell polymeric-based nanosystems: technology promise in tissue engineering, bioimaging and nanomedicine. *Polymers* 2: 323–352.

Hammerle, C.H., Chen, S.T., Wilson, T.G. Jr. et al. (2004). Consensus statements and recommended clinical procedures regarding the placement of implants in extraction sockets. *Int. J. Oral Maxillofac. Implants* 19 (Suppl): 26–28.

Hatcher, D.C., Dial, C., and Mayorga, C. (2003). Cone beam CT for pre-surgical assessment of implant sites. *J. Calif. Dent. Assoc.* 31 (11): 825–833.

Hislop, W.S., Finlay, P.M., and Moos, K.F. (1993). A preliminary study into the uses of anorganic bone in oral and maxillofacial surgery. *Br. J. Oral Maxillofac. Surg.* 31 (3): 149–153.

Hita-Iglesias, C. and Sanchez-Sanchez, F.J. (2016). Immediate implants placed in fresh sockets associated with periapical pathology: a split-mouth design and survival evaluation after 1 year follow up. *Clin. Implant. Dent. Relat. Res.* 18 (6): 1075–1083.

Hoang, T.N. and Mealey, B.L. (2012). Histologic comparison of healing after ridge preservation using human demineralized bone matrix putty with one versus two different-sized bone particles. *J. Periodontol.* 83 (2): 174–181.

Hoogeveen, E.J., Gielkens, P.F., Schortinghuis, J. et al. (2009). Vivosorb as a barrier membrane in rat mandibular defects. An evaluation with transversal microradiography. *Int. J. Oral Maxillofac. Surg.* 38: 870–875.

Hou, L.T., Yan, J.J., Tasi, A.Y.M. et al. (2004). Polymer-assisted regeneration therapy with Atrisorb® barriers in human periodontal intrabony defects. *J. Clin. Periodontol.* 31: 68–74.

Hultin-Mordenfeld, M., Johansson, A., Hedin, M. et al. (2004). A retrospective clinical study of wide-diameter implants used in posterior edentulous areas. *Int. J. Oral Maxillofac. Implants* 19: 387–392.

Hurzeler, M.B., Zuhr, O., Schupbach, P. et al. (2010). The socket shield technique: a proof of principle report. *J. Clin. Periodontol.* 37 (9): 855–862.

Iasella, J.M., Greenwell, H., Miller, R.L. et al. (2003). Ridge preservation with freeze-dried bone allograft and a collagen membrane compared to extraction alone for implant site development: a clinical and histologic study in humans. *J. Periodontol.* 74 (7): 990–999.

Ikada, Y. (2006). *Interface and Technology. Tissue Engineering Fundamentals and Applications*, 189–195. New York: Academic Press.

Ivanoff, C.J., Grondahl, K., Sennerby, L. et al. (1999). Influence of variations in implant diameters: a 3- to 5-year retrospective clinical report. *Int. J. Oral Maxillofac. Implants* 14: 173–180.

Jiansheng, H., Dongying, X., Xianfeng, W. et al. (2012). Clinical evaluation of short and wide diameter implants immediately placed into extraction sockets of posterior areas: a 2 year retrospective study. *J. Oral Implantol.* 38 (6): 729–737.

Jung, R.E., Schneider, D., Ganeles, J. et al. (2009). Computer technology applications in surgical implant dentistry: a systematic review. *Int. J. Oral Maxillofac. Implants* 24 (Suppl. 92): 109.

Kan, J.Y. and Rungcharassaeng, K. (2000). Immediate placement and provisionalization of maxillary anterior single implants: a surgical and prosthodontic rationale. *Prac. Periodontics Aesthet. Dent.* 12 (9): 817–824.

Kan, J.Y., Rungcharassaeng, K., and Lozada, J. (2003). Immediate placement and provisionalization of maxillary anterior single implants: 1-year prospective study. *Int. J. Oral Maxillofac. Implants* 18: 31–39.

Kan, J.Y., Rungcharassaeng, K., and Lozada, J. (2005). Bilaminar subepithelial connective tissue grafts for immediate implant placement and provisionalization in the esthetic zone. *J. Calif. Dent. Assoc.* 33 (11): 865–871.

Karoussis, I.K., Salvi, G.E., Heitz-Mayfield, L.J.A. et al. (2003). Long-term implant prognosis in patients with and without a history of chronic periodontitis: a 10-year prospective cohort study of the ITI Dental Implant System. *Clin. Oral Implants Res.* 14: 329–339.

Khayat, P.G., Hallage, P.G., and Toledo, R.A. (2001). An investigation of 131 consecutively placed wide screwed-vent implants.' *Int. J. Oral Max. Fac. Implants* 16 (6): 827–832.

Kikuchi, M., Koyama, Y., Yamada, T. et al. (2004). Development of guided bone regeneration membrane composed of β-tricalcium phosphate and poly(l-lactide-co-glycolide-co-ε-caprolatone) composites. *Biomaterials* 25: 5979–5986.

Kim, K. and Hun-Mo Sung, H. (2012). Outcomes of dental implant treatment in patients with generalized aggressive periodontitis: a systematic review. *J. Adv. Prosthodont.* 4 (4): 210–217.

Kim, Y.K., Yun, P.Y., Um, I.W. et al. (2014). Alveolar ridge preservation of an extraction socket using autogenous tooth bone graft material for implant site development: prospective case series. *J. Adv. Prosthodont.* 6: 521–527.

Kinoshita, Y. and Amagasa, A. (2002). Jawbone. In: *Methods of Tissue Engineering* (ed. A. Atala and R.P. Lanza), 1195–1204. New York: Academic Press.

Kois, J.C. (2001). Predictable single tooth peri-implants esthetics: five diagnostic keys. *Compend. Contin. Educ. Dent.* 22 (3): 199–206.

Krennmair, G., Seemann, R., Schmidinger, S. et al. (2010). Clinical outcome of root-shaped dental implants of various diameters: 5-year results. *Int. J. Oral Maxillofac. Implants* 25: 357–366.

Landsberg, C.J. (2008). Implementing socket seal surgery as a socket preservation technique for pontic site development: surgical steps revisited – a report of two cases. *J. Periodontol.* 79: 945–954.

Lazzara, R.J. (1989). Immediate implant placement into extraction sites: surgical and restorative advantages. *Int. J. Periodontics Restorative Dent.* 9: 333–343.

Lee, D.W., Pi, S.H., Lee, S.K., and Kim, E.C. (2009). Comparative histomorphometric analysis of extraction sockets healing implanted with bovine xenografts. Irradiated cancellous allografts and solvent-dehydrated allografts in humans. *Int. J. Oral Maxillofac. Implants* 24 (4): 609–615.

Lekovic, V., Camargo, P.M., Klokkevold, P.R. et al. (1998). Preservation of alveolar bone in extraction sockets using bioabsorbable membranes. *J. Periodontol.* 69: 1044–1049.

Liljenqvist, U., Lerner, T., Bullmann, V. et al. (2003). Titanium cages in the surgical treatment of severe vertebral osteomyelitis. *Eur. Spine J.* 12: 606–612.

Lindeboom, J.A., Tjiook, Y., and Kroon, F.H. (2006). Immediate placement of implants in periapical infected sites: a prospective randomized study in 50 patients. *Oral Surg. Oral Med. Oral Pathol. Oral Radiol. Endod.* 101: 705–710.

Lu, H.H., El-Amin, S.F., Scott, K.D., and Laurencin, C.T. (2003). Three-dimensional, bioactive, biodegradable, polymer-bioactive glass composite scaffolds with improved mechanical properties support collagen synthesis and mineralization of human osteoblast-like cells *in vitro*. *J. Biomed. Mater. Res. A* 64: 465–474.

Maksoud, M.A. (2001). Immediate implants in fresh posterior extraction sockets: report of two cases. *J. Oral Implantol.* 27: 123–126.

Malo, P., de Araujo Nobre, M., and Lopes, A. (2007). The use of computer-guided flapless implant surgery and four implants placed in immediate function to support a fixed denture: preliminary results after a mean follow-up period of thirteen months. *J. Prosthet. Dent.* 97: S26–S34.

Marconcini, S., Barone, A., Gelpi, F. et al. (2013). Immediate implant placement in infected sites: a case series. *J. Periodontol.* 84 (2): 196–202.

Matsusue, T., Hanafusa, S., Yamamura, T. et al. (1995). Tissue reaction of bioabsorbable ultra high strength poly (L-lactide) rod. A long-term study in rabbits. *Clin. Orthop. Relat. Res.* 317: 246–253.

Mechery, R., Thiruvalluvan, N., and Sreehari, A. (2015). Ridge split and implant placement in deficient alveolar ridge: case report and an update. *Contemp. Clin. Dent.* 6 (1): 94–97.

Meek, M.F., Jansen, K., Steendam, R. et al. (2004). *In vitro* degradation and biocompatibility of poly(DL-lactide-epsilon-caprolactone) nerve guides. *J. Biomed. Mater. Res.* 68: 43–51.

Mengel, R. and Flores-de-Jacoby, L. (2005). Implants in patients treated for generalized aggressive and chronic periodontitis: a 3-year prospective longitudinal study. *J. Periodontol.* 76 (4): 534–543.

Meredith, N., Alleyne, D., and Cawley, P. (1996). Quantitative determination of the stability of the implant-tissue interface using resonance frequency analysis. *Clin. Oral Implants Res.* 7: 261–267.

Misch, C. (2014). *Dental Implant Prosthetics*, 2e. Mosby Publishers.

Misch, C.E. and Dietsh, F. (1993). Bone-grafting materials in implant dentistry. *Implant Dent.* 2 (3): 158–167.

Misch, C.E., Dietsh-Misch, F., and Misch, C.M. (1999). A modified socket seal surgery with composite graft approach. *J. Oral Implantol.* 25 (4): 244–250.

Misch, C.E., Perel, M.L., Wang, H.L. et al. (2008). Implant success, survival and failure: the International Congress of Oral Implantologists (ICOI) Pisa Consensus Conference. *Implant Dent.* 17 (1): 5–15.

Moghadam, H.G. (2009). Vertical and horizontal bone augmentation with the intraoral autogenous J-graft. *Implant Dent.* 18: 230–238.

Neiva, R.F., Tsao, Y.P., Eber, R. et al. (2008). Effects of a putty-form hydroxyapatite matrix combined with the synthetic cell-binding peptide P-15 on alveolar ridge preservation. *J. Periodontol.* 79 (2): 291–299.

Neves, F.D., Mendonça, G., and Fernandes Neto, A.J. (2004). Analysis of influence of lip line and lip support in esthetics and selection of maxillary implant-supported prosthesis design. *J. Prosthet. Dent.* 91: 286–288.

Norton, M.R. (2011). The influence of insertion torque on the survival of immediately placed and restored single-tooth implants. *Int. J. Oral Maxillofac. Implants*, November–December 26 (6): 1333–1343.

Novaes, A.B. Jr. and Novaes, A.B. (1995). Immediate implants placed into infected sites: a clinical report. *Int. J. Oral Maxillofac. Implants* 10: 609–613.

Novaes, A.B. Jr., Marcaccini, A.M., Souza, S.L. et al. (2003). Immediate placement of implants into periodontally infected sites in dogs: a histomorphometric study of bone–implant contact. *Int. J. Oral Maxillofac. Implants* 18: 391–398.

Novaes, A.B. Jr., Vidigal, G.M. Jr., Novaes, A.B. et al. (1998). Immediate implants placed into infected sites: a histomorphometric study in dogs. *Int. J. Oral Maxillofac. Implants* 13: 422–427.

Nuss, K. and Rechenberg, B. (2008). Biocompatibility issues with modern implants in bone – a review for clinical orthopedics. *Open Orthop. J.* 2: 66–78.

O'Neal, R.B., Gound, T., Levin, M.P., and del Rio, C.E. (1978). Submergence of roots for alveolar bpne preservation. II. Reimplanted endodontically treated roots. *Oral Surg. Oral Med. Oral Pathol.* 46: 114–112.

Olate, S., Lyrio, M.C., de Moraes, M. et al. (2010). Influence of diameter and length of implant on early dental implant failure. *J. Oral Maxillofac. Surg.* 68 (2): 414–419.

Paolantonio, M., Dolci, M., Scarano, A. et al. (2001). Immediate implantation in fresh extraction sockets. A controlled clinical and histological study in man. *J. Periodontol.* 72 (11): 1560–1571.

Papaspyridakos, P., Chen, C.J., Chuang, S.K. et al. (2012). A systemic review of biologic and technical complications with fixed implant rehabilitations for edentulous patients. *Int. J. Oral Maxillofac. Implants* 27 (1): 102–110.

Parlar, A., Bosshardt, D.D., Unsal, B. et al. (2005). New formation of periodontal tissues around titanium implants in a novel dentin chamber model. *Clin. Oral Implants Res.* 16 (3): 259–267.

Patel, N. (2010). Integrating three-dimensional digital technologies for comprehensive implant dentistry. *J. Am. Dent. Assoc.* 141: 20S–24S.

Pennel, B.M., King, K.O., Wildermann, M.N., and Barron, J.M. (1967). A retrospective analysis of factors associated with multiple implant failures in maxillae. *J. Periodontol.* 38: 426–431.

Pommer, B., Hingsammer, L., Haas, R. et al. (2015). Denture related biomechanical factors for Fixed partial dentures retained on short dental implants. *Int. J. Prosthodont* 28 (4): 412–414.

Pontoriero, R., Wennström, J., and Lindhe, J. (1999). The use of barrier membranes and enamel matrix proteins in the treatment of angular bone defects. A prospective controlled clinical study. *J. Clin. Periodontol.* 26: 833–840.

Prakash, H. (2015). Computer aided implantology: changing trends. *Indian J. Dent. Res.* 26: 223–224.

Prosper, L., Crespi, R., Valenti, E. et al. (2010). Five-year follow-up of wide-diameter implants placed in fresh molar extraction sockets in the mandible: immediate versus delayed loading. *Int. J. Oral Maxillofac. Implants* 25: 607–612.

Quirynen, M., Vogels, R., Alsaadi, G. et al. (2005). Predisposing conditions for retrograde peri-implantitis, and treatment suggestions. *Clin. Oral Implants Res.* 16: 599–608.

Rabelo, G.D., de Paula, P.M., Rocha, F.S. et al. (2010). Retrospective study of bone grafting procedures before implant placement. *Implant Dent.* 19: 342–350.

Sapir, S. and Shapira, J. (2008). Decoronation for the management of an ankylosed young permanent tooth. *Dent. Traumatol.* 24 (1): 131–135.

Sarment, D.P., Sukovic, P., and Clinthorne, W. (2003). Accuracy of implant placement with a stereolithographic surgical guide. *Int. J. Oral Maxillofac. Implants* 18: 571–577.

Schulte, W. and Heimke, G. (1976). The Tübinger immediate implant. *Quintessenz* 27 (6): 17–23.

Sclar, A.G. (1999). Preserving alveolar ridge anatomy following tooth removal in conjunction with immediate implant placement. The Bio-Col technique. *Atlas Oral Max. Fac. Surg. Clin. N. Am.* 7 (2): 39–59.

Schnitman, P.A. and Hayashi, C. (2015). Papilla formation in response to computer-assisted implant surgery and immediate restoration. *J. Oral Implantol.* 41: 459–466.

Schulte, W. and Heimke, G. (1976). The Tubinger immediate implant. *Quintessence Int.* 27 (6): 17–23.

Schwartz, Z., Somers, A., Mellonig, J.T. et al. (1998). Addition of human recombinant bone morphogenic protein-2 to inactive commercial human demineralized freeze-dried bone allograft makes an effective composite bone inductive implant material. *J. Periodontol.* 69 (12): 1337–1345.

Schwartz-Arad, D. and Chausu, G. (1997). The ways and wherefores of immediate placement of implants into fresh extraction sites: a literature review. *J. Periodontol.* 68: 915–923.

Schwarz, F., Herten, M., Ferrari, D. et al. (2007). Guided bone regeneration at dehiscence-type defects using biphasic hydroxyapatite + beta tricalcium phosphate (cone ceramic) or a collagen-coated natural bone mineral (BioOss Collagen): an immunohistochemical study in dogs. *Int. J. Oral Maxillofac. Surg.* 36: 1198–1206.

Sela, M.N., Kohavi, D., Krausz, E. et al. (2003). Enzymatic degradation of collagen-guided tissue regeneration membranes by periodontal bacteria. *Clin. Oral Implants Res.* 14: 263–268.

Serino, G., Biancu, S., Iezzi, G., and Piattelli, A. (2003). Ridge preservation following tooth extraction using a polylactide and polyglycolide sponge as space filler: a clinical and histological study in humans. *Clin. Oral Implants Res.* 14 (5): 651–658.

Shapoff, C.A., Bowers, G.M., Levy, B. et al. (1980). The effect of particle size on the osteogenic activity of composite grafts of allogeneic freeze-dried bone and autogenous marrow. *J. Periodontol.* 51 (11): 625–630.

Shin, R.H., Friedrich, P.F., Crum, B.A. et al. (2009). Treatment of a segmental nerve defect in the rat with use of bioabsorbable synthetic nerve conduits: a comparison of commercially available conduits. *J. Bone Joint Surg. Am.* 91: 2194–2204.

Siegenthaler, D.W., Jung, R.E., Holderegger, C. et al. (2007). Replacement of teeth exhibiting periapical pathology by immediate implants: a prospective, controlled clinical trial. *Clin. Oral Implants Res.* 18: 727–737.

Sohrabi, K., Mushantat, A., Esfandiari, S., and Feine, J. (2012). How successful are small-diameter implants? A literature review. *Clin. Oral Implants Res.* 23 (5): 515–525.

Sonick, M. (1994). A comparison of the accuracy of periapical, panoramic and computed tomographic radiographs in locating the mandibular canal. *Int. J. Oral Maxillofac. Implants* 9: 455–460.

Sukovic, P. (2003). Cone beam computed tomography in craniofacial imaging. *Orthod. Craniofac. Res.* 6 (Suppl. 1): 31–36.

Taguchi, Y., Amizuka, N., Nakadate, M. et al. (2005). A histological evaluation for guided bone regeneration induced by a collagenous membrane. *Biomaterials* 26: 6158–6166.

Takata, T., Wang, H.L., and Miyauchi, M. (2001). Migration of osteoblastic cells on various guided bone regeneration membranes. *Clin. Oral Implants Res.* 12: 332–338.

Tallarico, M., Meloni, S.M., Canullo, L. et al. (2015). Five-year results of a randomized controlled trial comparing patients rehabilitated with immediately loaded maxillary cross arch fixed dental prosthesis supported by four or six implants placed using guided surgery. *Clin. Implant Dent. Relat. Res.* 18 (5): 965–972.

Tan-Chu, J.H., Tuminelli, F.J., Kurtz, K.S., and Tarnow, D.P. (2014). Analysis of buccolingual dimensional changes of the extraction socket using the "ice cream cone" flapless grafting technique. *Int. J. Periodontics Restorative Dent.* 34 (3): 399–403.

Ten Heggeler, J.M., Slot, D.E., and Van der Weijden, G.A. (2011). Effect of socket preservation therapies following tooth extraction in non-molar regions in humans: a systematic review. *Clin. Oral Implants Res.* 22 (8): 779–788.

Tolstunov, L. (2007). Implant zones of the jaws: implant location and related success rate. *J. Oral Implantol.* 33 (4): 211–220.

Turkyilmaz, I., Company, A.M., and McGlumphy, E.A. (2010). Should edentulous patients be constrained to removable complete dentures? The use of dental implants to improve the quality of life for edentulous patients. *Gerodontology* 27 (1): 3–10.

Valente, N. and Andreana, S. (2016). Peri-implant disease: what we know and what we need to know. *J. Periodontal Implant Sci.* 46 (3): 136–151.

Van Assche, N., van Steenberghe, D., Guerrero, M.E. et al. (2007). Accuracy of implant placement based on pre-surgical planning of three-dimensional cone-beam images: a pilot study. *J. Clin. Periodontol.* 34 (9): 816–821.

Van de Wiele, G., Teughels, W., Vercruyssen, M. et al. (2015). The accuracy of guided surgery via mucosa-supported stereolithographic surgical templates in the hands of surgeons with little experience. *Clin. Oral Implants Res.* 26 (12): 1489–1494.

Vandeweghe, S. and De Bruyn, H. (2012). A within implant comparison to evaluate the concept of platform switching: A randomised controlled trial. *Eur. J. Oral Implant.* 5 (3): 253–262.

Villa, R. and Rangert, B. (2005). Early loading of interforaminal implants immediately installed after extraction of teeth presenting endodontic and periodontal lesions. *Clin. Implant Dent. Relat. Res.* 7 (Suppl. 1): S28–S35.

Villa, R. and Rangert, B. (2007). Immediate and early function of implants placed in extraction sockets of maxillary infected teeth: a pilot study. *J. Prosthet. Dent.* 97 (Suppl. 6): S96–S108.

Villar, C.C. and Cochran, D.L. (2010). Regeneration of periodontal tissues: guided tissue regeneration. *Dent. Clin. N. Am.* 54: 73–92.

Waasdrop, J.A., Evian, C.I., and Mandracchia, M. (2010). Immediate placement of implants into infected sites: a systematic review of the literature. *J. Periodontol.* 81 (6): 801–808.

Weber, H.P., Crohin, C.C., and Fiorellini, J.P. (2000). A 5-year prospective clinical and radiographic study of non-submerged dental implants. *Clin. Oral Implants Res.* 11: 144–153.

Werbitt, M.J. and Goldberg, P.V. (1992). The immediate implant: bone preservation and bone regeneration. *Int. J. Periodontics Restorative Dent.* 12 (3): 206–217.

Wheeler, S.L., Vogel, R.E., and Casellini, R. (2000). Tissue preservation and maintenance of optimum esthetics: a clinical report. *Int. J. Oral Maxillofac. Implants* 15 (2): 265–271.

Wildermann, M.N. and Wentz, F.M. (1970). Repair of a dentogingival defect with a pedicle flap. *J. Periodontol.* 41: 551–565.

Wood, R.A. and Mealey, B.L. (2012). Histologic comparison of healing after tooth extraction with ridge preservation using mineralized versus demineralized freeze-dried bone allograft. *J. Periodontol.* 83 (3): 329–336.

Zaner, D.J. and Yukna, R.A. (1984). Particle size of periodontal bone grafting materials. *J. Periodontol.* 55 (7): 406–409.

Ziegler, C.M., Woertche, R., Brief, J., and Hassfeld, S. (2002). Clinical indications for digital volume tomography in oral and maxillofacial surgery. *Dentomaxillofac. Radiol.* 31 (2): 126–130.

5

Peri-implant Tissue Stability

Prevalence, Etiology, Prevention, and Treatment

5.1 Introduction

Over the past few years, all aspects of dentistry have undergone inspiration a advancements in the way that clinicians are not only required to treat disease and improve function but also to cope with the ever-increasing esthetic demands of their patients. To date, successful restorative dentistry can be best accomplished only when long term healthy and stable tissues surround either the natural teeth or their implant replacements. Therefore, accurate attention to both soft and hard tissue status around the natural teeth and implants before, during, and after the restorative procedures will not only enhance the treatment outcome but also minimize treatment complications. Implant retreated esthetics should involve a sold scientific base in its application, not only experience. All the different therapeutic modalities in the esthetic zone should be based on solid scientific research and clinical trials.

Achieving an esthetic outcome is always a new challenge to the clinician. The key points controlling the esthetic outcome include: the presence of healthy proximal papillae, an intact gingival form, and intact osseous architecture, while tissue phenotype influences not only the clinical result but also its longevity. Understanding the biological, microbiological, and physiological responses of the peri-implant tissues is an absolute prerequisite, and the peri-implant esthetic outcome is mainly determined by the patient's presented anatomical condition and the clinician's abilities. A thorough understanding of the anatomy of the supporting structures is essential for a correct diagnosis and treatment planning. For natural teeth, it has been estimated that over 60% of the population has at least one buccal recession defect and such defects are predominately seen in patients with good oral hygiene; in the USA, 23% of adults have one or more tooth surfaces with ≥3 mm gingival recession (Chan, Chun and MacEachern 2015) (see Figure 5.1a and b).

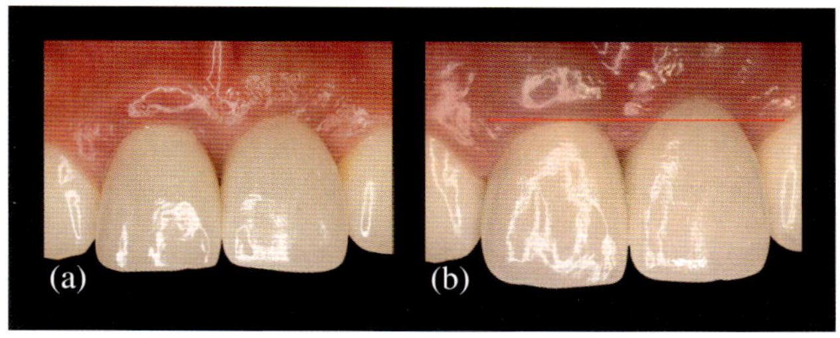

Figure 5.1 (a) Immediately restored implant, (b) One year post restorative showing the gingival recession around the margins.

The biologic width around a natural tooth and a dental implant differ, in height, histology, and vascularity. Histologically, there are more collagen fibers running parallel to the implant surface, so it is similar to mucosal scar tissue with a weak adherence around dental implant collars, which can make corrective procedures unpredictable and bacterial invasion greater and rapid. Peri-implant tissue stability in the esthetic zone helps provide and sustain long-term treatment success and depends on many factors that include: tissue phenotype, labial plate of bone thickness, alveolar crest height, prosthetic margins design, and other physiologic factors. Implant-related gingival stability can be influenced by many physiologic, anatomic or technical factors (Araujo and Lindhe 2005; Gracco et al. 2009; Yu, Ji and Shen 2009).

Other technical factors might affect peri-implant tissue stability such as the diameter of the implant used, the use of provisional restorations, the placement and timing of the final restoration delivery, and a lack of clinical experience. Buser et al. (2004) indicated that the use of wide diameter implants in the anterior zone induced labial plate bone resorption. Saadoun (2007) reported that soft tissue recession around a wide-diameter implant (≥5 mm) averaged 1.58 mm compared with 0.57 mm around a standard-diameter implant (<5 mm). It may be prudent to use standard-diameter implants in the esthetic zone.

Advances in Esthetic Implant Dentistry, First Edition. Abdelsalam Elaskary.

Companion website: www.wiley.com/go/elaskary/esthetic

Another contributing factor is implant position within the alveolar ridge and the time allowed for peri-implant tissue maturation (Kinsel and Capoferri 2008).

Gingival recession around natural teeth is defined as present when the location of the gingival margin is apical to the cemento-enamel junction (Peridontology AAP). A pre-clinical study (Baker and Seymour 1976) inducing gingival recession by replacing rat incisors with acrylic resin implants suggested that gingival recession is generally associated with (1) local inflammation characterized by mononuclear cells, (2) breakdown of connective tissue, and (3) proliferation of the oral and junctional epithelium into the site of connective tissue destruction. Other precipitating factors include traumatic forces (e.g. excessive brushing), habits (e.g., smoking, oral piercing), and plaque-induced inflammation (Chan et al. 2015).

5.2 Prevalence of Implant Related Tissue Migration

Gingival recession represents a clinical condition in adults frequently encountered in general dental practice. Society is evolving with more patients focusing on esthetic aspects of treatment outcome, which explains the growing interest by clinicians for observing soft tissue dynamics, objective esthetic ratings, and patient-centered outcomes. The progressive shortening of the treatment time from tooth loss to implant installation, has resulted in modifications of the classic immediate implant placement procedures, which may ultimately be a reflection of the patient's expectations (Araujo, Wennstrom and Lindhe 2006; Botticelli, Berglundh and Lindhe 2004) (see Figure 5.2a–e).

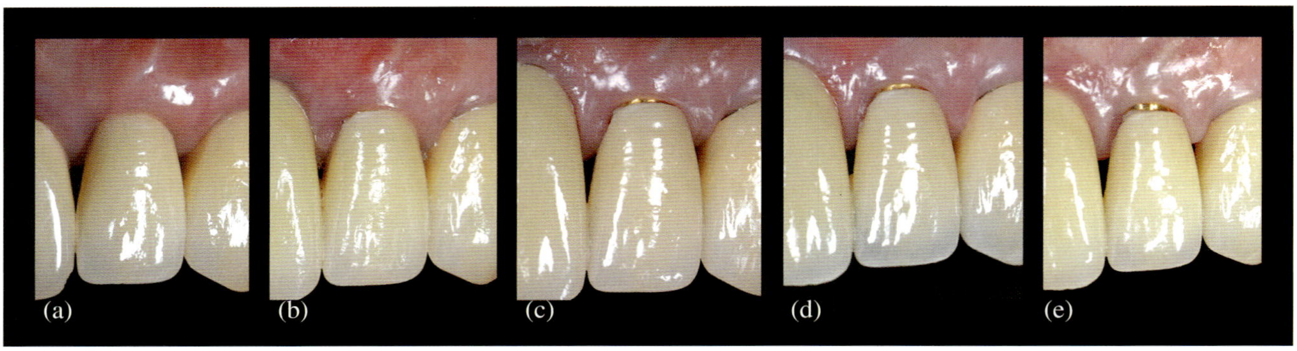

Figure 5.2 (a–e). Chronological (ascending) follow-up for apical tissue migration around implant supported restoration over a three year period.

According to various systematic reviews, single implant-supported restoration is predictable and successful following conventional implant surgery (Berglundh et al. 2002; Creugers et al. 2000; Jung et al. 2008). However, data on clinical response and parameters about response to trauma, prevalence implant related treatment complications, and bone remodeling rate may be considered limited. Various attempts have been made to evaluate the biologic scope of osseointegrated implants. Kan et al. (2009) clinically evaluated the dimensions of the peri-implant mucosa around two-stage maxillary anterior single implants in humans after one year of function and the influence of the peri-implant phenotype was also examined. It was concluded that the mean facial dimension of peri-implant mucosa of two-stage implants is slightly greater than the average dimension of that of the dentogingival complex. The level of the interproximal papilla of the implant is independent of the proximal bone level next to the implant but is related to the interproximal bone level next to the adjacent teeth. Greater peri-implant mucosal dimensions were noted in the presence of a thick peri-implant phenotype compared with a thin phenotype.

Kan et al. (2011) evaluated 35 patients, clinically and radiographically at presurgical examination, immediately after immediate implant placement, and at provisionalization, and recordings were made at one year after implant surgery and at the latest follow-up appointment. All implants retained their function. At the follow-up appointment, the mean mesial and distal marginal bone level changes were significantly greater than those observed at one year. At follow-up, the mean mesial and distal papilla (DP) level changes were significantly smaller than those observed at one year, whereas the mean facial gingival level change was significantly greater than that observed at one year. Sites with a thick gingival phenotype exhibited significantly minor changes on the facial gingival levels than sites with a thin gingival phenotype at both the appointments, with mean mid-facial recession being 1.13 mm. These findings were also confirmed from the work of Canullo and Rasperini (2007), who evaluated the soft tissue response to platform-switched implants after a mean of 22 months follow-up in a case series. During the follow-up period, the papillary level increased, with a mean value of 0.25 mm.

Thus, an intact facial bone wall thickness seems valuable for any successful esthetic procedure as it has a direct relationship to mid-facial recession (Kan et al. 2007). In a review article, Chen and Buser (2009) concluded that advanced mid-facial recession is common following immediate implant treatment. Other studies showed an advanced mid-facial recession occurred in <10% of the implants (Canullo, Iurlaro and Iannello 2009; Cosyn et al. 2012a, b; Raes et al. 2011).

Mean interproximal recession was frequently reported (11/13) and was low (<1 mm), suggesting a limited risk for advanced interproximal recession. In one study some tissue gain was observed (Canullo and Rasperini 2007). Lops et al. (2008) studied the interproximal recession with complete fill in nearly 70% of the cases; however, the changes in papilla height over time were found to be comparable for patients with a thick- and thin-scalloped gingival phenotype (Kan et al. 2011). Canullo et al. (2009) demonstrated significantly less prevalent interproximal recession for implants with a conical connection and platform switch when compared with implants with a flat-to-flat connection and without abutment diameter reduction.

De Rouck, Collys and Cosyn (2008) recorded on average 0.75 mm of advanced mid-facial recession and Cordaro, Torsello and Roccuzzo (2009), found advanced mid-facial recession in 38% and 85% of the patients with a thick- and thin-scalloped gingival phenotype, respectively. Tortamano et al. (2010) suggested that the need for socket grafting might limit the amount of mid-facial recession.

Small and Tarnow (2000) evaluated 63 implants in 11 patients. Baseline measurements were recorded at stage 2 surgery in two-stage implant systems and at stage 1 surgery in the one-stage system. Subsequent measurements were recorded at one week, one month, three months, six months, nine months, and one year after baseline measurements. The majority of the recessions occurred within the first three months, with 80% of all sites. It is therefore recommended that there should be a wait of three months for the tissue to stabilize before either selecting a final abutment or making a final impression.

In a systematic search by Cosyn et al. (2012a) it was concluded that the average interproximal tissue recession was 1 mm (less than 10% of the cases), suggesting that the risk of interproximal tissue drop and mid-facial recession is unlikely to occur, especially in patients with intact labial plate of bone, with thick overlaying soft tissues. (See Figure 5.3a and b).

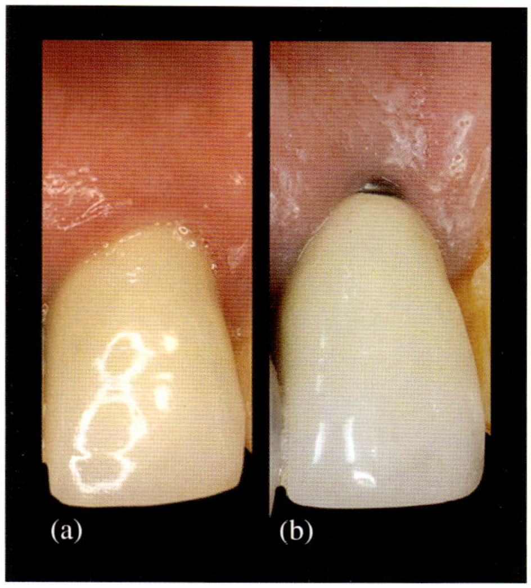

Figure 5.3 (a) Immediate implant placement and restoration of the maxillary left lateral incisor, (b) Six years follow up showing class I gingival recession occurred.

5.3 Factors that Lead to Implant-related Gingival Recession

5.3.1 Background

The preservation or reproduction of a healthy and stable mucogingival architecture surrounding dental implants placed in the anterior maxilla present esthetical challenges for the clinician that may arise for several reasons: the loss of soft tissue volume at the site, poor soft tissue quality at the site, and pre-existing bone loss after regular tooth extraction. While surgical reconstructive procedures have been proposed for the improvement of hard and soft tissue defects prior to implant placement, the preservation of appropriate soft tissue architecture around integrated implants remains challenging (Benic et al. 2012; Buser et al. 2004; Lang and Zitzmann 2012).

Factors that lead to implant related gingival recession can be classified as: physiological factors, which involve factors that influence recession via regular biologic processes, such as bone remodeling rate, tissue phenotype, and the influence of the thickness of the labial plate of bone; and technical factors, which deal with any technical errors that occur such as the use of wide implants, poor implant position, premature delivery of the final prosthetics, failing to use provisional restoration, and excessive cement located in the gingival sulcus around dental implants (see Figure 5.4).

It is commonly agreed that areas with less than 2 mm of attached gingiva and decreased buccolingual thickness are at a higher risk of recession (Lang and Zitzmann 2012).

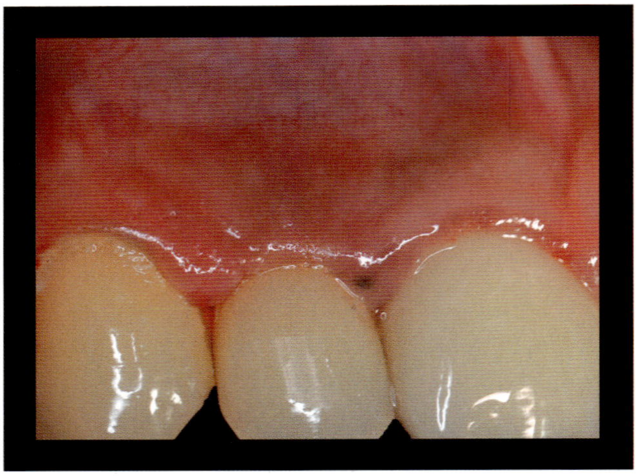

Figure 5.4 Implant supported restoration in thin scalloped tissue phenotype that requires immediate attention against recession.

Peri-implant tissue examination for mucogingival problems should therefore include assessment of the presence of local inflammation, the gingival thickness and the vestibular depth (Hall 1984). The clinician can also use a simple “tension test” (Vincent, Machen and Levin 1984), which involves pulling the cheeks or lips away from the teeth to assess whether there is adequate attached tissue. In areas of inadequate attached tissue there will be movement or blanching of the gingival margin.

5.3.2 Physiologic Factors

5.3.2.1 Influence of Thickness of the Labial Plate of Bone

Facial bone thickness is considered a crucial parameter for treatment planning decisions and predicting tissue stability in the anterior esthetic area. No consensus has yet been reached regarding the amount of buccal bone thickness that is needed when placing an implant to ensure a long-term satisfactory biologic and esthetic outcome but there are still certain guidelines that are proposed. Grunder, Gracis and Capelli (2005) emphasized the presence of an adequate facial bone thickness to ensure long-term peri-implant tissue stability. The buccal bone plate, especially in the anterior region, has been described as significantly thinner compared to the lingual and palatal components in animal and human studies (Buser et al. 2008; Hämmerle, Chen and Wilson 2004), probably making them more fragile and more easily resorbed. A study by Fu, Lee and Wang (2011) found a mean facial bone thickness of 0.83 mm (range, 0.3–1.60 mm) at 2 mm below the bone crest. Braut et al. (2012) found a mean bone thickness of 0.5 mm (range, 0–2.1 mm) at 4 mm apical from the CEJ and 0.6 mm (range, 0–2.8 mm) at the middle of the root. A similar study by Januário, Duarte and Barriviera (2011) on 250 subjects, found a mean bone thickness for the central and lateral incisors and canines of 0.6 (60.3) mm, 0.7 (60.3) mm, and 0.6 (60.3) mm, respectively, at 1 mm apical to the bone crest and of 0.6 (60.4) mm, 0.7 (60.4) mm, and 0.6 (60.4) mm at 3 mm apical to the bone crest. The mean overall thickness varied within 0.5 (60.4) mm and 0.7 (60.4) mm. A study by Huynh-Ba et al. (2016) in a sample of 93 sites showed a mean buccal bone thickness of 0.8 mm (range, 0.5–2 mm) for the maxillary anterior sites (canine to canine); 87.2% of the buccal bony walls had a width > 1 mm and only 2.6% of the walls were 2 mm wide. They postulated that a mean bone wall thickness for the anterior maxillary teeth at 4 mm apical to the CEJ of 1.19 mm (range, 0.30–3.30 mm) had a total of 43.3% with >1 mm of bone thickness and 0.82 mm (range, 0.20–1.60 mm) at the midpoint of the root had a total of 76.6% with <1 mm of bone thickness. For the mandibular teeth, the mean was 1.31 mm (range, 0.30–5.20 mm) with a total of 63.3% with >1 mm of bone thickness and 0.80 mm (range, 0.00–1.80 mm) with a total of 75.5% with <1 mm of bone thickness, respectively. The mean bone thickness at the apical area of the root was 1.80 mm (range, 0.20–3.60 mm) for the maxillary teeth and 3.78 mm (range, 0.00–7.90 mm) for the mandibular teeth.

Fuentes et al. (2015) have studied the anatomical dimensions of the buccal bone walls of the esthetic maxillary region for immediate implant placement, based upon cone-beam computed tomography (CBCT) scans in a sample of adult patients. They analyzed a sample of 50 CBCT scans, and concluded that less than 10% of sites showed more than a 2-mm thickness of the buccal bone wall, with the exception of the central incisor region, in which 14.4% of cases were ≥ 2 mm.

Le and Farahani (2012), who explored the relationship between the labial bone thickness (ILBT) and crestal labial soft tissue thickness for an implant, suggest that crestal labial soft tissue thickness around implants is significantly associated with the labial bone thickness in the anterior maxillary region. In other words, they concluded a direct relationship showing that the thicker the bone, the thicker the crestal labial soft tissue thickness around implants and vice versa. Kheur et al. (2015), suggested that there is a positive correlation between the labial and palatal bone and soft tissue thickness; and between the labial bone thickness and the labio-palatal socket thickness. No correlation was seen between the labial bone thickness and the labio-palatal tooth position. They also suggested that a minimum 2 mm thickness of bone is necessary to provide support to the supracrestal soft tissue, and that an accurate analysis with CBCT imaging before extraction is necessary for immediate implant placement. Wildermanm and Wentz (1965) and Pennel et al. (1967) histologically demonstrated a relationship between bone exposure and bone resorption in thin plates. Qahash, Susuin and Poolimeni (2008) demonstrated a correlation between the width of the buccal alveolar ridge and the extent of bone resorption using incandescent and fluorescent light microscopy analysis. They suggested that the width of the buccal alveolar ridge should be at least 2 mm to maintain the alveolar bone level, and the thicker lingual bone plate provided a larger wound space that was correlated to enhanced bone regeneration, whereas implants placed closer to the buccal plate were associated with increased crestal bone loss. If after implantation the buccal site thickness is less than 2 mm, vertical bone resorption is likely to occur (see Figures 5.5a, b and 5.6a, b).

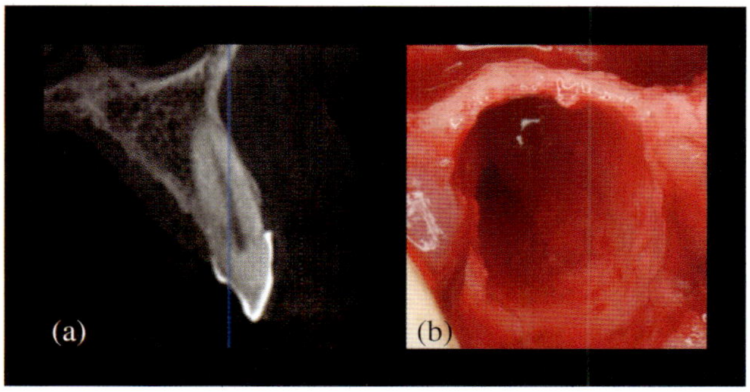

Figure 5.5 (a) and (b) Thin labial plate bone as a result of the labial position of the natural root.

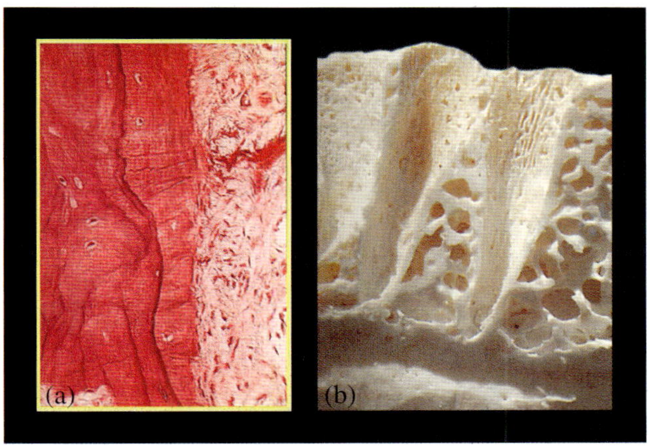

Figure 5.6 (a) Histological section of the periodontium stained with H and E showing the Sharpey's fibers and bundle bone, (b) Bundle bone type immediately at the time of tooth extraction.

5.3.2.2 Influence of Tissue Phenotype

Tissue phenotype is considered a major influencer in the overall prediction of the fate of an immediate implant placement procedure in the esthetic zone. It predicts to a great extent the future liability for implant related tissue migration and the overall possible tissue stability, so the clinician should identify the tissue phenotype prior to the start of the treatment, and identify the potential risks involved.

In tissue phenotype; the thin tissue seems to recede more often in response to inflammation and tissue manipulation. Gingival recessions confirm the relevance of an inflammatory infiltrate in the pathogenesis (Smukler and Landsberg 1984). In thin phenotype gingival recessions around natural teeth, the epithelium is acanthotic and proliferative and surrounded by an inflammatory infiltrate. In addition, necrotic cells can be found. Occasionally the dentogingival epithelium penetrates into the lamina propria, thereby decreasing the width of the lamina propria and allowing the dentogingival and oral epithelia to coalesce, resulting in loss of attachment to the tooth. The inflammatory infiltrate can span the entire thickness of the width of the gingiva thus promoting a further recession. In thicker gingiva, connective tissue free of inflammatory infiltrate may be interposed between the oral and junctional epithelia, preventing a recession (Baker and Spedding 2002; Miller 1985). Baldi et al. (1999) and Hwang and Wang (2006) stated that initial gingival thickness predicts the outcome of any root coverage procedures or any restorative treatments around natural teeth.

Claffey and Shanley (1986) defined the thin phenotype as having a gingival thickness ≤ 1.5 mm, and the thick as ≥ 2 mm or more. Clinical identification is important for better determination of the treatment outcome. Hirschfield (1923) was one of the earliest periodontists to comment on the relationships between alveolar anatomy and gingival form, noting that a thin alveolar contour was probably covered by a similar gingival form. It has been suggested that a direct correlation exists between gingival phenotype and the susceptibility to gingival recession following surgical and restorative procedures (see Figure 5.7). According to Evans and Chen (2008), the likelihood of gingival recession

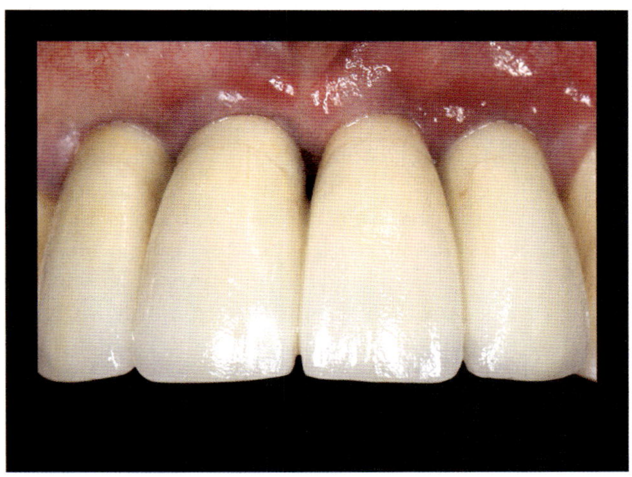

Figure 5.7 High risk thin scalloped tissue phenotype that most likely will induce post-restorative recession.

increases in patients with thin phenotypes present in immediate single implant-supported restorations. It is widely accepted that some gingival/periodontal problems are more likely to occur in patients with a thin phenotype. A 1991 animal study by Berglundh and colleagues concluded that thin gingival tissue can lead to marginal bone loss during formation of the peri-implant biologic width. Another study by Hwang and Wang (2006) reported that implant sites with thin mucosa were prone to angular bone defects, while stable crestal bone was maintained in implants surrounded by thick mucosa. According to Abrahamsson et al. (1998), thick tissues (i.e. ≥2.5 mm) can avoid significant crestal bone recession.

Fickl et al. (2008), in an interesting study that fully explained the reasons for the harmful effect of thin tissue phenotypes, stated that the thin periodontal phenotypes have an inherent osteoclastic activity that is signaled by any stimulus such as flap reflection; thus, osteoclastic activities occur at the internal and external sides and merge together, leading to a more pronounced loss of the buccal bone plate. Consequently, when the buccal bone plate is resorbed, the soft tissue complex can no longer be stabilized and will collapse into the newly formed defective space. As the buccal soft tissue occupies the place of the former buccal resorbed bone plate, the room for bone regeneration is reduced, leading to the observed major bucco-oral shrinkage, which is why serious esthetic changes in bone and mucosal anatomy may result after extraction in patients with thin-scalloped profiles.

Patients with a thick phenotype that consists of flat soft tissue form and a thick bony architecture are often found to be prevalent in the population. This type of tissue form, according to Kao, Fagan and Conte (2008), is dense and fibrotic with a large zone of attachment, thus making it more resistant to gingival recession (see Figure 5.8a and b).

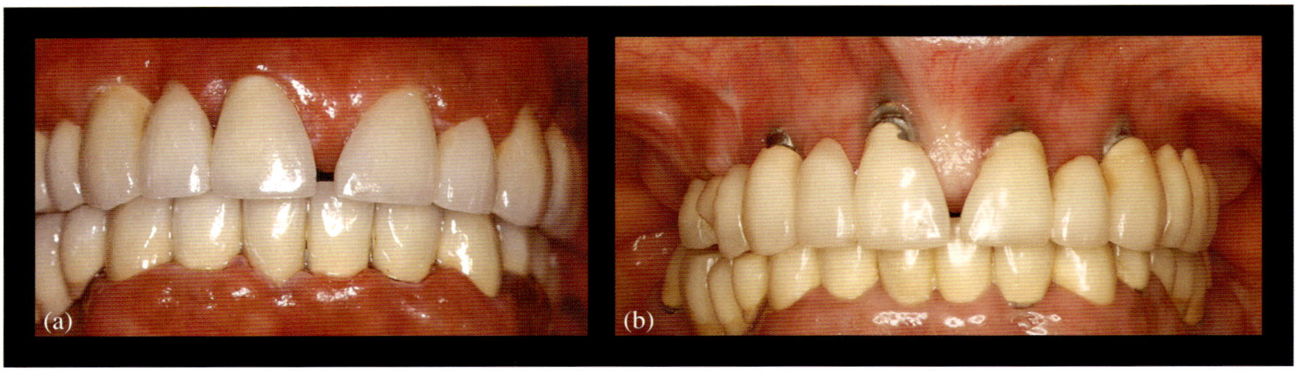

Figure 5.8 (a) and (b) Twelve years follow-up for implant supported restoration that shows related local gingival recession due to the poor soft tissue quality (lack of keratinized tissues) that indicates a thin tissue phenotype.

In contrast, thin gingival tissue tends to be delicate and almost translucent in appearance. The tissue appears friable with a minimal zone of attached gingiva. The soft tissue is highly accentuated and often suggestive of thin or minimal bone over the labial roots. Hwang and Wang (2006) documented that patients with a thin gingival phenotype were more likely to experience gingival recession following non-surgical periodontal therapy. The thinner periodontal phenotype needs more attention when an extraction is carried out owing to its thin alveolar plate (Kao et al. 2008). The hard and soft tissue contouring is more predictable after surgery for a thick phenotype. The value of a thick phenotype is emphasized by its increased wound coverage and site protection, and implant stability created by a predictable seal around the implants' collars. The thicker phenotype can resist mucosal recession, masks the restorative margins, and camouflages the titanium implant shadows. It also protects the biological seal around dental implants, thus reducing the tendency for crestal bone resorption. The amount of gingival thickness before regenerative surgery was found to be a predicting factor for the occurrence of further postoperative recession. However, in a thin phenotype, the mucogingival corrective surgical procedures can enhance the quality of tissue, resulting in a more favorable treatment outcome. A thick phenotype is more resistant to recession and more accommodating to different implant positions (Kao et al. 2008; Siegenthaler et al. 2007; Small, Tarnow and Cho 2001) (see Figure 5.9).

Dramatic alveolar bone resorption in the apical and lingual direction is possible in patients with a thin phenotype. The loss of peri-implant tissues may result in facial plate loss, revealing a grayish color underneath; additional bone and soft tissue grafting surgeries may be necessary (see Figure 5.10a and b).

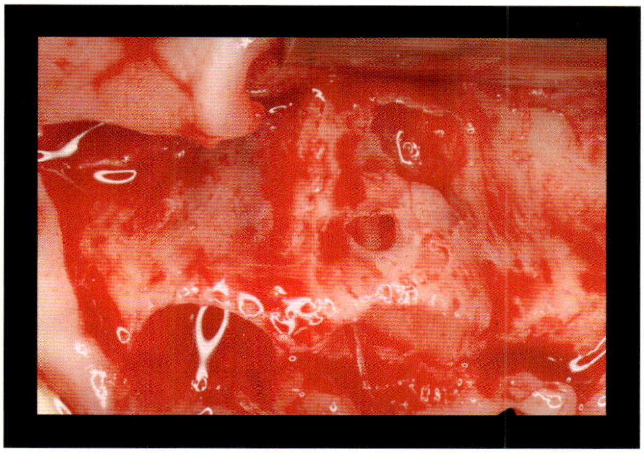

Figure 5.9 Socket labial wall that reveals apical fenestrations that indicated the typical osseous form of thin scalloped tissue phenotype.

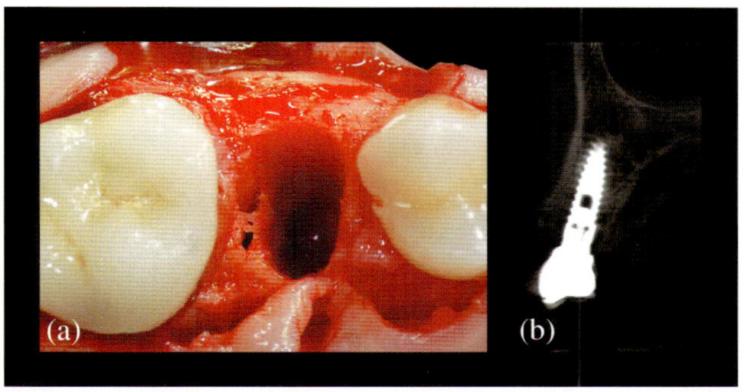

Figure 5.10 (a) and (b) Thick flat tissue phenotype with an excellent labial plate of bone thickness this would be in favor of any surgical maneuver.

Patients with thick and flat gingival phenotypes exhibit short papillae whereas thin-scalloped phenotypes have long papillae. This morphometric difference may be the cause of more papilla loss in the thin phenotype. Linkevicius et al. (2009) in their study concluded that the initial gingival tissue thickness at the crest may be considered as a significant predictor of marginal bone stability around implants. If the tissue thickness is 2.0 mm or less, crestal bone up to 1.45 mm may occur, despite a supracrestal position of the implant–abutment interface. Nisapakultorn et al. (2010), in their study on 40 patients, documented a thin phenotype being significantly associated with an increased risk of facial mucosal recession (see Figure 5.11a and b).

The thicknesses of the crestal bone on the buccal aspect significantly influence the bone remodeling rate during the initial four-month healing period after an immediate implant placement, while on the other hand, gingival thickness affects the treatment outcome possibly because of the difference in the amount of blood supply to the underlying bone and the susceptibility to resorption.

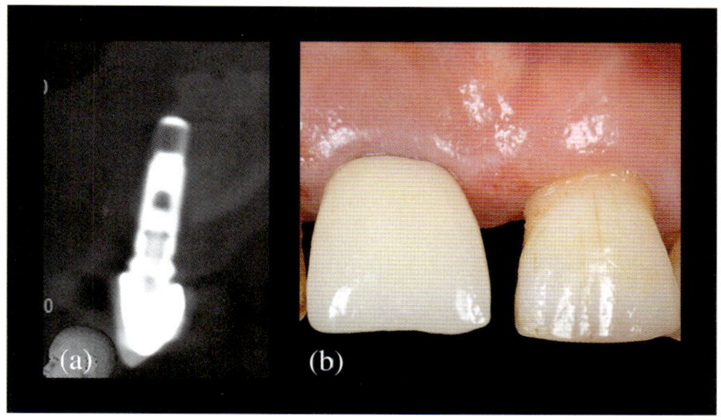

Figure 5.11 (a) Complete resorption of the labial plate of bone around previously restored dental implant, (b) Ten years follow-up where no recession is seen as a result of the thick tissue phenotype where abundance of keratinization exists.

Patients with a reduced mucosal thickness possess more dramatic alveolar resorption in the apical and lingual directions after tooth extraction. Therefore, special caution must be taken in the preoperative assessment of the mucosal thickness and the necessity for surgical enhancement of this mucosa (see Figure 5.12a and b).

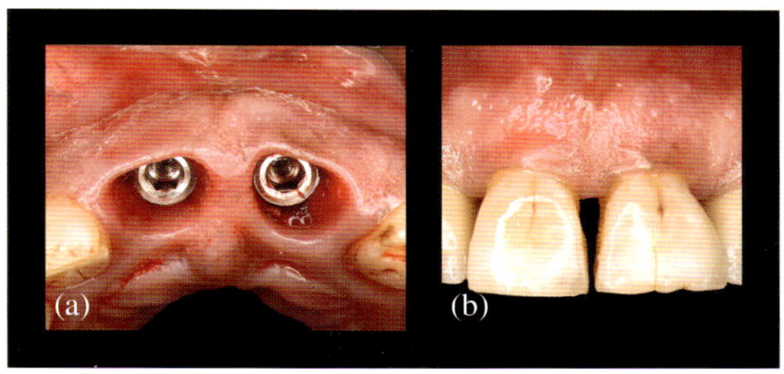

Figure 5.12 (a) Two implants Placed (Tapered Screw vent, Zimmer dental, Carlsbad, CA, USA) in thick flat tissue phenotype patient, (b) Case restored with no apical migration of the labial tissues that were recorded over six years.

A delayed implant placement might be considered when there is not enough soft and hard tissue thickness (Buser et al. 1991, 1999, 2008, 2013). However, a thin gingival phenotype is associated with a thin alveolar plate that makes the worst clinical outcome in the delayed immediate protocol; more ridge remodeling has been found in this phenotype when compared with a thick periodontal phenotype. Ridge preservation was should be considered for most thin phenotype cases (Ahmad 2010). Atraumatic natural tooth extraction is also necessary. It is the author's recommendation that a non-staged surgical approach in thin phenotype patients or those with a high-scalloped tissue profile should be undertaken whenever possible (whenever primary implant stability is achievable).

The reasons for this approach include: minimizing treatment time; decreasing the liability for scar tissue formation because multiple surgeries in the oral cavity will lead to further tissue shrinkage as well as scar tissue formation; and minimizing the likelihood of bone resorption after surgical intervention – in a staged approach, the main issue is the tendency for tissue to shrink, as happens whenever a surgical intervention is performed in thin tissue phenotype patients, which explains the preference of the non-staged treatment approach. Treatment should involve augmenting both bone and soft tissue together in the same treatment session, be cause the risk by that of a staged approach; the resultant tissue shrinkage is a major drawback of a staged approach (see Figure 5.13a and b).

Different gingival phenotypes are found between different age groups, with the thicker phenotype more prevalent in younger age groups. Vandana and Savitha (2005) showed thicker gingiva in a younger age group and stated that the decrease in keratinization and changes in the oral epithelium may be the contributing factors. Sanavi, Weisgold and Rose (1998) found that the inter-radicular bone is more abundant and thicker in the thinner phenotype. This in turn can cause more recession (see Figure 5.14a and b).

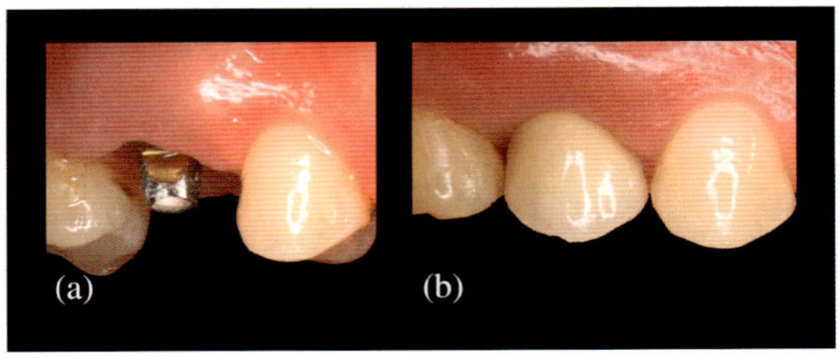

Figure 5.13 (a) and (b) Long term follow up of Pre and post-operative pictures of immediate implant placement in a thick flat tissue phenotype with no apical migration of the tissues.

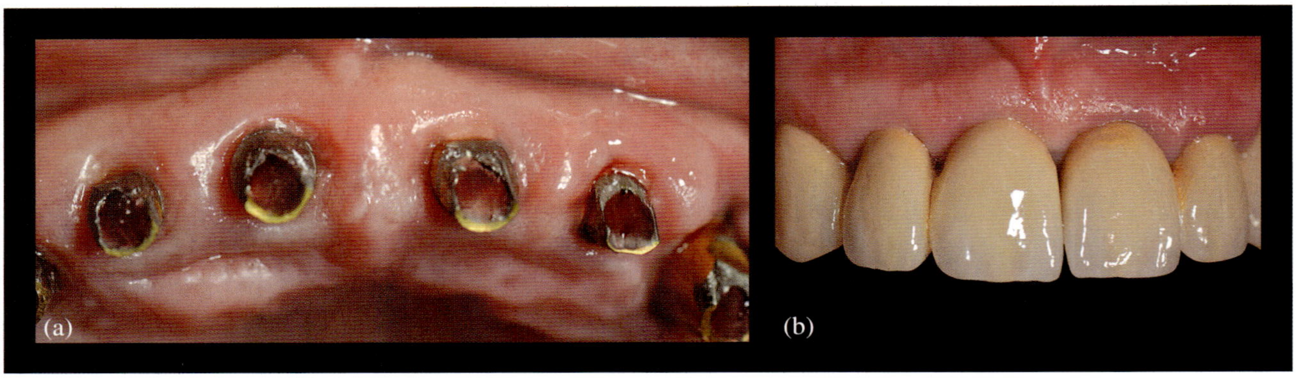

Figure 5.14 (a) and (b) Thick flat tissue phenotype that predicts positive clinical outcome with minimal or no soft tissue apical migration.

In a thin gingival phenotype, a faulty prosthetic margin invading the peri-implant tissue complex or extending beyond the implant collar might cause bone loss in this area. Thus, restoration going deeper into the sulcus will increase the risk of bone resorption as well as gingival recession via tissue displacement.

Residual cement also plays a role in the occurrence of implant related gingival recession specially in thin tissue phenotypes. It has been reported that excess luting cement can cause irritation to the gingival tissues leading to crestal bone loss and subsequent changes in the architecture of the soft tissue (Linkevicius et al. 2009). However, there is still no consensus about how excess cements cause tissue reactions and to what extent the excess cement contributes to peri-implantitis. Resin cements, with their high strength and non-soluble characteristics, are hard to detect and will not be dissolved by oral or sulcular fluids. Excess resin cements at the restoration margin are a major cause for soft tissue recession and inflammation. The authors contended that the primary retention of cemented implant prosthesis is not dependent on the type of cement used but more on the adaptation and seating of the prosthesis itself. Wilson (2009) demonstrated that suppuration or continued bleeding on probing around gingival margins of implant restorations had an 81% correlation to the presence of excess cement. Therefore, trapped cement would cause constant irritation to the gingival sulcus, which might induce recession.

5.3.2.3 Influence of the Underlying Periosteum

Periosteum can be described as an osteoprogenitor cell containing bone envelope, capable of being activated to proliferate by trauma, tumors, and lymphocyte mitogens. Periosteal cells secrete extracellular matrix and form a membranous structure so the periosteum offers a rich cell source for bone tissue engineering; hence, the regenerative potential of periosteum is immense (Mahajan 2012).

The periosteum is made up of three distinctive zones. Zone 1 has an average thickness of 10–20 μm consisting predominantly of osteoblasts representing 90% of the cell population, while collagen fibrils comprise 15% of the volume. The majority of cells in zone 2 are fibroblasts, with endothelial cells. Zone 3 has the highest volume of collagen fibrils and fibroblasts among all the three zones. Fibroblasts make up more than 90% of the cells in zone 3 (Reynders, Becker and Broos 1998; Mahajan 2012).

The structure of periosteum varies with age. In infants and children it is thicker, more vascular, active, and loosely attached as compared to adults, where it is thinner, less active, and firmly adherent (Tran Van, Vignery and Baron 1982). The periosteum has a rich vascular plexus of capillaries supplying blood to bone that reside within the cortex, linking the medullary and periosteal vessels which promote revascularization during wound healing. Studies have reported the existence of osteogenic progenitors, similar to mesenchymal stem cells (MSCs), in the periosteum (Wang et al. 2013).

Studies have shown promising results with the use of periosteum to treat gingival recession defects (Mahajan 2010). Periosteum-derived progenitor cells may serve as an optimal cell source for tissue engineering based on their accessibility, ability to proliferate rapidly, and capability to differentiate into multiple mesenchymal lineages (Taba et al. 2005). A study by De Bari, Dell'Accio and Vanlaume (2006) indicates that periosteal progenitor cells are able to differentiate not only into bone and cartilage cells but also into adipocyte and skeletal myocyte cells.

Nobuto et al. (2005) have suggested a role for the periosteum in tissue healing and postoperative angiogenesis and concluded that after mucoperiosteal flap elevation, the periosteal vascularity exhibited potent blood vessel-forming activity through various angiogenic mechanisms and through repair activity. Therefore, clinicians should minimize periosteal trauma and manipulation as much as possible during surgery to maintain the maximum tissue reparative capacity.

The higher bone loss rate with classic incision sites occurred when a papilla detached from bone, where the interdental bone in proximity to the adjacent tooth is denuded from the periosteum, the bone blood supply can be affected (Evian, Corn and Rosenberg 1985). Therefore, excluding interproximal papillae from the mucoperiosteal flap (papillae preservative flaps) might help to minimize postoperative tissue recession (see Figures 5.15a, b and 5.16a–c).

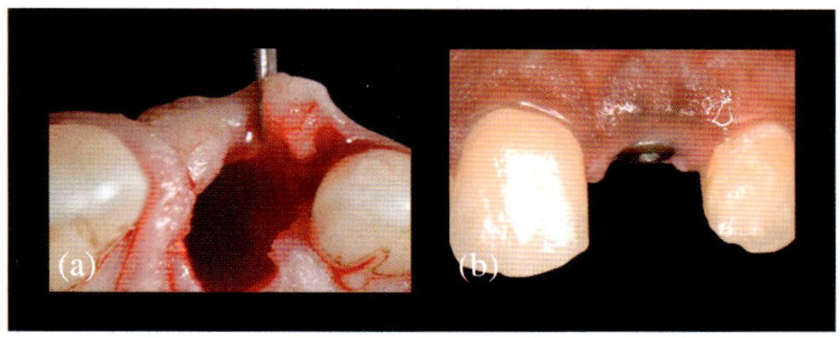

Figure 5.15 (a) Mucosal reflection at the area of the interdental papilla at the time of implant placement, (b) Post-operative drop of the interdental papilla height as a result of periosteal reflection.

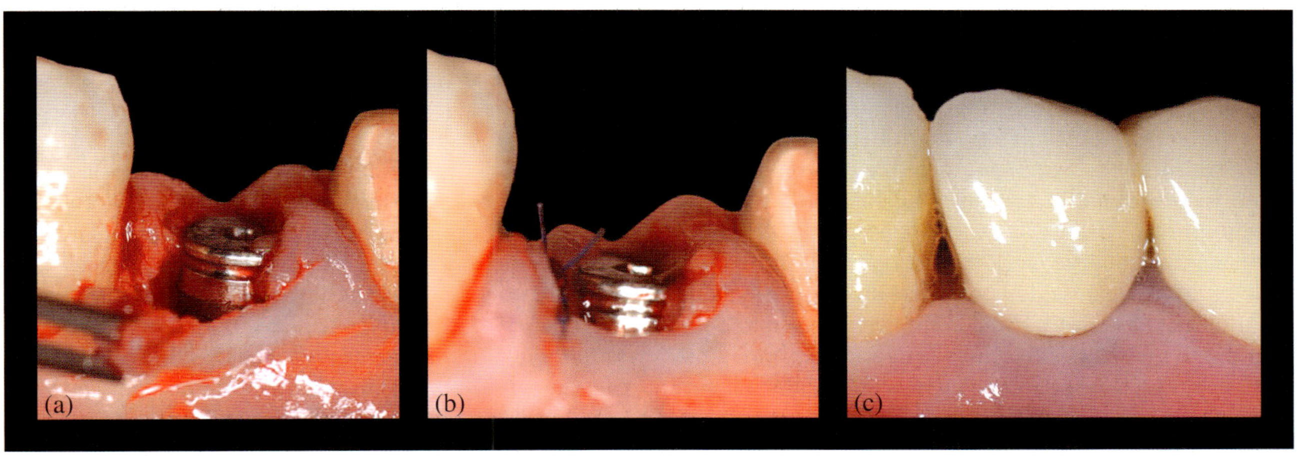

Figure 5.16 (a) Periosteal reflection and cutting of the mesial papilla, (b) Suturing, (c) Drop of the papillary height as a result of a periosteal reflection (blunting).

Excessive periosteal stripping not only jeopardizes the soft tissue flap vascularity but may also lead to postoperative tissue necrosis, while incomplete mucoperiosteal management can lead to improper soft tissue closure or a closure under tension. It is the author's opinion that flapless implant placement intervention could be highly valuable (whenever indicated) to the overall treatment outcome for many obvious reasons. However, a strict protocol should be implemented that includes the mandatory use of CBCT along with a CAD/CAM surgical guide.

5.3.2.4 The Influence of the Immediate Implant Placement on Alveolar Bone Remodeling

Tooth extraction will be followed by marked change in the tissue volume of the alveolar ridge. In a clinical study, Schropp, Wenzel and Kostopoulos (2003) demonstrated that the loss of volume horizontally amounts to 5–7 mm within the first 12 months after tooth extraction. This corresponds to approximately 50% of the original width of the alveolar bone. Cardaropoli et al. (2005) and Araujo and Lindhe (2005) stated that the coronal thin part of the buccal bone wall of the extraction socket is often comprised solely of bundle bone. The bundle bone loses its function after tooth extraction and is resorbed by osteoclastic activity, which might affect the bone remodeling process. Additionally, most of the experimental studies utilized mucoperiosteal flaps exposing the buccal bone, which might have further detrimental effects on the resorption process occurring after tooth extraction (Araujo and Lindhe 2005; Cardaropoli et al. 2005). Araujo et al. (2006) studied the histological effects of surgical trauma on soft- and hard-tissue remodeling and concluded that all test teeth demonstrated signs of attachment loss and bone loss.

Araujo and Lindhe (2005) stated that osteoclasts were indeed present in the exposed area of the alveolar ridge, which exhibited signs of surface resorption. Fickl et al. (2008) stated that when the buccal bone plate is resorbed, the soft tissue complex can no longer be stabilized and will collapse into the newly formed space. As the buccal soft tissue occupies the place of the former buccal bone plate, the room for bone regeneration is reduced, leading to the observed major shrinkage, especially in thin phenotypes.

During the healing period, the buccal crestal bone undergoes variable degrees of resorptive and modeling changes characterized by a combination of bone fill within the original peri-implant defect, resorption of the buccal plate of bone of approximately 50% of the original width, and approximately 1 mm loss of crestal bone height (Botticelli et al. 2004; Araujo and Lindhe 2005; Araujo et al. 2006; Sanz et al. 2015). This situation may be unstable and may predispose the mucosa to recession (Hermann, Schenk ad Schoolfield 2001). Araújo and Lindhe suggested that following tooth extraction, the blood vessels in the periodontium supplying the thin bone walls are severed, thereby causing facial bone plate resorption (Araujo and Lindhe 2005).

A study by Araujo et al. (2006) to evaluate tissue remodeling in fresh extraction sockets, showed that the buccal and lingual bone walls underwent marked surface resorption and the height of the thin buccal hard tissue wall was reduced at the end of four weeks. As the process of healing continued and the buccal bone crest shifted further in the apical direction, the buccal crest was located >2 mm apical of the marginal border of the SLA surface at 12 weeks. Thus, it was concluded that the bone-to-implant contact established during the early phase of socket healing following implant installation was in part lost when the buccal bone wall underwent continued resorption.

Araujo et al. (2006) explained that the modeling in the marginal defect region was accompanied by marked attenuation of the dimensions of both the delicate buccal and the wider lingual bone walls. Bone loss at molar sites was more pronounced than at the premolar locations. Implant placement failed to preserve the hard tissue dimension of the ridge following tooth extraction. The buccal as well as the lingual bone walls were resorbed, although some marginal loss of osseointegration was also evident.

Araujo et al. (2006) demonstrated that the resorption of the buccal/lingual walls of the extraction site occurred in two overlapping phases. During phase 1, the bundle bone was resorbed and replaced with woven bone. Since the crest of the buccal bone wall comprised solely bundle bone, this modeling resulted in substantial vertical reduction of the buccal crest. Phase 2 included resorption that occurred from the outer surfaces of both bone walls.

Schropp et al. (2003) reported a reduction of 50% of the width of the alveolar ridge at 12 months after tooth extraction. Hence, preservation of the alveolus at the time of extraction of prominent roots in the anterior maxilla is crucial. A study by Ferrus et al. (2010) confirmed that the position of the implant, the size of the horizontal buccal gap, and the buccal bone crest thickness significantly influenced the remodeling rate of the hard tissue during a four-month period of healing after immediate implant placement into an extraction socket. Also, the sites where the buccal bone wall was thicker than 1 mm showed a better gap filling and minimal vertical resorption of the buccal crest when compared to sites with thinner bone (<1 mm). The possible relationship between gingival tissue form and the underlying bone was previously analyzed by Fu et al. (2011), showing a moderate correlation between soft and hard tissues in the anterior region.

It seems that there is a need to preserve or increase the hard and soft tissue thickness using different types of interventions (Chen et al. 2009), which often might reduce and sometimes eliminate the need for subsequent augmentation procedures. Wildermanm and Wentz (1965) when explaining histogenesis of repair, observed different healing patterns of buccal and lingual plates of the anterior mandibular region of dogs. A mean labial gingival recession of 0.5–1 mm around single implants, due the bone remodeling after implant surgery, seems to be a common finding after implant restorations. Also, at one year between single implant placement and the second-stage surgery, a mean reduction in facial bone thickness and facial bone height of 0.4 and 0.7 mm have been reported.

With a thorough understanding of the available literature, it may be concluded that irrespective of the simultaneous placement of dental implants in fresh extraction sites, there are variable degrees of bone remodeling that in turn influence the occurrence of implant related gingival recession, and apical migration of implant related tissues can occur due to many other variables. This warrants the clinician attention to take these facts into consideration when deciding upon any treatment plan that has a high esthetic demand.

5.3.2.5 Other Related Factors

Several regenerative techniques have been proposed to increase the alveolar volume both vertically and horizontally to prepare the alveolar ridge for correct placement of oral implants. Each of these grafting modalities has its own inherited remodeling rate that might be followed by soft tissue drop. Various authors have reported average amounts of autogenous bone block resorption varying from 20 to 50% in the absence of complications during healing. In a study by Cordaro, Amadé and Cordaro (2002), 45% resorption of autogenous onlay grafts was reported (see Figure 5.17a and b).

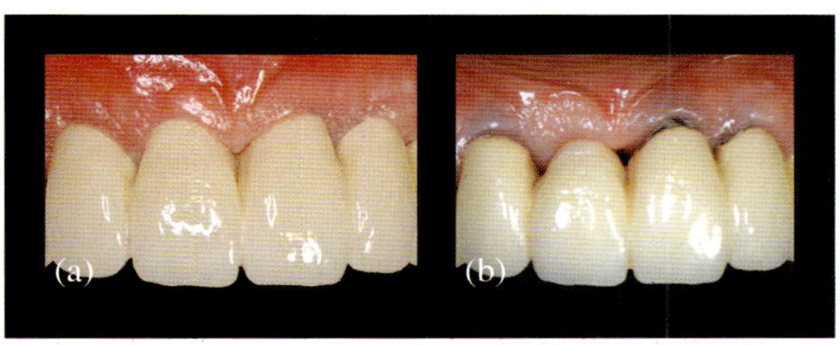

Figure 5.17 (a) and (b) clinical example of post regenerative gingival recession as a result of post-operative remodeling, this one year comparative view warrants the attention to allow a sufficient time for the provisional restoration.

A systematic review by Rocchietta, Fontana and Simion (2008) recorded different resorption values considering vertical bone augmentation procedures. Various recommendations have been made to reduce post-regenerative bone resorption, one of which is to overbuild or over-contour the defect site to compensate for future grafted bone resorption. However, excessive over-contouring of the defect site may present challenges to an optimal soft tissue closure, risking soft tissue dehiscence. Another approach is to combine bone blocks with various bone substitutes and barrier membranes during augmentation of implant sites, which might reduce resorption of block grafts. A monocortical bone graft placed with the osseointegrated fixtures were found to provide acceptable degrees of resorption during a five year period and prevented failure of the prosthetic rehabilitation (Liu and Kerns 2014). Another study conducted by Gultekin et al. (2016), compared the remodeling rate and the volumetric changes after autogenous ramus block bone grafting (RBG) or guided bone regeneration (GBR) in horizontally deficient maxilla before implant placement. They concluded that both RBG and GBR hard-tissue augmentation techniques provide adequate bone graft volume and stability for implant insertion. However, GBR causes greater resorption at maxillary augmented sites than RBG, which clinicians should consider during treatment planning.

Gingival recession occurring around dental implants could also be because of continuous muscular activity from the labial frenum attachment, which induces continuous apical pull on the gingival margin (see Figure 5.18).

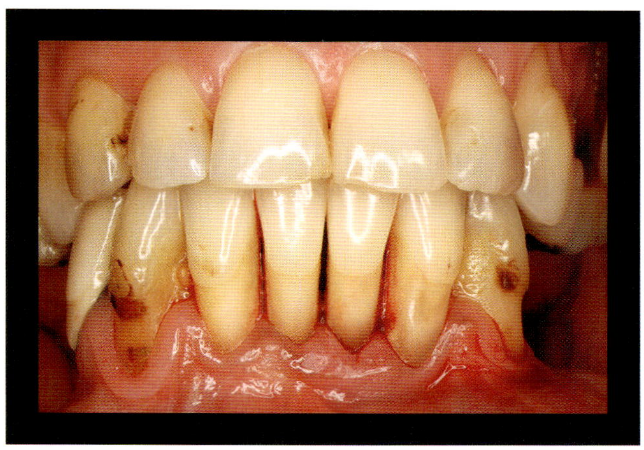

Figure 5.18 Reduced band of keratinized tissue as a result of muscular pulling effect.

A muscle pull on the gingival of the implant site will lead to continuous, steady gingival recession and action must be taken to relieve the implant from that tension. In some cases, a frenectomy few weeks before the implant surgical procedure may need to be carried out to eliminate the muscle pull, as shown in Figure 5.19a and b.

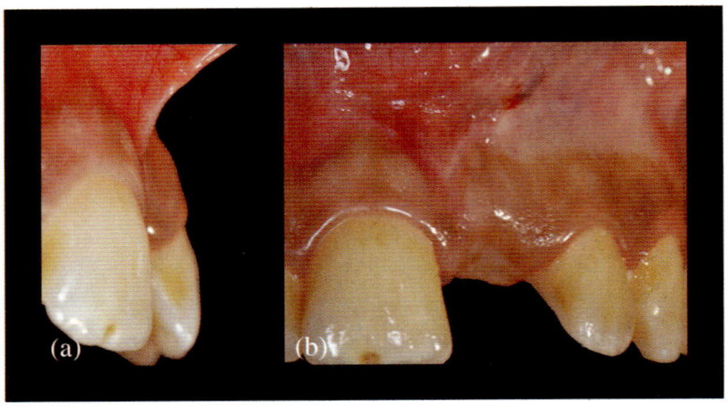

Figure 5.19 (a) and (b) A frenectomy procedure performed with laser to prevent the pulling effect of the tissue apically, it is highly suggested to perform frenectomy regularly prior to performing any reconstructive surgery.

5.3.3 Technical Factors

5.3.3.1 Implant Positioning Errors

Implant fixture position has a direct impact on many aspects of the future outcome of the implant supported restoration, and subsequently peri-implant tissue violation. For instance, placing the implants too far labially will also lead to resorption of the thin labial plate followed by apical displacement of labial tissue complex, as shown in Figure 5.20a and b.

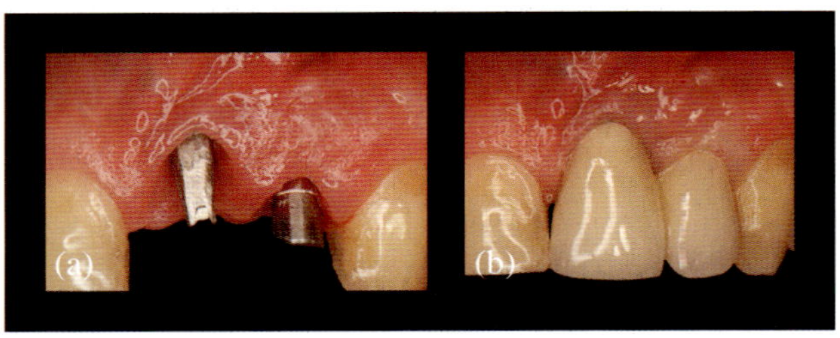

Figure 5.20 (a) Gingival recession related to the implant replacing maxillary left central incisor as a result of too deep and too far labial placement, (b) Case restored with asymmetrical gingival contours.

The extent of resorption appears more pronounced when the implant shoulder is placed less than half a millimeter from the crestal plate buccolingually (Ramanauskaite and Juodzbalys 2016).

Incorrect implant position in the alveolar ridge may occur because of many factors, such as not using a surgical guide, imprecise fabrication of a surgical guide, lack of control during the drilling procedure, poor pre-surgical planning, poor armamentarium, incomplete knowledge, and in experience. A minor deviation from the standard known clinical guidelines for esthetic implant positioning in any dimension will surely result in esthetic fallout, as shown in Figure 5.21a and b.

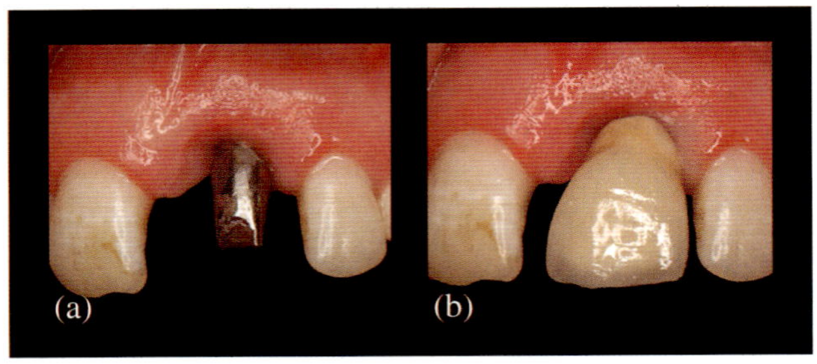

Figure 5.21 (a) Gingival recession related to the implant replacing maxillary left central incisor as a result of too deep and too far palatal placement, (b) Case restored with asymmetrical gingival contours.

To establish and maintain an ideal soft tissue architecture, implants should be positioned at the correct distance to the adjacent dentition, at the correct depth, and more palatally positioned (Choquet et al. 2001; Grunder et al. 2005; Kan et al. 2003). When dealing with anterior single implant supported restorations, the thickness of facial bone as well as the dimensions of the facial peri-implant mucosa are critical for the achievement and long-term stability of good esthetics, with a reduced risk of future tissue recession (Buser et al. 2004; Grunder et al. 2005). When implants are incorrectly angled or improperly positioned, various prosthodontic techniques have been reported, including the use of a gingiva-colored acrylic resin façade, a flexible silicone-based tissue-colored material, or removable prostheses (Cura, Saraçoglu and Cötert 2002; Everhart and Cavazos 1983; Gardner and Stankewitz 1982; Greene 1998).

Juodzbalyus and Wang (2007) stated that a natural buccal and proximal restorative contour can be ensured by correctly orienting the implant in a buccopalatal position. A minimum space of 2 mm should be maintained on the buccal side in front of the external implant collar surface, and correct three-dimensional implant positioning has been considered important for long term maintenance of soft tissue levels (Buser et al. 2004). An association of buccal implant malpositioning and mid-facial recession has been described (Chen et al. 2007, 2009) and should be considered by surgeons when pursuing immediate implant placement. Studies identified the tooth-to-implant distance and the level of the contact point in relation to the bone crest as key factors for maintaining healthy papillae (Lops et al. 2008; Romeo et al. 2008).

It is essential that the clinician is familiar with the various unfortunate clinical situations that may arise due to misplacement and the ways to solve them. The axial misplacement of the dental implant within its hosing can be damaging to the overall health of the soft and hard tissues surrounding the implant, as a resulting deep gingival sulcus with a long junctional epithelium can be a serious consequence due to the further deep positioning of the implant and the failure of hygiene practice. This creates a favorable environment for several types of bacteria, including anaerobic bacteria, to colonize and populate. The deeper an implant is inserted into the bone, the more bone will be resorbed around the implant following second-stage surgery with an abutment connection. This bone resorption is not a pathological condition but a physiological reaction to the implant misplacement. Inflammation and gingival bleeding usually occur as a result of the inaccessibility for hygiene measures from one side and bacterial endotoxins from another side. It becomes increasingly urgent to ensure complete removal of the excess luting cement from the interface between the abutment and the restoration. Correction of this clinical dilemma is almost impossible to achieve unless supragingival margins of the prosthesis are fabricated.

The failure to position the implant at its optimal depth, such as being placed too shallow, often results in a short crown with constricted margins due to the absence of the "running room." This makes stacking the prosthetic components supragingival. This clinical predicament is impossible to amend or rectify. The difficulty remains in handling the margins of the final prosthesis and hiding the abutment collar sublingually. In this particular condition, implant removal can be the treatment of choice. The improper mesiodistal positioning of the implant might lead to the total absence of restorative possibilities, and if the implant is placed in the interdental papilla space or is placed too mesialized or leaving no or a minimal space for restoration, it becomes impossible to restore. Violating the labial plate of bone or the labial soft tissues might constitute a major clinical dilemma that is impossible to correct even with the use of the angulated abutments. The consequences of violating the labial plate integrity goes beyond the teeth to the lip support, as it might impinge on lip harmony. Placing the implant angulation in a too-far lingual position might result in tongue crowding, because to impinge on the tongue space can significantly compromise speech and mastication.

A fair number of clinical approaches have been described to resolve misaligned and malpositioned dental implants if an unfavorable inclination of the implant fixture is the only problem. The use of angulated abutments can often improve the prosthetic results of an implant-supported restoration. Even using the preangulated abutments in too-far labial implant placement cases will not be effective in most clinical situations because the preangled abutment usually requires a larger restorative dimension than other types and the gingival collar of the preangled abutment will encroach upon the peri-implant soft tissue and violate its natural contours. The use of the angled abutments will not ensure any protection against recession.

Several factors have been proposed as being important in determining the stability of the peri-implant marginal mucosa, including the implant shoulder position in a buccolingual and apicocoronal plane (Buser et al. 2004; Garber 1981). In relation to the optimal buccolingual position, Buser et al. (2004) recommended that the implant shoulder should be placed 1–2 mm lingual to the emergence of the adjacent teeth to ensure maintenance of an adequate width of buccal bone and stable mucosa over the buccal implant surface. Evans and Chen (2008) suggested that the buccolingual position of the implant shoulder is a highly significant factor in determining the degree of buccal marginal tissue recession. Implants with a shoulder position at or buccal to a line drawn between the cervical margins of adjacent teeth demonstrated three times more recession than implants with a shoulder position lingual to this line.

5.3.3.2 The Influence of the Implant Collar Design

The peri-implant crest module is the collar portion of the dental implant creating a transition zone between the prosthetic part and the implant body. Its design and position in relation to the alveolar crest is critical and its relationship to the abutment implant interface plays a major role in overall harmonious integration and soft tissue health. Early tissue breakdown leading to soft tissue and hard tissue loss starts at the crest module. Misch, Qu and Bidez (1999) have studied the influence of the implant crest components and their angulation in relation to the shear and compressive loading. Smooth surface implant collars have been extensively used in past decades; however, a significant drawback of the smooth collar stems from its questionable integration with the surrounding hard tissues. When the smooth collar of an implant is placed under the crest of the bone, increased shear forces are created to the adjacent bone, and eventually bone is resorbed, leading to a marginal bone loss with a long junctional epithelium (Hermann et al. 2001). Hermann et al. (2001) examined the peri-implant soft tissue dimensions at varying locations of a rough/smooth implant border in one-piece and two-piece implants in relation to the crest of the bone, when submerged and non-submerged techniques were employed. Crestal bone changes around two types of implants with varying smooth collar lengths (2.8 and 1.8 mm) were evaluated. Their findings suggest an absence of bone loss was observed when the implants with rough crest modules were placed at the level of crestal bone, exhibiting a shorter (1.8 mm) as opposed to a slightly larger (2.8 mm) machined collar portion.

Weiner, Somin and Ehrenberg (2008) observed that initially the experimental implants showed greater bone attachment along the laser microtextured collar. However, the controls had more soft tissue downgrowth, greater osteoclastic activity, and increased saucerization compared with sites adjacent to experimental implants. There was closer adaptation of the bone to the laser microtextured collars. It was concluded that the use of tissue engineered collars with micro-grooving seems to promote bone and soft tissue attachment along the collar and facilitate development of a biological width (see page 158) (Nevins et al. 2008).

In a clinical study evaluating laser micro-texturing for soft tissue and bone attachments to dental implants, Pecora et al. (2009) incorporated a tapered dental implant (Laser-Lok surface treatment) with a 2 mm wide collar, to accomplish bone and connective tissue attachment while inhibiting epithelial downgrowth in a prospective, controlled, multicenter clinical trial. A consistent difference in the probing depth between Laser-Lok and the control implant demonstrated the formation of a stable soft tissue seal above the crestal bone. Laser etched collars limited the crestal bone loss to the 0.59 mm range as opposed to the 1.94 mm crestal bone loss reported for the control implant (Elaskary 2009; Pecora et al. 2009; Ricci and Alexander 2001) (see Figure 5.22a and b).

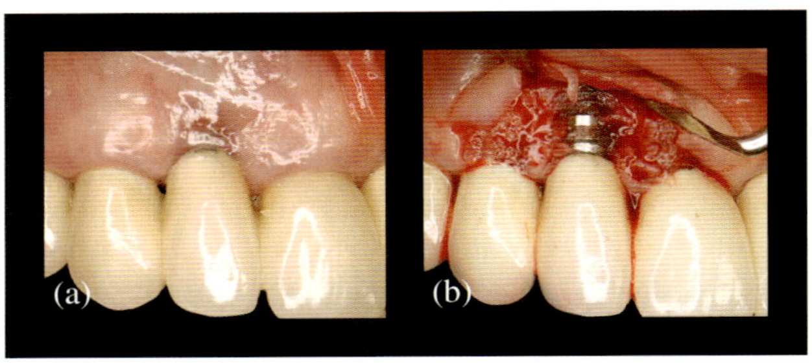

Figure 5.22 (a) and (b) Implant supported restoration revealing soft tissue thinning and bone resorption as a result of using an implant with smooth collar component.

A study of the effect of a machined/rough implant collar on the osseous crest has shown that the least marginal bone loss with each implant occurred when the collar of the implant was placed above the alveolar crest (Alomrami et al. 2005). A change in implant design towards a scalloped collar to mirror the bone and soft tissue topography with rough surfaces and grooves did not prove to be practical (Wöhrle 2003). Also, it did not show any clinical benefits and made implant position orientation difficult. The last thread location of the implant determines the effective level of remodeling after loading, and this is perhaps even more important than the position of the implant/abutment microgap (Rompen, Touati and Van Dooren 2003). It is the author's opinion that implants with microthreads reaching the collar do not seem to prevent bone resorption from occurring (see Figure 5.23a and b).

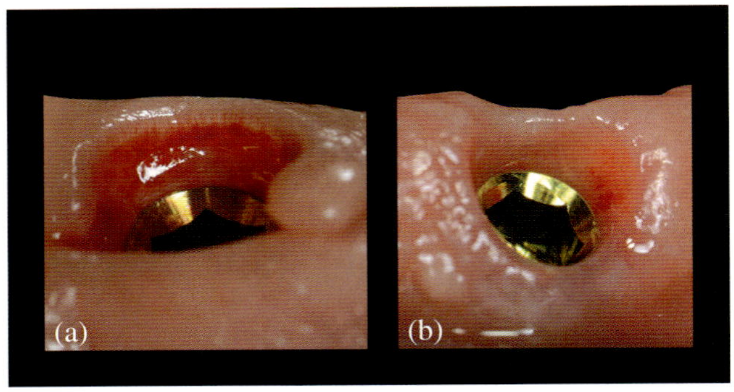

Figure 5.23 (a) and (b) Effect of laser lock etched collar showing tissue tags and epithelial attachment (left side) versus regular smooth collar (right side).

5.3.3.3 The Influence of the Provisional and Prosthetic Designs

The role of interim dental restorations used for optimizing the final result of the restorative and prosthodontic procedures has changed dramatically in the past few years. These restorations are no longer regarded as temporary restorations but rather as provisional restorations with distinct functions and purposes. Provisional restorations have become a vital diagnostic and assessment tool to evaluate function color, shape, contour, occlusion, periodontal response, implant healing, and overall esthetics. With increased demands placed on provisional restorations, new materials and techniques are being developed and some existing protocols are being refined to accomplish the desired goals. Provisional restorations are often in the oral environment for several weeks, requiring a precise fabrication. An adequate understanding of the relationship between periodontal tissues and restorative dentistry is paramount to ensure adequate form, function, and esthetics, as well as comfort of the dentition (Nugala, Kumar and Krishna 2012).

With dental implants, the clinical scenario is significantly different from that of a natural dentition, with the implant and/or abutment surface being a non-vital structure without a blood supply. Dental implant design and surface improvements have helped clinicians direct their treatment approach towards a more immediate timetable as well as a more esthetically driven one (Smeets, Stadlinger and Schwarz 2016).

Many factors play a role in the emergence profile: (1) the smoothness and degree of finish of the temporization, (2) venting of the temporization to avoid excessive cement in the gingival crevice, (3) continuous changing of the prosthetic margins in accordance with soft tissue maturation to provide steady soft tissue support, and (4) the cleanness and purity of the provisional materials. Using the provisional restoration for a sufficient time (four to six weeks) allows the soft tissue to reach its final healing stage and optimal maturation. Then when final prostheses are inserted, minimal or no tissue remodeling or migration occurrs.

The prosthetic stage is highly influential in the maintenance of peri-implant tissue stability. It involves, the use of accurate provisional restorations, optimal final prosthetic fabrication, and a precise duration of the provisional restoration, which are all factors that need full attention. Implant provisional restorations provide significant and invaluable benefits such as enhanced patient comfort and satisfaction, as well as the ability to contour peri-implant tissues (Botticelli et al. 2004). This is critical in the esthetic zone, where the contouring of the soft tissues provide an ideal emergence profile to aid in both esthetics and phonetics (Neale and Chee 1994; Chu et al. 2012; Hui et al. 2001).

The interfaces between the gingival unite and the implant collar is mainly composed of the epithelium and connective tissue, which forms the biological width (Abrahamsson et al. 1997; Berglundh et al. 1991; Hermann et al. 2000). The tissue at the most coronal aspect and adjacent to the implant abutment consists of the free gingival margin, which is covered by stratified squamous epithelium. As the epithelium progresses down the implant it becomes non-keratinized, below the junctional epithelium attachment lies the connective tissue attachment (McKinney et al. 1985). Current attention is driven towards the influence of the provisional restorations to the overall stability of the gingival tissues, and the optimal requirements of the provisional subgingival margins were described by (Luchinskaya et al. 2017).

Long-term use of a provisional restoration should precede the insertion of the final prosthesis. This will help the maturation of the soft tissue during the provisionalization stage (Lazzara 1993), thus minimizing the tendency for future exposure of the final implant-supported components. Especially in the esthetic zone, placing the provisional restoration for a period of four to six weeks will provide the clinicians with the final mature gingival margin level after soft tissue remodeling has been finalized. In addition, long-term temporization will help to guide the soft tissues to mature and remodel, preventing eventual collapse. The rush for premature delivery of a prosthesis will lead to recession of the gingival tissue as the peri-implant soft tissue continues to remodel (see Figure 5.24a and b).

In order to allow stable soft and hard tissue margins around the dental implant abutment, the transmucosal area of the abutment design should not be oversized and expanded but rather stay narrow and concave to thicken and immobilize the circular connective tissue around the connection. This induces thickening of the connective tissue zone, which will ensure long-term stability of the marginal tissues (Touati, Rompen and Van Dooren 2005) (see Figure 5.25a and b).

The material composition of the implant transmucosal area, surface topography, surface tension, and surface energy

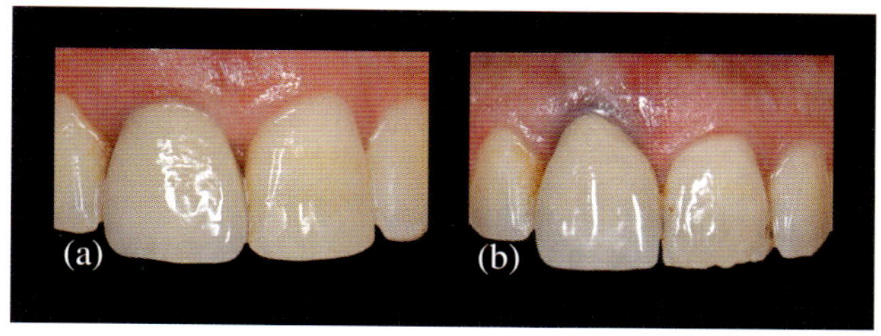

Figure 5.24 (a) Maxillary right central incisor restored with an implant supported restoration, (b) Two years post restorative result showing apical migration of the related tissues as a result of the too deeply placed margins of the restoration under gingival margin.

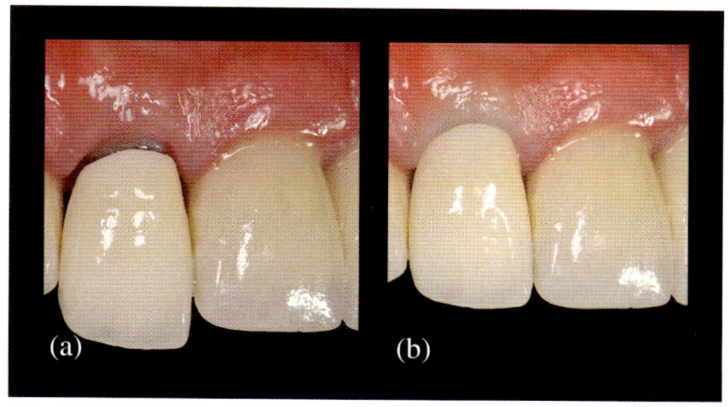

Figure 5.25 (a) and (b) Pre and post crown cementation on an implant, note the pressure induced on the gingival margins that might induce apical tissue migration.

have been studied over the years. Gittens et al. (2013) investigated the influence of surface hydrophilicity of titanium implant surfaces on the behavior and differentiation of the epithelial cells. Spriano et al. (2017) suggested that surface hydrophilicity might positively influence the epithelial seal around dental implants. Proliferation, spreading, and moving of the epithelial cells were enhanced on hydrophilic titanium surfaces compared with hydrophobic titanium surfaces. In addition, relatively smoother surfaces were preferred (Novaes et al. 2010). Few articles have been found in the literature regarding cell adhesion or cell proliferation on to permanent abutment materials such as titanium, gold alloy, and ceramics (Abdulmajeed and Willberg 2015; Gasik 2016, 2017); however, we are expecting a huge leap in this path to develop in the near future that will help increase peri-implant tissue stability around dental implant prosthetics. The prosthetic margins should be designed to avoid inducing too much pressure to the overlying soft tissues, as any extra pressure induced to the transmucosal area will be translated into apical migration of this tissue, especially in a thin tissue phenotype. The more pressure that is induced, the more liability there is for recession. Labial prosthetic margins should be either equi-gingival slightly below gingival margin and the abutment shoulder should also be brought up to this level to allow the prosthetic margins to rest on it, leaving the transmucosal area intact and undisturbed (Neale and Chee 1994) (see Figure 5.26).

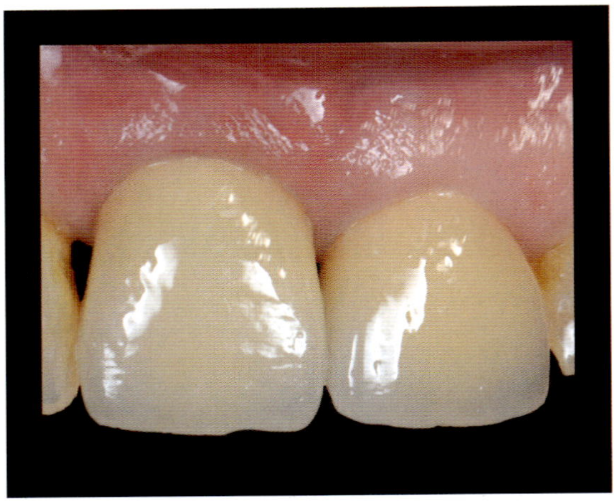

Figure 5.26 Final implant supported prosthesis delivery revealing excessive pressure on the tissue to the gingival margin leading to recession.

5.3.3.4 Miscellaneous Factors

In natural dentition, gingival morphology is partly related to the tooth shape and form (Dhir 2011). Tooth crown morphology can be triangular, ovoid, or square shaped with a long, narrow, or short form. Olson and Lindhe (1991) in their study reported that individuals with a long narrow tooth form demonstrated a thin free gingiva, shallow probing depth, and pronounced scalloped contour of the gingival margin. Similarly, the tooth shape and form can influence the peri-implant soft tissue architecture. Tooth shape is one of the five essential diagnostic key factors for peri-implant esthetics (Garber, Salama and Salama 2001; Kois and Kan 2001). These key factors include the relative tooth position, form of the periodontium, phenotype of the periodontium, tooth shape, and position of the osseous crest. According to Garber et al. (2001), subjects with a long narrow form of the upper central incisors experienced more recession of the gingival margin at buccal surfaces than subjects who had a short wide tooth form. Individuals with square-shaped teeth have more favorable esthetic outcomes because of the long proximal contact and less papillary tissue, whereas the triangular tooth shape has a proximal contact located more incisally needing more tissue height to fill in and is therefore at a high risk of "black hole formation" (Dhir 2011) (see Figure 5.27a–d).

Others also suggested that morphologic characteristics of the periodontium are partly related to the shape and form of the teeth (Hirschfeld et al. 1923; Wheeler 1961; Seibert 1993; Seibert). Weisgold (1977) considered that a long tapering (triangular) crown shape was more susceptible to recession, while flat (square) teeth seemed to have greater bands of keratinized gingival, which were more resistant to recession. Olsen and Lindhe (1991) also found that the central incisors with a narrow tooth form had a greater amount of recession when compared to incisors with a square shape.

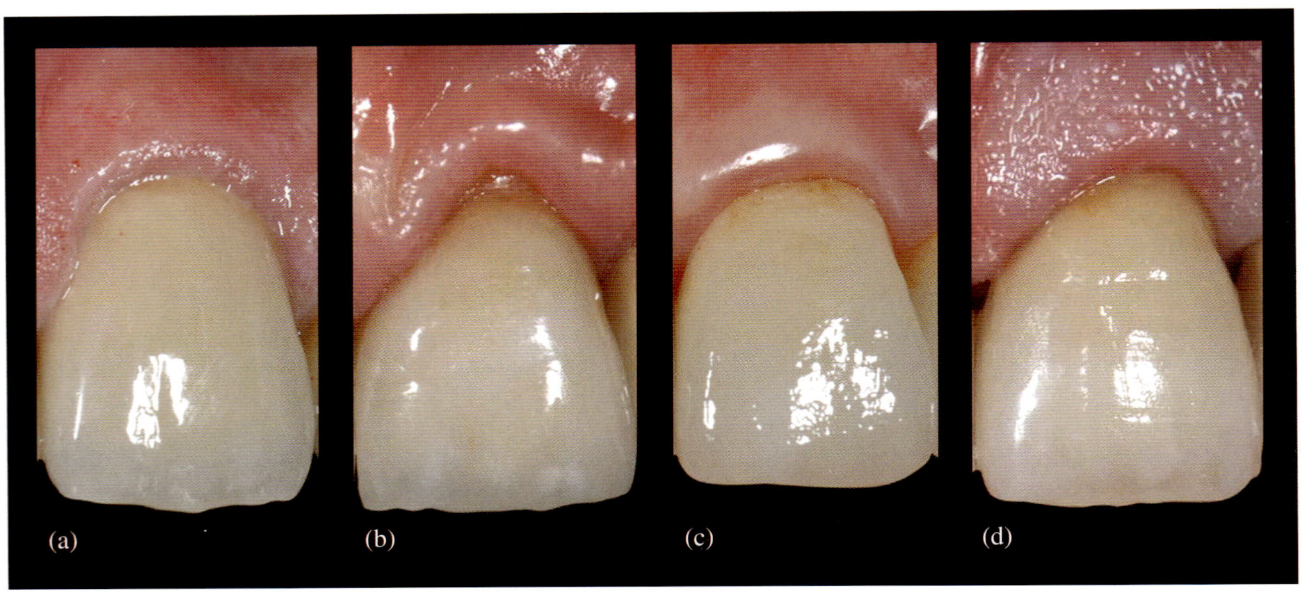

Figure 5.27 (a–d) Different teeth morphology determines the soft tissue liability to apical migration, longer and triangular crowns are more liable to recession.

The contribution of oral hygiene practices to the occurrence of gingival recession remains a major consideration in our understanding of the etiology, the prognosis, and the treatment. It is important to recognize that gingival recession may be associated with both extremes; poor oral hygiene, and extremely good oral hygiene. In the former type, meticulous brushing is thought to introduce trauma to the gingiva leading to recession (Addy, Mostafa and Newcombe 1987; Niemi, Sandholm and Ainamo 1984). This type of recession is commonly seen on the facial side of canines and premolars and associated with overzealous brushing habits. Poor oral hygiene is associated with recession due to plaque-induced inflammation and subsequent attachment loss. It appears that many factors related to tooth brushing may contribute to recession. These factors include brushing force and brush hardness, frequency and duration of tooth brushing, as well as frequency of changing tooth brushes and the brushing techniques and types of manual or electric brushes used (Rajapakse, McCracken and Gwynnett 2007). For both overzealous and insufficient oral hygiene, an underlying inflammatory response is likely to contribute to tissue destruction resulting in gingival recession.

On the other hand, Strub, Gaberthüel and Grunder (1991) stated that the keratinized mucosa or dental plaque does not seem to be related to implant failure but that its presence might facilitate the patient's hygienic procedures. Wennstrom, Bengazi and Lekholm (1994) in his study concluded that the absence of keratinized mucosa was associated with a higher plaque index and gingival index, but not with annual bone loss, while Chung et al. (2006) stated that an increased width of keratinized mucosa around implants was associated with a lower mean alveolar bone loss and improved indices of soft tissue health. Zigdon and Machtei (2008) stated that a narrow band of keratinized mucosa may lead to increased recession, and the absence of adequate keratinized mucosa around implants was associated with higher plaque accumulation, gingival inflammation, bleeding on probing, and mucosal recession (Adibrad, Shahabuei and Sahabi 2009). Kim et al. (2009) also supported the fact that decreased keratinized mucosa width was associated with recession and marginal bone resorption. The existence of at least 2 mm of keratinized mucosa was also beneficial for reduced plaque accumulation and bleeding (Schrott et al. 2009). Thus, it was concluded that keratinized mucosa was not a critical factor in the maintenance of interproximal bone, but less keratinized mucosa was associated with more gingival inflammation, plaque accumulation, and recession (Crespi, Capparè and Gherlone 2010).

5.4 Classification of Implant-related Gingival Recession

Replacement of the natural dentition in the esthetic zone often requires a prosthesis of optimal form and shade, which, in turn, necessitates the establishment of natural and harmonious gingival architecture surrounding the prosthesis. Moreover, Chen and Buser (2009) concluded that advanced mid-facial recession is common following immediate implant placement (see Figure 5.28a–c).

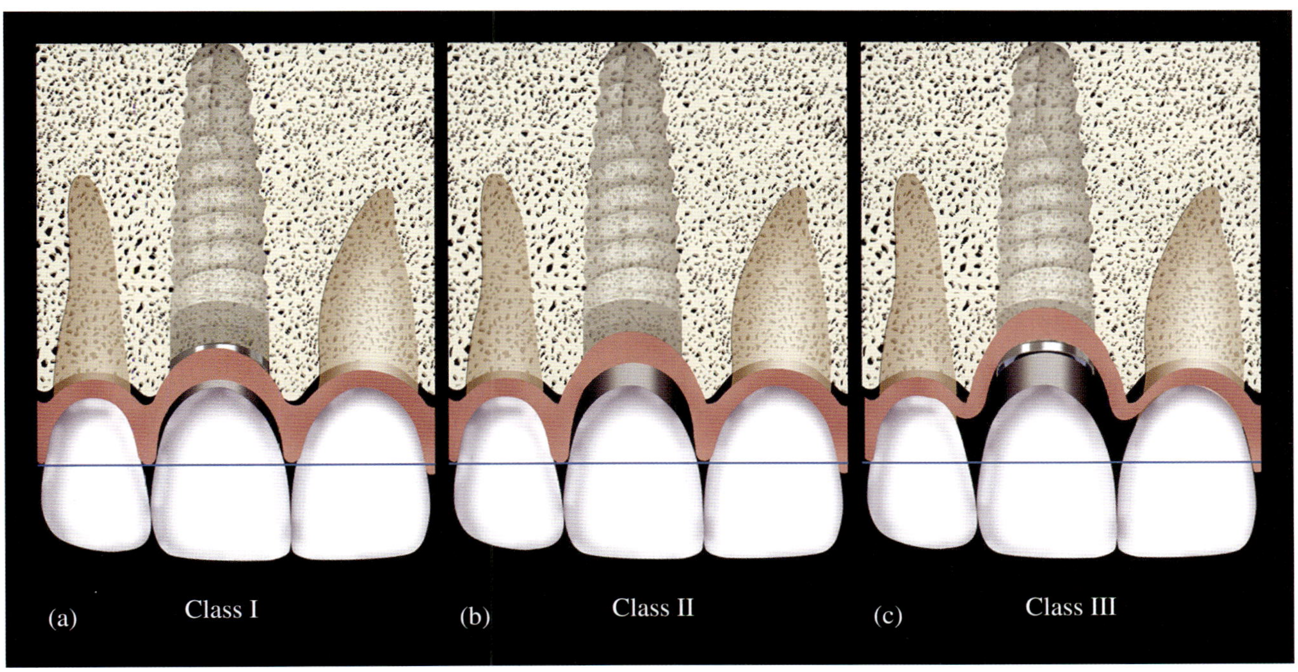

Figure 5.28 (a) Class I mild gingival recession that does not exceed 1 mm, (b) Moderate recession more than 1 mm with intact a papillary height, (c) Severe gingival recession exposing part of the implant fixture with drop of papillary levels.

There are many clinical pictures of implant related gingival recession, therefore it would be invaluable to present a classification system that helps communication between the dental team as well as presenting a proposed clinical intervention for each classification.

Accordingly, the author introduced a new basic classification system for implant-related gingival recession. Class I (minor recession) presents less than 1 mm of recession from the mid-facial aspect with the height of interdental papillae intact. Class II (moderate recession) may be categorized as: class II is an implant-related gingival recession that ranges between 1 and 2 mm from the mid-facial aspect, with both proximal papillae heights intact; it has two subdivision class II division 1, where the labial plate of bone is resorbed while the palatal plate of bone is intact, and class II division 2, where both plates of bone (labial and palatal) are resorbed, confirmed by the CBCT scan. Class III (severe recession) presents more than 2 mm recession from the mid-facial aspect, where one or both peri-implant papillae have lost height (see Figure 5.29a–c and Table 5.1) (Elaskary et al. 2016).

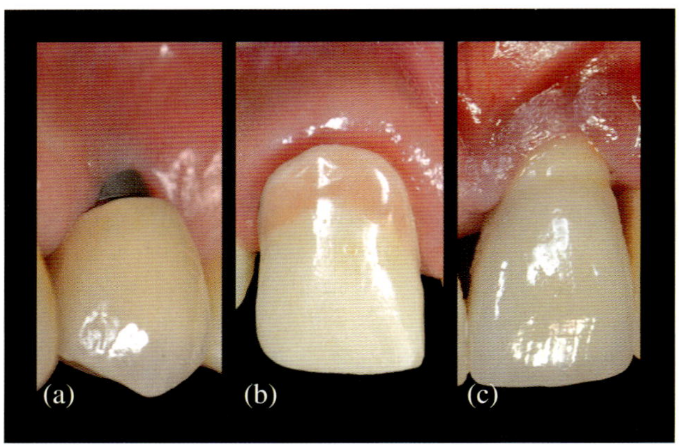

Figure 5.29 (a–c) A Clinical example of Class I, II, and II recession.

5.5 Recession Scoring Template

Several attempts have been made to measure apical tissue migration around natural teeth. Cabello, Rioboo and Fabrega (2012) observed the soft tissue level changes in relation to immediate implant placement using a rigid acrylic stent overlapping the incisal edges of the adjacent teeth with three reference dimples placed in the stent corresponding to the mesial and distal interdental papilla and the level of the gingival zenith. An electronic caliber was then used to measure the distance approximated to a tenth of a millimeter.

On the study cast, a rigid stent is prepared with light-cured resin, covering the incisal edges of at least one adjacent tooth on each side of the target tooth. The stent is >2 mm thick so can be modified to allow seating over the final restoration. Distances are found from the stent to the distal papilla (DP), the mesial papilla (MP), and the gingival zenith (Z). Distances are measured using a precision digital caliper. Three dimples are ditched in the stent, approximately in the vertical projection of the papillae and zenith.

Elaskary et al. (2016) introduced an innovative easy to use scoring method for assessing the level of peri-implant soft tissue mid-buccal gain, to be used before and after treatment to assess the progress of the treatment using a custom fabricated acrylic resin template. The device consists of a custom-designed template that rests on the incisal edges of the maxillary teeth adjacent to the dental implant and has an acrylic extension protruding to the mid-buccal gingival contour of the affected implant-supported crown and its adjacent teeth. The template is used to record implant-related gingival recession, as it reflects the amount of existing recession prior to treatment as a base line to indicate the amount of soft-tissue correction needed, which is represented by a line connecting the mid-buccal point of the two adjacent teeth. This method is subjective because it involves an observer who grades the amount of recession on a 0-to-2 scoring system.

After treatment of the gingival recession, the same acrylic template will be used again to compare the difference in the levels of the gingival margin and to follow

Table 5.1 Classification of implant-related gingival recession.

Class 1	Minor recession	Less than 1 mm recession from the mid-facial aspect with the interdental intact
Class 2	Moderate recession	
Class 2 division 1		There is 1–2 mm recession from the mid-facial aspect with both interdental papilla and palatal plate of bone intact whereas the buccal plate of bone is deficient >3 mm
Class 2 division 2		There is 1–2 mm recession from the mid-facial aspect with interdental papilla intact whereas both buccal and palatal plates of bone are deficient >3 mm
Class 3	Severe recession	More than 2 mm recession from the mid-facial aspect with the peri-implant papillae level dropped apically

the stability of tissue margins over the years. This is assessed by measuring the deepest point in the mid-buccal curve around the old implant-supported restoration and comparing it with the soft tissue margin around the new implant-supported restoration after completion of the treatment. This offers a simple and accurate method to measure the gingival recession treatment outcome. After the recession treatment is completed, the acrylic template can be placed again and the difference in the gingival margin levels compared. This technique focuses mainly on monitoring implant-related gingival recession (see Figures 5.30a and b, 5.31a and b, and 5.32a and b).

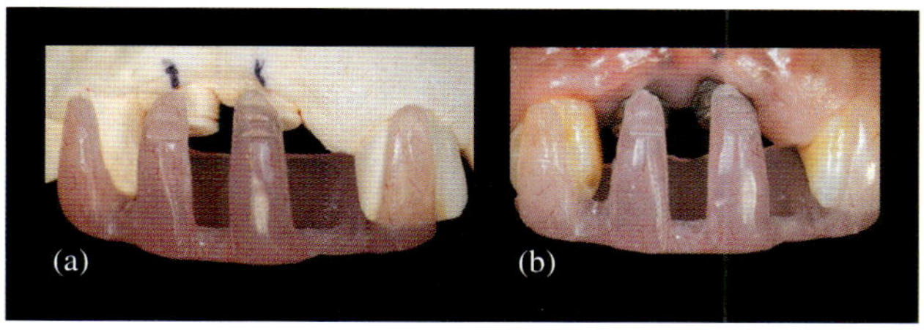

Figure 5.30 (a) and (b) The scoring template that measures the amount of tissue gain (regenerated) post treatment of recession.

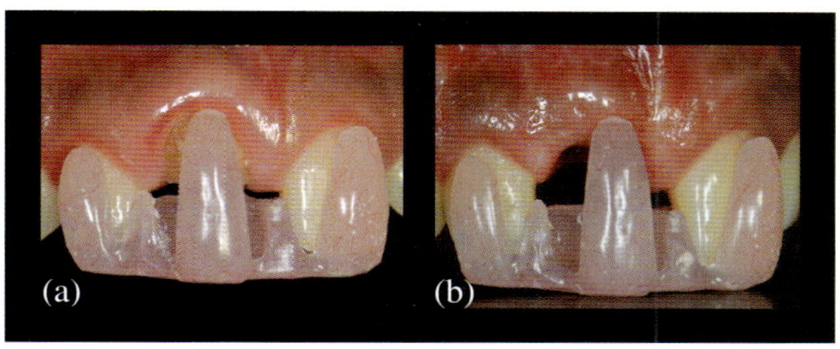

Figure 5.31 (a) and (b) The scoring template that measures the amount of tissue gain (regenerated) post treatment of recession.

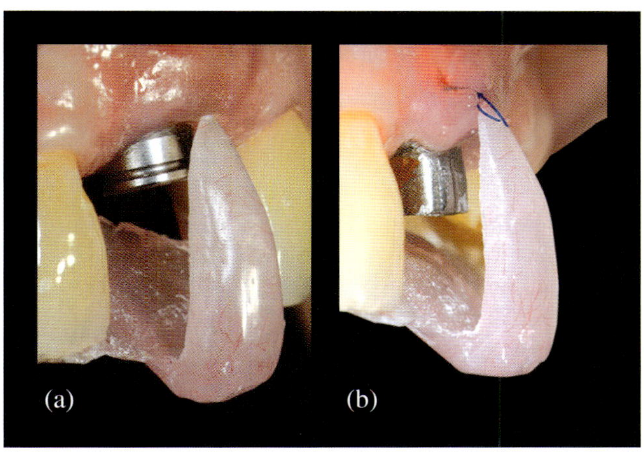

Figure 5.32 (a) and (b) Pre- and post operative picture of the scoring template showing 1.5 mm tissue gain incisally.

5.6 Treatment of Implant-related Gingival Recession

The treatment of implant-related recession has not been studied as much as the causes for it (Zucchelli et al. 2013). Peri-implant tissue architecture thus takes a major share in the esthetic set-up of any implant-supported restoration (Buser et al. 1991; Hansson, Albrektsson and Brånemark 1983; Strid 1985). Many authors (Cardaropoli, Lekholm and Wennstrom 2006; De Rouck et al. 2008; Evans and Chen 2008; Juodzbalys and Wang 2007; Kan et al. 2003; Small and Tarnow 2000) have reported various degrees of implant-related mid-facial gingival recession; however, proposed repair attempts have been limited mainly to connective tissue grafts (CTGs) (Garber 1981; Lai et al. 2010; Seibert 1993; Shibli, d'Avila and Marcantonio 2004; Wennstrom 1996) or acellular dermal matrix grafts (Mareque-Bueno 2011).

Investigating the etiology of implant-related tissue migration is becoming a cornerstone in setting the treatment protocol, because if the reason behind recession is not allocated then any treatment used will be valueless. Another significant factor is the armamentarium available for the clinician to use when considering esthetic zone. Maximum results are obtained with microsurgical instruments that are sharp and precise, and the use of loupes, microscopes, etc. The surgical skills of the clinician is yet another important factor that will ultimately predict the success or failure of the treatment, and which involves the ability to manage both soft and hard tissue components. Selecting the right candidate for the procedure is important because not all candidates are suitable to receive the treatment.

Several other factors that contribute to the selection of the correct treatment are the degree of recession, oral hygiene level, the intellectual level of the patient to understand the complexity of the treatment, patient willingness to treatment commitment, and financial considerations; for instance, the additional fees of the treatment.

5.6.1 Preventive Treatment Options

Nowadays practitioners must comprehend and manage an extremely esthetically aware population. Often unreasonable demands from patients and occasionally unrealistic promises by practitioners can lead to unsatisfactory experiences for all parties. The main goal of preventive measures is to decrease the possibility of recession occurring.

5.6.1.1 Innovative Implant-related Designs

The currently available micro and macro designs of implant fixtures have offered many advantages for keeping bone loss at minimal levels or allowing epithelial attachment to the neck of the implant fixture and thus minimizing the recession tendency. One examples of a breakthrough in implant fixture microdesign is laser etching of the implant collar, which was developed to create the optimal implant surface design. It includes a series of precision-engineered cell-sized channels that are laser-machined on to the surface of the dental implant's collar (Nevins et al. 2006). Hermann et al. (2001) described surface micro channels as micro-grooves with a specific size and depth. Nevins et al. (2006) reported eight micrometer microchannels that are 6 μm deep and are present in the upper zone of an implant collar that has limited epithelial cell down-growth along the implant surface by inhibiting cell migration and enhanced soft tissue attachment, 12 μm microchannels that are 12 μm deep present in the lower zone of implant collar that inhibited the fibrous tissue growth, and an enhanced proliferation of osteoblastic cells. Weiner et al. (2008) demonstrated limited epithelial downgrowth due to closer adaptation of the bone to the laser microtexture collars.

In the study undertaken by Nevins et al. (2006), they described supracrestal oriented collagen fibers running towards microgrooves using polarized light microscopy, whereas micro-computerized tomography demonstrated a higher bone implant contact covering all threads of the implant (see Figure 5.33a–c).

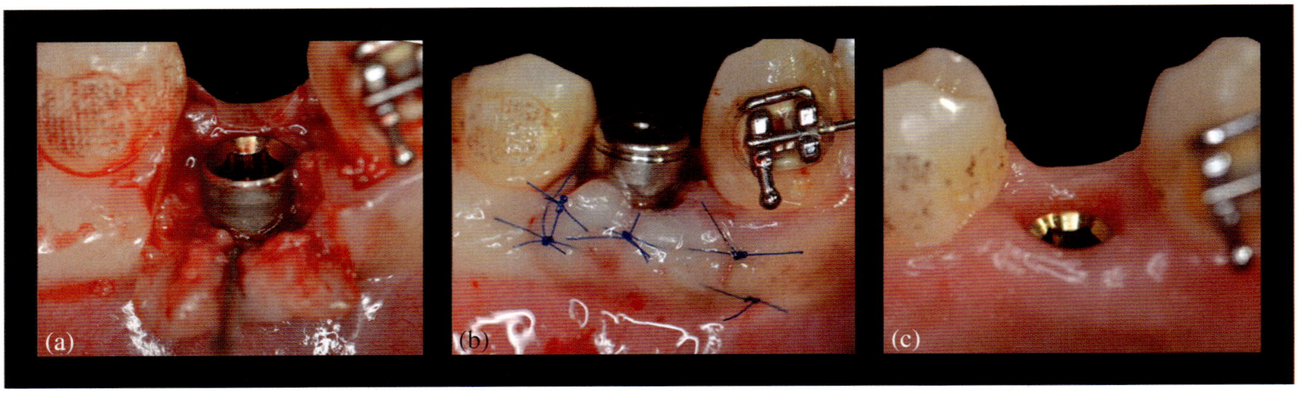

Figure 5.33 (a–c). Note the effect of the laser etching on the implant fixture collar in relation to soft tissue stability (Laser lok, BioHorizons, Birmingham, AL, USA).

Iezzi et al. (2006) carried out a histological evaluation of three immediately loaded Laser-Lok implants and demonstrated a more stable crestal bone level after four months. Shapoff et al. (2010) have also proved the role of laser etching in preventing crestal bone loss and concluded that it minimized bone loss of up to 0.46 mm. Pecora et al. (2009) concluded that Laser-Lok implants showed a reduction in bone loss of 70% (1.35 mm) compared to adjacent conventional implants after 37 months of their placement and no clinical difference was noted between mandible and maxilla. Nevins et al. (2006) infer that until now Laser-Lok has been the only surface treatment that has shown a true physical connective tissue attachment of implant to bone. Therefore, using a laser-etched implant collar might halt implant recession by stopping crestal bone resorption, and stabilize soft tissue margins.

Yet another factor that aims to minimize bone loss around the implant fixture is platform switching of the prosthetic components. A traditional horizontally matching implant–abutment connection is less reliable in keeping bone stable compared to implants with a platform-switched connection. Implants with a traditional platform are positioned equally with the bone crest where a microgap is located near the bone and bone resorption may start. In implants with platform switching, the microgap is horizontally moved away from the bone; thus, less bone loss occurs (Lazzara and Portar 2006). Ericsson et al. (1992) proved that the microgap is contaminated and inflammatory cell infiltrate forms in the connective tissue zone, contacting the implant–abutment interface.

Lazzara and Portar (2006) studied the biologic process that resulted in the loss of crestal bone height, which may be altered when the outer edge of the implant abutment interface is horizontally repositioned away from the outer edge of the implant platform. Towards the mid axis, a radiographic follow-up over the years demonstrated a smaller than expected vertical change in osseous height. A study found a mean bone loss of 0.7 mm for 30 platform-switched implants compared to 2.5 mm bone loss for 30 control implants, carried out six months after attachment of the abutment. Another study examined the biomechanical advantage of platform switching using three-dimensional finite element models. They found that the stress concentration at the cervical bone interface was greatly reduced when a narrow diameter abutment was connected. Canullo and Rasperini (2007) performed a study where in limited cases, implants were placed in the extraction sockets and it was observed that immediate loading with platform-switched implants provided peri-implant hard tissue stability and papilla preservation.

Degidi et al. (2008) examined histologically removing a human implant two months after placement and speculated that an inward shift of the inflammatory connective tissue zone at the implant–abutment junction could be the reason for bone preservation. Degidi et al. (2008) reported no resorption of coronal bone at a human implant one month after loading. Hürzeler et al. (2007) performed a study including 15 patients who received 14 wide-diameter implants with platform-switched abutments and 8 implants with a regular diameter. Lesser mean crestal bone resorption (0.12 versus 0.29 mm) of 0.12 ± 0.40 mm was observed in platform-switched cases compared to 0.29 ± 0.34 mm in control cases, one year after final restoration. Cappiello et al. (2008) observed that one year after loading, a vertical bone loss in 75 platform-switched implants varied between 0.6 and 1.2 mm (mean: 0.95 ± 0.32 mm), while for 56 control implants, the bone loss was between 1.3 and 2.1 mm (mean: 1.67 ± 0.37 mm). A two-year follow-up revealed a mean bone loss of 0.04 ± 0.22 mm on 60 platform-switched implants, while for 60 control implants the mean was 0.27 ± 0.46 mm.

Another study looked at the effect of microthreads and platform switching on crestal bone stress levels using finite element analysis. This study showed that when the abutment diameter decreased from 5.0 to 4.5 mm and then to 4.0 mm, the microthread model showed a reduction of stress at the crestal bone level from 6.3 to 5.4% after vertical loading. Therefore, the value of using platform switching in minimizing apical tissue migration around dental implants was found to be high. Using platform-switched implants definitely minimizes the bone resorption and hence implant-related gingival recession; those platform-switched surfaces are proven to improve the peri-implant mucosa condition.

5.6.1.2 Thickness Doubling of the Labial Tissue Volume

It may not be an overstatement that the majority of surgical implant procedures in the esthetic region include an indication for soft tissue grafting. The inevitable alteration of alveolar ridge dimensions that follows a tooth extraction often results in the placement of the implant in a site that has undergone a reduction in soft and hard tissue volume in comparison to its neighboring dentate sites. This discrepancy is even more pronounced in single-implant sites where a concavity forms between the edentulous site and the root prominences of the neighboring dentition (Ioannou et al. 2015). The long-term stability of pink esthetics around dental implant-supported prostheses has been strongly correlated with adequate peri-implant soft tissue thickness, that is, a thick peri-implant phenotype (Fu et al. 2011; Geurs, Vassilopoulos and Reddy 2010; Kan et al. 2011).

Factors that should be considered when evaluating the need for soft tissue grafting include the level of clinical attachment on an adjacent tooth to support papillary height, the thickness of the coronal soft tissue margin to ensure a proper emergence profile, the thickness of labial soft tissue to simulate root eminence and prevent transillumination of underlying metallic structure show up, and the position of the mucogingival junction and amount of keratinized tissue to produce a harmonious blend with that of the adjacent teeth. It was proposed that if tissue thickness is 2 mm or less, the formation of biological width around implants will involve bone loss (Grunder 2011). Later, this statement was confirmed clinically in a study by Linkevicius et al. (2011) showing that up to 1.35 mm of bone loss might be expected if implants are placed in thin mucosal tissues. As a possible solution, Linkevicius et al. (2009) suggested investigating the option to thicken soft tissues before or during implant placement to reduce crestal bone loss. First described by Edel (1974), the technique of autologous CTG emerged steadily as an indispensable therapeutic tool. Subepithelial connective tissue grafts (SCTGs) or free gingival grafts (FGGs) can be employed to reconstruct the buccal dimensions of the site, improving the tissue thickness and also the esthetic outcome. These grafts create the illusion of root prominence and increase the width of the crestal peri-implant mucosa to provide an emergence profile for the restoration and to enable the constructed site to closely resemble a natural tooth (Farmer and Darby 2014; Schropp et al. 2003).

When a thin phenotype is diagnosed, an SCTG or an FGG can be used to prevent potential long-term recession of the facial mucosal margin or permeation of a gray color from the implant transmucosal components (Cosyn et al. 2012a) and by increasing the gingival thickness. Gingival thickness augmented with a CTG has been proven to be a successful procedure in preserving soft tissue levels and improving clinical attachments and overall tissue stability when performed in conjunction with implant placement. The use of connective tissue autografts or allografts for thickening the mucosa might add 1.3 mm to tissue thickness. Each graft has its indications and clinical applications. For example, thickening of thin tissues might have an impact on reducing crestal bone loss by an average of 1.8 mm after a one year follow-up (Strub and Gaberthuel 1992; Grunder 2000; Hermann et al. 2007) (see Figure 5.34).

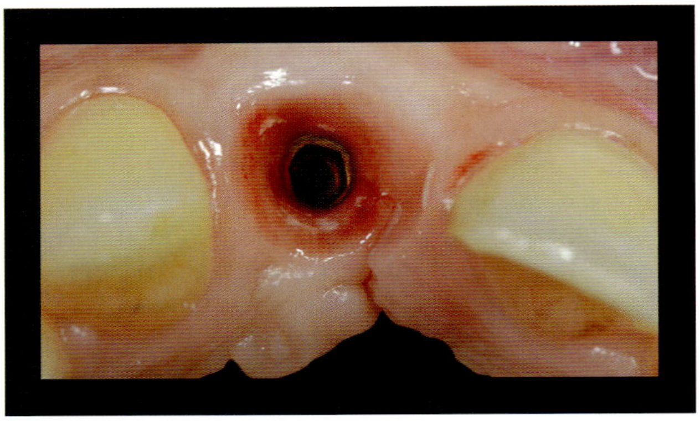

Figure 5.34 The effect of the use of platform switched implant on the soft tissue margin, bulking the biological width in a horizontal direction.

Covani et al. (2004) reported the use of free CTG as a biologic barrier to cover residual alveolar defects associated with an immediate implant to allow undisturbed healing of peri-implant deep tissue. Studies have shown that this protocol is a valuable procedure to obtain excellent function and cosmetic implant restoration. Bianchi and Sanfilippo (2004) reported that the newly created soft tissue graft was well maintained for up to two years and that the facial gingival margin receded on an average of 0.4 mm in two years. Kan et al. (2011) reported mid-facial margin recession of approximately 0.5 mm even after one year of immediate implant placement with placing CTG. Papilla levels showed slightly increased tendencies in height of 0.5 mm mesially and 0.3 mm distally from the time the prosthesis was in place. The cumulative implant success rate following single immediate tooth replacement with dental implants and a SCTG was 90% after a one-year follow-up. Shibli et al. (2004) studied the use of a SCTG to augment a soft tissue margin discrepancy for a single-implant crown in the anterior maxilla and concluded that the use of soft tissue grafts to correct an esthetic deficiency may be considered a feasible approach to establish new and stable peri-implant soft tissue contours. Covani et al. (2007) and Marconcini et al. (2013) both conducted a study on 10 patients (5 men and 5 women) in the age group of 42–55 years. The teeth were extracted and implants were placed without consideration of a mucoperiosteal flap. Immediately after implantation, a CTG was placed over the implants to treat the gingival recession. The second stage of surgery was performed six months after the initial procedure. Esthetic outcomes were evaluated using the measurements before implant placement and 12 months after surgery for the width of the keratinized mucosa, the emergence profile of the crown, and patient satisfaction. It was concluded that the surgical approach used can be considered as a treatment option in cases with non-salvageable teeth showing gingival recession and the absence of attached gingiva.

However, the timing of implant placement following tooth removal may be important to take advantage of soft tissue healing without losing bone volume. Thickening of the connective tissue interface between the implant and the soft tissue seems to ensure long-term stability of the biologic width and thus the esthetic profile (see Figure 5.35a–l).

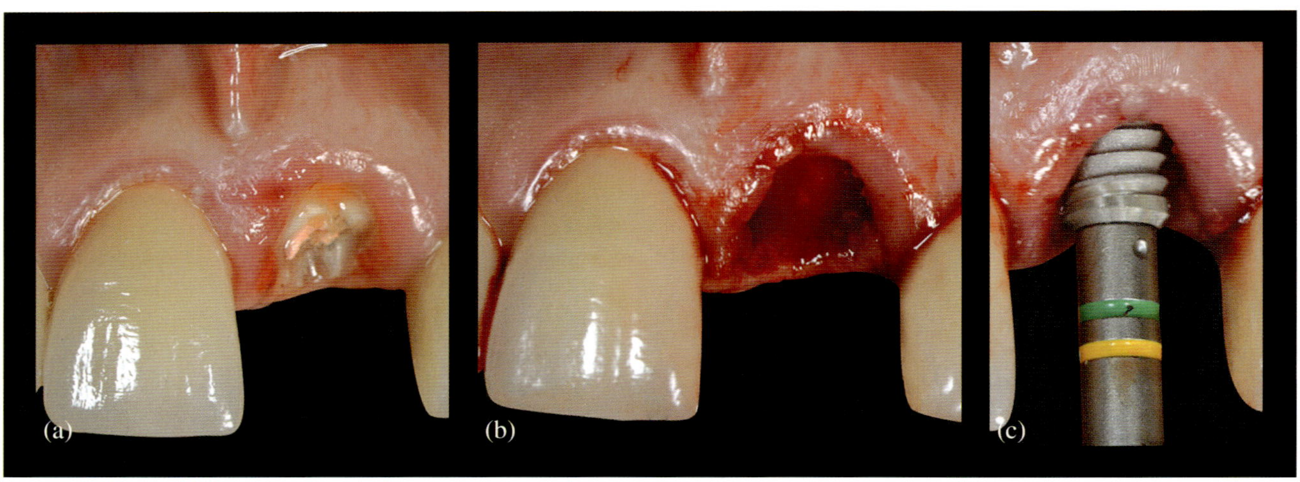

Figure 5.35 (a) Preoperative view of broken hopeless root in a thin scalloped tissue phenotype, (b) Root extracted atraumatically, (c) Tapered plus (Laser lok, BioHorizons, Birmingham, AL, USA) emphasizing the value of Platform switching is inserted.

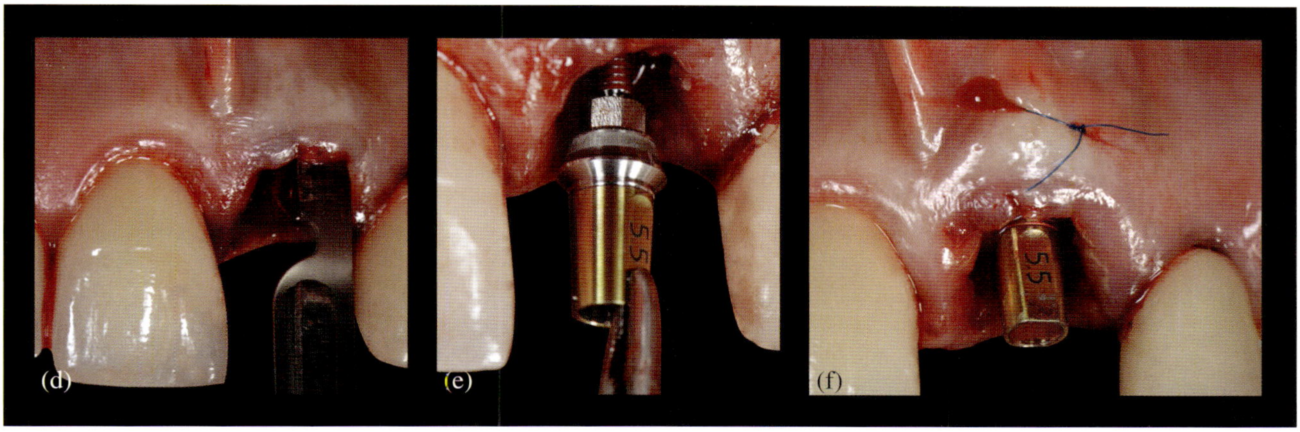

Figure 5.35 (d) Cervicular incision is being made to insert the connective tissue graft, (e) Laser etched base one time abutment being inserted for immediate loading, (f) Connective tissue graft is introduced and stabilized by 1–0 proline sutures.

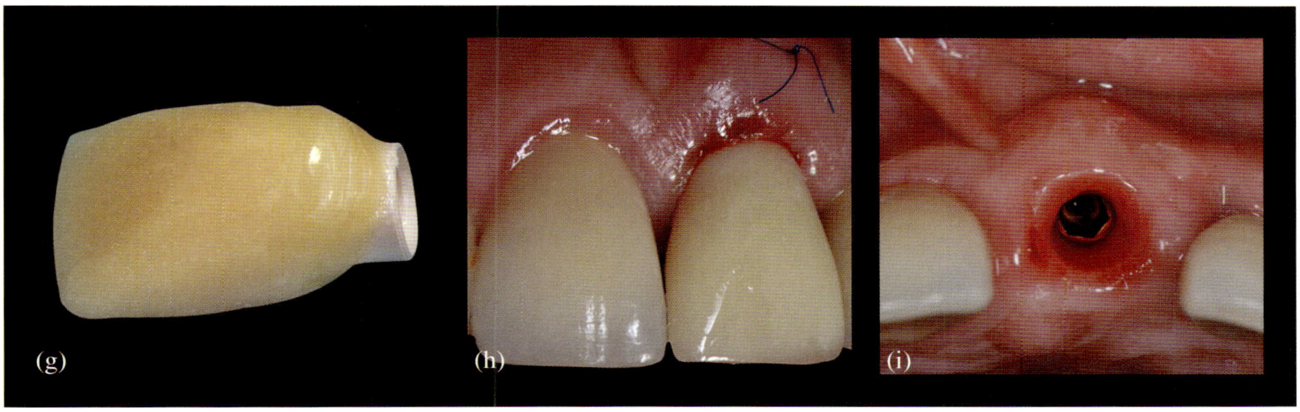

Figure 5.35 (g). Provisional restoration is prepared, (h) Provisional restoration intra-operatively, (i) Tissue is over profiled as result of using connective tissue graft.

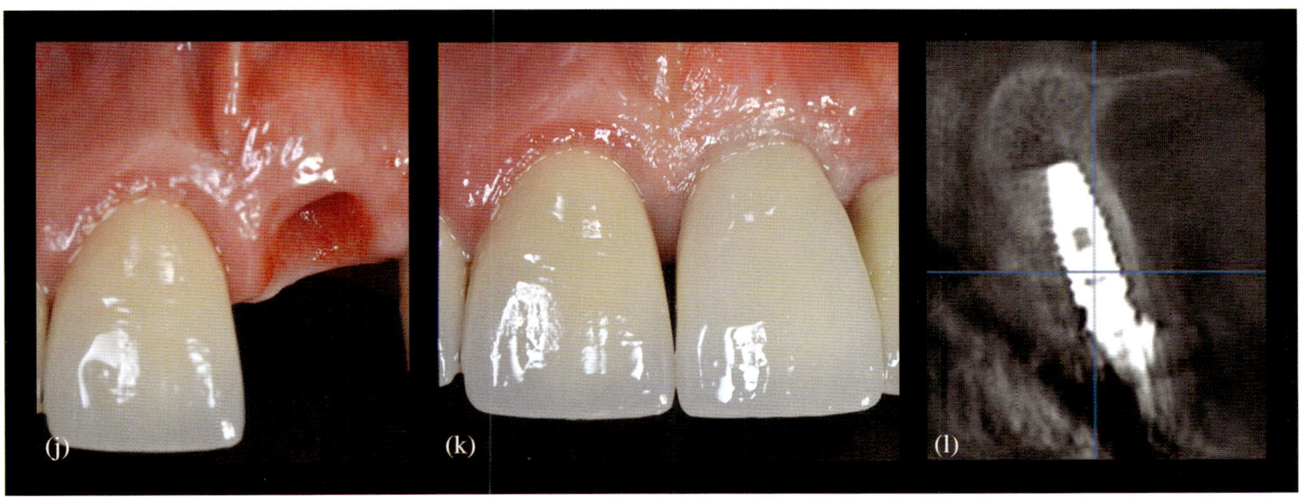

Figure 5.35 (j) Three weeks post-operative showing remarkable tissue position, (k) Case finally restored with zirconia crown, (l) Six months cone beam follow up CT scan showing intact labial plate of bone.

Tsuda et al. (2011) conducted a study on 10 patients (4 men, 6 women) with a mean age of 48 years (range from 35 to 70) who underwent extraction and immediate tooth replacement with SCTG. It was found that at one year, all implants remained osseointegrated, with an overall mean marginal bone change of +0.10 mm and a mean facial gingival level change of −0.05 mm. Papilla Index scores indicated that at 12 months more than a 50% papilla fill was observed in 80% of all sites. The results of this case series suggest that, in addition to a favorable implant success rate and peri-implant tissue response, the facial gingival level around single immediately placed implants can also be maintained following connective tissue grafting when proper three-dimensional implant positioning is achieved and bone is grafted into the implant socket gap.

In a study by Grunder et al. (2010), 24 patients were treated consecutively with implants placed in the maxillary anterior area at the time of tooth extraction. Among the study subjects, 12 patients were treated without raising a flap, whereas the remaining 12 patients were treated with a subepithelial connective graft that was placed using the tunnel technique in the labial area at the time of tooth extraction and implant placement. An average loss of soft tissue volume in the non-grafted group was 1.063 mm, whereas in the grafted group there was a slight gain of 0.34 mm.

It is the author's opinion that with any thin tissue phenotype, a CTG should be undertaken routinely to stabilize peri-implant tissues, to minimize bone resorption, and to prevent possible future recession.

In cases with a thin or fenestrated facial plate wall in the anterior maxilla mostly due to the facial position of anterior teeth roots, undergoes substantial resorption following tooth extraction (Araujo and Lindhe 2005; Cardaropoli et al. 2005). Preoperative diagnostic procedures and risk assessments should include CBCT scan, because it yields submillimeter accuracy for linear measurements (Loubele et al. 2008).

The facial bone wall should ideally measure at least 2 mm thick to ensure proper soft tissue support and to avoid resorption of the facial wall following restoration (Buser et al. 2006, 2009; Grunder et al. 2005). Whenever labial plate bone is deficient or thin, bone augmentation procedures are recommended to achieve an adequate bony contour (Belser et al. 2009) (see Figure 5.36a–k).

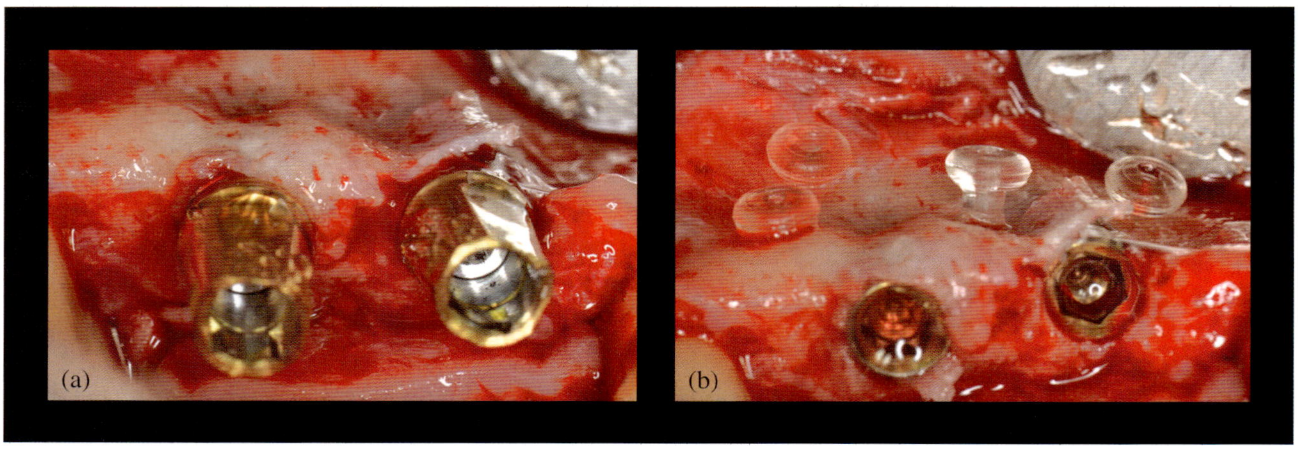

Figure 5.36 (a) Two implants were placed restoring the missing teeth, note the thin nature of the related labial plate of bone that warrants thickening, (b) Poly-DL-lactic acid membrane (PDLLA) screws used to tent the bone graft to double the thickness of the labial plate of bone.

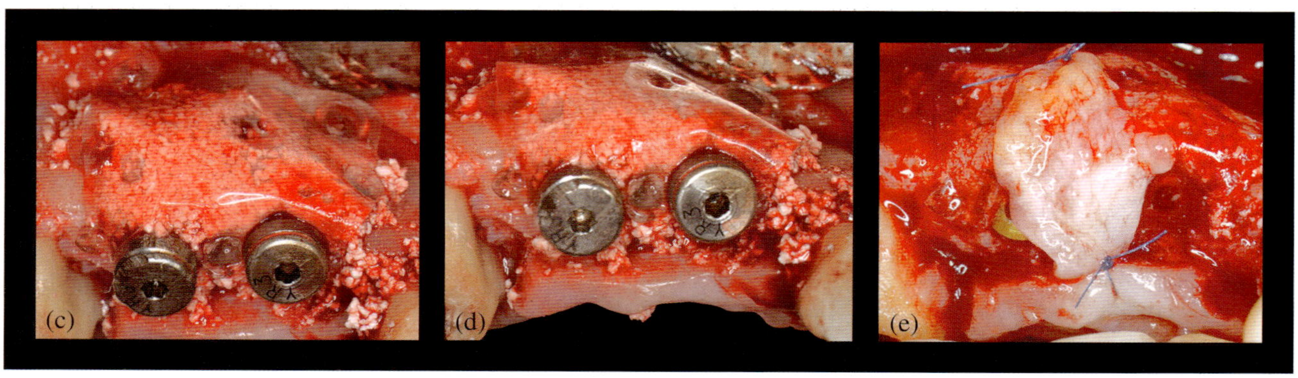

Figure 5.36 (c) and (d) A PDLLA membrane was used, fitted and stabilized, (e) Connective tissue graft stabilized to enhance tissue profile.

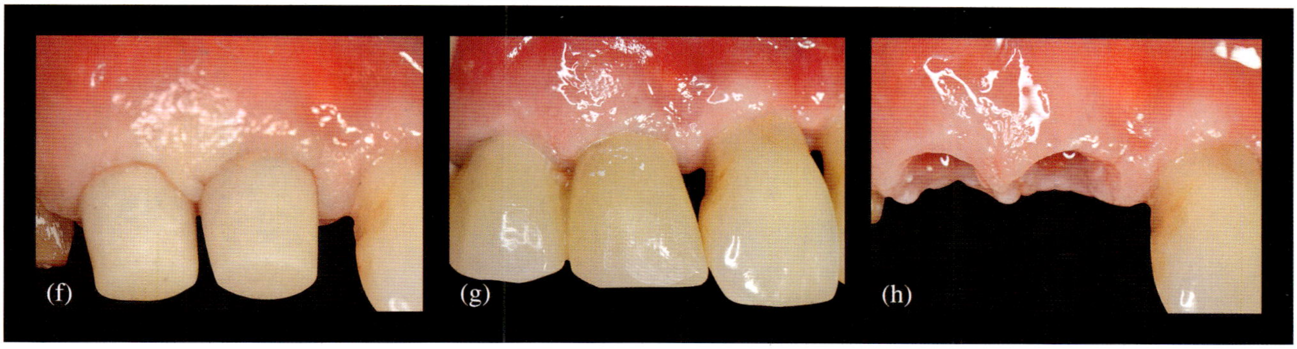

Figure 5.36 (f) and (g) Provisional crowns in position, (h) Tissue profile being developed using the temporary crowns.

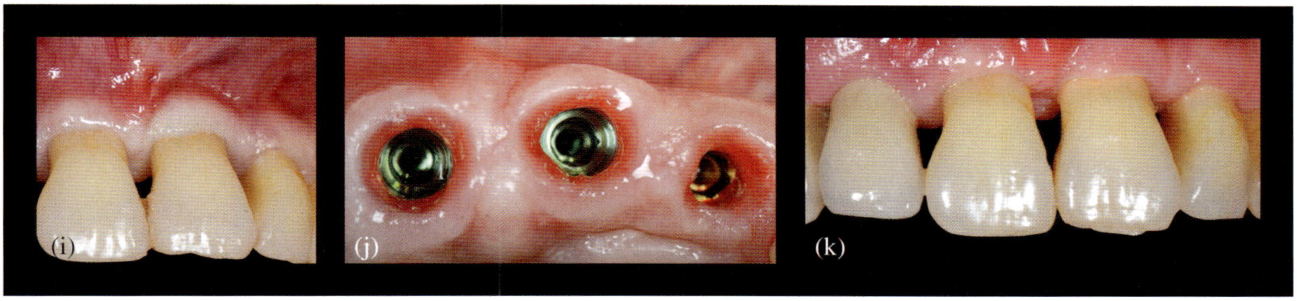

Figure 5.36 (i) One Week post healing showing an excellent soft tissue margins and highly ecstatic contours, (j) Soft tissue margins showing an exact duplication of the original emergence profile of natural teeth before extraction, (k) Case finally restored.

In a study by Braut et al. (2012), CBCT was used to examine the facial bone wall of teeth in the anterior maxilla. The results indicated that the facial bone wall in the anterior maxilla is mostly thin, with a mean thickness between 0.5 and 0.7 mm. The analysis yielded a trend towards decreasing thickness from posterior (first premolars) towards anterior tooth positions (central incisors).

A thin facial bone wall undergoes a substantial resorption process within the first four to eight weeks following tooth extraction, leading to a reduction in bone height of approximately 2–3 mm on the facial aspect (Araujo and Lindhe 2005). This bone resorption is a biologic phenomenon, caused mainly by the interruption of blood supply through blood vessels within the periodontal ligament. Nevins et al. (2006) confirmed these results in their study, where the ridges of non-grafted extraction sockets showed a more than 20% loss of crest height. In consequence, an implant site with a missing or a thin facial bone wall requires a bone augmentation procedure if a reasonable esthetic and functional outcome are desired. The goal of such a procedure is to build up the bony contour necessary to resist against recession for adequate support of esthetically pleasing soft tissues (Buser et al. 2008, 2009).

Several treatment modalities have been described for osseous augmentation of the labial plate of bone prior to or along with implant placement (thickness doubling). These include GBR (Buser 1993) with or without particulate bone grafting with bone blocks harvested intraorally or extraorally. The mandibular symphysis and ramus buccal shelf are excellent intraoral sources to obtain a corticocancellous or pure mono-cortical bone block, respectively, for alveolar ridge augmentation.

The symphysis has been reported to provide sufficient bone to augment a deficient ridge by 4–6 cm in the horizontal dimension and up to 4 mm of thickness covering a length of up to a three-tooth defect (Pikos 2000; Schwartz-Arad and Chausu 1997). With an average bone volume of approximately 860 mm (Buser 1993; Wang, Misch and Neiva 2004) (see Figure 5.37a–d).

The symphysis offers a larger graft volume of over 50% than can be obtained from the mandibular ramus, with much easier surgical access (Wang et al. 2004). The average symphysis graft is composed of 65% cortical bone and 36% cancellous bone, as opposed to the mandibular ramus, which is nearly 100% cortical (Schwartz-Arad and Chausu 1997).

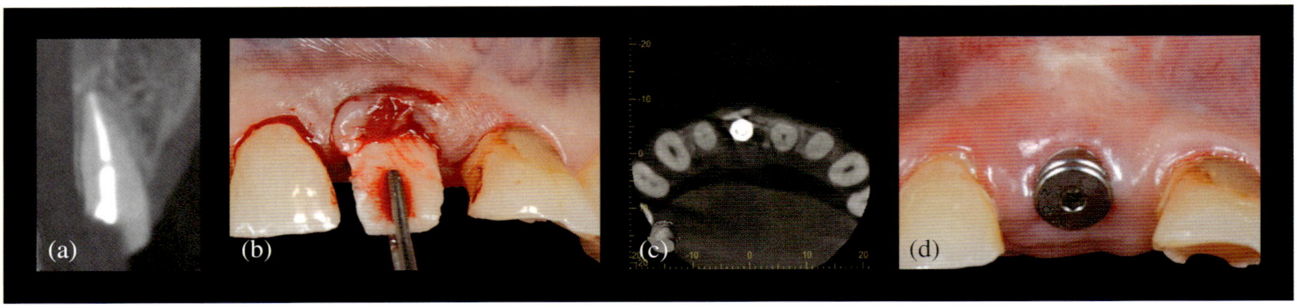

Figure 5.37 (a) Cone-beam computed tomography (CBCT) scan showing very thin labial plate of bone that might lead to future recession, (b) Mono-cortical autograft being harvested from the chin, thinned to 0.5 mm thick and adjusted to fit the recipient site, then introduced from the crest area after releasing the soft tissues and decorticating the host site and stabilized from the apical area with a micro screw via sulcular incision, (c) CBCT scan showing the thickening of labial plate of bone after the enhancement, (d) two weeks post-operative view showing excellent healing.

The corticocancellous nature of bone harvested from this site facilitates faster vascular in-growth once the block has been placed, resulting in more rapid integration and less potential resorption during healing (Hammack and Enneking 1960). However, for thickening a thin plate of bone, only a small bone graft size is required. Most cases can be resolved with a 1 mm thick monocortical block. As these monocortical block grafts compensate for the lost ridge width successfully, lamellar bone sheaths may be used to augment the ridge width and replace or thicken the resorbed bone plates (see Figures 5.38a–c and 5.39a–l).

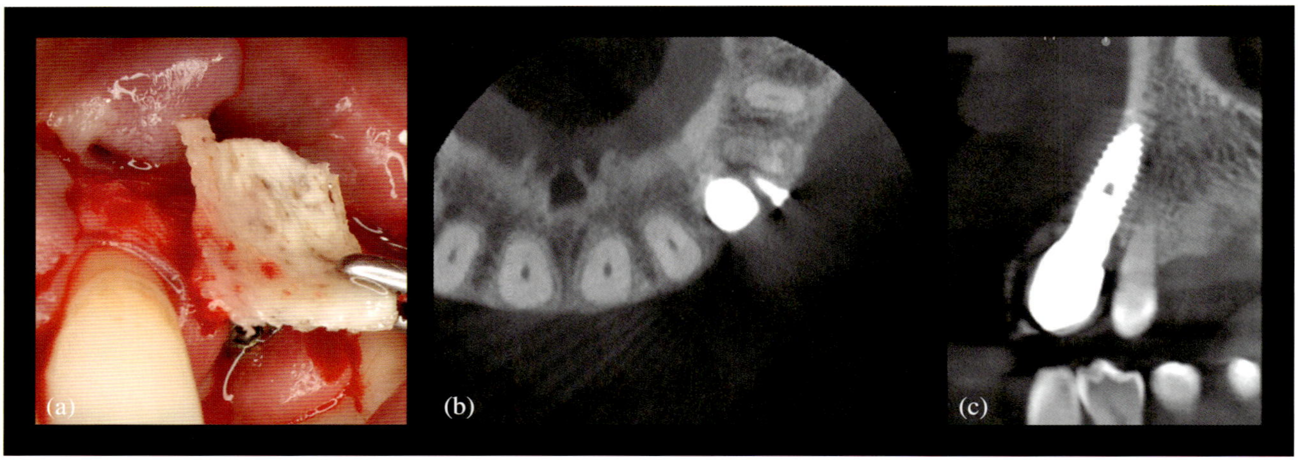

Figure 5.38 (a) An autograft cancellous bone sheet bone sheet is introduced to the site to treat the defect, (b) and (c) Three years post-surgery showing the resorption of the cancellous sheet that indicates the superiority of the cortical sheets.

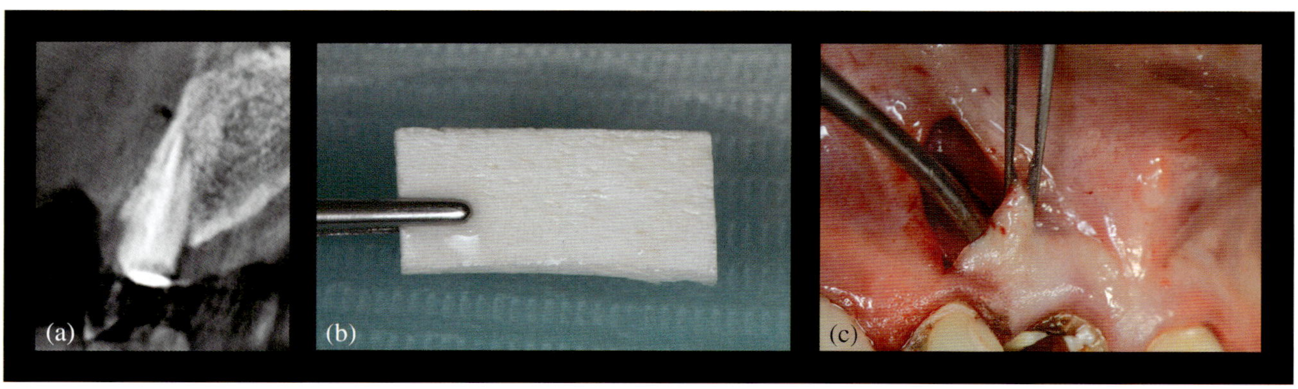

Figure 5.39 (a) Cone-beam computed tomography (CBCT) scan of central incisor showing the thin labial plate of bone, (b) Laminar xenograft bone sheet being hydrated, (c) Vertical full mucoperiosteal flap reflected to allow access to the labial plate of bone.

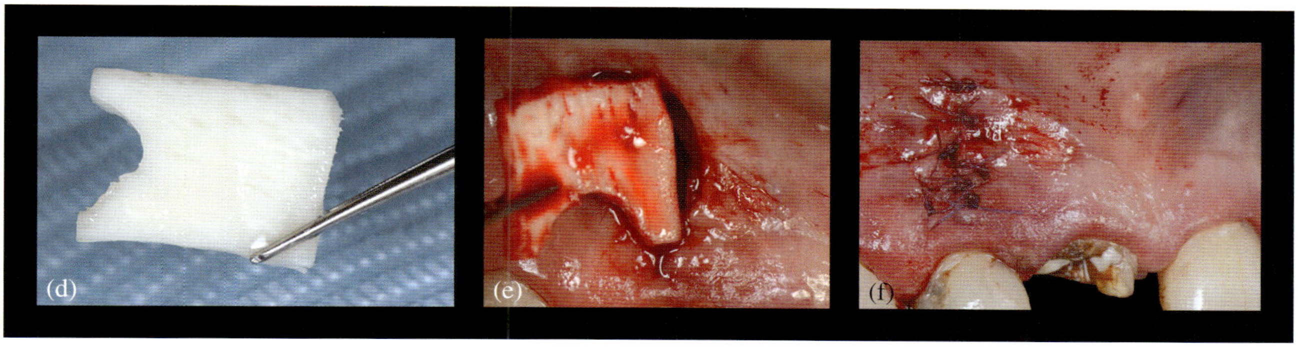

Figure 5.39 (d) The sheet is being tailored to fit the recipient site, (e) the sheet is being introduced, (f) incision line closed.

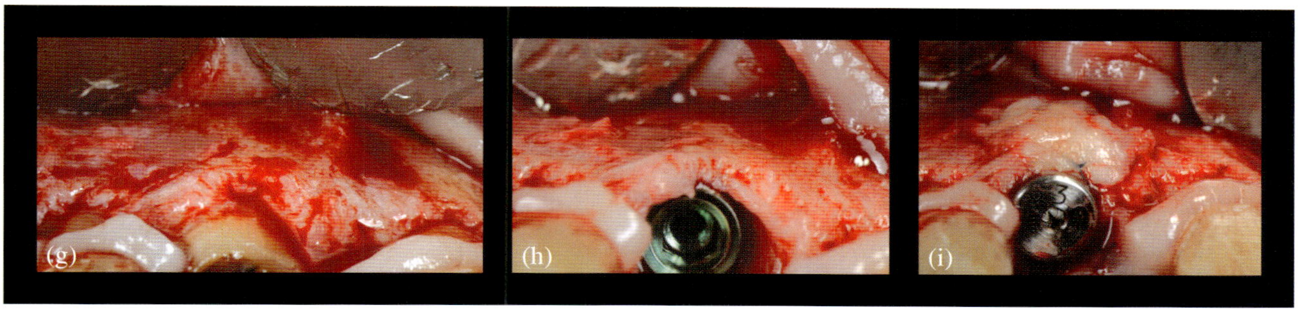

Figure 5.39 (g) three months post grafting showing doubling the thickness of the labial plate of bone, (h) An implant is placed, (i) a connective tissue graft is used to enhance the overall soft tissue profile.

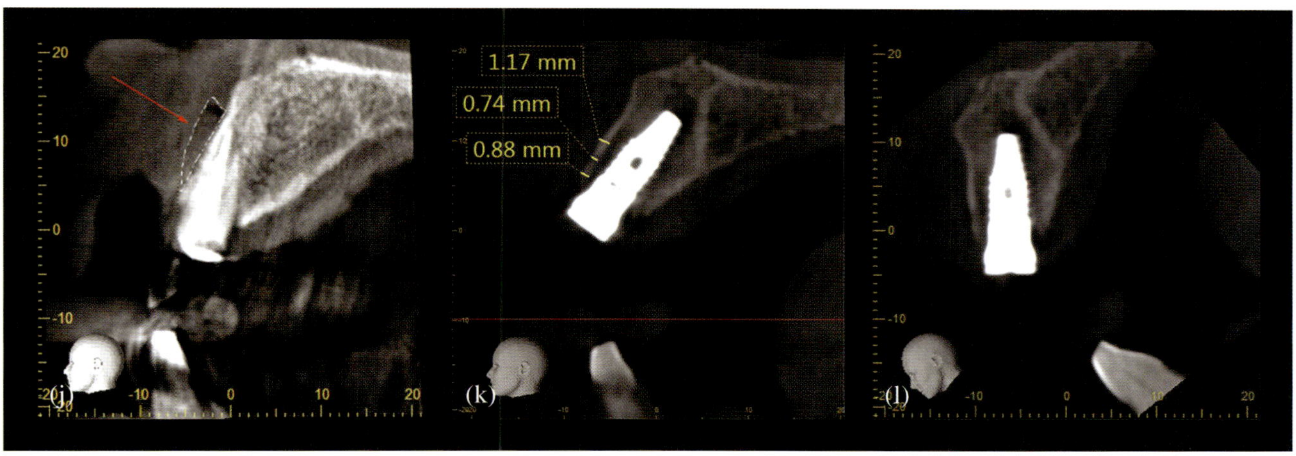

Figure 5.39 (j) Showing preoperative radiographic picture of the sheet in place, (k) and (l) Radiographic pictures showing the enhancement of the overall labial plate of bone quality and quantity.

In a study by Hämmerle, Araújo and Simion (2012), bone growth along the implant surface achieved using lamellar bone sheath along with a membrane to act as a scaffold, measured 91% for the membrane only group, 52% for the lamellar bone group, and 42% for the non-grafted group. The width of the regenerated bone was 1.5 mm above the bottom of the original defect. In conclusion, the lamellar bone sheets exhibited osteoconductive properties and hence can be recommended for GBR procedures in dehiscence defects (see Figure 5.40a–o).

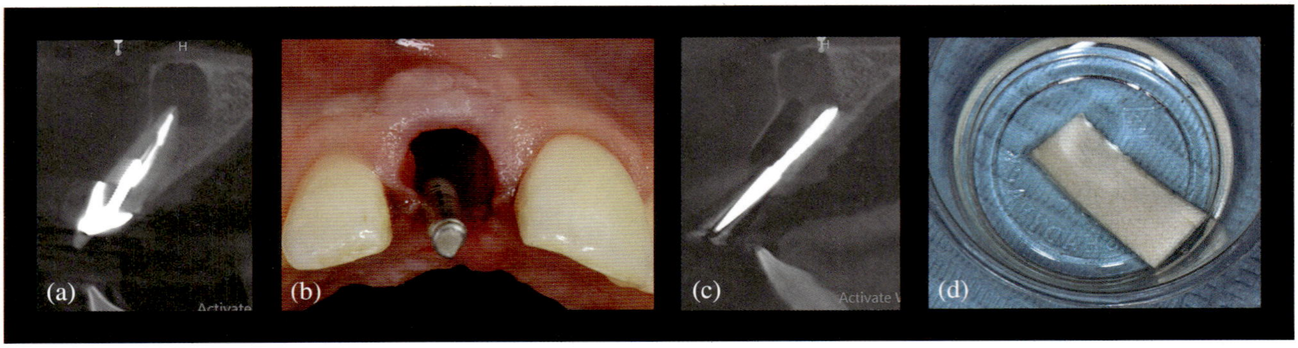

Figure 5.40 (a) Preoperative radiographic view of failed central incisor presented with a very thin labial plate of bone and periapical infection, (b) and (c) A platally directed pilot drilling position is made to avoid the proximity to the labial plate of bone, (d) Xenograft laminar bone sheet is dehydrated half an hour before placement.

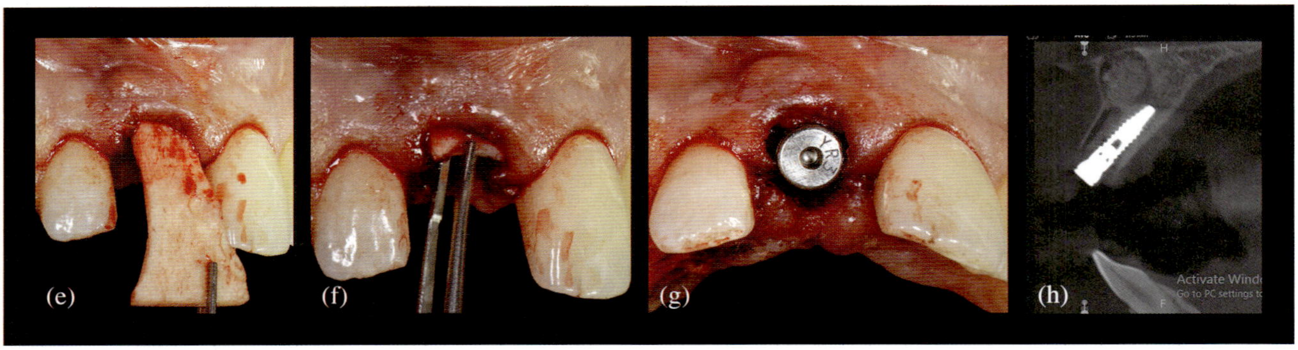

Figure 5.40 (e–g) The socket was cleaned off the granulation tissues, using curretts then irrigated, then a diode laser used to sterilize the local tissues, the sheet is tailored and introduced from the socket orifice above the labial plate of bone and seated all the way, the socket voids grafted with particulated grafting mix, the implant was inserted in the correct position, (h) Cone-beam computed tomography (CBCT) scan showing immediate post-operative result.

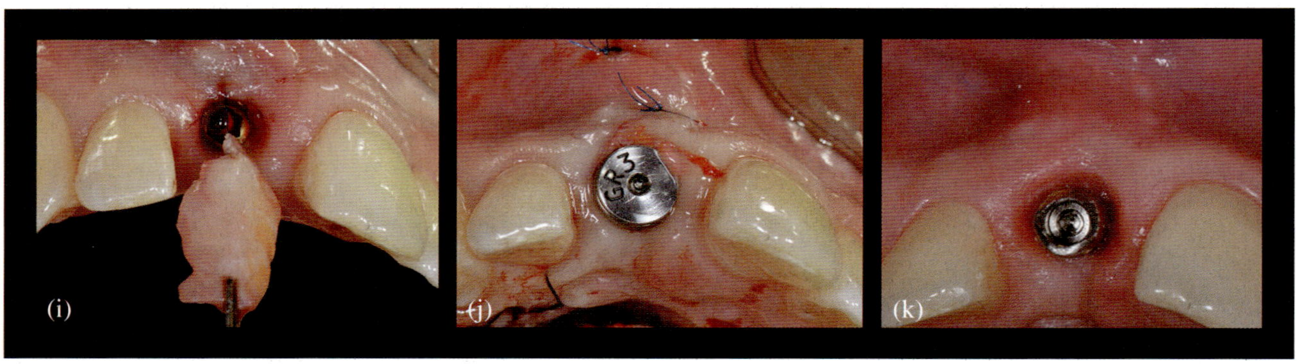

Figure 5.40 (i–k) Connective tissue graft is stabilized in place.

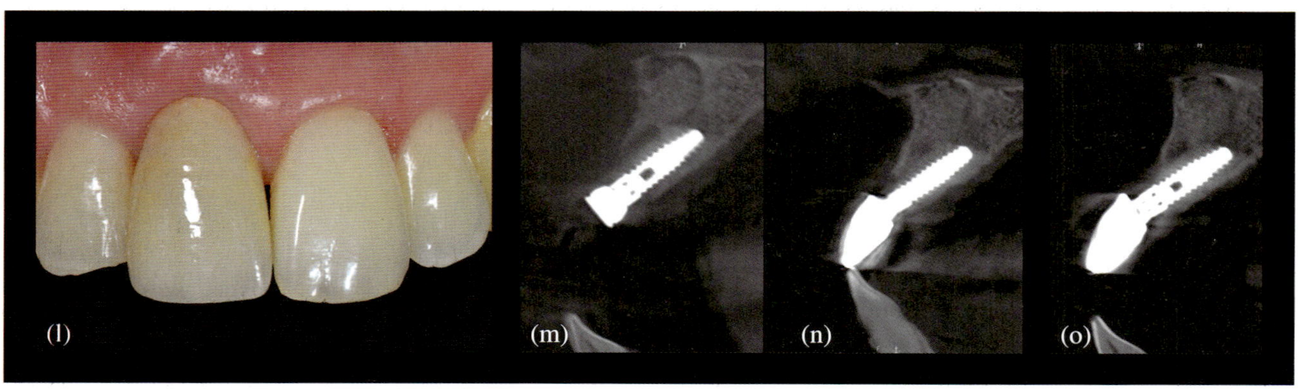

Figure 5.40 (l) Case finally restored, showing stable tissue margins, (m) Six month post-operative CBCT scan showing the labial plate of bone condition, (n) One year post-operative showing improved labial plate of bone thickness and over all tissue stability, (o) One year and a half post-operative showing improved labial plate of bone thickness and over all tissue stability.

5.6.1.3 Subcrestal Implant Placement

Many authors have advocated subcrestal positioning of dental implants to minimize the future potential for recession. Barros, Novaes and Korn (2015), in a histologic study in dogs, found that vertical bone resorption was decreased in the subcrestal groups compared to the equicrestal groups. Weng, Nagata and Bell (2008) and Welander, Abrahamsson and Berglundh (2009), in two different experiments in dogs, found that healing of implants placed in a subcrestal position could result in osseointegration to the abutment region of the implant (i.e. coronal to the IAJ). The location of the implant shoulder subcrestally avoids metal exposure and allows an adequate vertical dimension with an esthetic emergence profile. Changes in the buccal soft tissue margin were observed by Chen et al. (2007), with a mean follow-up of 18 months, marginal tissue recession of greater than 1 mm occurred in 33% of the sites. The occurrence of recession was significantly associated with the position of the implant shoulder in relation to the buccal bone plate. Recession of 16.7% occurred in the position of the implant shoulder and 58.3% in the buccal bone plate. Thicker bone and soft tissue around an implant is essential for ensuring long-term success. Placing an implant >2 mm from the facial bone and 1 mm subcrestally has resulted in greater preservation of the crestal bone. However, it is the author's recommendation that subcrestal implant positioning needs to be performed with extreme caution to avoid implant positioning that might be too deep; future peri-implant soft tissue thickness should be properly calculated prior to undertaking this maneuver.

5.6.2 Treatment for Class I Recession

Marginal soft tissue stability is considered to be a significant factor for achieving any esthetic outcome with implant-supported restorations (Zucchelli et al. 2013) for which a stable architecture of the peri-implant soft tissues plays a pivotal role in the esthetic outcome. The facial gingival margin around the restored dental implant must be of the same emergence as that of the contralateral tooth, that is, in harmony with the adjacent teeth. The occurrence of gingival recession related to dental implant-supported restoration in the facial aspect becomes a dilemma for both patients and clinicians (Gracco et al. 2009). Moreover, the thin gingival phenotype fails to act as a strong barrier against bacterial invasion of the peri-implant tissue (Cairo, Pagliaro and Nieri 2008). In contrast, the thick gingival tissue phenotype will eventually resist against future gingival recession due to the enhanced quality of soft and hard tissue (Linkevicius et al. 2010) and will react to trauma by forming a periodontal pocket (Fu et al. 2011). It has also been observed that the influence of tissue phenotype on a peri-implant tissue response seemed to be limited only to facial gingival recession and does not influence interproximal papilla or proximal marginal bone levels (Kan et al. 2011). Thus, the clinician must identify the type of tissue phenotype at the implant site before starting treatment so likelihood of soft tissue recession can be minized.

Long-term changes have been reported in the position of the facial soft tissue margins following restoration of 106 stage I ITI implants in 39 patients, in both maxillary and mandibular anterior regions. After two years, a 1 mm mid-facial soft tissue recession was present in 61% of the patients (see Figure 5.41a, b).

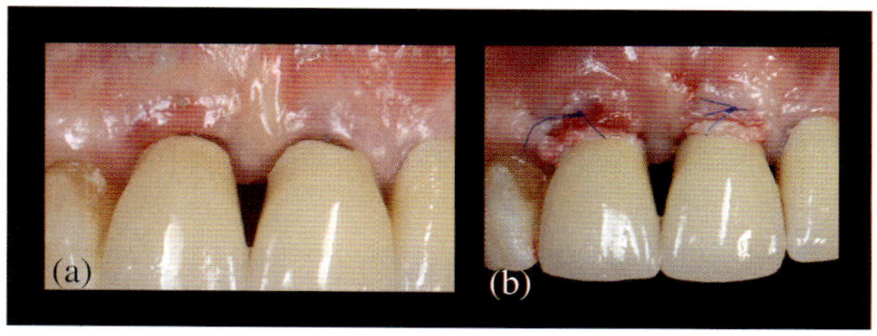

Figure 5.41 (a, b) Correcting Class I recession type, thin mucosa by using a-cellular dermal graft.

Unlike natural teeth where a minimal recession of 1–2 mm might not always produce esthetic discomfort, a minimal amount of titanium exposure can jeopardize the overall treatment outcome, as it may be unacceptable to the patient. Ideally, clinicians should select the technique for treating these situations (class I implant-related gingival recessions) based on the best available evidence. Unfortunately, most systematic reviews on mucogingival therapy (Cairo et al. 2008; Oates, Robinson and Gunsolley 2003; Roccuzzo et al. 2002) have not presented information regarding the treatment of peri-implant soft tissue recession. They managed recession reduction on natural teeth, which represents the mean percentage of root coverage. Depending on the surgical technique utilized, it is within the 50–90% range, the latter value being considered clinically satisfying (see Figure 5.42a–e).

At the 6th European Workshop on Periodontology, Cairo et al. (2008) presented a narrative review, based mainly on expert opinions, case reports, and case series. Literature analysis showed that (1) the width of keratinized tissues did not influence the survival rate of dental implants; (2) there is no evidence to recommend a specific technique to preserve/augment keratinized tissue; and (3) factors including bone level, keratinized tissue, and implant features have not been shown to be associated with future mucosal recession around dental implants. The only possible conclusion, approved by the Consensus Report (Palmer and Cortellini 2008), was that although scientific evidence in most part is lacking, soft tissue augmentation at implant sites may be considered in some clinical situations (see Figure 5.43a–e).

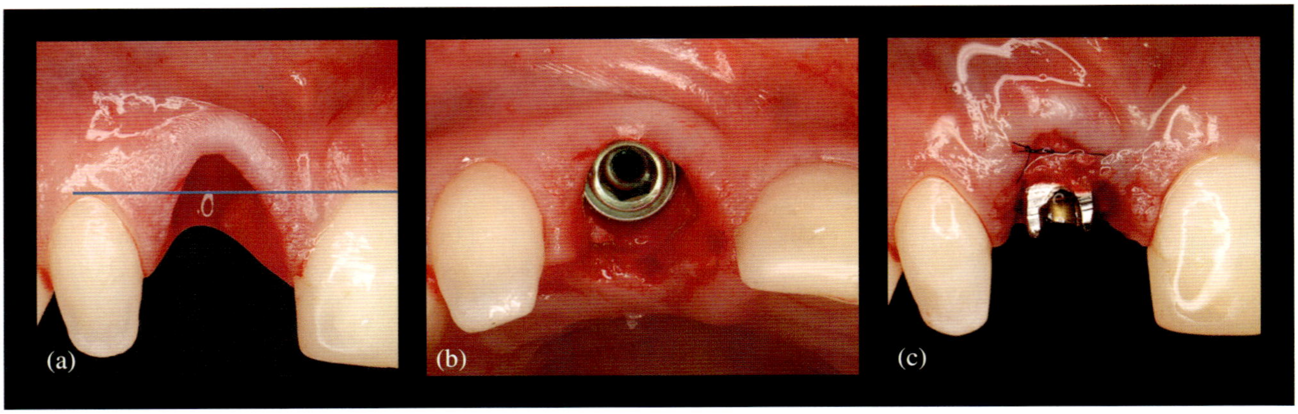

Figure 5.42 (a) Class I recession type, (b) Implant fixture placed (Tapered Internal, BioHorizons, Birmingham, AL, USA), (c) Connective tissue graft is placed.

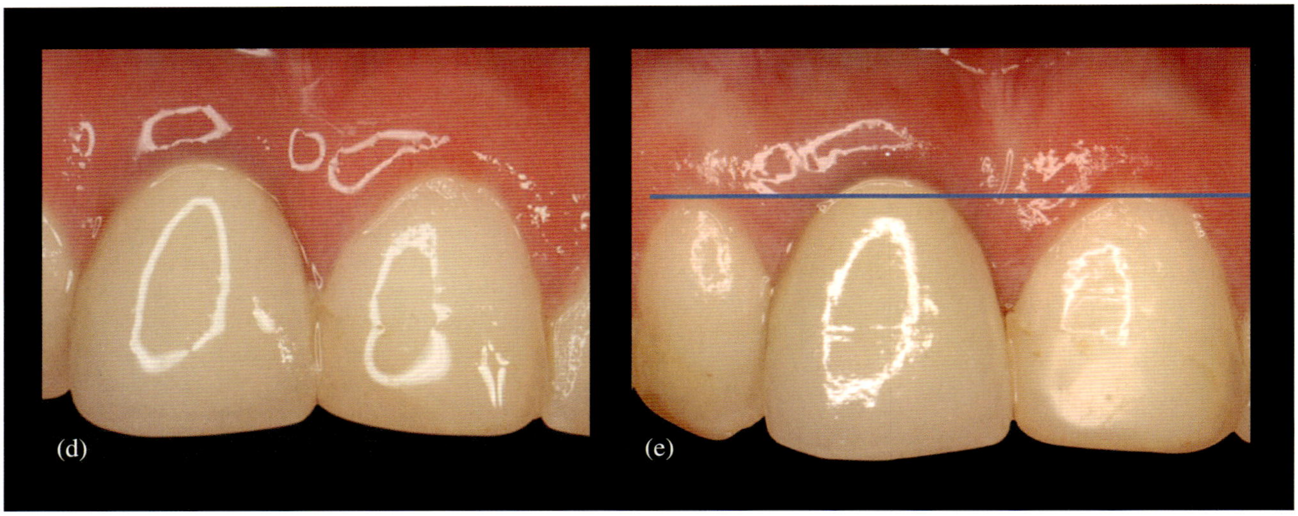

Figure 5.42 (d) Case finally restored, (e) the connective tissue graft augmentation procedure was able to improve class I recession case with minor recession.

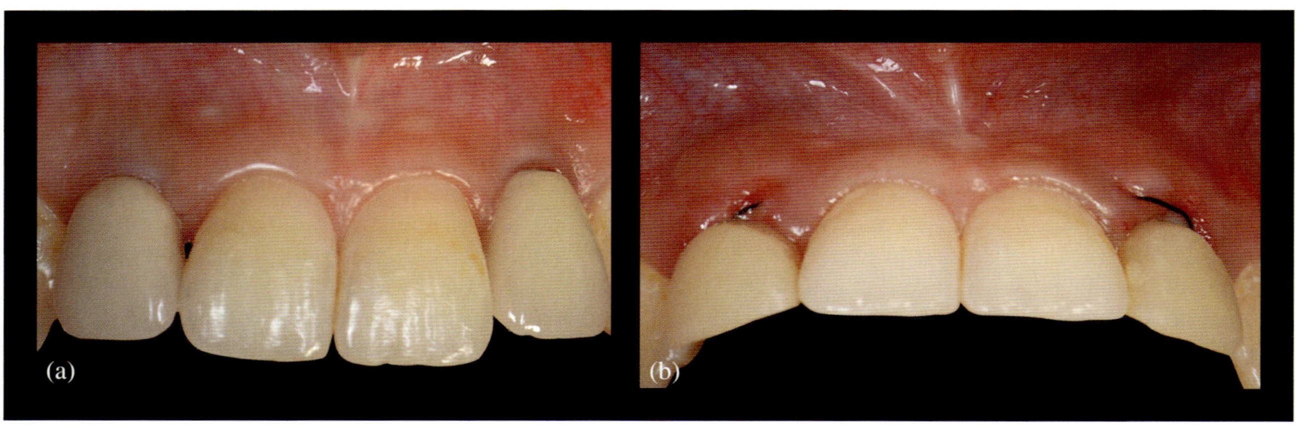

Figure 5.43 (a) Preoperative view of class I gingival recession around right and left central incisor, (b) Incisal view at the time of healing.

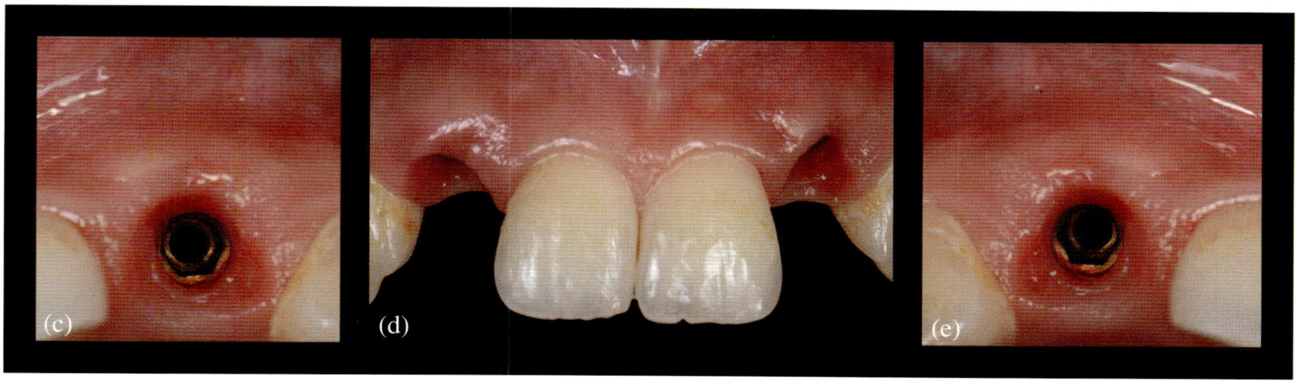

Figure 5.43 (c–e) Soft tissue maturation and profiling using provisional restoration showing enhanced tissue keratinization and treating the recession.

One prospective cohort study (Burkhardt, Joss and Lang 2008) tried to evaluate the outcome of soft tissue dehiscence coverage around single-implant restoration. A coronal advanced flap (CAF) with CTG techniques was used to treat 10 patients and they evaluated healing up to six months. After one month, the mean of soft tissue dehiscence coverage was 75%, 70% at three months, and 66% at six months. They concluded that a clinically significant improvement of soft tissue dehiscence was obtained with a combination of CAF and CTG, but complete "recession" coverage was not possible.

Shibli et al. (2004) described the use of a subepithelial CTG to repair a soft tissue margin discrepancy for a single-implant crown in the anterior maxilla. Lai et al. (2010) presented a resubmerged implant technique with connective tissue grafting for implant coverage around a maxillary left central incisor of a 39-year-old woman. Mareque-Bueno (2011) described a surgical procedure for coronally advancing the peri-implant mucosa to treat a soft tissue dehiscence in a single-tooth implant-supported restoration. The results for all these reported the possibility of achieving only partial soft tissue coverage over an implant-supported restoration with the combined use of an acellular dermal matrix and a coronally positioned flap (see Figure 5.44a–d).

In a study on 20 patients, Zucchelli et al. (2012) presented a treatment consisting of the removal of the implant-supported crown, reduction in the implant abutment, a coronally advanced flap in combination with CTG, and final restoration. At one year the mean coverage was 96.3% and complete coverage was achieved in 75% of the treated sites. Esposito et al. (2012) attempted a systematic review for the Cochrane Collaboration Group, but he was not able to find a single acceptable randomized control trial in the literature to provide recommendations on which would be the best incision/suture techniques/materials to correct/augment peri-implant soft tissues (see Figure 5.45a–g).

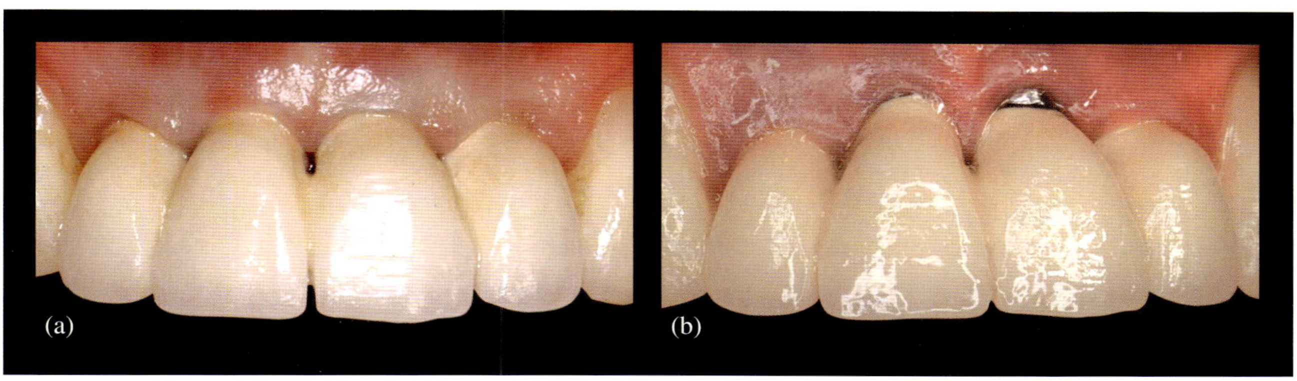

Figure 5.44 (a) Implant supported restoration replacing four maxillary anterior teeth in place two months post implant insertion, (b) Two year post restorative result showing apical soft tissue migration around the two maxillary central incisors.

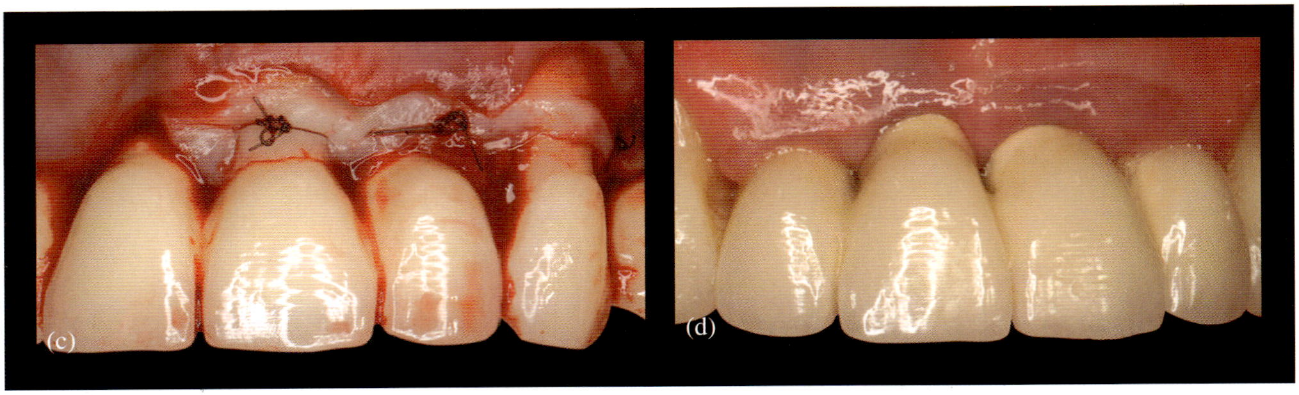

Figure 5.44 (c) Sub-epithelial connective tissue graft is secured in place to treat the recession, (d) Three years result post connective tissue grafting.

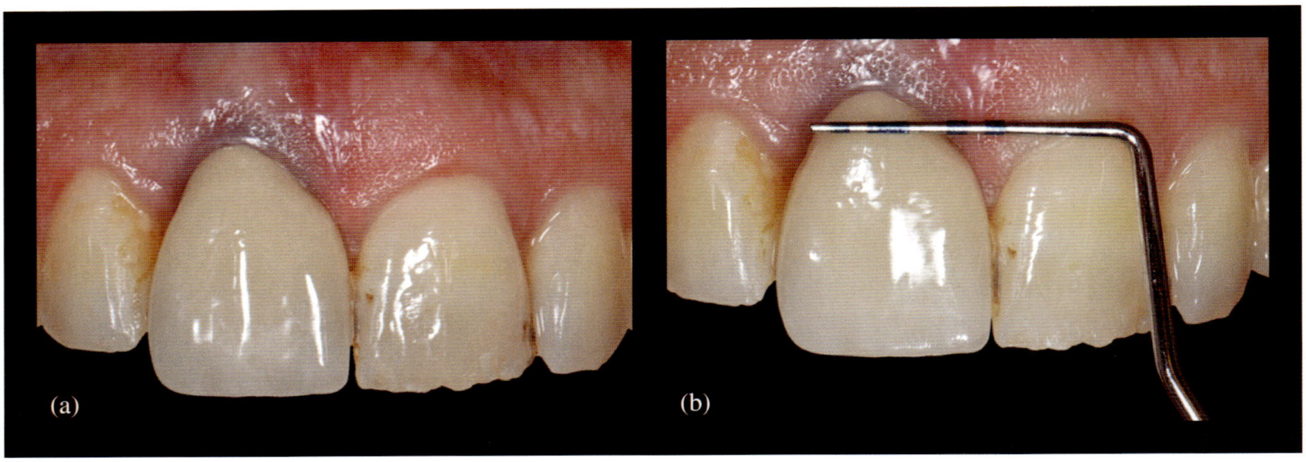

Figure 5.45 (a) and (b) Pre-operative view of a class 1 recession case limited to the right maxillary central incisor.

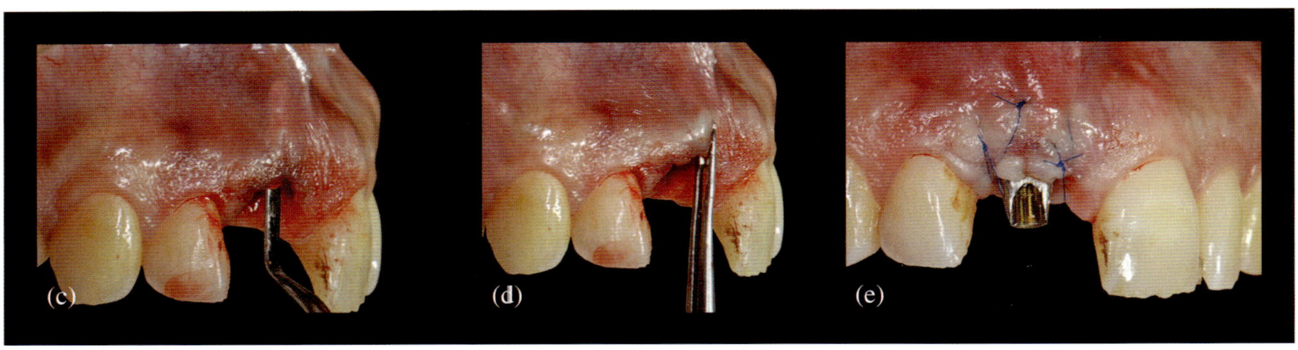

Figure 5.45 (c) Blunt dissection of the soft tissues to allow complete mobility or the flap, (d) Flap finally mobilized, (e) Connective tissue graft is introduced to treat the recession.

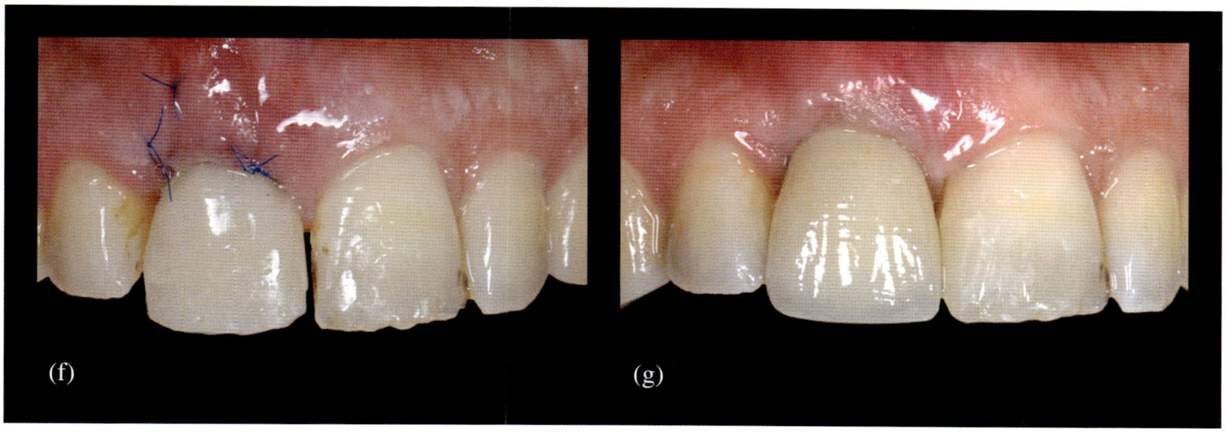

Figure 5.45 (f) One week post-operative healing, (g) Final case restored with a new zirconia crown and the recession were completely treated.

Wilson et al. (2013) performed a study with 16 patients, who presented a peri-implant buccal soft tissue recession and consequent exposure of the collar of the implant. A thick gingival cuff of the maxillary tuberosity area was selected as the donor site. After local anesthesia of the recipient and donor sites with mepivacaine plus epinephrine 1:100000, an intracrevicular incision was performed and a partial thickness flap was elevated. After preparing the recipient site, the gingival cuff was excised. The donor soft tissue was de-epithelialized and trimmed with a mucotome to give a U-shape to facilitate an optimal adaptation to the collar of the implant. The prepared connective tissue was placed in the recipient bed and immobilized. Complete coverage was achieved in 9 of the 16 cases (56.3%) (see Figure 5.46a and b).

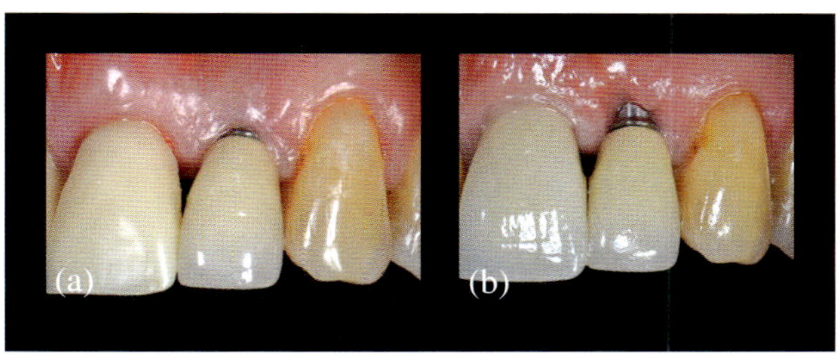

Figure 5.46 (a) and (b) Pre and post-operative Clinical examples that shows the failure of connective tissue grafts to treat recession.

A modified socket seal surgery has been developed by Misch et al. (1999). A composite autograft made of connective tissue periosteum and bone is used to seal the socket. A CTG has the advantage over a keratinized graft by blending into the surrounding attached gingival regions offering similar color and texture of the epithelium. The composite graft also contains autogenous bone. The major advantage of autologous bone is a more rapid and predictable osteogenic activity. The composite graft technique is indicated when a non-infected tooth is extracted with defective socket walls and an implant is planned as a replacement. It is not indicated for infection in the socket area or if bone removal was required to extract the tooth (see Figure 5.47a and b).

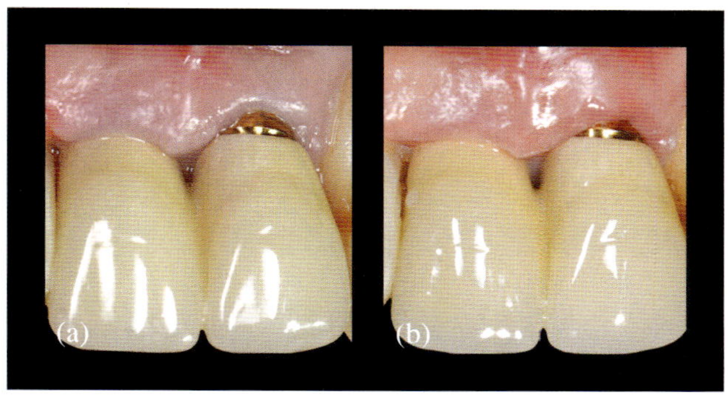

Figure 5.47 (a) and (b) Pre and post-operative Clinical examples that shows the failure of connective tissue grafts to treat recession.

In conclusion, CTGs can treat minimal tissue discrepancies, provided that the implant is in the correct 3D position. However, the use of CTGs to treat class 1 recession is not as successful as when used with anural teeth, because they don't offer a high success rate. The smaller the recession size, the more chances for CTG to succeed.

5.6.3 Treatment for Class II Recession

Class II (*moderate recession*) is an implant-related gingival recession that ranges between 1 and 2 mm from the mid-facial aspect, with both proximal papillae intact heights. It has two subdivisions: class II division 1, where the labial plate of bone is resorbed while the palatal plate of bone is intact, and class II division 2, where both plates of bone (labial and palatal) are resorbed and confirmed by the CBCT scan (see Figure 5.48a–d).

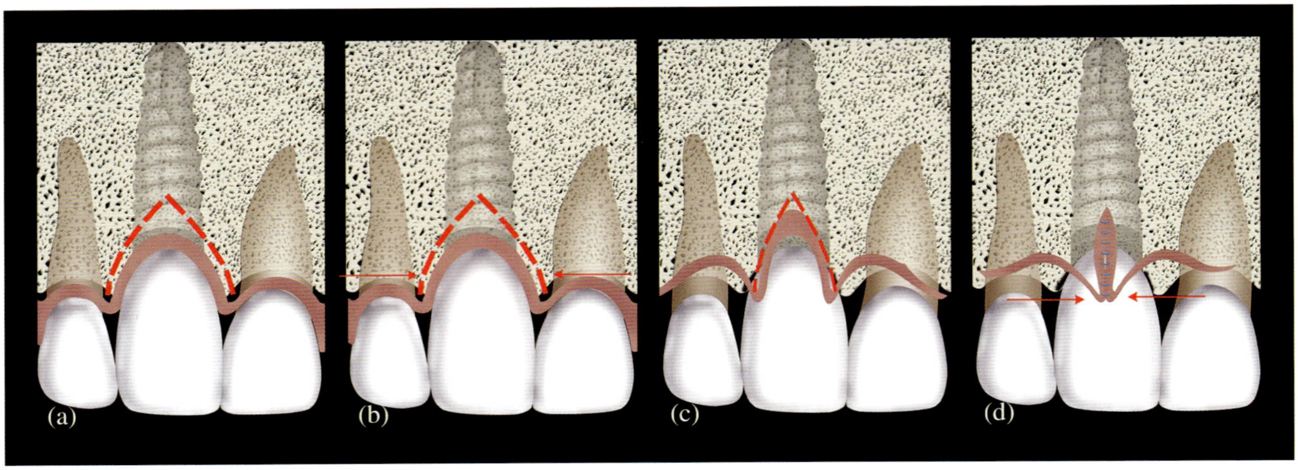

Figure 5.48 (a–d) A schematic drawing showing the steps of performing double papillary flap approximation.

The author introduced a novel proposed treatment protocol called the combo protocol, since it is a combination of two soft tissue procedures: (1) the double papilla approximation flap and (2) the subepithelial pedicle palatal flap. The combo protocol is used in conjunction with any osseous grafting technique, no matter what the osseous corrective procedure is. In other words, it is a pure soft tissue discipline with a complementary osseous grafting of the defective socket walls. Before starting with the correction procedure, the availability and quality of the soft tissue should be inspected. The partial-thickness palatal pedicle graft technique was first proposed by Cohen and Ross (1968) who reported more than an 85% success rate in covering denuded roots. The double papilla approximation flap also gives predictable useful results (see Figures 5.49a, b, 5.50a and b, and 5.51a–d).

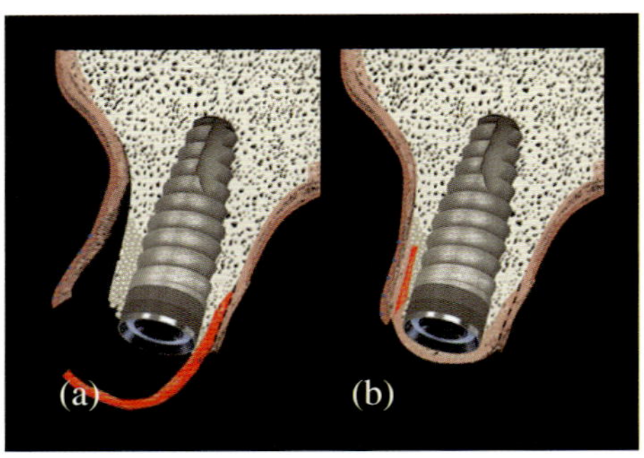

Figure 5.49 (a) and (b) A schematic drawing showing a sub epithelial connective tissue graft pedicle rotated from the palate.

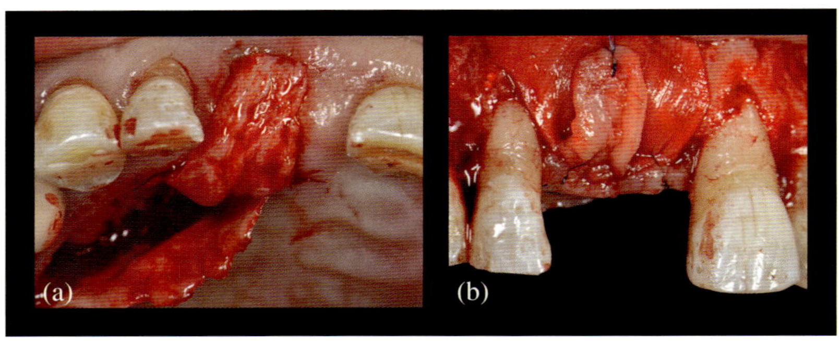

Figure 5.50 (a) and (b) Rotated sub epithelial connective tissue graft stabilized towards the labial side.

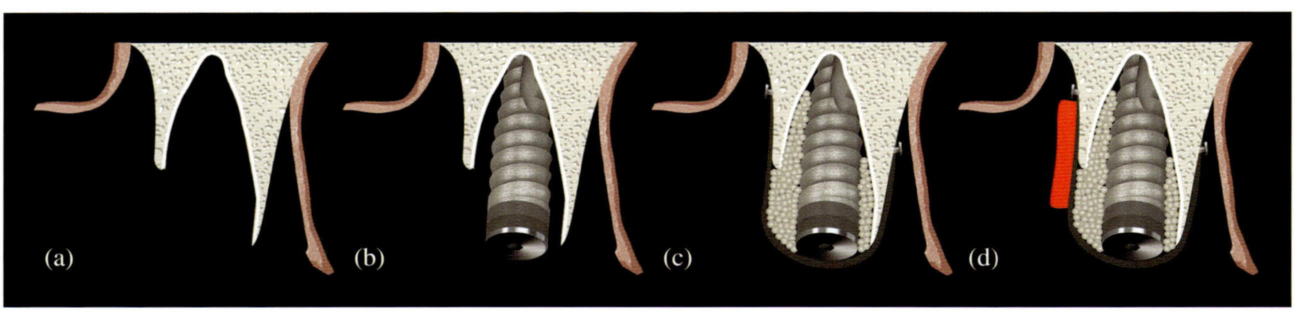

Figure 5.51 (a–d) A diagram showing step by step protocol of treating class II gingival recession.

Burkhardt and Lang (2005) investigated the surgical coverage of reseeded roots caused by trauma or inflammatory reactions that seem to be a common feature of the buccal tissue morphology. Mathews (2000) demonstrated that, for immediate implants, the palatal subepithelial connective tissue pedicle provides an underlying tissue bed for the double papilla approximated flaps in the presented combo protocol. All the prosthetic parts should be removed at the time of surgery to allow the optimal graft positioning (see Figures 5.52a, b, 5.53a–i, and 5.54a–g).

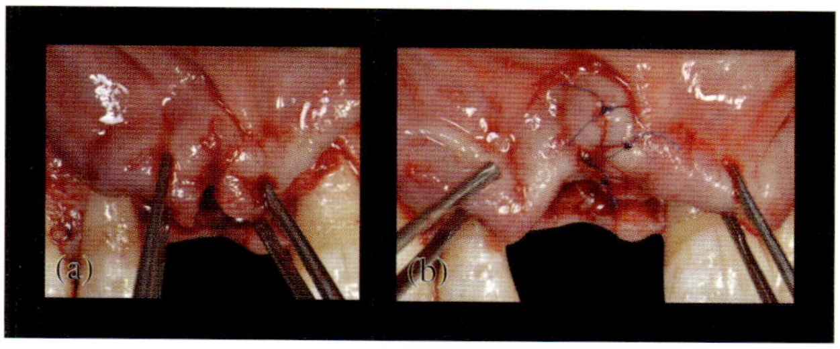

Figure 5.52 (a) and (b) Double papillary flap approximation steps.

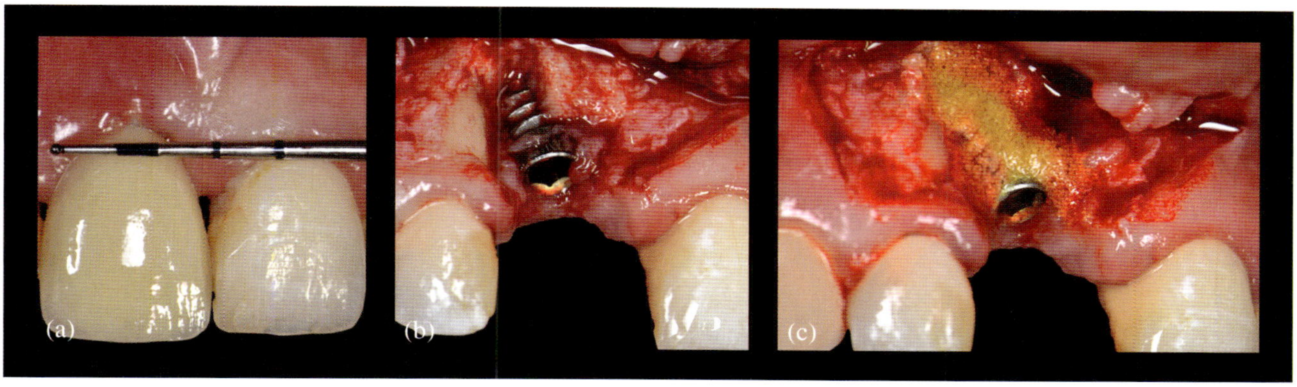

Figure 5.53 (a) Class II recession around implant supported restoration, (b) Bone reveal defect after flap reflection, (c) Decontaminate of the implant surface with tetracycline slurry for two minutes.

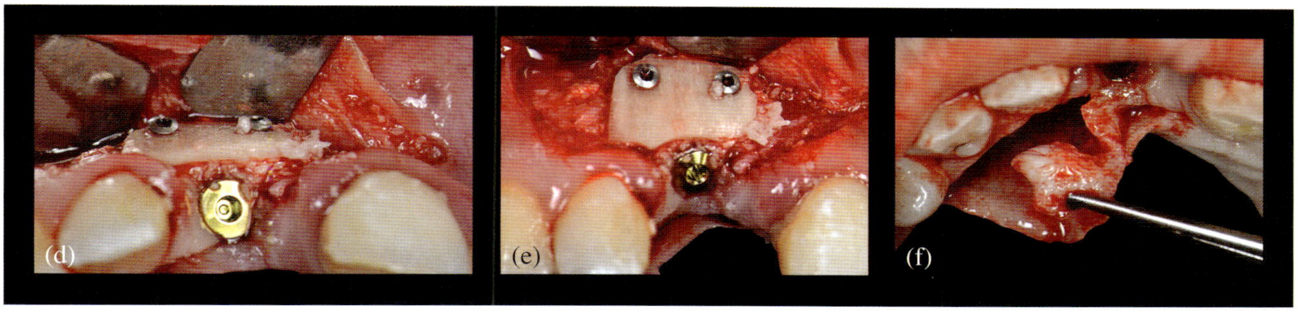

Figure 5.53 (d) and (e) Monocortical allograft sheet stabilized with two micro screws, (f) Sub epithelial connective tissue graft rotated from the palate.

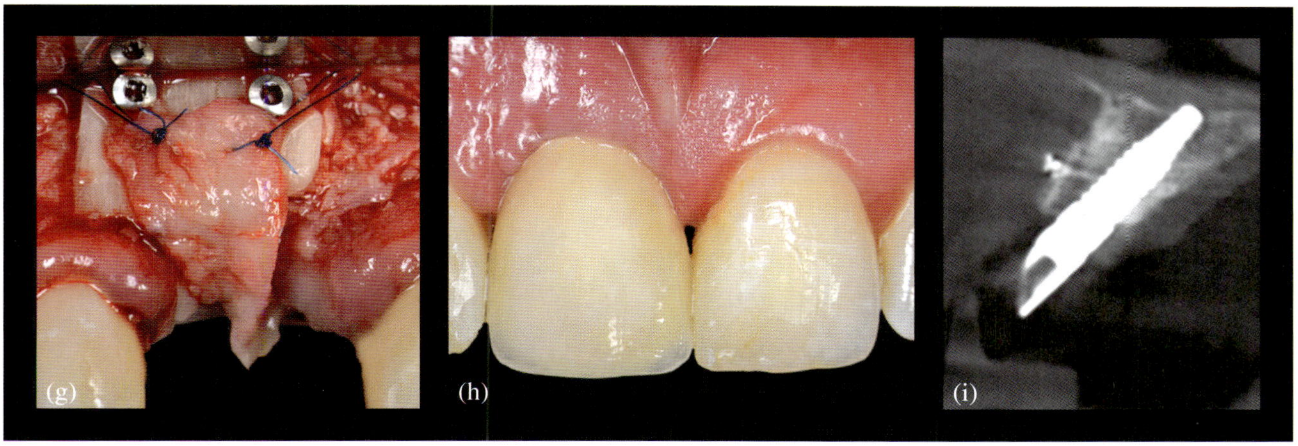

Figure 5.53 (g) Rotated palatal flap stabilized to the labial side, (h) Final case restored, (i) Cone-beam computed tomography (CBCT) scan showing the implant position in place.

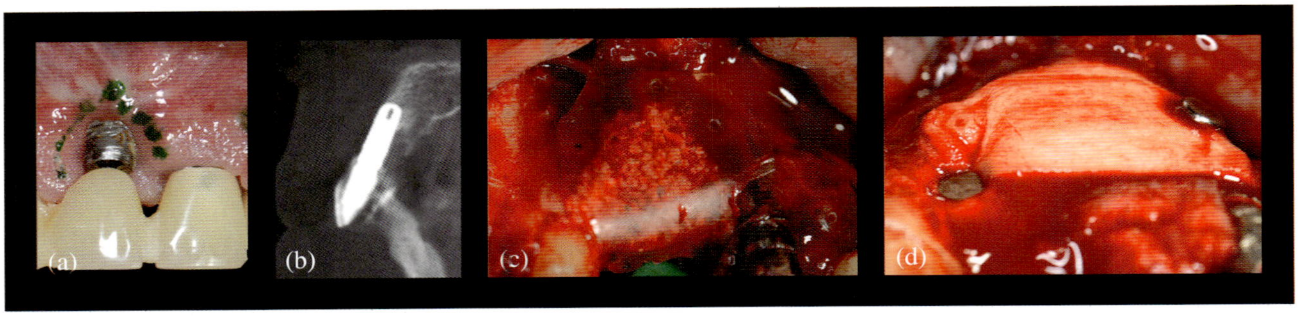

Figure 5.54 (a) Class II gingival recession, double papillary flap outlines planned for the surgery, (b) Cone-beam computed tomography (CBCT) scan showing both labial and palatal bone resorption, (c) Intra-operative view showing the new implant being placed and the area is grafted with a particulate bone graft and covered with a PDDLA membrane, (d) Collagen membrane stabilized with two membrane tacs.

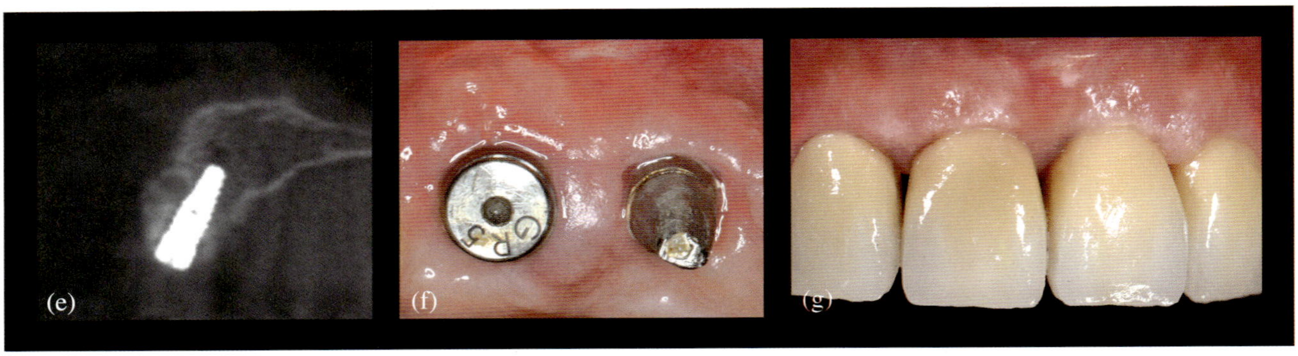

Figure 5.54 (e) CBCT scan showing the new implant with new regenerated bone around its labial surface, (f) Healing abutment connected for tissue profiling, (g) Case finally restored.

In the study by Elaskary et al. (2016), 10 patients (5 females and 5 males) between 24 and 63 years of age presented with *class II division 2* gingival recession (1–2 mm recession from the mid-facial aspect with interdental papilla intact, where both buccal and palatal plates of bone are deficient by >3 mm. Detailed medical histories were obtained, and exclusion criteria included smoking and alcoholism. Informed consent forms were signed after an explanation was given of the procedure. All 10 patients received preoperative clinical and radiographic examinations (CBCT) and baseline plaque index scores were documented. Baseline markings of gingival recession were recorded using a specially designed acrylic template. Measurements were again recorded at four, six, and nine months, postoperatively. The protocol used involved a double papillary flap approximation and rotated palatal subepithelial connective tissue pedicle graft used together and covering any particulated or autogenous bone graft material (Elaskary and Pipco 2000) (see Figures 5.55a–i and 5.56a–e).

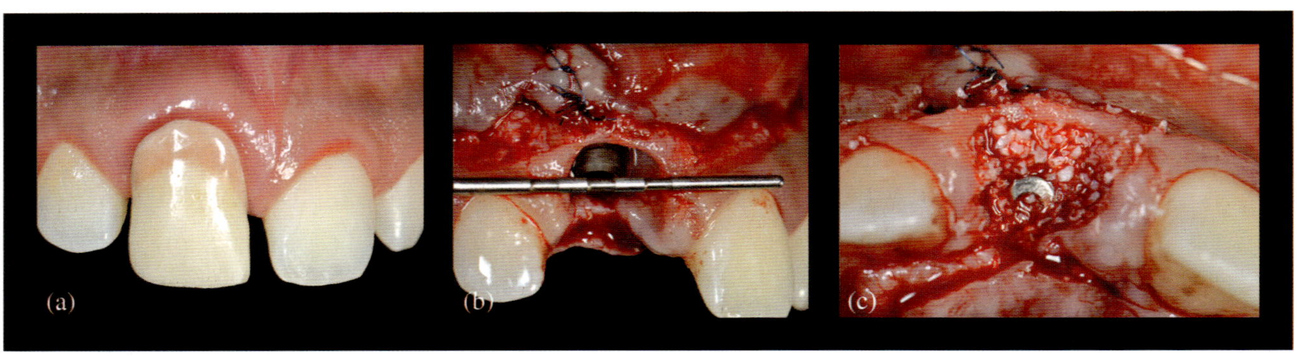

Figure 5.55 (a) Class II gingival recession, (b) A new implant is placed according to the three dimensional esthetic positioning protocol, (c) Intra-operative view showing the implant in place and the area grafted with particulated bone graft,

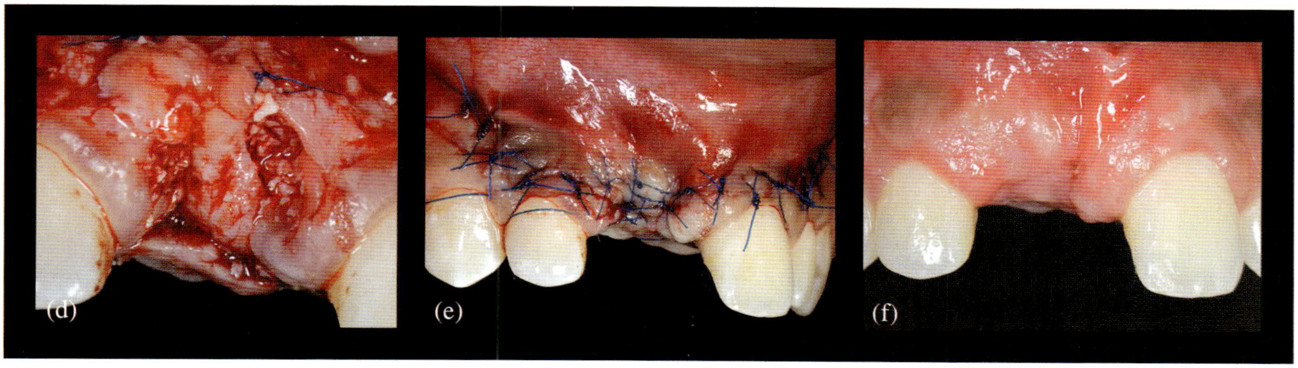

Figure 5.55 (d) Rotated pedicle connective tissue graft is rotated to the labial side and stabilized, (e) Flap sutured, (f) Four weeks post-operative showing uneventful healing.

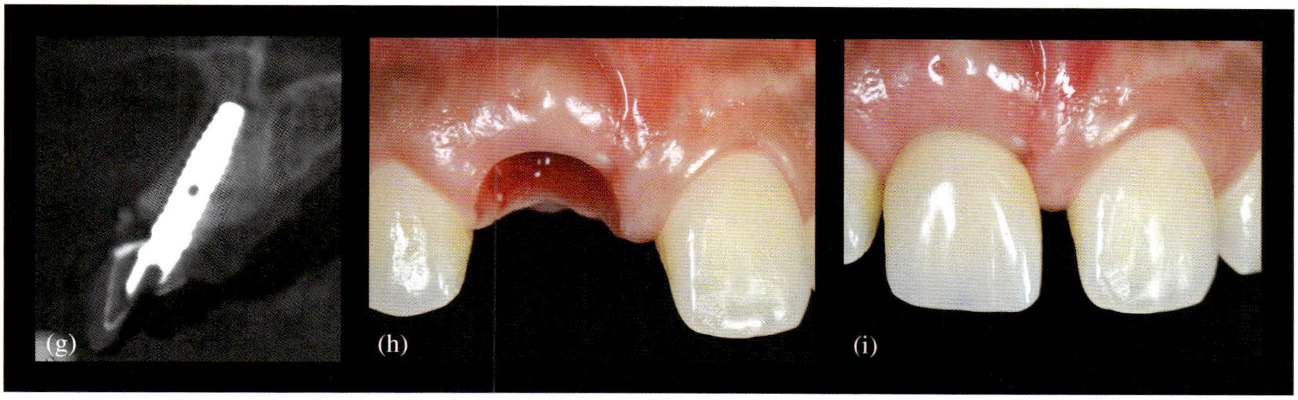

Figure 5.55 (g) Cone-beam computed tomography (CBCT) scan showing implant with new regenerative bone, (h) Soft tissue profile, (i) Finally case restored showing 90% improved recession.

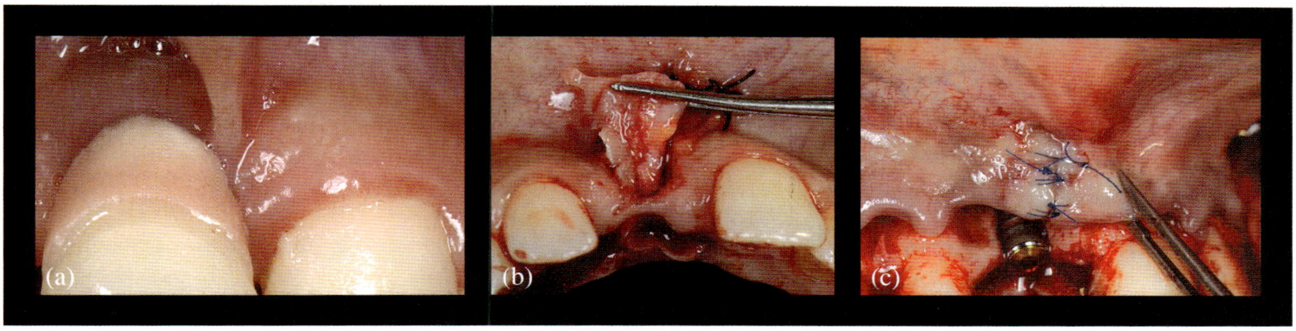

Figure 5.56 (a) Intra-operative view of Class II gingival recession, (b) Pedicle sub-epithelial connective tissue graft is rotated, (c) Double papillary flap sutured.

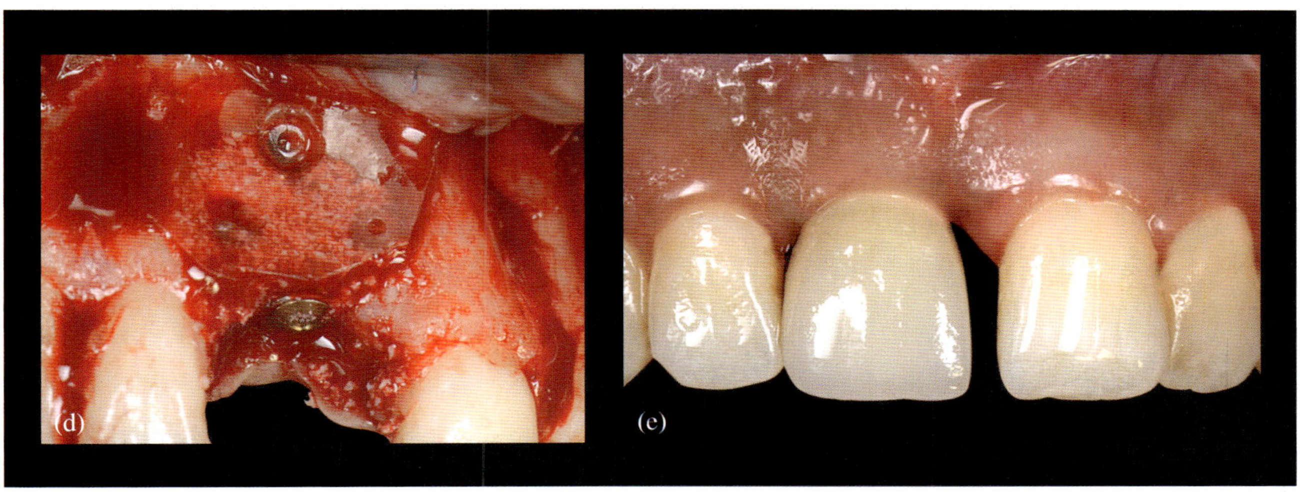

Figure 5.56 (d) Particulated bone graft is placed under the poly-DL-lactic acid membrane (PDLLA) membrane, (e) Case finally restored.

All surgeries were performed under local anesthesia after removing all existing prosthetic parts. The surgery involved three stages: soft-tissue preparation, implant removal and replacement with a new implant, and finally bone grafting of the osseous defect.

The double papillary approximation flap was performed buccally and a No. 15c blade was used to make a V-shaped incision labially around the recession location, following the outline of the gingival recession. This incision provided a fresh wound surface for tissue approximation. Two relaxing horizontal incisions were made on the adjacent mesial and distal interdental papilla coronally parallel to the cementoenamel junction with a No. 15c blade to allow better relaxation of the flap, followed by two releasing oblique incisions made at the line angles of the adjacent teeth and extended beyond the mucogingival junction. At the base of the flap, the periosteum was scored to prepare a tension-free flap closure. The V-section was then raised together and sutured together using a suture needle 6–0 proline interrupted sutures (Ethicon, Agnthos AB, Sweden). A palatal flap was dissected to obtain SCTG directly opposite to the recession location, which would be later rotated to the buccal recession area labially. Dissection of the mucoperiosteal flap and the underlying preparation of a subepithelial connective tissue flap to a depth of 5–8 mm were then performed (Khoury and Happe 2000). A sharp incision of the subepithelial tissues was then made parallel to the first incision to harvest a SCTG, but leaving it attached in the anterior region as a pedicle (see Figure 5.57a–e).

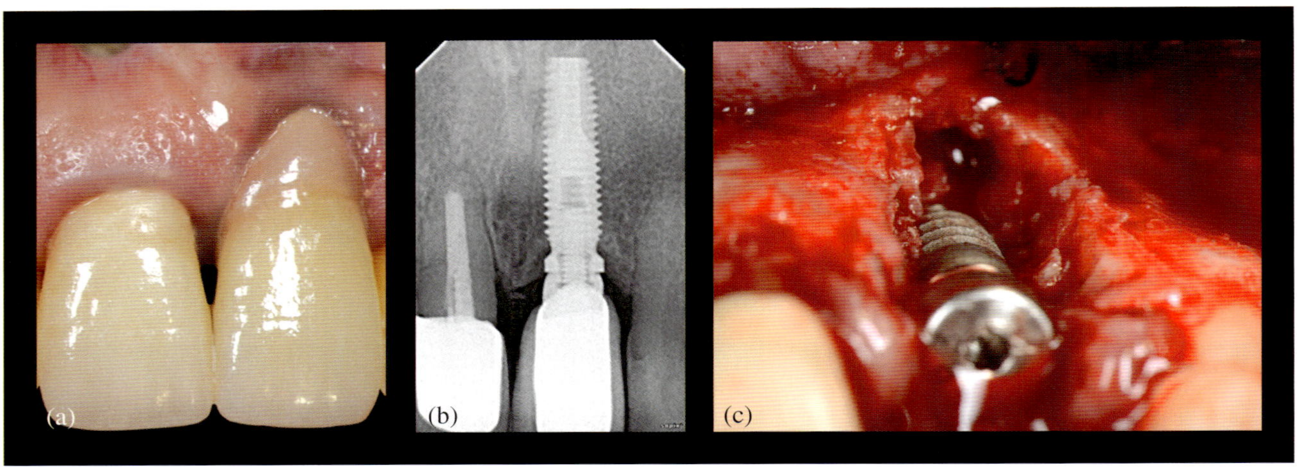

Figure 5.57 (a) Pre-operative view of Class II gingival recession, (b) Peri-apical radiographic view showing too deep implant position, (c) A new implant in place.

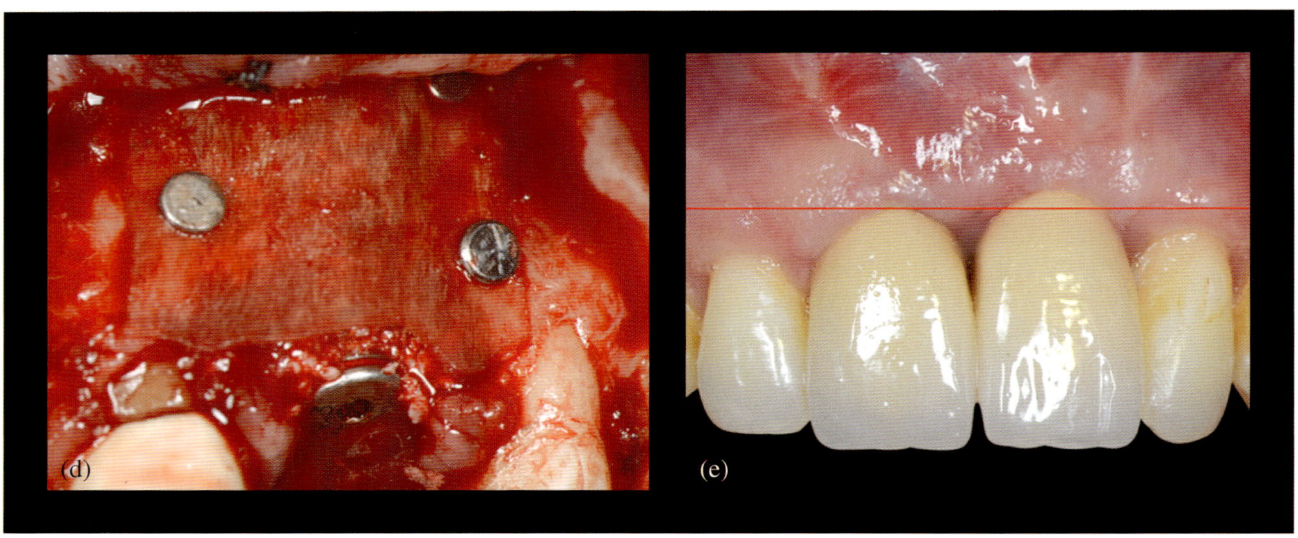

Figure 5.57 (d) Xenograft Lamellar bone sheet is placed and stabilized with membrane tacs, (e) Case finally restored showing 85% of treatment success.

The failed implant was then removed and followed by inserting a new implant (BioHorizons, Birmingham, Alabama, USA) simultaneously. Then the osseous defect around the new implant was grafted with a particulated autogenous bone grafting mix. The bone graft mix was formed of autogenous bone chips harvested from the operating site using bone scraper and bone allograft particles. The particulated bone graft was then stabilized and covered with a poly-DL-lactic acid membrane (PDLLA) (KLS Martin, Germany) and four thermal screws (see Figure 5.58a–v).

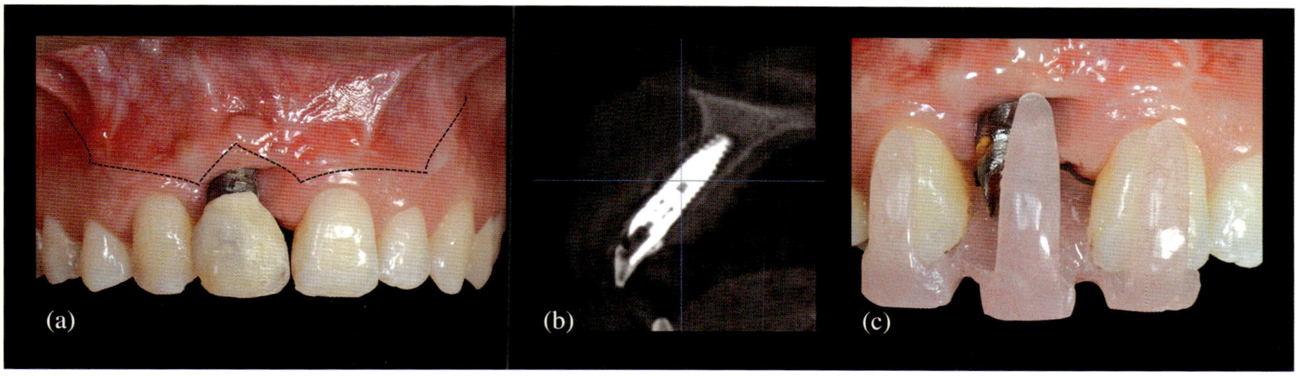

Figure 5.58 (a) Preoperative view outlining the incision line for a class II recession case, (b) CBCT scan showing failed implant with labial plate of bone resorption, (c) Scoring template in place.

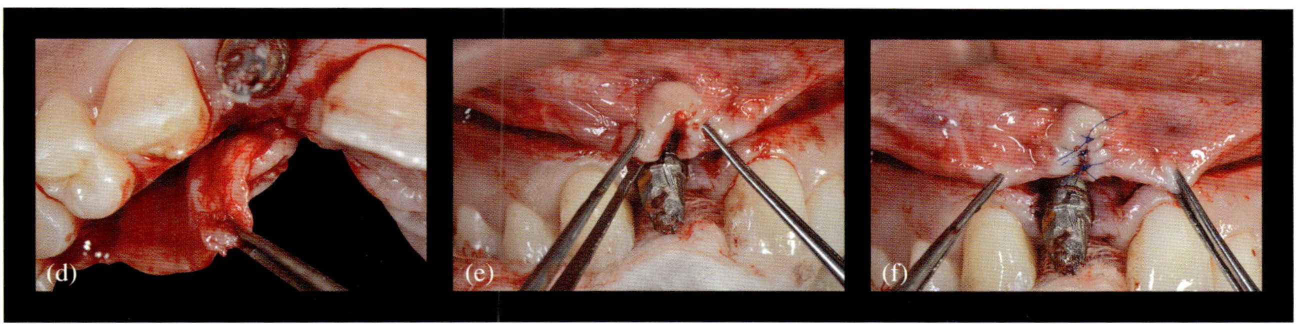

Figure 5.58 (d) Harvesting the rotated palatal connective tissue flap, (e) and (f) Double papillary flap sutured.

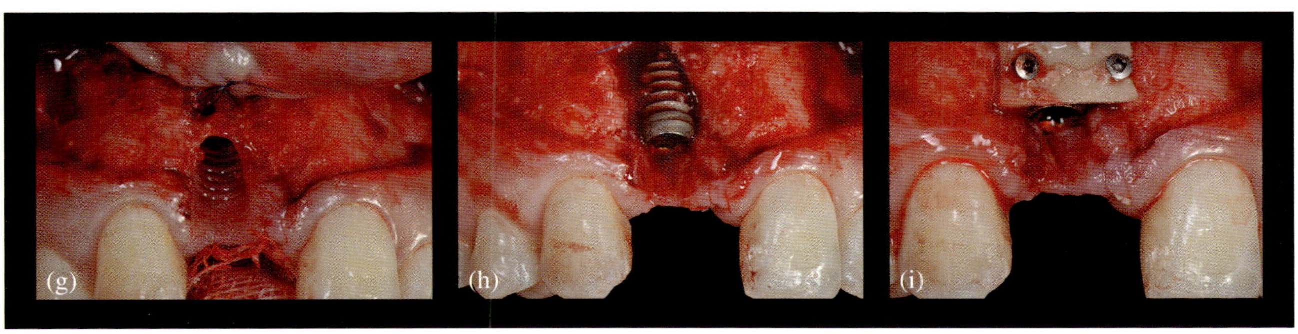

Figure 5.58 (g) The implant was removed, (h) a new implant was placed, (i) Cortico-cancellous block graft (harvested from the chin) is stabilized with two titanium micro screws.

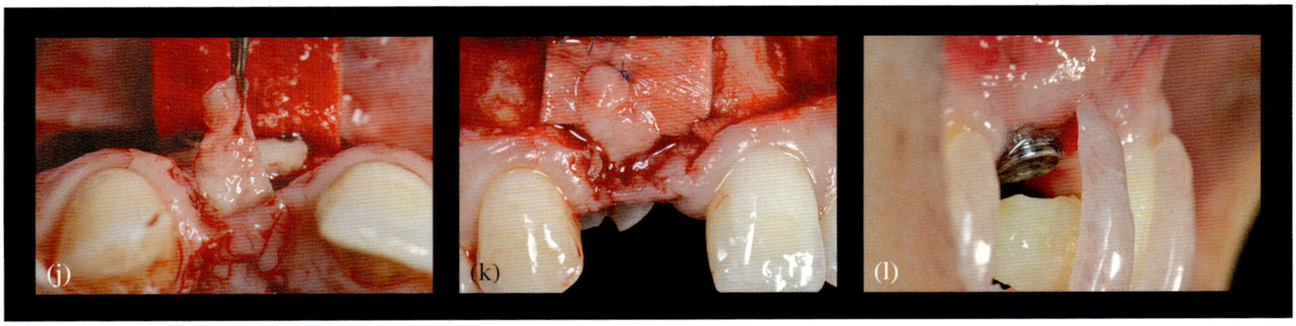

Figure 5.58 (j) and (k) The pedicle connective tissue graft is rotated labially and secured to the collagen membrane, (l) Scoring template showing 1 mm tissue gain incisally, indicating that more soft tissue height is needed due to the lack of soft tissue resiliency.

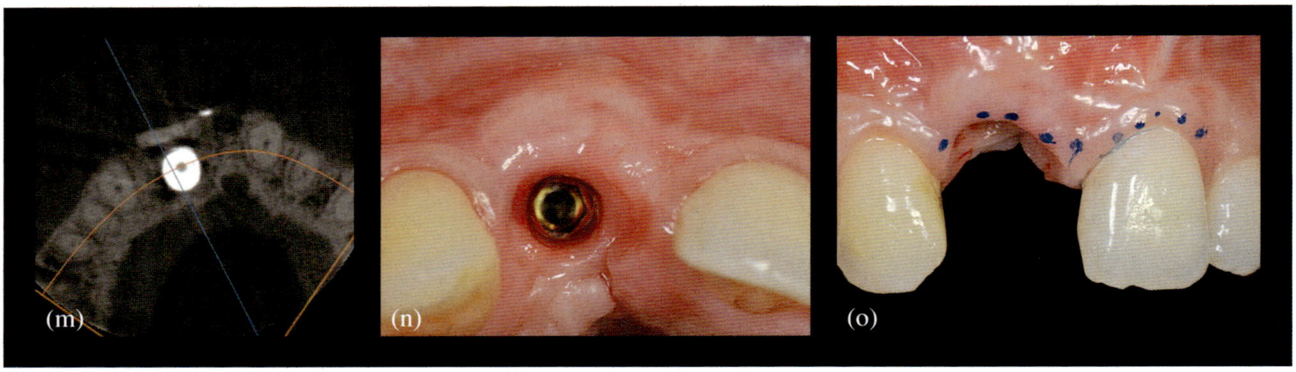

Figure 5.58 (m) CBCT showing the re-gain of labial contour, (n) Soft tissue profiling, (o) Case showing that it still requires more tissue to completely treat the recession.

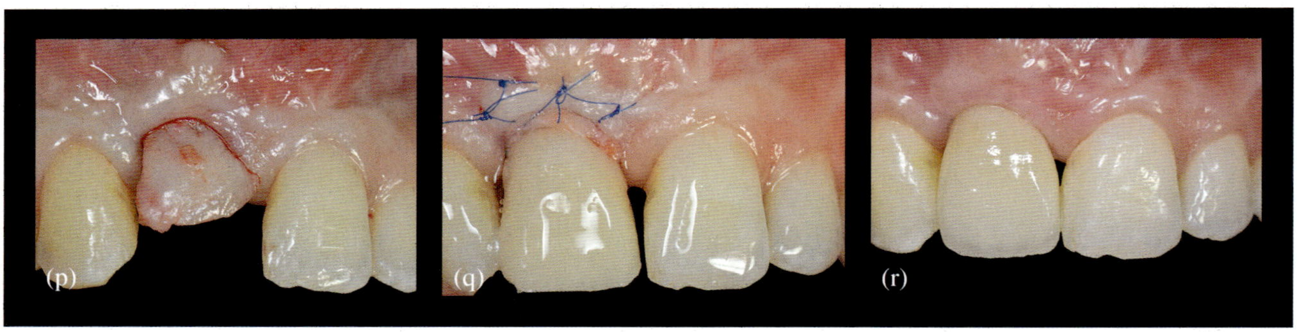

Figure 5.58 (p) Connective tissue graft is used to compensate with the tissue discrepancy, (q) Connective tissue graft sutured, (r) Case finally restored showing completely treated gingival recession.

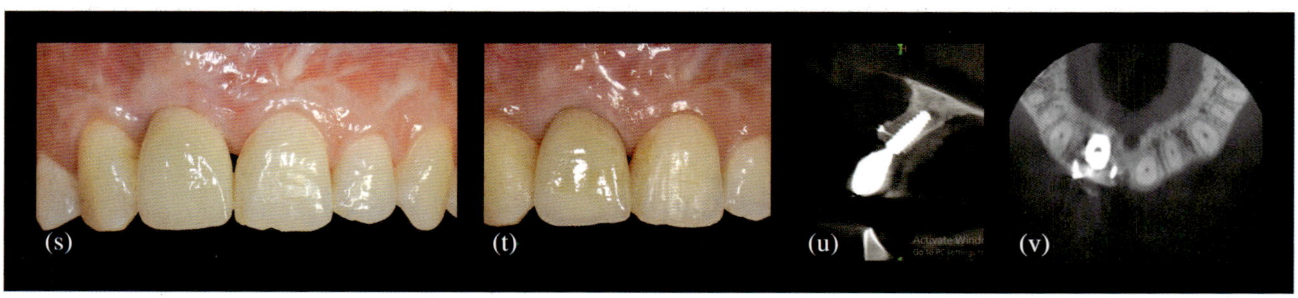

Figure 5.58 (s) and (t) One year follow up showing stable marginal tissue, (u) and (v) Two years follow up radiographic view and clinical view showing highly improved soft and hard tissue thickness.

The palatal subepithelial connective tissue pedicle was then rotated labially to cover the bone graft and sutured to the shield membrane using a 6–0 coated VICRYL™ (Ethicon, Agnthos AB, Sweden). The palatal wound at the donor site is then sutured along with the labial flap using 6.0 proline (Ethicon, Agnthos AB, Sweden). The new implant was left submerged during the healing period and a resin-bonded bridge was used as a provisional prosthesis. Postoperative instructions were given to the patients along with postoperative antibiotics (see Figure 5.59a–h).

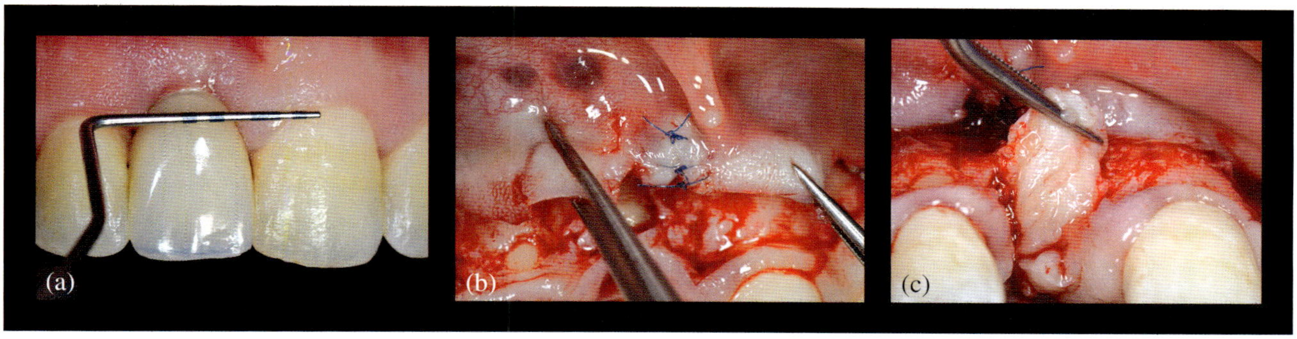

Figure 5.59 (a) Class II gingival recession, (b) Double papillary flap adjusted, (c) Rotated connective tissue palatal flap.

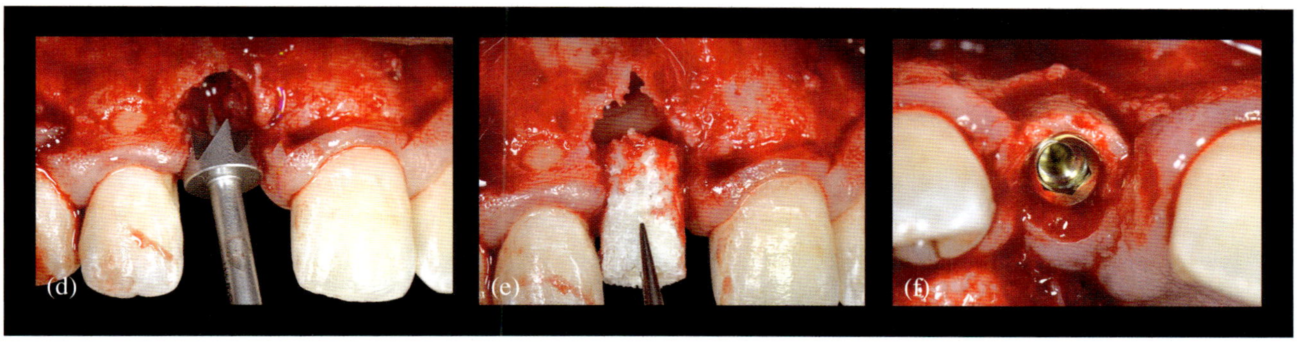

Figure 5.59 (d) Recipient site preparation to receive an allograft bone ring, (e) The bone ring is being fitted in place, (f) Incisal view showing the implant stabilizing the bone ring in place.

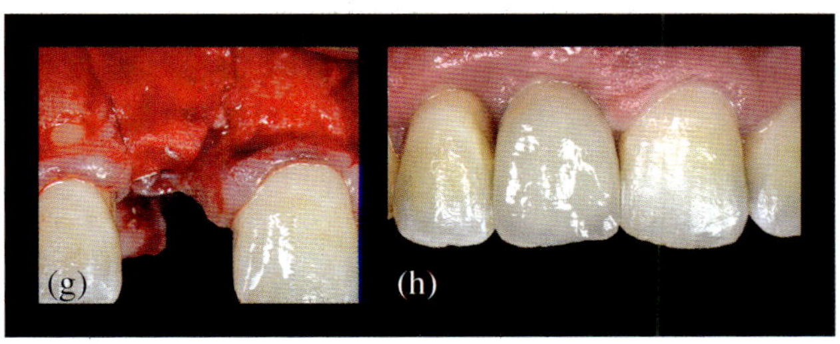

Figure 5.59 (g) Collagen membrane is being placed, (h) Case finally restored with 90% successes.

All patients, were followed for four, six, and nine months after surgical recession coverage. Table 5.2 presents the recordings of the presurgical degree of implant-related gingival recessions (mm) and postoperative amount of soft-tissue gain (mm) throughout the study period. Moreover, the mean ± SD amount of implant-related gingival recession (mm) at different follow-up periods is represented in Table 5.3. On average, the baseline gingival recession was 1.9 ± 0.5 mm, which decreased significantly ($P < 0.05$) during the study to reach 0.6 ± 0.9 mm after four months. Furthermore, at six and nine months postoperative, gingival recession observed was 0.7 ± 0.9 mm, which was also statistically significant compared to baseline values ($P < 0.05$). On comparing gingival recession values at four, six, and nine months postoperatively, no statistically significant difference was evident, proving that the amount of soft tissue gained after the surgical procedure did not deteriorate and showed good stability during the follow-up period.

At the end of the nine-month follow-up period, all cases showed improved soft tissue coverage of the recession area (Table 5.4) except two patients who failed to show soft tissue gain, one was a smoker and the other had a higher plaque index with a score of 2.

Table 5.2 Presurgical amount of implant-related gingival recessions (mm) and postoperative amount of soft tissue gain (mm) throughout the study period recorded by the acrylic template.

Case no.	Presurgical amount of gingival recession	Soft tissue gain at 4 months	Soft tissue gain at 6 months	Soft tissue gain at 9 months
1	1.5	1.30	1.30	1.40
2	2.5	2.50	2.30	2.30
3	2.0	1.80	1.80	1.80
4	1.0	1.00	1.00	1.00
5	1.5	1.20	1.10	1.00
6	1.3	1.20	1.25	1.25
7	1.8	1.57	1.56	1.57
8	2.5	2.00	1.80	1.80
9	2.5	0.00	0.00	0.00
10	2.0	−0.10	−0.10	−0.20

Table 5.3 Results of repeated measures (ANOVA) test for comparison between mean ± SD amount of implant-related gingival recession (mm) at different follow-up periods.

Period	Mean ± SD	*P* value
Baseline gingival recession	1.9[a] ± 0.5	
Gingival recession after 4 months	0.6 ± 0.9	
		0.001[b]
Gingival recession after 6 months	0.7 ± 0.9	
Gingival recession after 9 months	0.7 ± 0.9	

Adjusted *P* value for repeated measures (ANOVA).
[a] Significantly different.
[b] Significant at $P \leq 0.05$.

At the early clinical attempts to search for the best clinical protocol offering a high clinical predictably, it has been found that using coronal repositioning flaps alone does not offer any improvement of recession around dental implant sites. The discipline of the combo proposed clinical protocol offers mainly a soft tissue solution to provide an optimal and adequate housing for the bone graft of your choice. That means that the soft tissue provides the optimal housing for any bone graft to be used, which favors the improvement of the receded areas. The decision to remove or retain the implant depends on the degree of bone resorption around the implant. In class II division 1, the implant should not be removed; in such case, the exposed threads get decontaminated and then grafted. In class II division 2, the implant must be completely removed and replaced with a new one (if the bone resorption is more than 4 mm on the platal side). Identifying the tissue phenotype and the reason for the implant-related gingival recession becomes a vital part of the treatment. CTG solutions alone usually offer less consistent success rates for the treatment of class I implant-related gingival recession (see Figure 5.60a–c).

Each time a soft tissue surgery is performed, soft tissue scarring and soft tissue stiffness will be anticipated. This explains the benefit of the non-staged grafting approach where soft and hard tissue are augmented and repaired in one session, along with the complete removal of the inflammatory tissue in the site (see Figure 5.61 a and b).

5.6.4 Treatment for Class III Recession

Class III implant-related gingival recession presents more than a 2-mm recession from the mid-facial aspect where the peri-implant papillae vertical height is dropped. A customized treatment approach is proposed for class III recession. The available options involve inlay grafts, interposition grafts, biocritical grafts, and onlay grafts. Below are some treatment suggestions for class III recessions. All the cases presented with class III recession should have a customized approach, no single protocol is described for these cases, because it has variable degrees of tissue damage and profile collapse (Jensen and Terheyden 2009).

To increase the vertical height of mandibular and maxillary edentulous ridges, onlay grafting using bone blocks was first introduced in the early 1990s (Pikos 2000). The classic block augmentation technique involves the use of an autologous bone block fixed to the recipient ridge with osteosynthesis screws or dental implants (Cordaro et al. 2010). After performing recipient site corticotomy

Table 5.4 Patients' characteristics and percentage of improvement reported nine months after surgical procedure.

Characteristics	Not improved (No.)	Not improved (%)	Improved (No.)	Improved (%)	P value
Gender					0.114[a]
Male	2	40.0	3	60.0	
Female	0	0.0	5	100.0	
Plaque Index Score					0.784[b]
0	0	0.0	6	100.0	
1	0	0.0	2	100.0	
2	2	100.0	0	0.0	
Systemic Condition					0.784[b]
Free	2	28.6	5	71.4	
Controlled diabetes	0	0.0	1	100.0	
Mild hypertension	0	0.0	1	100.0	
Stomach ulcer	0	0.0	1	100.0	
Intraoral habits					0.035[a,c]
Nonsmoking	1	11.1	8	88.9	
Smoking	1	100.0	0	0.0	

[a] *P* value based on Fischer exact probability.
[b] *P* value based on Monte Carlo exact possibility.
[c] Significant at $P \leq 0.5$.

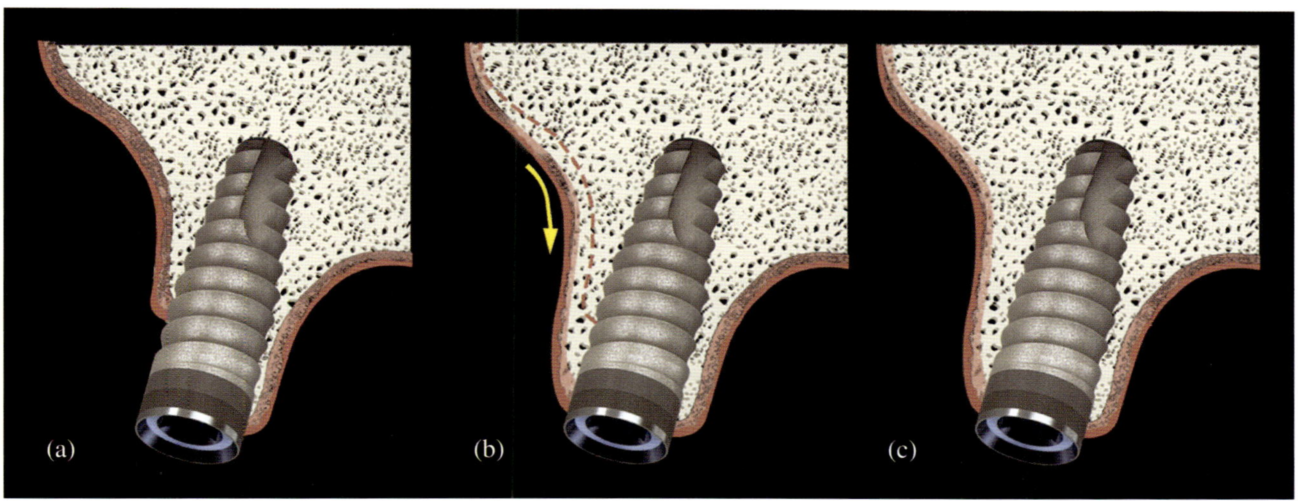

Figure 5.60 (a–c) Coronal repositioning flap will never attain any success in treating class II recession.

to encourage nourishment the graft, the latter is laid over the defective recipient bed and immobilized (Levin, Nitzan and Schwartz-Arad 2007).

Onlay autogenous grafts can be used to treat horizontal ridge deficiencies; however, when used to treat vertical ridge defects, it would be used from both aspects of the defective ridge labial and palatal plates. The bone healing cascade occurs with the infiltration of inflammatory cells, followed by in-growth of new vessels and the replacement of necrotic tissues (Lee and Butler 1997). These events vary depending on the status of graft vascularity, the characteristics of the graft, and the condition of the recipient bed. Nonvascularized grafts undergo necrosis, as only the osteocytes on the surface re-establish blood supply and survive (Manson 1994). The remainder of the graft is infiltrated by blood vessels from the recipient site and repopulated by recipient MSCs (Lee and Butler 1997) (see Figure 5.62a–e).

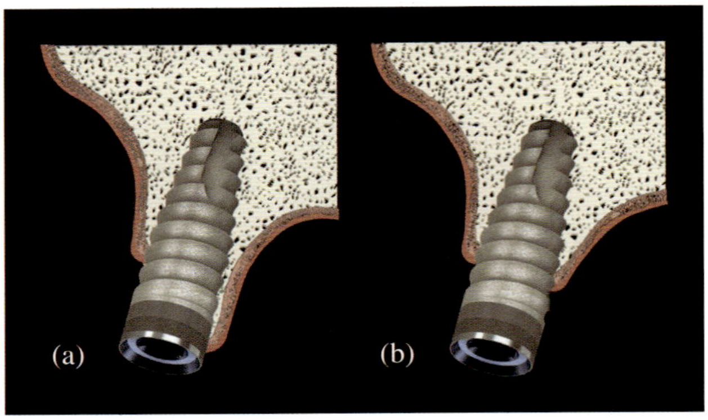

Figure 5.61 (a) In case of labial plate resorption only while the palatal plate is intact, the implant could be saved, decontaminated and grafted, (b) In case of both labial and palatal bone plate loss the implant should be removed and replaced by a new one.

For larger defects, cortical bone shells can be used to augment both labial and palatal sides. Bone shells are harvested with a special cutting wheel from the retromolar region, then the bone granules inserted between the two shells from resorption. Additional harvesting of bone chips is also necessary (Khoury and Khoury 2007). A corticocancellous bone block was harvested from the lateral side of retromolar area using piezosurgery and had a thickness of about 3 mm. A bone mill was used to produce bone chips, then the block spliced into two pieces with a cutting wheel and used as the shells (Stimmelmayr et al. 2012). The milled bone chips were mixed with autogenous blood and placed between the shells after fixation, and collagen fleece placed to fill the donor site defect (Khoury and Khoury 2006) (see Figure 5.63a–q).

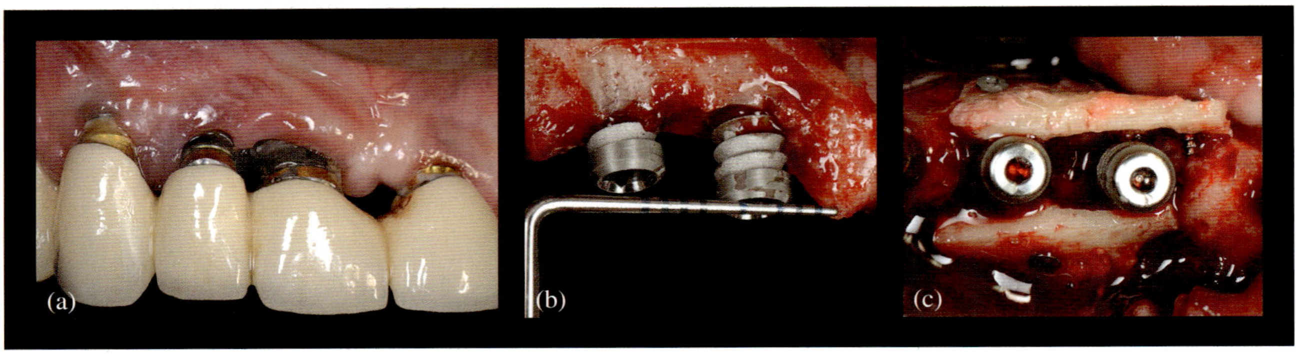

Figure 5.62 (a) Pre-operative view of contiguous implants with class III recession, (b) Two implants (Tapered plus, BioHorizons) are placed according to the esthetic protocol, (c) Bi-Cortical stabilization of two mono-cortical autograft blocks to the labial and palatal bone defects.

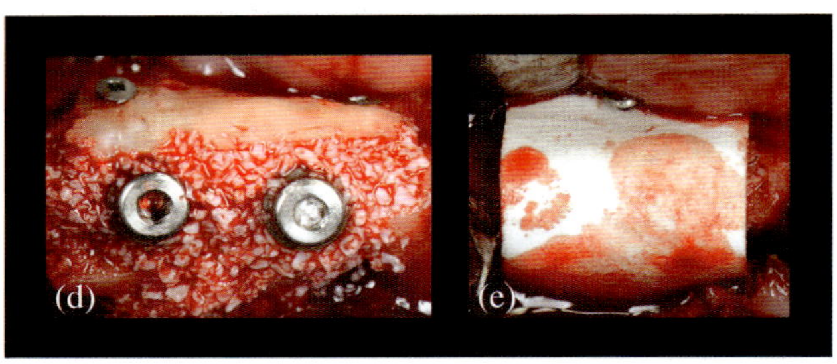

Figure 5.62 (d) Gaps filled with allografts, (e) Collagen membrane is stabilized by two auto tacs.

By elevating a full-thickness flap with a crestal incision, it is shifted palataly and two further vertical relieving incisions, allows complete visibility and access.

The bone shells were trimmed and adjusted with a round bur and anchored in the host bone with titanium micro screws. Space between two shells and the alveolar bone can be filled with a mix of milled bone chips and blood or allograft alone, or particulate allograft. The bone graft was covered with a resorbable collagen membrane then flap closure performed. The major advantage of this technique is the abundant restoration of the natural bone architecture, with a minimal resorption rate (see Figure 5.64a–o).

Another clinical application that can increase the vertical dimension of the alveolar bone is the use of sandwich-interpositional osteoplasties. When compared to onlay grafts, there is a major advantage because the soft tissue remains attached to the alveolar ridge of the place to be grafted (Kawakami et al. 2013), thus minimizing the tendency for wound-related complications. Sandwich osteotomies present the possibility for the good healing tendencies of inlay and interpositional osteoplasties (sandwich) with angiogenesis from all sides of the graft, i.e. closed compartment (see Figure 5.65a–f).

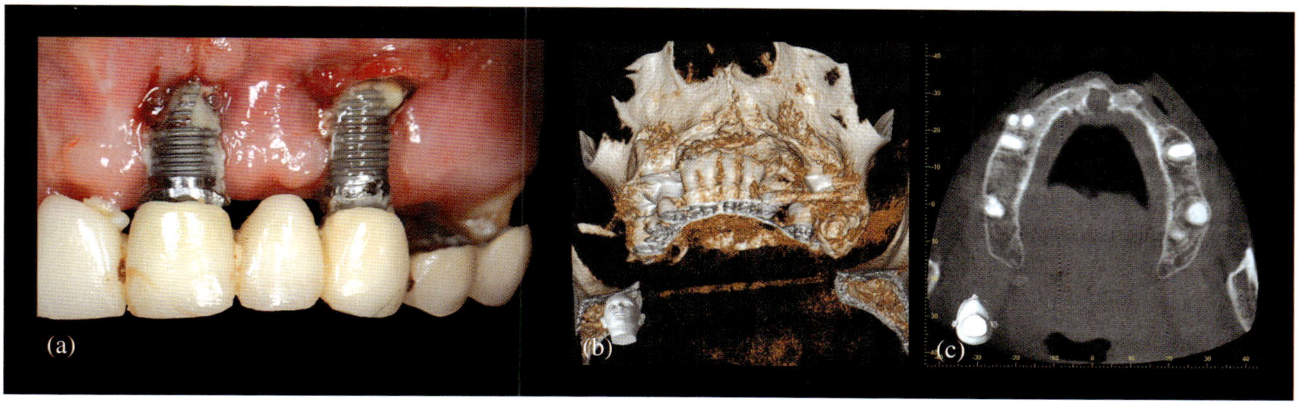

Figure 5.63 (a) Sever gingival recession around dental implants supported restoration, (b) and (c) cone-beam computed tomography (CBCT) showing extreme alveolar bone resorption after implant being removed.

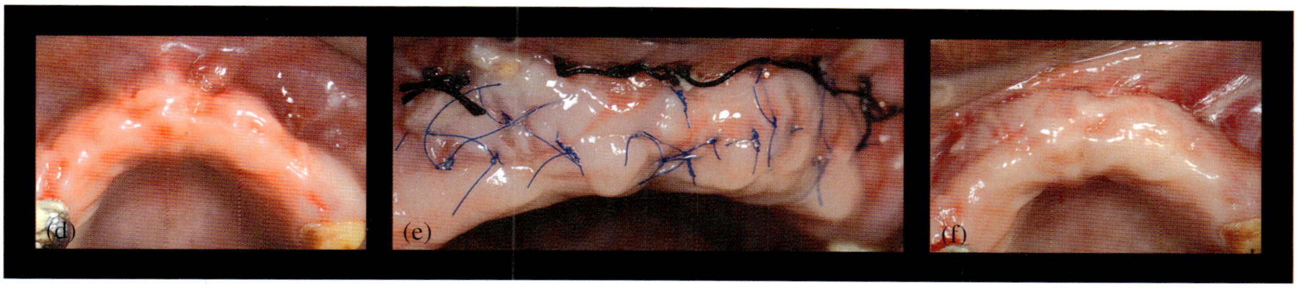

Figure 5.63 (d) Three weeks post implant removal showing heal ridge with deficient keratinized mucosa, (e) Onlay connective tissue graft with vestibuloplasty, (f) Five weeks post vestibuloplasty.

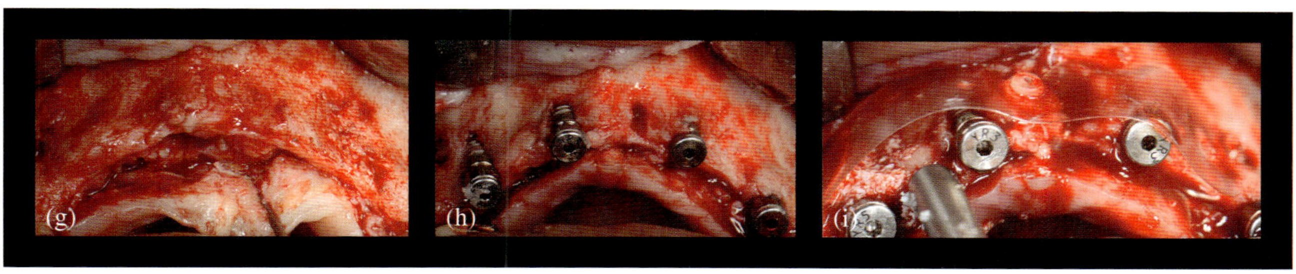

Figure 5.63 (g) Intra-operative view showing thin alveolar ridge that is planned for non-staged implant placement approach, (h) Implants placed with excellent pr mary stability revealing bone deficiency, (i) poly-DL-lactic acid membrane (PDLLA) membrane stabilized.

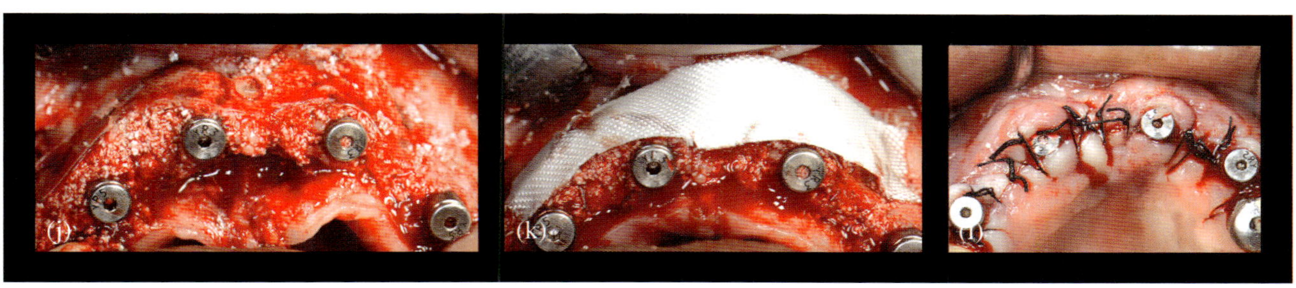

Figure 5.63 (j) Particulate bone graft was filled between implant and the membrane, (k) Surgi seal membrane placed on top the PDLLA membrane to enhance the adherence of the flap, (l) Healing abutment connected and flap sutured.

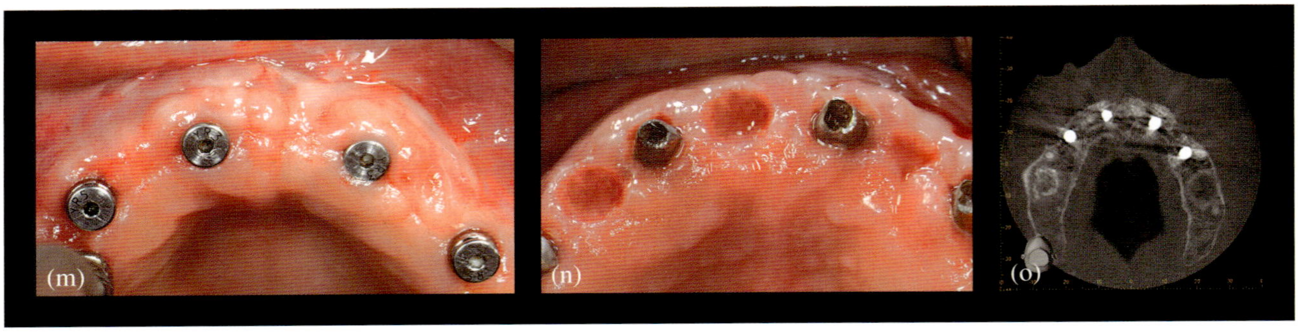

Figure 5.63 (m) Two moths post implant insertion showing excellent tissue width and quality, (n) Pontic development method, (o) CBCT showing the amount of regenerated bone around implants five months post-operative.

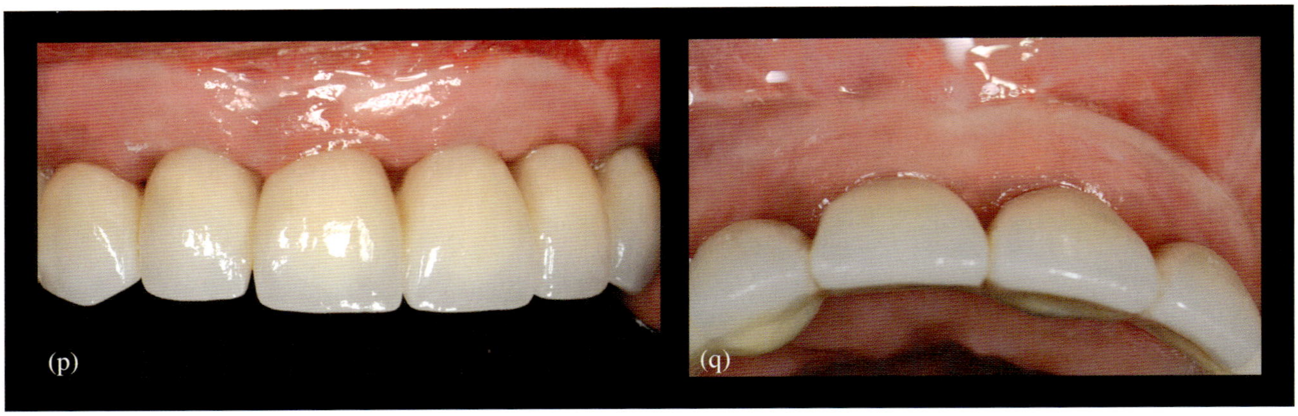

Figure 5.63 (p) and (q) Final case restored showing abundance of keratinized mucosa and regenerated alveolar bone.

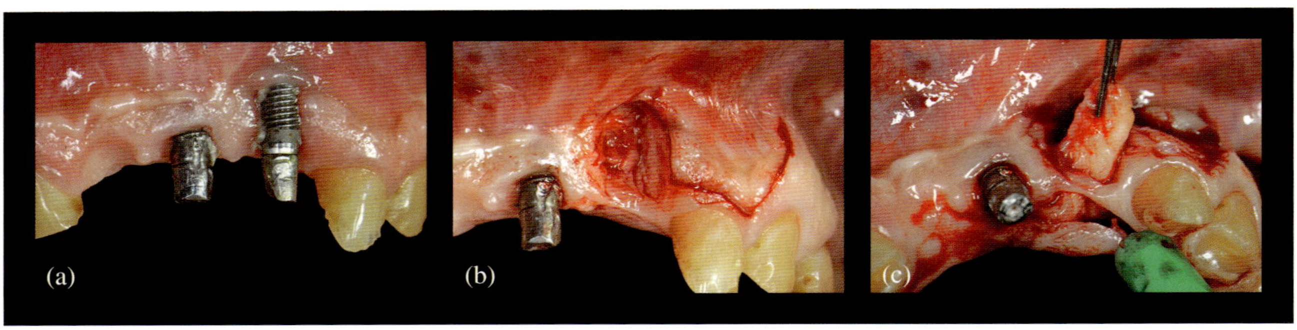

Figure 5.64 (a) Restoration removed, (b) One implant removed, (c) Sub epithelial connective tissue graft.

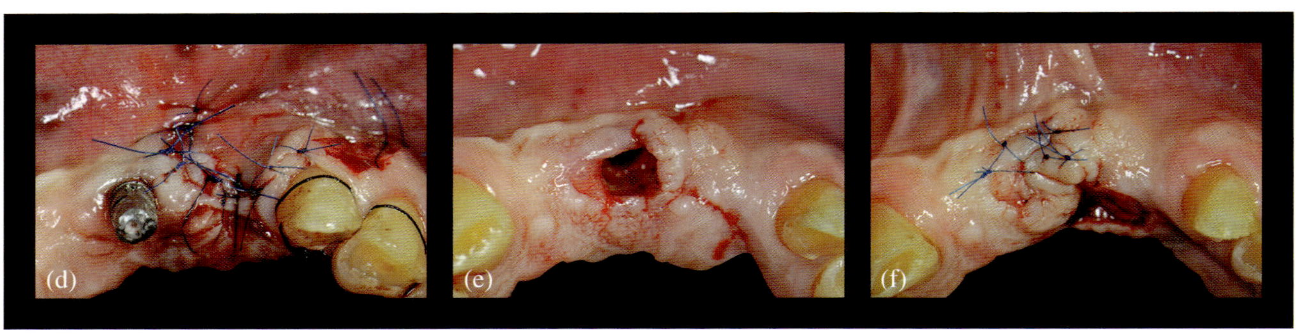

Figure 5.64 (d) Rotated buccal flap, (e) The second implant was removed, (f) Rotated palatal flap.

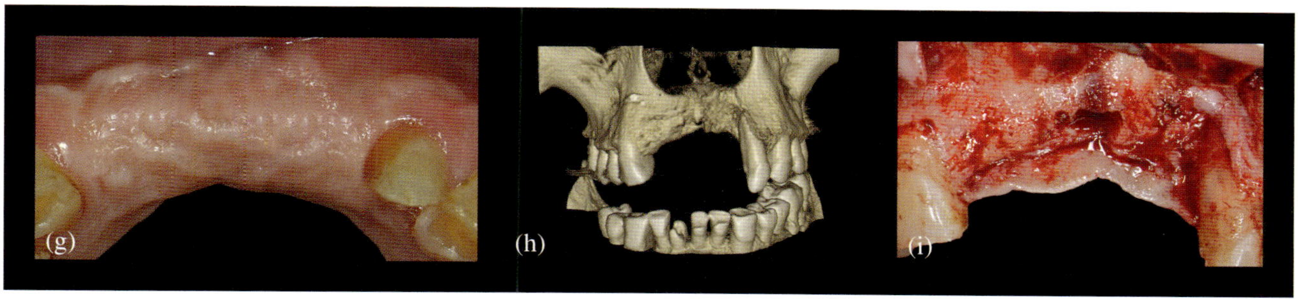

Figure 5.64 (g) Final ridge healed with improved keratinization, (h) 3D view showing osseous defect, (i) Intra operative view showing defect. size.

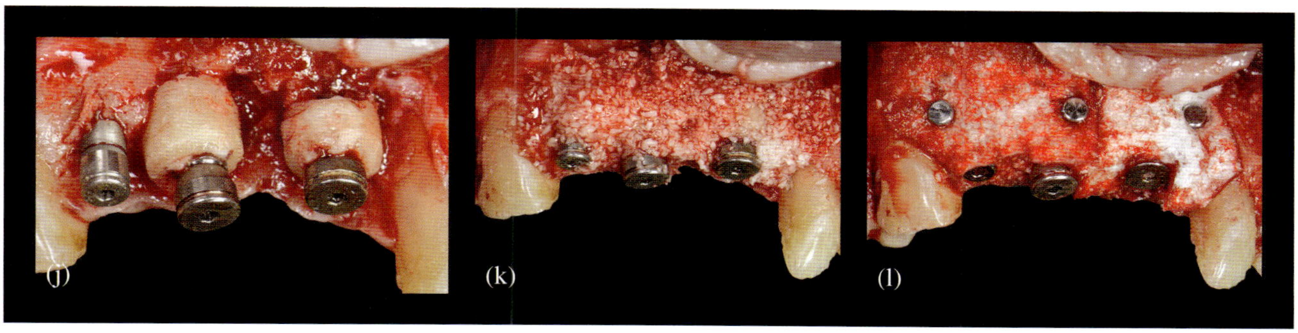

Figure 5.64 (j) Three implants placed with two of them grafted with autogenous bone ring harvested from the patient chin, (k) Voids filled with particulated graft, (l) Collagen membrane stabilized.

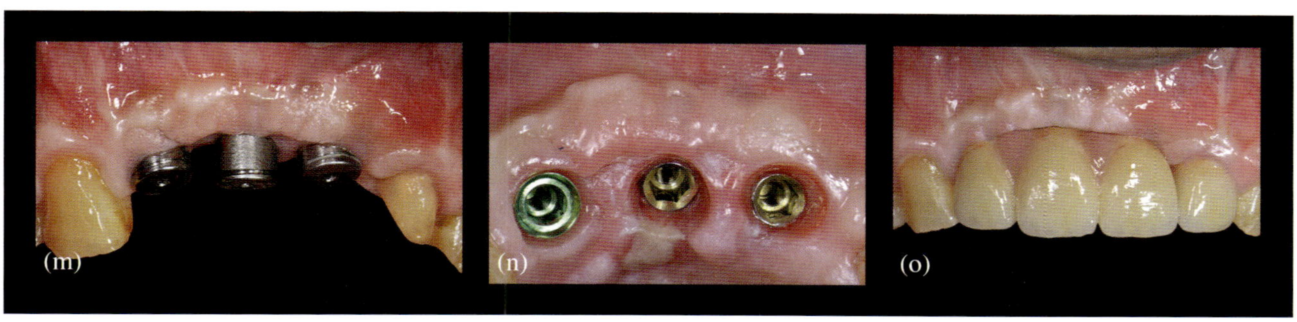

Figure 5.64 (m) Final tissue maturation around healing abutments, (n) Optimal labial tissue bulk is obtained, (o) Final case restored.

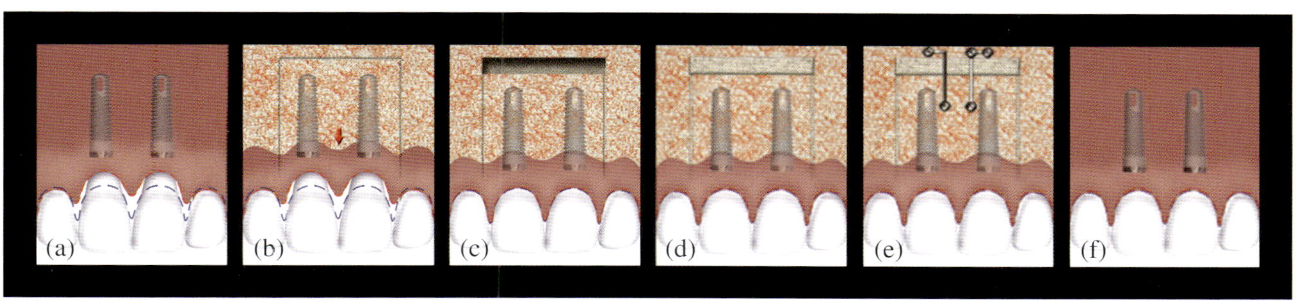

Figure 5.65 (a–f) Schematic drawing showing the stages of using Sandwich Osteotomy (Interpostional Grafts).

The sandwich technique, which uses a bone block graft positioned between osteotomized bony segments, was successfully combined with the visor osteotomy to augment a severely atrophic edentulous mandible (Stoelinga et al. 1986) (see Figure 5.66a–d).

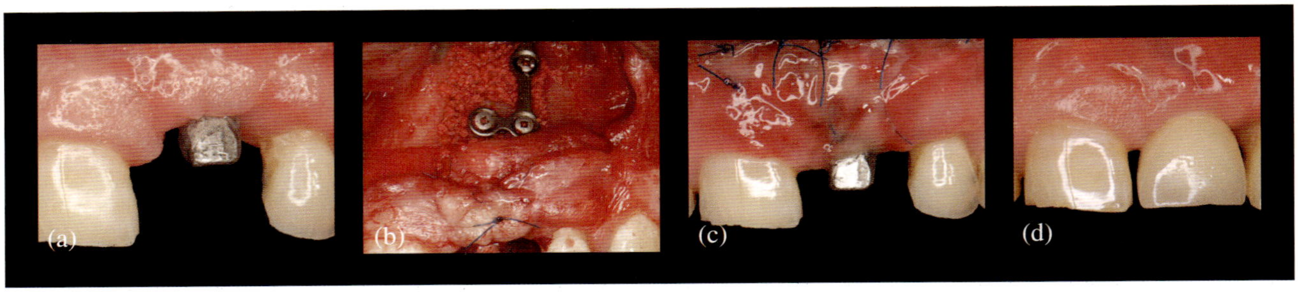

Figure 5.66 (a) Class III recession as a result of too deep implant position, (b) Sandwich osteotomy is performed along with an Interposition graft stabilized with micro titanium plate, (c) One week post healing, (d) The case finally restored with almost 90% improvement of the recession.

This surgical method implies filling the osteotomy cavity with a material – autologous bone or any other filling biomaterial. Interpositional or inlay grafts as a "sandwich" involve the placement of graft material within a three-walled cancellous compartment. This allows the recipient sites to contain and stabilize the graft material, and the circulating blood flow between the osteotomized bony blocks provide cells, soluble regulators, and nourishment (Kraut 1985) (see Figure 5.67a–l).

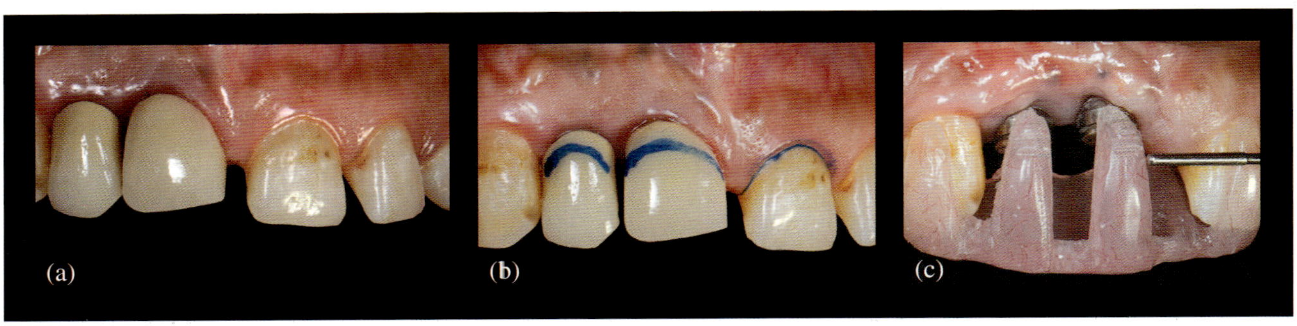

Figure 5.67 (a) Preoperative view of class III gingival recession, (b) Markings of the required tissue future levels, (c) Scoring template in place.

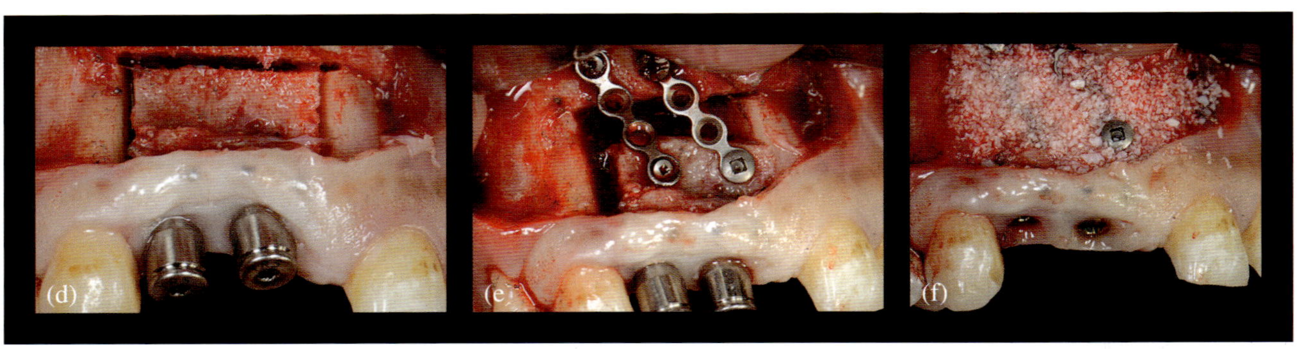

Figure 5.67 (d) Sandwich Osteotomy is undertaken, (e) The mobilized bone block is moved incisally along with implants in place, (f) Bone allografts is used to fill the gap.

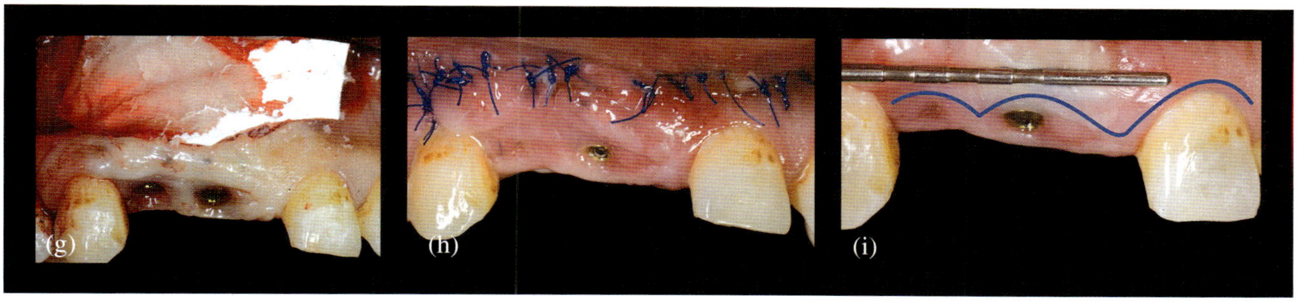

Figure 5.67 (g) Collagen membrane was used to cover the grafted bone, (h) Case finally sutured, (i) Marked outlines showing the improvement of the clinical situation.

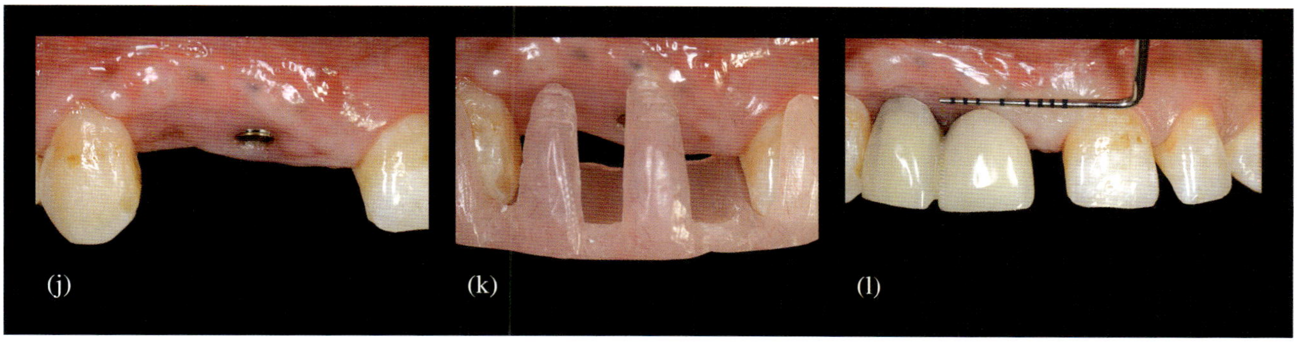

Figure 5.67 (j) Three months post healing, (k) Scoring template showing the amount of tissue gain from Sandwich Osteotomy procedure, (l) The case is temporized showing 85% of improvement.

The surgical procedure involves an elliptical incision of 10–12 mm from the ridge bone in the labiobuccal gingiva of the edentulous area. A full thickness flap is raised without detaching the lingual and the crestal mucoperiosteum to expose the labiobuccal cortical bone of the posterior atrophic mandible and the mental nerve. Two vertical and one horizontal osteotomies are made with a surgical burr and saws The horizontal osteotomy was located at least 2 mm below the ridge bone and 2 mm above the mandibular canal. The osteotomized segment was then raised in the coronal direction, sparing the lingual periosteum (see Figure 5.68a–c).

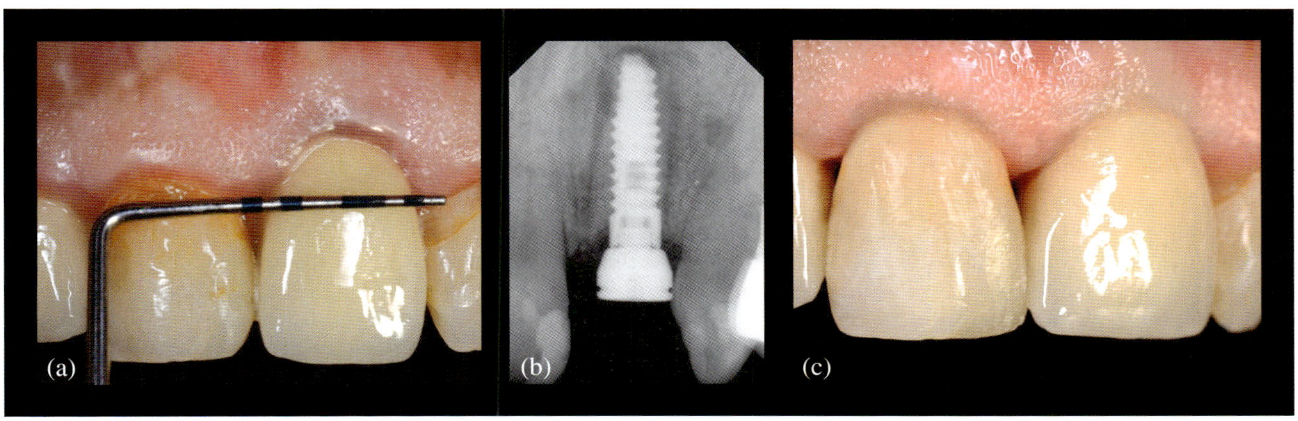

Figure 5.68 (a) Class III gingival recession around the Implant replacing the maxillary left central incisor, (b) Peri-apical radiographic view showing the mobilized osteotomy in place, (c) Case finally restored.

A block autograft or xenograft block might be placed as an interpositional graft between the mobilized bone block and the basal bone; a particulated autograft can fill in the gaps around the interpositional graft. The bone block is them stabilized to the basal bone titanium miniplates and miniscrews. The grafts can be covered with a collagen resorbable membrane. A flap was sutured in two layers, the inner layer submucosal mattress sutures and the outer layer suturing mucosa. After six months, all the space was filled with viable bone, the moved osteotomy block was stable to place an implant, with an average gain ranged between 5 and 8 mm of vertical gain (Kawakami et al. 2013) (see Figure 5.69a and b).

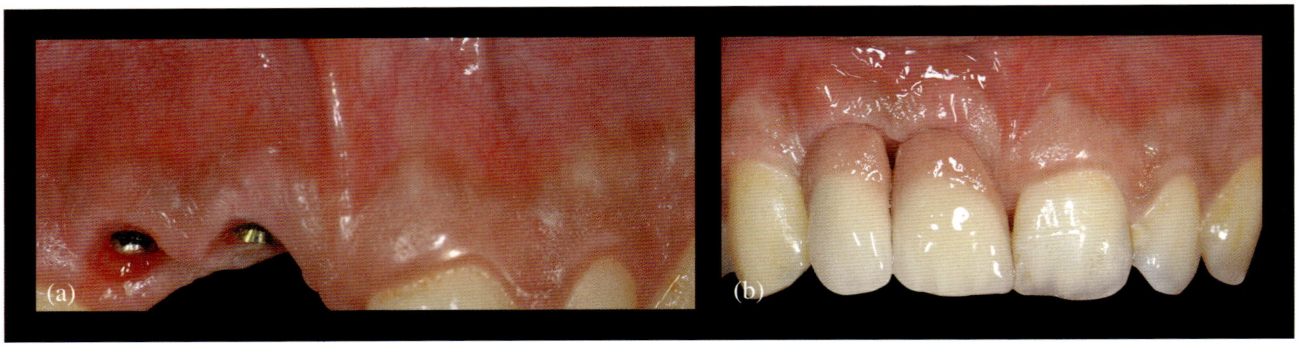

Figure 5.69 (a) and (b) In class III recession pink porcelain could be a minimal invasive solution.

A similar approach to sandwich osteotomy is the osteoperiosteal flap (OPF) that is achieved through a vascularized segmental moving osteotomy. The biologic principles are acquired from Le Fort I techniques in craniomaxillofacial surgery. This technique depends on maintenance of vascularization in bone fragments from the periosteum. The OPF technique has made a strong contribution towards management of these defects. Mobilizing a segment of alveolus attached to the overlying soft tissue can obtain uni- or bi-directional augmentation (Jenson 2010). OPFs through segmental osteotomies are used in combination with interpositional grafts in the gap generated by transposition of the flap in the desired position to achieve a vertical ridge gain. The preoperative planning included fabrication of two surgical splints. The first splint was fabricated for transmucosal positioning of the implant osteotomy sites in the existing alveolus position. The second splint was fabricated from the predetermined augmented vertical position of the dentoalveolar segment with ideal inter-occlusal clearance (Tsegga and Wright 2017). The OPF combined with interpositional (inlay) grafts are increasingly being used more for implant site development in ridges with height deficiencies. The main advantage of osteotomy-based techniques is the preservation of the attached gingiva and even the papillae in some cases (Kramer, Dempf and Bremer 2005).

Sandwich techniques are similar to distraction osteogenesis in terms of the surgical approach and having similar healing patterns and end results expected for the soft tissue aspect; as with distraction osteogeneses, the liability of soft tissue scar formation is high (Scipioni, Bruschi and Calesini 1994). Distraction osteogenesis is a technique used in craniomaxillofacial surgery to achieve high bone volume gain in a vertical axis. It is based on the biological principle of bone callus mechanical elongation through slow and progressive separation under tension of two bone fragments surrounding the callus to achieve new bone formation (Cheung et al. 2013). The technique includes three phases: (1) the latency phase of seven days, when soft tissues heal around the surgical site where the distractor is placed; (2) the distraction phase, when the two bone fragments are separated incrementally at a rate of 0.5–1 mm day^{-1}; and (3) the consolidation phase, when the newly formed bone mineralizes and matures (Vega and Bilbao 2010). The potential is to achieve significant vertical bone augmentation to adverse recession. Devices utilized can be of intraosseous or extraosseous configuration. An intraosseous approach with a small-diameter device that achieved vertical bone augmentation of 9 mm and provided a gain of 4–6 mm of vertical height was reported with prosthetic restorable distractors (Chiapasco et al. 2004).

There are many instances when extensive surgery is refused by patients, in these cases the option of another resolution is also important. Lost peri-implant tissues can also be corrected by applying gingiva-colored porcelain on the cervical portion of implant-supported ceramic restorations, thus saving the hardship of performing complex surgical interventions.

5.7 Conclusion

The management of gingival recession and its sequelae is based on a thorough assessment of the etiological factors, the skills of the clinician, the status of the local tissues, the systemic condition of the patient, and the readiness of the patient to undergo such surgical procedures. Preventive measures should be taken prior to starting the treatment to avoid complications.

Selection of the appropriate treatment modality for implant-related gingival recession demands knowledge about the underlying causes of the recession. The diagnosis of the etiology enables a clinician to treat the cause rather than only the manifestation.

Factors like gingival phenotype and labial bone thickness should be well studied and managed, soft tissue augmentation procedures can be carried out before or simultaneously with the implant placement. Soft tissue correction should be considered as soon as the clinician recognizes the soft tissue deficiencies at any stage of the implant treatment. The selection of the surgical techniques should be dictated by several factors, including the anatomy of the defect site, such as the extent of the recession defect, the presence or absence of keratinized tissue adjacent to the defect, the width and height of the interproximal soft tissue, the operator skills, and the depth of the vestibule or the presence of labial frenum (Zucchelli et al. 2013). Moreover, the selection of the shortest treatment path is advisable (Kerner and Migonney 2010). Attempts to reduce the number of surgeries and intraoral surgical sites, must be considered together. The surgeon's clinical experience may be a potential factor influencing judgments, case selection, and surgical skills. However, accurate case selection has proven to enhance a long-term clinical outcome (Haghighati et al. 2009).

References

Abdulmajeed, A.A. and Willberg, J. (2015). In vitro assessment of the soft tissue / implant interface using porcine gingival explants. *J. Mater. Sci. Mater. Med.* 26: 1–7.

Abrahamsson, I., Berglundh, T., Glantz, P.O., and Lindhe, J. (1998). The mucosal attachment at different abutments: an experimental study in dogs. *J. Clin. Periodontol.* (25): 721–727.

Addy, M., Mostafa, P., and Newcombe, R.G. (1987). Dentine hypersensitivity: the distribution of recession, sensitivity and plaque. *J. Dent.* 15 (6): 242–248.

Adibrad, M., Shahabuei, M., and Sahabi, M. (2009). Significance of the width of keratinized mucosa on the health status of the supporting tissue around implants supporting overdentures. *J. Oral Implantol.* 35: 232–237.

Abrahamson, I., Berglundh, T., and Lindhe, J. (1997). The mucosal barrier fillowing abutmnet dis/reconnection. An experimental study in dogs. *J. Clin. Periodontol.* 24 (8): 568–572.

Ahmad, I. (2010). Risk management in clinical practice. Part 5. Ethical considerations for dental enhancement procedures. *Br. Dent. J.* 209: 207–214.

Alomrami, A., Hermann, J., Jones, A. et al. (2005). The effect of a machined collar on coronal hard tissue around titanium implants: a radiographic study in the canine mandible. *Int. J. Oral Maxillofac. Implants* 20 (5): 677–686.

Araujo, M.G. and Lindhe, J. (2005). Dimensional ridge alterations following tooth extraction: an experimental study in the dog. *J. Periodontol.* 32: 212–218.

Araujo, M.G., Wennstrom, J.L., and Lindhe, J. (2006). Modelling of the buccal and lingual bone walls of fresh extraction sites following implant installation. *Clin. Oral Implants Res.* 17 (6): 606–614.

Baker, D.L. and Seymour, G.J. (1976). The possible pathogenesis of gingival recession. A histological study of induced recession in the rat. *J. Clin. Periodontol.* 3 (4): 208–219.

Baker, P. and Spedding, C. (2002). The aetiology of gingival recession. *Dent. Update.* 29 (2): 59–62.

Baldi, C., Pini-Prato, G., Nieri, M. et al. (1999). Coronally advanced flap procedure for root coverage. Is flap thickness a relevant predictor to achieve root coverage? A 19-case series. *J. Periodontol.* 70: 1077–1084.

Barros, R.M., Novaes, A.B. Jr., and Korn, P. (2015). Bone formation in a local defect around dental implants coated with extracellular matrix components. *Clin. Implant. Dent. Relat. Res.* 17 (4): 742–757.

Belser, U.C., Vailati, F., Bornstein, M.M. et al. (2009). Outcome evaluation of early placed maxillary anterior single tooth implants using objective esthetic criteria: a cross-sectional, retrospective study in 45 patients with a 2- to 4-year follow-up using pink and white esthetic scores. *J. Periodontol.* 80: 140–151.

Benic, G.I., Wolleb, K., Sancho-Puchades, M., and Hämmerle, C.H. (2012). Systematic review of parameters and methods for the professional assessment of aesthetics in dental implant research. *J. Clin. Periodontol.* 39 (Suppl. 12): 160–192.

Berglundh, T., Lindhe, J., Ericsson, I. et al. (1991). The soft tissue barrier at implants and teeth. *Clin. Oral Implants Res.* 2 (2): 81–90.

Berglundh, T., Persson, L., and Klinge, B. (2002). A systematic review of teh incidence of biological and technical complications in implant dentistry reported in prospective longitudinal studies of at least 5 years. *J. Clin. Periodontol.* 29 (Suppl. 3): 197–212.

Bianchi, A.E. and Sanfilippo, F. (2004). Single tooth replacement by immediate implant and connective tissue graft: 1 1–9 year clinical evaluation. *Clin. Oral Implants Res.* 15 (3): 269–277.

Botticelli, D., Berglundh, T., and Lindhe, J. (2004). Hard-tissue alterations following immediate implant placement in extraction sites. *J. Clin. Periodontol.* 31: 820–828.

Braut, V., Bornstein, M.M., Lauber, R., and Buser, D. (2012). Bone dimensions in the posterior mandible: a retrospective radiographic study using cone beam computed tomography. Part 1: analysis of dentate state. *Int. J. Periodontics Restorative Dent.* 32 (2): 175–184.

Burkhardt, R. and Lang, N.P. (2005). Coverage of localized gingival recessions: comparison of micro- and macrosurgical techniques. *J. Clin. Periodontol.* 32: 87–93.

Burkhardt, R., Joss, A., and Lang, N.P. (2008). Soft tissue dehiscence coverage around endosseous implants: a prospective cohort study. *Clin. Oral Implants Res.* 19 (5): 451–417.

Buser, D.A. (1993). Localized ridge augmentation using GBR. I. Surgical procedures in the maxilla. *Int. J. Periodontics Restorative Dent.* 1993: 29–45.

Buser, D., Chappuis, V., Kuchler, U. et al. (2013). Long-term stability of early implant placement with contour augmentation. *J. Dent. Res.* 92 (12 Suppl): 176S–182S.

Buser, D., Chen, S.T., Weber, H.P., and Belser, U.C. (2008). Early implant placement following single-tooth extraction in the esthetic zone: biologic rationale and surgical procedures. *Int. J. Periodontics Restorative Dent.* 28: 441–451.

Buser, D., Halbritter, S., Hart, C. et al. (2009). Early implant placement with simultaneous guided bone regeneration following single-tooth extraction in the esthetic zone: 12-month results of a prospective study with 20 consecutive patients. *J. Periodontol.* 80 (1): 152–162.

Buser, D., Martin, W., and Belser, U.C. (2004). Optimizing esthetics for implant restorations in the anterior maxilla: anatomic and surgical considerations. *Int. J. Oral Maxillofac. Implants* 19 (Suppl): 43–61.

Buser, D., Martin, W.D., and Bleser, U.C. (2006). Surgical considerations with regard to single-tooth replacements in the esthetic zone: standard procedure in sites without bone deficiencies. In: *ITI Treatment Guide, Vol 1: Implant Therapy in the Esthetic Zone – Single-Tooth Replacements* (ed. D. Buser, U. Belser and D. Wismeijer), 26–37. Berlin: Quintessence.

Buser, D., Mericske-Stern, R., Dula, K., and Lang, N.P. (1999). Clinical experience with one-stage, non-submerged dental implants. *Adv. Dent. Res.* 13: 153–161.

Buser, D., Schenk, R.K., Steinemann, S. et al. (1991). Influence of surface characteristics on bone integration of titanium implants. A histomorphometric study in miniature pigs. *J. Biomend. Mater. Res.* 25: 889–902.

Cabello, G., Rioboo, M., and Fabrega, J.G. (2012). Immediate placement and restoration of implants in the aesthetic zone with a trimodal approach: soft tissue alterations and its relation to gingival biotype. *Clin. Oral Implants Res.* 24 (10): 1094–1100.

Cairo, F., Pagliaro, U., and Nieri, M. (2008). Soft tissue management at implant sites. *J. Clin. Periodontol.* 35 (8 Suppl): 163–167.

Canullo, L., Iurlaro, G., and Iannello, G. (2009). Double-blind randomized controlled trial study on post-extraction immediately restored implants using the switching platform concept: soft tissue response. Preliminary report. *Clin. Oral Implants Res.* 20: 414–420.

Canullo, L. and Rasperini, G. (2007). Preservation of peri-implant soft and hard tissues using platform switching of implants study placed in immediate extraction sockets: with 12 to 36- month follow-up. *Int. J. Oral Maxillofac. Implants* 22: 995–1000.

Cappiello, M., Luongo, R., Di Lorio, D. et al. (2008). Evaluation of peri-implant bone loss around platform-switched implants. *Int. J. Periodontics Restorative Dent.* 28 (4): 347–355.

Cardaropoli, G., Araujo, M., Hayacibara, R. et al. (2005). Healing of extraction sockets and surgically produced, augmented and non-augmented, defects in the alveolar ridge. An experimental study in the dog. *J. Clin. Periodontol.* 32: 35–44.

Cardaropoli, G., Lekholm, U., and Wennstrom, J.L. (2006). Tissue alterations at implant-supported single-tooth replacements: a 1-year prospective clinical study. *Clin. Oral Implants Res.* 17 (2): 165–171.

Chan, H.L., Chun, Y.P., and MacEachern, M. (2015). Does gingival recession require surgical treatment? *Dent. Clin. North. Am.* 59 (4): 981–996.

Chen, S.T. and Buser, D. (2009). Clinical and esthetic outcomes of implants placed in post-extraction sites. *Int. J. Oral Maxillofac. Implants* 24: 186–217.

Chen, S.T., Darby, I.B., and Reynolds, E.C. (2007). A prospective clinical study of non-submerged immediate implants: clinical outcomes and esthetic results. *Clin. Oral Implants Res.* 18: 552–562.

Chen, S.T., Darby, I.B., Reynolds, E.C., and Clement, J.G. (2009). Immediate implant placement postextraction without flap elevation. *J. Periodontol.* 80: 163–172.

Cheung, L.K., Chua, H.D., Hariri, F. et al. (2013). Alveolar distraction osteogenesis for dental implant rehabilitation following fibular reconstruction: a case series. *J. Oral Maxillofac. Surg.* 71 (2): 255–271.

Chiapasco, M., Romeo, E., Casentini, P., and Rimondini, L. (2004). Alveolar distraction osteogenesis vs. vertical guided bone regeneration for the correction of vertically deficient edentulous ridges: a 1–3-year prospective study on humans. *Clin. Oral Implants Res.* 15 (1): 82–95.

Choquet, V., Hermans, M., Adriaenssens, P. et al. (2001). Clinical and radiographic evaluation of the papilla level adjacent to single-tooth dental implants. A retrospective study in the maxillary anterior region. *J. Periodontol.* 72: 1364–1371.

Chu, C.M., Huang, H.L., Hsu, J.T., and Fuh, L.J. (2012). Influences of internal tapered abutment designs on bone stresses around a dental implant: three-dimensional finite element method element with statistical evaluation. *J. Periodontal.* 83: 111–118.

Chung, D.M., Oh, T., Shotwell, J. et al. (2006). Significance of keratinized mucosa in maintenance of dental implants with different surfaces. *J. Periodontol.* 77: 1410–1420.

Claffey, N. and Shanley, D. (1986). Relationship of gingival thickness and bleeding to loss of probing attachment in shallow sites following nonsurgical periodontal therapy. *J. Clin. Periodontol.* 13: 654–657.

Cohen, D.W. and Ross, S.E. (1968). The double papillae repositioned flap in periodontal therapy. *J. Periodontol.* 39 (2): 65–70.

Cordaro, L., Amadé, D.S., and Cordaro, M. (2002). Clinical results of alveolar ridge augmentation with mandibular block bone grafts in partially edentulous patients prior to implant placement. *Clin. Oral Implants Res.* 13 (1): 103–111.

Cordaro, L., Torsello, F., Accorsi Ribeiro, C. et al. (2010). Inlay-onlay grafting for three-dimensional reconstruction of the posterior atrophic maxilla with mandibular bone. *Int. J. Oral Maxillofac. Surg.* 39: 350–357.

Cordaro, L., Torsello, F., and Roccuzzo, M. (2009). Clinical outcome of submerged vs. non-submerged implants placed in fresh extraction sockets. *Clin. Oral Implants Res.* 20: 1307–1313.

Cosyn, J., Eghbali, A., Hanselaer, L. et al. (2012a). Predictors of inter-proximal and midfacial recession following single implant treatment in the anterior maxilla: a multivariate analysis. *J. Clin. Periodontol.* 39: 895–903.

Cosyn, J., Hooghe, N., and De Bruyn, H. (2012b). A systematic review on the frequency of advanced recession following single immediate implant treatment. *J. Clin. Periodontol.* 39 (6): 582–589.

Covani, U., Bortolaia, C., Barone, A., and Sbordone, L. (2004). Bucco-lingual crestal bone changes after immediate and delayed implant placement. *J. Periodontol.* 75 (12): 1605–1612.

Covani, U., Marconcini, S., Gallasini, G. et al. (2007). Connective tissue graft as a biologic barrier to cover an immediate implant. *J. Periodontol.* 78: 1644–1649.

Crespi, R., Capparè, P., and Gherlone, E. (2010). Fresh-socket implants in periapical infected sites in humans. *J. Periodontol.* 81: 378–383.

Creugers, N.H., Kreulen, C.M., Snoeck, P.A., and De Kanter, R.J. (2000). A systematic review of single-tooth restorations supported by implants. *J. Dent.* 28: 209–217.

Cura, C., Saraçoglu, A., and Cötert, H.S. (2002). Alternative method for connecting a removable gingival extension and fixed partial denture: a clinical case. *J. Prosthet. Dent.* 88: 1–3.

De Bari, C., Dell'Accio, F., and Vanlaume, J. (2006). Mesenchymal multipotency of adult human periosteal cells demonstrated by single-cell lineage analysis. *Arthritis Rheum.* 54 (4): 1209–1221.

De Rouck, T., Collys, K., and Cosyn, J. (2008). Immediate single-tooth implants in the canterior maxilla: a 1-year case cohort study on hard and soft tissue response. *J. Clin. Periodontol.* 35: 649–657.

Degidi, M., Novaes, A.B. Jr., Nandi, D., and Piattelli, A. (2008). Outcome analysis of immediately placed, immediately restored implants in the esthetic area: the clinical relevance of different interimplant distances. *J. Periodontol.* 79: 1056–1061.

Dhir, S. (2011). The peri-implant esthetics: an unforgettable entity. *J. Indian Soc. Periodontol.* 15 (2): 98–103.

Edel, A. (1974). Clinical evaluation of free connective tissue grafts used to increase the width of keratinized gingival. *J. Clin. Periodontol.* 1 (4): 185–196.

Elaskary, A.S. (2009). Dental implants: aesthetic complications. *Implants* 10 (4): 26–29.

Elaskary, A.S., Ghallab, N.A., Tan, S.-C. et al. (2016). Implant-related gingival recession: pilot case series presents novel technique and scoring template. *Compendium* 37: 468–480.

Elaskary, A.S. and Pipco, D.J. (2000). Autogenous and allogenous bone grafting techniques to maximize esthetics. *J. Prosthet. Dent.* 83: 153–157.

Ericsson, I., Berglundh, T., Marinello, C. et al. (1992). Long-standing plaque and gingivitis at implants and teeth in the dog. *Clin. Oral Implants Res.* 3 (3): 99–103.

Esposito, M., Maghaireh, H., Grusovin, M.G. et al. (2012). Soft tissue management for dental implants: what are the most effective techniques? A Cochrane systematic review. *Eur. J. Oral Implantol.* 5: 221–238.

Evans, C.D. and Chen, S.T. (2008). Esthetic outcomes of immediate implant placements. *Clin. Oral Implants Res.* 19 (1): 73–80.

Everhart, R.J. and Cavazos, E. Jr. (1983). Evaluation of a fixed removable partial denture: Andrews Bridge System. *J. Prosthet. Dent.* 50: 180–184.

Evian, C.I., Corn, H., and Rosenberg, E.S. (1985). Retained interdental procedures for maintaining anterior esthetics. *Compend. Contin. Educ. Dent.* (1): 58–65.

Farmer, M. and Darby, I. (2014). Ridge dimensional changes following single-tooth extraction in the aesthetic zone. *Clin. Oral Implants Res.* 25 (2): 272–277.

Ferrus, J., Cecchinato, D., Pjetursson, E.B. et al. (2010). Factors influencing ridge alterations following immediate implant placement into extraction sockets. *Clin. Oral Implants Res.* 21 (1): 22–29.

Fickl, S., Zuhr, O., Wachtel, H. et al. (2008). Hard tissue alterations for socket preservation: an experimental study in the beagle dog. *Clin. Oral Implants Res.* 19: 1111–1118.

Fu, J.H., Lee, A., and Wang, H.L. (2011). Influence of tissue biotype on implant esthetics. *Int. J. Oral Maxillofac. Implants* 26 (3): 499–508.

Fuentes, R., Flores, T., Navarro, P. et al. (2015). Assessment of buccal bone thickness of aesthetic maxillary region: a cone-beam computed tomography study. *J. Periodontal. Implant Sci.* 45 (5): 162–168.

Garber, D.A. (1981). The edentulous ridge and fixed prosthodontics. *Compend. Contin. Educ. Dent.* 2: 212.

Garber, D.A., Salama, M.A., and Salama, H. (2001). Immediate total tooth replacement. *Compend. Contin. Educ. Dent.* 22 (3): 210–216. 218.

Gardner, F.M. and Stankewitz, C.G. (1982). Using removable gingival facades with fixed partial dentures. *J. Prosthet. Dent.* 47: 262–264.

Gasik M.. 2016 'Advances in biomaterials simulation and evaluation procedures.' Proc 1st Intern Symp On Creation of Life Innovation Materials, JWRI, Osaka, Japan;3:3–4.

Gasik, M. (2017). Understanding biomaterial-tissue interface quality: combined in vitro evaluation. *Sci. Technol. Adv. Mater.* 18 (1): 550–562.

Geurs, N.C., Vassilopoulos, P.J., and Reddy, M.S. (2010). Soft tissue considerations in implant site development. *Oral Maxillofac. Surg. Clin. North Am.* 22 (3): 387–405.

Gittens, R.A., Olivares-Navarrete, R., Cheng, A. et al. (2013). The roles of titanium surface micro/nanotopography and wettability on the differential response of human osteoblast lineage cells. *Acta Biomater* 9: 6268–6277.

Gracco, A., Lombardo, L., Mancuso, G. et al. (2009). Upper incisor position and bony support in untreated patients as seen on CBCT. *Angle Orthod.* 79 (4): 692–702.

Greene, P.R. (1998). The flexible gingival mask: an aesthetic solution in periodontal practice. *Brit. Dent. J.* 184: 536–540.

Grunder, U. (2000). Stability of the mucosal topography around single tooth implants and adjacent teeth: 1-year results. *Quintessence Int.* 17: 11–17.

Grunder, U. (2011). Crestal ridge width changes when placing implants at the time of tooth extraction with and without soft tissue augmentation after a healing period of 6 months: report of 24 consecutive cases. *Int. J. Periodontics Restorative Dent.* 31 (1): 9–17.

Grunder, U., Gracis, S., and Capelli, M. (2005). Influence of the 3D bone to implant relationship on esthetics. *Int. J. Periodontics Restorative Dent.* 25 (2): 113–119.

Grunder, U., Spielmann, H.P., and Snétivy, D. (2010). Development, *in vitro* testing, and clinical use of a 3.5 mm-diameter zirconia abutment. *Eur. J. Esthet. Dent.* 5 (2): 158–170.

Gultekin, G., Bedeloglu, E., Kose, E., and Mijiritsky, E. (2016). Comparison of bone resorption rates after intraoral block bone and guided bone regeneration augmentation for the reconstruction of horizontally deficient maxillary alveolar ridges. *Biomed. Res. Int.* 2016: 4987437.

Haghighati, F., Mousavi, M., Moslemi, N. et al. (2009). A comparative study of two root-coverage techniques with regard to interdental papilla dimension as a prognostic factor. *Int. J. Periodontics Restorative Dent.* 29: 179–189.

Hall, W.B. (1984). Can attached gingival be increased non-surgically? *J. Clin. Periodontol.* 11: 95–103.

Hammack, B.L. and Enneking, W.F. (1960). Comparative vascularization of autogenous and homogenous bone transplants. *J. Bone Joint Surg.* 42A: 811.

Hämmerle, C.H., Araújo, M.G., and Simion, M. (2012). Osteology Consensus Group 2011. Evidence-based knowledge on the biology and treatment of extraction sockets. *Clin. Oral Implants Res.* 23: 80–82.

Hämmerle, C.H., Chen, S.T., and Wilson, T.G. Jr. (2004). Consensus statements and recommended clinical procedures regarding the placement of implants in extraction sockets. *Int. J. Oral Maxillofac. Implants* 19 (Suppl): 26–28.

Hansson, H.A., Albrektsson, T., and Brånemark, P.I. (1983). Structural aspects of the interface between tissue and titanium implants. *J. Prosthet. Dent.* 50 (1): 108–113.

Hermann, J.S., Buser, D., Schenk, R.K. et al. (2000). Biologic width arounf titanium implants. A physiologically formed and stable diemnsion over time. *Clin. Oral Implants Res.* 11 (11): 1–11.

Hermann, F., Henriette, L., and Palti, A. (2007). Factors influencing the preservation of the peri-implant marginal bone. *Implant. Dent.* 11: 162–169.

Hermann, J.S., Schenk, R.K., and Schoolfield, J.D. (2001). Biologic width around one- and two-piece titanium implants. A histometric evaluation of unloaded

nonsubmerged and submerged implants in the canine mandible. *Clin. Oral Implants Res.* 12: 559–571.
Hirschfield, I. (1923). A study of skulls in the American Museum of Natural History in relation to periodontal disease. *J. Dent. Res.* 5: 251–265.
Hui, E., Chow, J., Ji, D. et al. (2001). Immediate provisional for single tooth implant replacement with the Brånemark system: Preliminary report. *Clin. Imp. Dent. & Rel. Res.* 3 (2): 79–86.
Hürzeler, M., Fickl, S., Zuhr, O., and Wachtel, H.C. (2007). Peri-implant bone level around implants with platform-switched abutments: preliminary data from a prospective study. *J. Oral Maxillofac. Surg.* July 65 (7 Suppl. 1): 33–39.
Huynh-Ba, G., Meister, D.J., Hoders, A.B. et al. (2016). Esthetic, clinical and patient-centered outcomes of immediately placed implants (Type 1) and early placed implants (Type 2): preliminary 3-month results of an ongoing randomized controlled clinical trial. *Clin. Oral Implants Res.* 27 (2): 241–252.
Hwang, D. and Wang, H.L. (2006). Flap thickness as a predictor of root coverage: a systematic review. *J. Periodontol.* 77: 1625–1634.
Iezzi, G., Pecora, G., Scarano, A. et al. (2006). Histologic evaluation of 3 retrieved immediately loaded implants after a 4-month period. *Implant. Dent.* 15 (3): 305–312.
Ioannou, A.L., Kotsakis, G.A., McHale, M.G. et al. (2015). Soft tissue surgical procedures for optimizing anterior implant esthetics. *Int. J. Dent.* 2015: 740764.
Januário, A.L., Duarte, W.R., Barriviera, M. et al. (2011). Dimension of the facial bone wall in the anterior maxilla: a cone-beam computed tomography study. *Clin. Oral Implants Res.* 22: 1168–1171.
Jensen, S.S. and Terheyden, H. (2009). Bone augmentation procedures in localized defects in the alveolar ridge: clinical results with different bone grafts and bone-substitute materials. *Int. J. Oral Maxillofac. Implants* 24 (Suppl): 218–236.
Jenson, O.T. (2010). *The Osteoperiosteal Flap: A Simplified Approach to Alveolar Bone Reconstruction*. Quintessence Pub.
Jung, R., Pjetursson, B., Glauser, G. et al. (2008). A systematic review of teh 5-year survival and complication rates of implant-supported single crowns. *Clin. Oral Implants Res.* 19: 1135–1140.
Juodzbalys, G. and Wang, H.L. (2007). Soft and hard tissue assessment of immediate implant placement: a case series. *Clin. Oral Implants Res.* 18 (2): 237–243.
Kan, J.Y., Rungcharassaeng, K., and Lozada, J. (2003). Immediate placement and provisionalization of maxillary anterior single implants: 1-year prospective study. *Int. J. Oral Maxillofac. Implants* 18: 31–39.
Kan, J.Y., Rungcharassaeng, K., Lozada, J.L., and Zimmerman, G. (2011). Facial gingival tissue stability following immediate placement and provisionalization of maxillary anterior single implants: a 2- to 8-year follow-up. *Int. J. Oral Maxillofac. Implants* 26: 179–187.
Kan, J.Y., Rungcharassaeng, K., Sclar, A., and Lozada, J.L. (2007). Effects of the facial osseous defect morphology on gingival dynamics after immediate tooth replacement and guided bone regeneration: 1-year results. *Int. J. Oral Maxillofac. Surg.* 65: 13–19.
Kan, J.Y.K., Rungcharassaeng, K., Morimoto, T., and Lozada, J.L. (2009). Facial gingival tissue stability after connective tissue graft with single immediate tooth replacement in the esthetic zone: consecutive case report. *J. Oral Maxillofac. Surg.* 67 (11 Suppl): 40–48.
Kao, R.T., Fagan, M.C., and Conte, G.J. (2008). Thick vs. thin gingival biotypes: a key determinant in treatment planning for dental implant. *J. Calif. Dent. Assoc.* 36: 193–198.
Kawakami, P.Y., Dottore, A.M., Bechara, K. et al. (2013). Alveolar osteotomy associated with resorbable non-ceramic hydroxylapatite or intra-oral autogenous bone for height augmentation in posterior mandibular sites: a split-mouth prospective study. *Clin. Oral Implants Res.* 24 (9): 1060.
Kerner, S. and Migonney, V. (2010). Bone tissue response to titanium implant surfaces modified with carboxylate and sulfonate groups. *J. Mater. Sci. Mater. Med.* 21 (2): 707–715.
Kheur, M., Kheur, S., Kantharia, N., and Le, B. (2015). Three dimensional evaluation of alveolar bone, soft tissue dimensions of maxillary incisors for immediate implant placement: a CBCT assisted analysis. *Clin. Oral Implants Res.* 26 (Suppl. 12): 407–415.
Khoury, F. and Happe, A. (2000). The palatal subepithelial connective tissue flap method for soft tissue management to cover maxillary defects: a clinical report. *Int. J. Oral Maxillofac. Implants* 15 (3): 415–418.
Khoury, F. and Khoury, C. (2006). Mandibular bone block grafts: diagnosis, instrumentation, harvesting techniques and surgical procedures. In: *Bone Augmentation in Oral Implantology* (ed. F. Khoury, H. Antoun and P. Missika), 115–212. Chicago, IL: Quintessence.
Khoury, F. and Khoury, C.H. 2007. 'Mandibular bone block grafts: diagnosis, instrumentation, harvesting techniques and surgical procedures,' in F. Khoury, H. Antoun, and P. Missika (eds.) *Bone Augmentation in Oral Implantology*. Quintessence, Berlin., pp. 115–212.
Kim, B.S., Kim, Y.K., Yun, P.Y. et al. (2009). Evalutaion of peri-implant tissue response according to the presence of keratinized mucosa. *Oral Surg. Pral. Med. Oral Pathol. Oral Radiol. Endod.* 107: e24–e28.
Kinsel, R.P. and Capoferri, D. (2008). A simplified method to develop optimal gingival contours for the single implant-supported, metal–ceramic crown in the

aesthetic zone. *Pract. Proced. Aesthet. Dent.* 20 (4): 231–236. quiz 7.

Kois, J.C. and Kan, J.Y.K. (2001). Predictable peri-implant gingival aesthetics: surgical and prosthodontic rationales. *Pract. Proced. Aesthet. Dent.* 13: 691–698.

Kramer, F.J., Dempf, R., and Bremer, B. (2005). Efficacy of dental implants placed into fibula-free flaps for orofacial reconstruction. *Clin. Oral Implants Res.* 16 (1): 80–88.

Kraut, R.A. (1985). Composite graft for mandibular alveolar ridge augmentation: a preliminary report. *J. Oral Maxillofac. Surg.* 43 (11): 856–859.

Lai, Y.L., Chen, H.L., Chang, L.Y., and Lee, S.Y. (2010). Resubmergence technique for the management of soft tissue recession around an implant: case report. *Int. J. Oral Maxillofac. Implants* 25 (1): 201–204.

Lang, N.P. and Zitzmann, N.U. (2012). Working Group 3 of the VIII European Workshop on Periodontology. Clinical research in implant dentistry: evaluation of implant-supported restorations, aesthetic and patient-reported outcomes. *J. Clin. Periodontol.* 39 (Suppl. 12): 133–138.

Lazzara, R.J. (1993). Effect of implant position on implant restoration design. *J. Esthet. Restor. Dent.* 5 (6): 265–269.

Lazzara, R.J. and Portar, S.S. (2006). Platform switching: a new concept in implant dentistry for controlling post-restorative crestal bone levels. *Int. J. Periodontics Restorative Dent.* 26: 9–17.

Le, B.T. and Farahani, A. (2012). Labial bone thickness in area of anterior maxillary implants associated with crestal labial soft tissue thickness. *Implant. Dent.* 21: 406–410.

Lee, W.P.A. and Butler, P.E.M. (1997). Transplant biology and applications to plastic surgery. In: *Grabb and Smith's Plastic Surgery* (ed. S.J. Aston, R.W. Beasley and C.H.M. Thorn), 27. Philadelphia, PA: Lippincott–Raven.

Levin, L., Nitzan, D., and Schwartz-Arad, D. (2007). Success of dental implants placed in intraoral block bone grafts. *J. Periodontol.* 78 (1): 18–21.

Linkevicius, T., Apse, P., Grybauskas, S., and Puisys, A. (2009). The influence of soft tissue thickness on crestal bone changes around implants: a 1 year prospective controlled clinical trial. *Int. J. Oral Maxillofac. Implants* 24 (4): 712–719.

Linkevicius, T., Apse, P., Grybauskas, S., and Puisys, A. (2010). Influence of thin mucosal tissues on crestal bone stability around implants with platform switching: a 1-year pilot study. *J. Oral Maxillofac. Surg.* 68 (9): 2272–2277.

Linkevicius, T., Vindasiute, E., Puisys, A., and Peciuliene, V. (2011). The influence of margin location on the amount of undetected cement excess after delivery of cement-retained implant restorations. *Clin. Oral Implants Res.* 22 (12): 1379–1384.

Liu, J. and Kerns, D. (2014). Mechanisms of guided bone regeneration: a review. *Open Dent. J.* 8: 56–65.

Lops, D., Chiapasco, M., Rossi, A. et al. (2008). Incidence of inter-proximal papilla between a tooth and adjacent immediate implant placed into a fresh extraction socket: 1-year prospective study. *Clin. Oral Imp. Res.* 19: 1135–1140.

Loubele, M., Van Assche, N., Carpentier, K. et al. (2008). Comparative localized linear accuracy of small-field cone beam CT and multislice CT for alveolar bone measurements. *Oral Surg Oral Med. Oral Pathol. Oral Radiol. Endod.* 105: 512–518.

Luchinskaya, D., Du, R., Owens, D.M. et al. (2017). Various surface treatments to implant provisional restorations and their effect on epithelial cell adhesion: A comparative in vitro study. *Implant Dent.* 26 (1): 12–23.

Mahajan, A. (2010). Treatment of multiple gingival recession defects using periosteal pedicle graft: a case series. *J. Periodontol.* 81 (10): 1426–1431.

Mahajan, A. (2012). Periosteum: a highly underrated tool in dentistry. *Int. J. Dent.* 2012: 717816.

Manson, P.N. (1994). Facial bone healing and bone grafts. A review of clinical physiology. *Clin. Plast. Surg.* 21 (3): 331–348.

Marconcini, S., Barone, A., Gelpi, F. et al. (2013). Immediate implant placement in infected sites: a case series. *J. Periodontol.* 84 (2): 196–202.

Mareque-Bueno, S. (2011). A novel surgical procedure for coronally repositioning of the buccal implant mucosa using acellular dermal matrix: a case report. *J. Periodontol.* 82 (1): 151–156.

Mathews, D.P. (2000). Soft tissue management around implants in the esthetic zone. *Int. J. Periodontics Restorative Dent.* 20: 141–149.

McKinney, R.V. Jnr, Steflik, D.E., and Koth, D.L. (1985). Evidence for a junctional epithelial attachment to ceramic dental implants. A transmission electron microscopic study. *J. Periodontol.* 56 (10): 579–591.

Misch, C.E., Qu, Z., and Bidez, M.W. (1999). Mechanical properties of trabecular bone in the human mandible: implications for dental implant treatment planning and surgical placement. *J. Oral Maxillofac. Surg.* 57 (6): 700–706.

Miller, P.D. (1985). Root coverage using the free soft tissue autograft following citric acid application. III. A successful and predictable procedure in areas of deep-wide recession. *Int. J. Periodontics Restorative Dent.* 5 (2): 14–37.

Neale, D. and Chee, W.W.L. (1994). Development of soft tissue emergence profile: a technique. *J. Prosthet. Dent.* 71: 364–368.

Nevins, M., Camelo, M., de Paoli, S. et al. (2006). A study of the fate of the buccal wall of extraction sockets of teeth with prominent roots. *J. Periodontol.* 26: 19–29.

Nevins, M., Nevins, M.L., Camelo, M. et al. (2008). Human histologic evidence of a connective tissue attachment to a dental implant. *Int. J. Periodontics Restorative Dent.* 28: 111–121.

Niemi, M.L., Sandholm, L., and Ainamo, J. (1984). Frequency of gingival lesions after standardized brushing as related to stiffness of toothbrush and abrasiveness of dentifrice. *J. Clin. Periodontol.* 11 (4): 254–261.

Nisapakultorn, K., Suphanantachat, S., Silkosessak, O., and Rattanamongkolgul, S. (2010). Factors affecting soft tissue level around anterior maxillary single-tooth implants. *Clin. Oral Implants Res.* 21 (6): 662–670.

Nobuto, T., Suwa, F., Kono, T. et al. (2005). Microvascular response in the periosteum following mucoperiosteal flap surgery in dogs: 3-dimensional observation of an angiogenic process. *J. Periodontol.* 76: 1339–1345.

Novaes, A. Jr., de Souza, S.L., de Barros, R.R. et al. (2010). Influence of implant surfaces on osseointegration. *Braz. Dent. J.* 21 (6)): 471–481.

Nugala, B., Kumar, S., and Krishna, P.M. (2012). Biologic width and its importance in periodontal and restorative dentistry. *J. Conserv. Dent.* 15: 12–17.

Oates, T.W., Robinson, M., and Gunsolley, J.C. (2003). Surgical therapies for the treatment of gingival recession. A systematic review. *Ann. Periodontol.* 8 (1): 303–320.

Olsen, M. and Lindhe, J. (1991). Periodontal characteristics in individuals with varying form of the upper central incisor. *J. Clin. Periodontol.* 18: 78–82.

Palmer, R.M. and Cortellini, P. (2008). Group B of European Workshop on Periodontology. Periodontal tissue engineering and regeneration: consensus report of the Sixth European Workshop on Periodontology. *J. Clin. Periodontol.* 35 (8): 83–86.

Pecora, G.E., Ceccarelli, R., Bonelli, M. et al. (2009). Clinical evaluation of laser microtexturing for soft tissue and bone attachment to dental implants. *Implant Dent.* 18 (1): 57–66.

Pennel, B.M., King, K.O., Wilderman, M.N., and Barron, J.M. (1967). Repair of the alveolar process following osseous surgery. *J. Periodontol.* 38 (5): 426–431.

Periodontology AAP. (2001). Glossary of Periodontal Terms.

Pikos, M.A. (2000). Block autografts for localized ridge augmentation: part II. The posterior mandible. *Implant. Dent.* 9 (1): 67–75.

Qahash, M., Susuin, C., and Poolimeni, G. (2008). Bone healing dynamics at buccal peri-implant sites. *Clin. Oral Implants Res.* 19 (2): 166–172.

Raes, F., Cosyn, J., Crommelinck, E. et al. (2011). Immediate and conventional single implant treatment in anterior maxilla: one-year results of a case series on hard and soft tissue response and aesthetics. *J. Clin. Periodontol.* 38: 385–394.

Rajapakse, P.S., McCracken, G.I., and Gwynnett, E. (2007). Does tooth brushing influence the development and progression of non-inflammatory gingival recession? A systematic review. *J. Clin. Periodontol.* 34 (12): 1046–1061.

Ramanauskaite, A. and Juodzbalys, G. (2016). Diagnostic principles of peri-implantitis: a systematic review and guidelines for peri-implantitis diagnosis proposal. *J. Oral Maxillofac. Res.* 7 (3): e8.

Reynders, P., Becker, J., and Broos, P. (1998). The osteogenic potential of free periosteal autografts in tibial fractures with severe soft tissue damage: an experimental study. *Acta Orthop. Belg.* 64 (2): 184–192.

Ricci, J.L. and Alexander, H. (2001). Laser microtexturing of implant surfaces for enhanced tissue integration. *Key Eng. Mater.* 198–199: 179–202.

Rocchietta, I., Fontana, F., and Simion, M. (2008). Clinical outcomes of vertical bone augmentation to enable dental implant placement: a systematic review. *J. Clin. Periodontol.* 35 (8 Suppl): 203–215.

Roccuzzo, M., Bunino, M., Needleman, I., and Sanz, M. (2002). Periodontal plastic surgery for treatment of localized gingival recessions: a systematic review. *J. Clin. Periodontol.* 29 (Suppl. 3): 178–194.

Romeo, E., Lops, D., Rossi, A. et al. (2008). Surgical and prosthetic management of interproximal region with single-implant restorations: 1-year prospective study. *J. Periodontol.* 79: 1048–1055.

Rompen, E., Touati, B., and Van Dooren, E. (2003). Factors influencing marginal tissue remodeling around implants. *Pract. Proced. Aesthet. Dent.* 15 (10): 754–761.

Saadoun, A.P. (2007). Soft tissue recession around implants: is it still unavoidable? *Pract. Proced. Aesthet. Dent.* 19 (1): 55–62.

Sanavi, F., Weisgold, A.S., and Rose, L.F. (1998). Biologic width and its relation to periodontal biotypes. *J. Esthet. Dent.* 10 (3): 157–163.

Sanz, M., Ivanoff, C.J., Weingart, D. et al. (2015). Clinical and radiologic outcomes after submerged and transmucosal implant placement with two-piece implants in the anterior maxilla and mandible: 3-year results of a randomized controlled clinical trial. *Clin. Implant Dent. Relat. Res.* 17 (2): 234.

Schropp, L., Wenzel, A., and Kostopoulos, L. (2003). Bone healing and soft tissue contour changes following single-tooth extraction: a clinical and radiographic 12-month prospective study. *Int. J. Periodontics Restorative Dent.* 23: 313–323.

Schrott, A.R., Jimmenez, M., Hwang, J.W. et al. (2009). Five-year evaluation of the influence of keratinized mucosa on peri-implant soft tissue health and stability around implants supporting full-arch mandibular fixed prostheses. *Clin. Oral Implants Res.* 20 (10): 1170–1177.

Schwartz-Arad, D. and Chausu, G. (1997). The ways and wherefores of immediate placement of implants into fresh extraction sites: a literature review. *J. Periodontol.* 68: 915–923.

Scipioni, A., Bruschi, G.B., and Calesini, G. (1994). The edentulous ridge expansion technique: a five-year study. *Int. J. Periodontics Restorative Dent.* 14: 451–459.

Seibert, J. (1993). Reconstruction of the partially edentulous ridge: gateway to improved prosthetics and superior aesthetics. *Pract. Periodontics Aesthet. Dent.* (5): 47–55.

Shapoff, C.A., Lahey, B., Wasserlauf, P.A., and Kim, D.M. (2010). Radiographic analysis of crestal bone levels around Laser-Lok collar dental implants. *Int. J. Periodontics Restorative Dent.* 30 (2): 129–132.

Shibli, J.A., d'Avila, S., and Marcantonio, E. Jr. (2004). Connective tissue graft to correct peri-implantsoft tissue margin: a clinical report. *J. Prosthet. Dent.* 91: 119–122.

Siegenthaler, D.W., Jung, R.E., Holderegger, C. et al. (2007). Replacement of teeth exhibiting periapical pathology by immediate implants: a prospective, controlled clinical trial. *Clin. Oral Implants Res.* 18 (6): 727–737.

Small, P.N. and Tarnow, D.P. (2000). Gingival recession around implants: a 1-year longitudinal prospective study. *Int. J. Oral Maxillofac. Implants* 15: 527–532.

Small, P.N., Tarnow, D.P., and Cho, S.C. (2001). Gingival recession around wide-diameter versus standard-diameter implants: a 3- to 5-year longitudinal prospective study. *Pract. Proced. Aesthet. Dent.* 13 (2): 143–146.

Smeets, R., Stadlinger, B., and Schwarz, F. (2016). Impact of dental implant surface modifications on osseointegration. *Biomed. Res. Int.* 6285620. doi: 10.1155/2016/6285620.

Smukler, H. and Landsberg, J. (1984). The toothbrush and gingival traumatic injury. *J. Periodontol.* 55 (12): 713–719.

Spriano, S., Sarath Chandra, V., Cochis, A. et al. (2017). How do wettability, zeta potential and hydroxylation degree affect the biological response of biomaterials? *Mater. Sci. Eng. C Mater. Biol.* 74 (1): 542–555.

Stimmelmayr, M., Güth, J.F., Schlee, M. et al. (2012). Use of a modified shell technique for three-dimensional bone grafting: description of a technique. *Aust. Dent. J.* 57: 93–97.

Stoelinga, P.J., Blijdorp, P.A., Ross, R.R. et al. (1986). Augmentation of the atrophic mandible with interposed bone grafts and particulate hydroxylapatite. *J. Oral Maxillofac. Surg.* 44 (5): 353–360.

Strid, K.G. 1985. 'Radiographic procedures,' in P.I. Brånemark, K.G. Zarb, and T. Albrektsson (eds.) *Tissue Integrated Prostheses. Osseointegration in Clinical Dentistry*, Quintessence, Chicago, IL.pp. 259–265.

Strub, J. and Gaberthüel, T. (1992). The role of attached gingival. I. The health of the peri-implant tissue in dog. *Int. J. Periodontics Restorative Dent.* 12: 415–425.

Strub, J.R., Gaberthüel, T.W., and Grunder, U. (1991). The role of attached gingiva in the health of peri-implant tissue in dogs. 1. Clinical findings. *Int. J. Periodontics Restorative Dent.* 11 (4): 317–333.

Taba, M. Jr., Jin, Q., Sugai, J.V., and Giannobile, W.V. (2005). Current concepts in periodontal bioengineering. *Orthod. Craniofacial Res.* 8: 292–302.

Tortamano, P., Camargo, L.O., Bello-Silva, M.S., and Kanashiro, L.H. (2010). Immediate implant placement and restoration in the esthetic zone: a prospective study with 18 months of follow-up.' *Int. J. Oral Maxillofac. Implants* 25 (2): 345–350.

Touati, B., Rompen, E., and Van Dooren, E. (2005). A new concept for optimizing soft tissue integration. *Pract. Proced. Aesthet. Dent.* 17 (10): 711–712. 714–715.

Tran Van, P.T., Vignery, A., and Baron, R. (1982). Cellular kinetics of the bone remodeling sequence in the rat. *Anat. Rec.* 202 (4): 445–451.

Tsegga, T. and Wright, T. (2017). Maxillary segmental osteoperiosteal flap with simultaneous placement of dental implants: case report of a novel technique. *Int. J. Implant Dent.* 3: 2.

Tsuda, H., Rungcharassaeng, K., Kan, J.Y. et al. (2011). Peri-implant tissue response following connective tissue and bone grafting in conjunction with immediate single-tooth replacement in the esthetic zone: a case series. *Int. J. Oral Maxillofac. Implants* 26: 427–436.

Vandana, K.L. and Savitha, B. (2005). Thickness of gingival in association with age, gender and dental arch location. *J. Clin. Periodontol.* 32 (7): 828–830.

Vega, L.G. and Bilbao, A. (2010). Alveolar distraction osteogenesis for dental implant preparation: an update. *Oral Maxillofac. Surg Clin. North. Am.* 22 (3): 369–385.

Vincent, J.W., Machen, J.B., and Levin, M.P. (1984). Assessment of attached gingiva using the tension test and clinical measurements. *J. Prosthet. Dent.* 52 (6): 781–786.

Wang, H.L., Misch, C., and Neiva, R.F. (2004). "Sandwich" bone augmentation technique: rationale and report of pilot cases. *Int. J. Periodontics Restorative Dent.* 24 (3): 232–245.

Wang, X., Wang, Y., Gou, W. et al. (2013). Role of mesenchymal stem cells in bone regeneration and fracture repair: a review. *Int. Orthop.* 37 (12): 2491–2498.

Weiner, S., Simon, J., and Ehrenberg, D.S. (2008). The effects of laser microtextured collars upon crestal bone levels of dental implants. *Implant. Dent.* 17 (2): 217–228.

Weisgold, A.S. (1977). Contours of the full crown restoration. *Alpha Omegan* 70: 77–89.

Welander, M., Abrahamsson, I., and Berglundh, T. (2009). Subcrestal placement of two-part implants. *Clin. Oral Implants Res.* 20 (3): 226–231.

Weng, D., Nagata, M.J., and Bell, M. (2008). Influence of microgap location and configurationon the peri-implnat bone morphology in submerged implants. An experimental study in dogs. *Clin. Oral Implants Res.* 19 (11): 1141.

Wennstrom, J.L. (1996). Mucogingival therapy. *Ann. Periodontol.* 1 (1): 671–701.

Wennstrom, J.L., Bengazi, F., and Lekholm, U. (1994). The influence of the masticatory mucosa on the peri-implant soft tissue condition. *Clin. Oral Implants Res.* 5: 1–8.

Wheeler, R.C. (1961). Complete crown form and the periodontium. *J. Prosthet. Dent.* 11: 722–734.

Wildermanm, M.N. and Wentz, F.M. (1965). Repair of a dentogingival defect with a pedicle flap. *J. Periodontol.* 36: 218–223.

Wilson, T.G. Jr. (2009). The positive relationship between excess cement and peri-implant disease: a prospective clinical endoscopic study. *J. Periodontol.* 80 (9): 1388–1392.

Wilson, T.G. Jr., Roccuzzo, M., Ucer, C., and Beagle, J.R. (2013). Immediate placement of tapered effect (TE) implants: 5-year results of a prospective, multicenter study. *Int. J. Oral Maxillofac. Implants* 28 (1): 261–269.

Wöhrle, P.S. (2003). Nobel perfect esthetic scalloped implant: rationale for a new design. *Clin. Implant Dent. Relat. Res.* 5 (Suppl. 1): 64–73.

Yu, Q.P.X., Ji, G.P., and Shen, G. (2009). The association between lower incisal inclination and morphology of the supporting alveolar bone – a cone-beam CT study. *Int. J. Oral Sci.* 1: 217–223.

Zigdon, H. and Machtei, E.E. (2008). The dimensions of keratinized mucosa around implants affect clinical and immunological parameters. *Clin. Oral Implants Res.* 19: 387–392.

Zucchelli, G., Mazzotti, C., Bentivogli, V. et al. (2012). The connective tissue platform technique for soft tissue augmentation. *Int. J. Periodontics Restorative Dent.* 32 (6): 665–675.

Zucchelli, G., Mazzotti, C., Mounssif, I. et al. (2013). A novel surgical–prosthetic approach for soft tissue dehiscence coverage around a single implant. *Clin. Oral Implants Res.* 24 (9): 957–962.

6

Revisiting Guided Bone Regeneration in the Esthetic Zone

Rawad Samarani

Department of Periodontology, Saint-Joseph University, Beirut, Lebanon

6.1 Introduction

From a functional point of view, the need for adequate bone volume is a prerequisite for stable long-term implant survival. In the esthetic zone however, the need for bone volume to establish proper ridge contour and height, and for proper papillary support is even greater. This becomes especially important in patients with high lip line. Hence the need for re-establishing a proper bone volume and contour in cases of deficient alveolar ridges. For this purpose, several approaches have been proposed with varying levels of documentation and evidence. Among these approaches, the guided bone regeneration (GBR) principle is the most documented (Aghaloo and Moy 2007; Benic and Hämmerle 2014). It is a well-established procedure for the augmentation of deficient alveolar ridges, with more than 25 years of clinical documentation.

But despite the relatively abundant amount of literature on GBR, the evidence is sometimes weak in several aspects, notably the comparative performance of the different biomaterials available for GBR, the factors affecting outcome variability, the long-term results, and the predictability in challenging defects like the esthetic defect; the vertical defect; and the complete atrophic jaw.

The purpose of this chapter is to briefly review the GBR principle and technique, to look into special considerations for the esthetic zone in terms of surgical technique, choice of biomaterials, need for optimal ridge volume, need for appropriate soft tissue quality and quantity, need to differentiate between different defect types, and need to understand and manage possible complications.

6.2 Biological Rationale and Historic Overview

The biological basis of GBR has its roots in what was conceived in the early 1980s as a technique for periodontal regeneration, termed Guided Tissue Regeneration (GTR) (Nyman et al. 1982). The GTR used a physical barrier, notably an expanded polytetrafluoroethylene (e-PTFE) membrane, to shield the periodontal defect from the surrounding epithelium and connective tissues, giving way for periodontal ligament and alveolar bone cells to selectively populate the defect. Histological proof of regeneration of the cementum, the periodontal ligament, and the alveolar bone along with improved clinical parameters made GTR successful (Gottlow 1993). This success fueled the efforts to apply the same principle of using a physical barrier for a supposedly easier task of shielding a bony-only defect from fibroblastic invasion, giving way for bone cells to populate the defect (Dahlin et al. 1988). This approach was termed guided bone regeneration (GBR). The GBR rationale would be based on using the characteristic spontaneous healing capacity of bone, guided by the presence of a physical barrier. The regeneration would follow the pattern of bone formation occurring during development and growth (Schenk et al. 1994).

After an initial developmental clinical phase where only membranes were used for GBR, the addition of bone fillers was later proposed to reduce membrane collapse and to optimize the amount of bone formation underneath the membrane.

In the initial clinical applications, GBR was used to regenerate bone defects around implants placed in

Advances in Esthetic Implant Dentistry, First Edition. Abdelsalam Elaskary.

Companion website: www.wiley.com/go/elaskary/esthetic

post-extraction sites (Becker and Becker 1990) and to regenerate peri-implant dehiscence-type defects (Jovanovic, Spiekermann and Richter 1992). Later, GBR became the standard of care in treating localized alveolar ridge defects whether simultaneously with implant placement or in a separate preceding surgery. More extensive and challenging defects were also addressed, like vertical ridge augmentations (Simion, Trisi and Piattelli 1994).

6.3 Surgical Protocol and Special Considerations for the Esthetic Zone

GBR is a rather advanced surgical procedure and necessitates proper surgical skills and trainings. The following gives a detailed descriptions of the surgical steps. Special considerations for the esthetic zone are discussed.

6.3.1 Flap Design

Proper access to the surgical site is of paramount importance. Large trapezoidal or triangular mucoperiosteal flaps encompassing one or two adjacent teeth have been advocated. Flap advancement is performed to allow coronal flap mobilization and tension-free closure. Wound closure favoring primary intention wound healing is essential in the GBR procedure to protect the graft site from bacterial invasion and to allow undisturbed healing (Wang and Boyapati 2006).

6.3.1.1 Incisions at the Edentulous Site

In the early clinical applications of GBR, mid-crestal incisions were believed to result in more soft tissue dehiscences. Consequently, the use of para-crestal incisions was advocated (Buser et al. 1993). In the mandible, a vestibular or mucobuccal fold incision was used. In the maxilla, mucobuccal fold and palatal incisions were used. The amount of palatal off-set ranged from a couple of millimeters from the mid-crest to incision lines placed distantly in the palate. In later applications, paracrestal incisions were abandoned because of their tendency to heal more slowly than crestal incisions (Cranin et al. 1998) and because they are associated with increased pain, inflammation, and edema (Scharf and Tarnow 1993). It was also believed that the risk of dehiscence is associated with inappropriate flap advancement, the failure to achieve tension free closure, and inadequate suturing techniques, rather than the position of the incision line. In the maxilla, however, it is believed that a slight off-set, either vestibular or palatal, can have some advantages in specific situations. Even though no comparative studies have been conducted to test the superiority of one approach over another, the following differentiation can be relevant, especially in the esthetic zone.

6.3.1.1.1 Mid-crestal Incision

This type of incision respects the vascular network of the mucosa, and ideally should be positioned in the avascular zone located on the ridge crest (Casino et al. 1997; Kleinheinz et al. 2005). The buccal and lingual aspects of the mucosa covering the alveolar ridge have separate vascular networks running in a postero-anterior direction. The crestal area of the edentulous alveolar ridge is covered by a relatively avascular zone of 1–2 mm wide with no anastomoses crossing the alveolar ridge (Kleinheinz et al. 2005; Koymen et al. 2009). Consequently, para-midline incisions would leave a terminal part of one of the flaps with no blood supply from its corresponding vascular network. The blood supply of this flap edge will be hindered by the presence of the avascular zone, leading to a potential necrosis of this flap edge and a possible wound dehiscence.

The disadvantage of the mid-crestal incision is that it usually extends to the middle of the papilla adjacent to the edentulous site. Cutting through a papilla of a thin scalloped periodontium in the esthetic zone can cause papilla cratering and/or collapse, leading to an unfavorable papilla at the end of the treatment.

A mid-crestal incision would preferably be used in cases of thin mucosa (Park and Wang 2007) and/or in patients who systemically are at an increased risk of ischemic wound dehiscence (e.g. patients who smoke, have diabetes, or are of an advanced age) to reduce the risk of flap edge necrosis (Table 6.1). The mean width of keratinized gingiva on adjacent teeth may be used as a guide to determine the initial incision location (Park and Wang 2007).

6.3.1.1.2 Slightly Palatal Incision

The advantage of this type of incision is that it leaves an adequate width of unscarred keratinized tissue buccally to the incision line. This band of tissue will be transposed facially at the abutment connection surgery and will constitute an unscarred, esthetically pleasing band of keratinized gingiva on the buccal aspect of the implant. Another advantage is the fact that it spares the adjacent papilla and it cuts at its palatal base, rather than cutting through it. The entire papilla will be reflected with the buccal flap.

A slightly palatal incision would preferably be used for small edentulous spaces of the anterior maxilla (Table 6.1).

Table 6.1 Recapitulative table on the various types of horizontal incisions at the edentulous site.

	Advantages	Disadvantages	Indications
Mid-crestal	• Respects the primary blood supply	• Cuts through the middle of the adjacent papilla, thereby increasing the risk of papillary sloughing	• Thin mucosa • Patients at increased risk of ischemic wound dehiscence (smokers, diabetes, advanced age,…)
Slightly palatal	• Unscarred band of keratinized gingiva present buccally to the implant restoration at the end of the treatment • Does not cut through the adjacent papilla thereby reducing the risk of papillary sloughing	• Risk of buccal flap edge necrosis in susceptible patients	• Small edentulous spaces of the anterior maxilla
Slightly vestibular	• Reduces palatal shifting of the soft tissue, thereby facilitating buccal transpositioning of the keratinized gingiva at the abutment connection surgery	• Risk of palatal flap edge necrosis in susceptible patients	• Big three-dimensional ridge augmentations in the maxilla

6.3.1.1.3 *Slightly Vestibular Incision*

This type of incision is favored in cases where a large bone graft volume is anticipated in the maxilla, notably in vertical augmentations. The advantage of this incision is that it reduces palatal shifting of the soft tissues after wound approximation, thus facilitating the buccal transpositioning of the keratinized tissue at the abutment connection surgery (Table 6.1).

6.3.1.2 Incisions at the Adjacent Teeth and Vertical Releasing Incisions

The incision should extend from the edentulous area to encompass at least one or two (exceptionally more) adjacent teeth in an intrasulcular fashion on both the buccal and palatal/lingual aspects. At the papillae level, and especially in the esthetic zone, we favor a papilla preserving incision similar to that termed the simplified papilla preservation flap for flap surgery using periodontal access (Cortellini, Prato and Tonetti 1999). The advantage of this incision design over the classical full papilla reflection is the reduction of papillary sloughing and collapse, especially in thin scalloped periodontium.

Vertical releasing incisions are placed on the buccal aspect, whereas on the palatal side a large envelope flap is advised. Exceptionally, vertical releasing incisions can be placed palatally. On the buccal aspect, the vertical releasing incision should follow a "J" pattern, starting at the line angles of the tooth (Simion et al. 1994), slightly diverging outward, and extending into the alveolar mucosa. In esthetic areas, beveled incision through the keratinized gingiva has the potential to reduce postoperative scarring. When possible, vertical incisions should not be placed in the front visible area; they should be placed on the distal aspects of the canines or more distally.

6.3.1.3 Flap Advancement

Advancement flaps are common practice in oral surgery. Actually used for various applications, they have their roots in the advancement flap described by Rehrmann (1936) for the closure of oro-antral communications. The Rehrmann-plasty uses two vertical releasing incisions and a periosteal incision to allow coronal advancement of the buccal flap. In the GBR procedure, periosteal incisions alone cannot satisfy the need for the advanced flap mobilization that is required to treat severe bone defects. Elongation of the submucosa and flap separation from the underlying muscles should also be performed, depending on the severity of the defect, the vestibular depth, and the presence of scar tissues.

A typical full-thickness mucoperiosteal flap is bound externally by the mucosa and internally by the periosteum. The intermediate part is the submucosal tissue. The periosteum is a dense and thin tissue layer less than 0.4 mm thick. It makes up the most rigid part of the flap due to the lack of elastic fibers. The submucosa, in contrast, is a loose connective tissue of varying thicknesses containing numerous elastic fibers (contains also adipose tissue, minor salivary glands, blood vessels, and nerves). Although generally loose, it contains strands of densely grouped collagenous fibers. More apically, the submucosa becomes attached to the adjacent muscles: orbicularis oris in the anterior parts of the mouth, mentalis in the anterior mandible area, buccinators in the posterior buccal areas and mylohyoid in the lingual aspect.

When *minor flap advancement* is desired, severing the periosteum with a superficial incision running parallel to the bone surface is able to sufficiently release the flap. The cut should be performed at a level apical to the mucogingival junction to avoid flap perforation (Table 6.2).

Table 6.2 Recapitulative table on the various degrees of flap advancement.

Flap advancement	Recommended technique	Instrument used	Dissection plane and directions	Indications
Minor	• Superficial periosteal incision	• Blade	• Apical to the muco-gingival junction • Runs parallel to the bone surface	• Small dehiscence-type defects
Moderate	• Add: Localize and cut the dense strands of collagen fibers in the submucosa	• Blade	• Outward direction	• Knife edge ridge defect
	• Add: Stretch the submucosa	• Wide end of a periosteal elevator (blunt)	• Stretch apart the flap by pushing in coronal direction	
Major	• Add: Separate the submucosa from the underlying muscles	• Blade or Curved Scissors	• Runs parallel to the outer surface of the flap	• Three-dimensional or vertical defects
Additional	• Add: *Superficial extension of the vertical releasing incisions*	• *Blade*	• *Follows the direction that would liberate the flap from its corners*	• *Applicable for all defects*

When *moderate advancement* is desired, localizing and severing the dense strands of collagen fibers located in the submucosa will liberate the flap even further. This should be performed with a scalpel blade. A good approach is to explore and localize the strands of collagen with the tip of the blade and to cut in an outward motion. The advantage of this approach is a selective cutting in the submucosal plane, thus minimizing injury to the blood vessels. The alternative approach is to blindly deepen, with the scalpel blade, the initial periosteal cut at the expense of possible vessel injury. This approach is sometimes inevitable due to the difficulty of adequately visualizing and localizing the strands of collagen. Another approach proposed for the posterior mandible, consisted of using the blade edge in a horizontal brushing motion (Ronda and Stacchi 2015). After cutting in the submucosa, an additional flap elongation can be achieved by stretching the submucosal tissue. This can be attained by inserting closed blunt scissors or a hemostat into the incision line. The instrument is opened vertically to stretch apart the two sides of the incision line (Greenstein et al. 2009). Another way to stretch the submucosa that we favor over the previous one is to insert the wide end of a periosteal elevator (e.g. Prichard) into the incision line and push it in a coronal direction (Table 6.2).

When *major flap advancement* is desired, separating the submucosa from the surrounding muscles (Romanos 2010) or cutting through the muscles advised (Kim, Kim and Leem 2015). The first approach is preferable for being less morbid. In the specific case of the anterior maxilla, we believe that the first approach also has a decreased risk of upper lip paresthesia. The upper lip takes its sensory innervation through branches of the infra-orbital nerve. The orbicularis oris muscle has its motor innervation from the buccal branch of the facial nerve. These nerve branches run through the thickness of the orbicularis oris muscle. A deep cut into the muscle thickness can potentially sever some nerve endings, potentially leading to upper lip paresthesia or to reduced lip mobility. In the orbicularis oris and the buccinators regions, separating the submucosa from the adjacent muscle fibers should be performed with curved dissecting scissors. The dissection plane should follow the outer surface of the flap and the path of least resistance, trying to avoid cutting through the muscles as much as possible (Table 6.2). Care must be taken not to perforate the flap. On the lateral sides of the maxilla, the dissection should never go as far as the parotid duct.

If *additional advancement* is desired after executing all of the above, a superficial extension of the vertical releasing incisions will liberate the flap from its corners (Fugazzotto 1999; Sclar 2003) (Table 6.2).

More advancement can be also performed by combining the coronal advancement of the flap with lateral sliding resulting in papillary shifting on the adjacent teeth. A more distant vertical releasing incision encompassing at least two adjacent teeth should be anticipated (Urban et al. 2016a).

Alternative techniques to the coronal buccal flap advancement described above have been proposed, consisting of elongating the buccal or the palatal flaps.

The buccal mucoperiosteal flap can be extended by creating a pedicled periosteal flap with a coronal base.

The periosteal flap is reflected over the alveolar crest and used for primary intention wound closure (Triaca et al. 2001). To extending the palatal flap, a similar technique of flap extension was also proposed (Fugazzotto 1999). Another technique for extending the palatal flap uses two superimposed split thickness incisions to create a further extension of the palatal flap (Tinti and Parma-Benfenati 1995). These two techniques of palatal flap elongation pose a risk of potential flap necrosis and should only be performed when the thickness of the palatal tissues is greater than 5 mm. All these alternative techniques have the advantage of reducing the need for buccal flap advancement and thereby minimizing the reduction of vestibular depth.

6.3.2 Recipient Site Preparation

The cortical surface of the recipient site should be scraped with a sharp instrument to clean any remnants of periosteal tissue (Simion et al. 1994). Then, cortical perforation of the recipient site with a small bur (around 1 mm) is performed (Figures 6.1j and 6.2f). In a GBR rat calvarial model, cortical perforations were responsible for significantly increased bone formation (172.8%) compared to an intact osseous surface (Rompen et al. 1999). The perforations of cortical bone at the recipient site may facilitate the migration of osteoprogenitor cells from the bone marrow into the isolated space. Also, it may allow bleeding from the marrow spaces, favoring the development of blood capillaries (Majzoub et al.

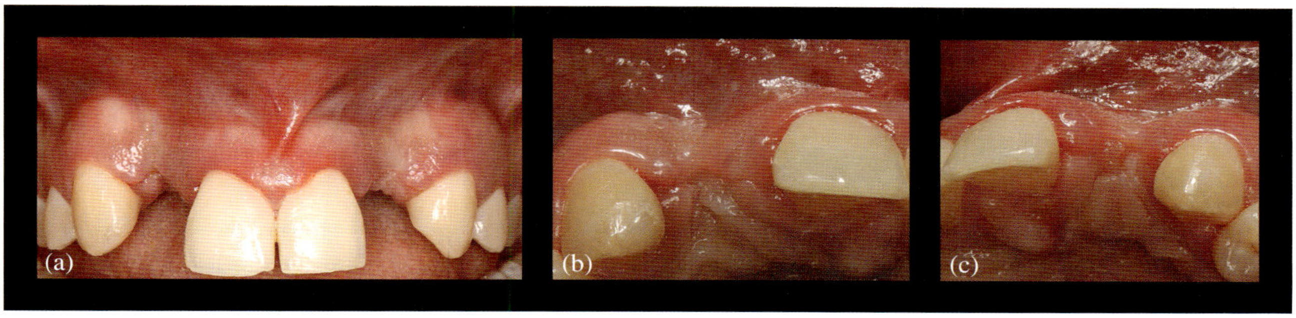

Figure 6.1 (a) Vertical and lateral defect at the lateral incisors due to previous implant failure. (b) Occlusal view of the right lateral incisor site. (c) Occlusal view of the left lateral incisor site.

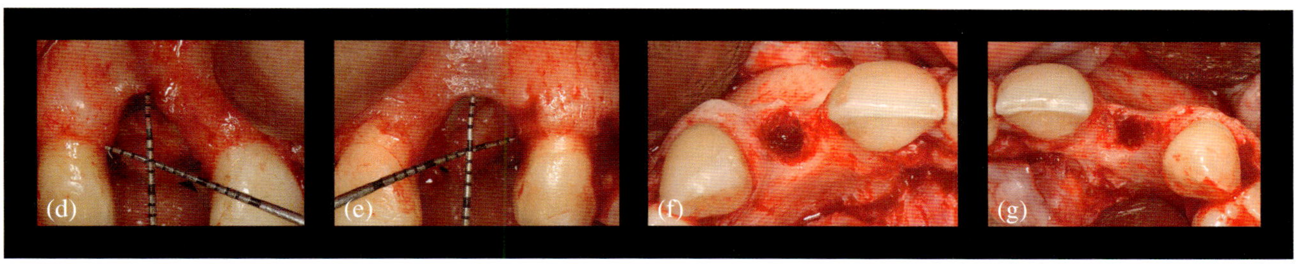

Figure 6.1 (d) Vertical component of the defect at site 12 amounting to more than 6 mm. (e) Vertical component of the defect at site 22 amounting to 5 mm. (f) Horizontal component of the defect at site 12. (g) Horizontal component of the defect at site 22.

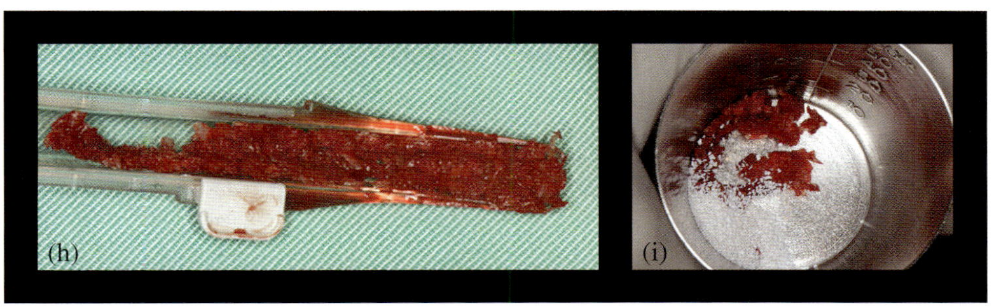

Figure 6.1 (h) Cortical bone shavings collected with a bone scraper. (i) 1 : 1 mixture of autogenous bone and anorganic bovine bone.

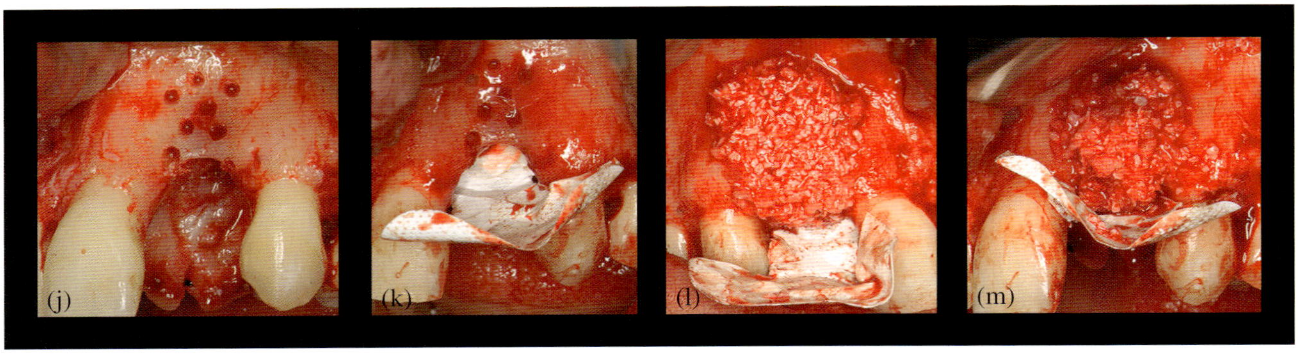

Figure 6.1 (j) Cortical perforations. (k) Stabilization of titanium-reinforced d-PTFE (Cytoplast®) membrane with mini-screws on the palatal side. (l) Composite bone graft in place at 12. (m) Composite bone graft in place at 22.

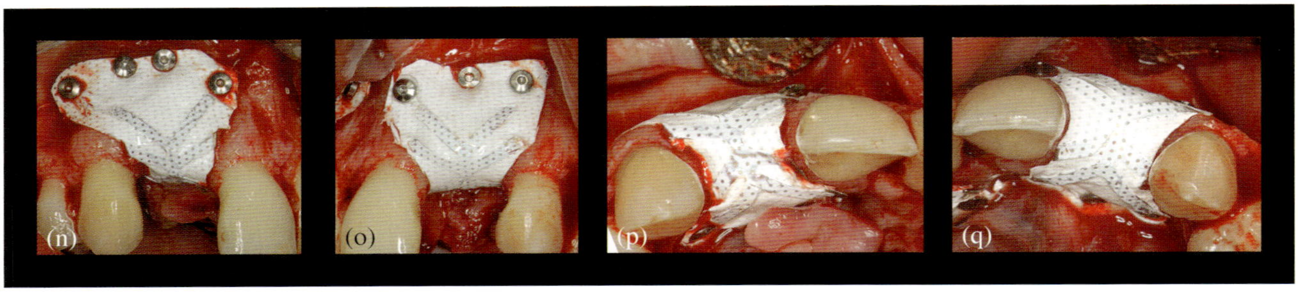

Figure 6.1 (n) Membrane secured buccally with pins at 12 and adapted to the alveolar contour. (o) Membrane secured buccally with pins at 22 and adapted to the alveolar contour. (p) Occlusal view of the membrane in place at 12. (q) Occlusal view of the membrane in place at 22.

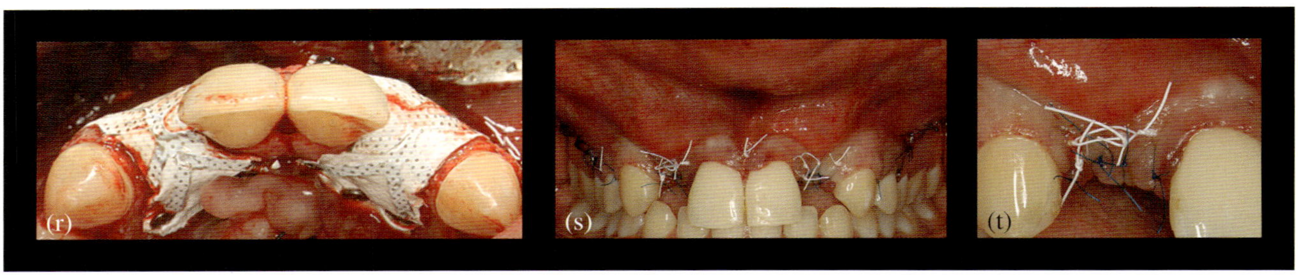

Figure 6.1 (r) The membrane is kept at a distance of 1–1.5 mm from the adjacent tooth root. (s) Sutures. (t) Site 12: close up view showing the d-PTFE thread (white) used to close the horizontal incision at the deeper level and the polypropylene thread (blue) used to close the superficial level.

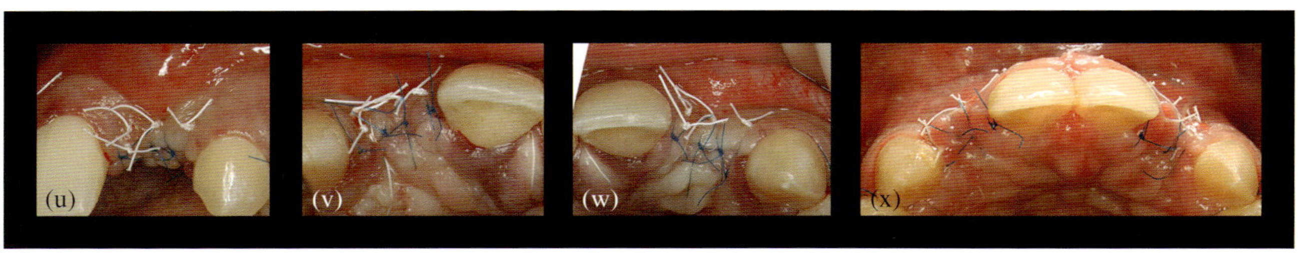

Figure 6.1 (u) Site 22: close up view showing the d-PTFE thread (white) used to close the horizontal incision at the deeper level and the polypropylene thread (blue) used to close the superficial level. (v) Site 12: close up view showing the d-PTFE thread (white) used to close the horizontal incision at the deeper level and the polypropylene thread (blue) used to close the superficial level. (w) Site 22: close up view showing the d-PTFE thread (white) used to close the horizontal incision at the deeper level and the polypropylene thread (blue) used to close the superficial level. (x) Soft tissue healing at two weeks.

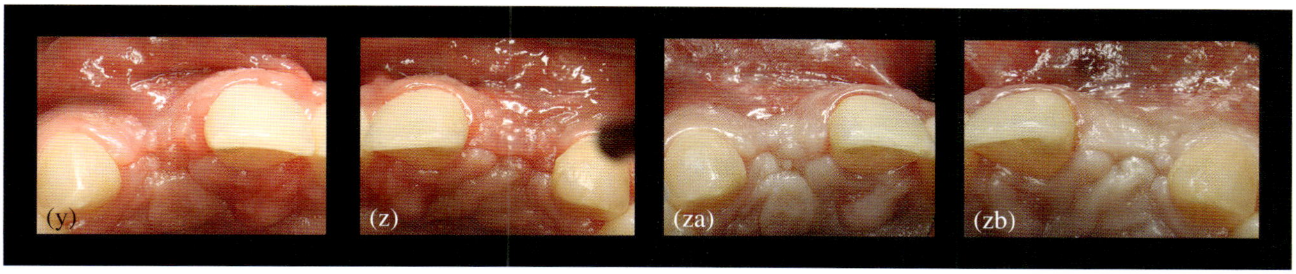

Figure 6.1 (y) Site 12: soft tissue healing at six weeks. (z) Site 22: soft tissue healing at six weeks. (za) Site 12: soft tissue healing at nine months. (zb) Site 22: soft tissue healing at nine months.

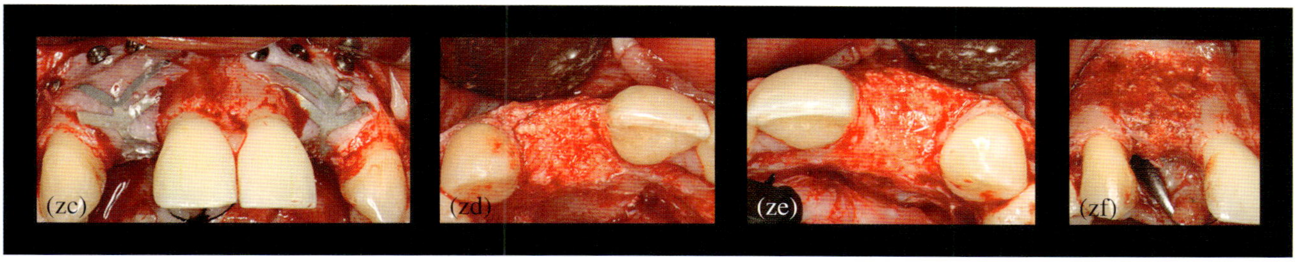

Figure 6.1 (zc) Full thickness flap elevation at nine months. (zd) Site 12: occlusal view of the regenerated area. (ze) Site 22: occlusal view of the regenerated area. (zf) Site 12: buccal view of the regenerated area.

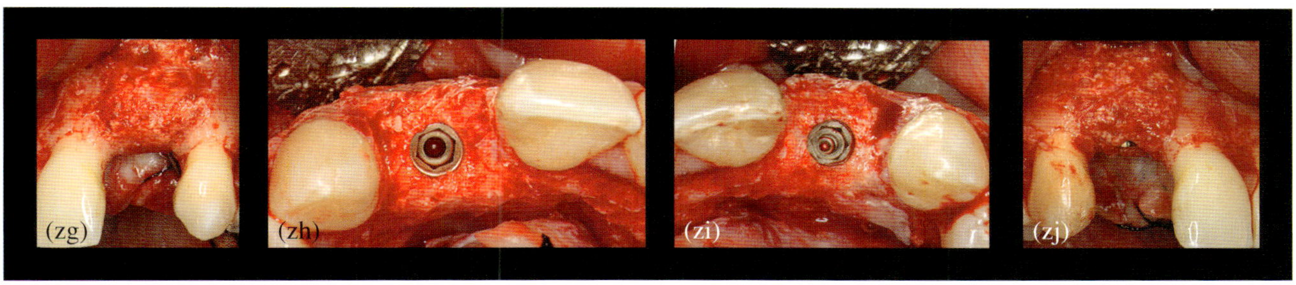

Figure 6.1 (zg) Site 22: buccal view of the regenerated area. (zh) Site 12: implant placement of 3.7 mm of diameter. (zi) Site 22: implant placement of 3.7 mm of diameter. (zj) Site 12: buccal view at implant placement.

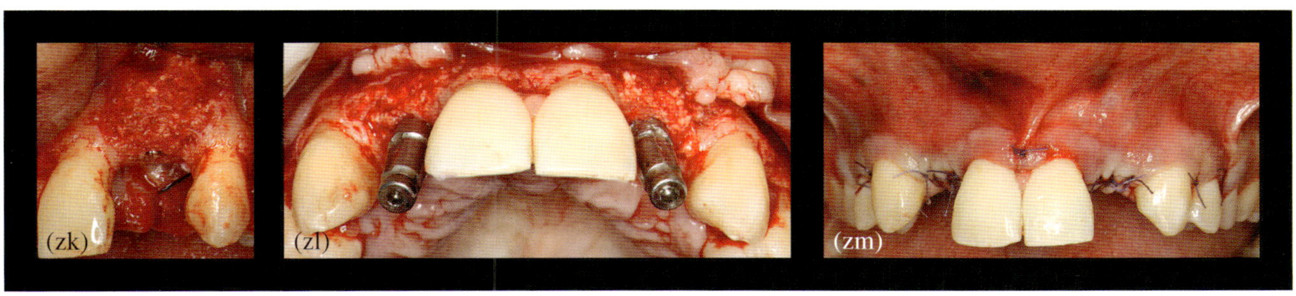

Figure 6.1 (zk) Site 22: buccal view at implant placement. (zl) Indexing at implant placement to allow temporary crown insertion at abutment connection surgery. (zm) Submerged healing of the inserted implants.

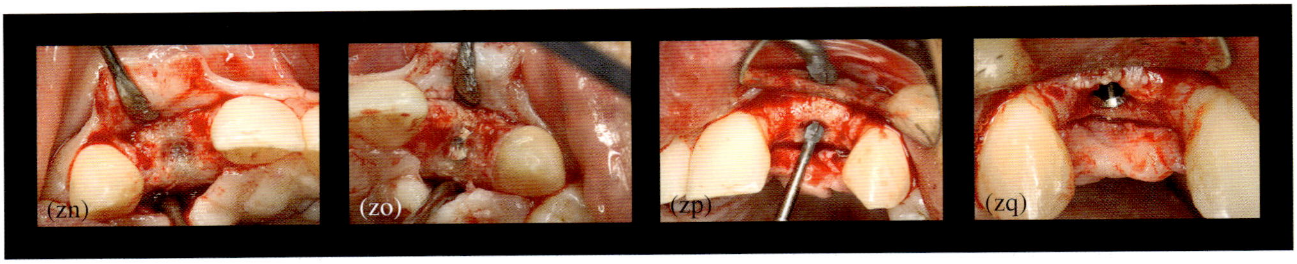

Figure 6.1 (zn) Site 12 at second stage surgery. No the bone overgrowth on the cover-screw. (zo) Site 22 at second stage surgery. No the bone overgrowth on the cover-screw. (zp) Bone removal with a surgical bur to allow access to the cover-screw. (zq) Site 12: buccal view after bone reduction.

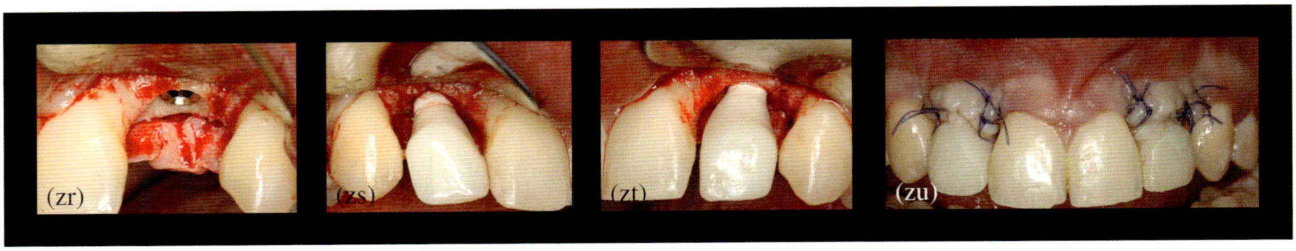

Figure 6.1 (zr) Site 22: buccal view after bone reduction. (zs) Site 12: screw-retained temporary crown fabricated on a PEEK abutment. Note the concave emergence profile. (zt) Site 22: screw-retained temporary crown fabricated on a PEEK abutment. Note the concave emergence profile. (zu) Sutures. Note the buccal increase in the ridge volume.

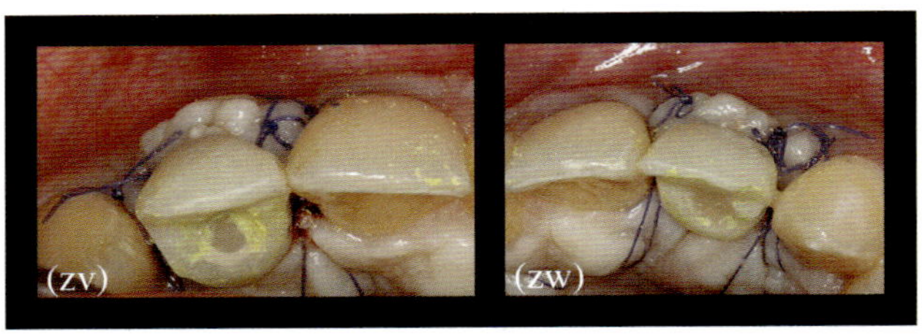

Figure 6.1 (zv) Sutures. Note the buccal increase in the ridge volume. (zw) Sutures. Note the buccal increase in the ridge volume.

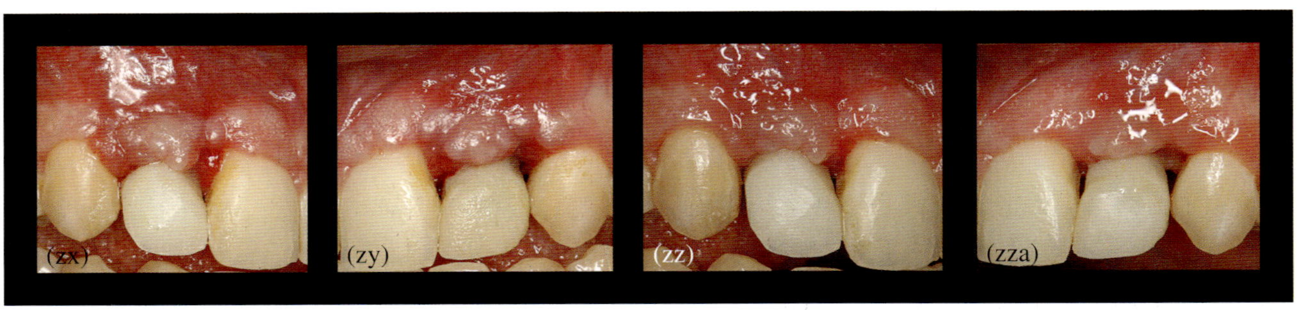

Figure 6.1 (zx) Soft tissue healing at two weeks. (zy) Soft tissue healing at two weeks. (zz) Soft tissue healing at eight weeks. (zza) Soft tissue healing at eight weeks.

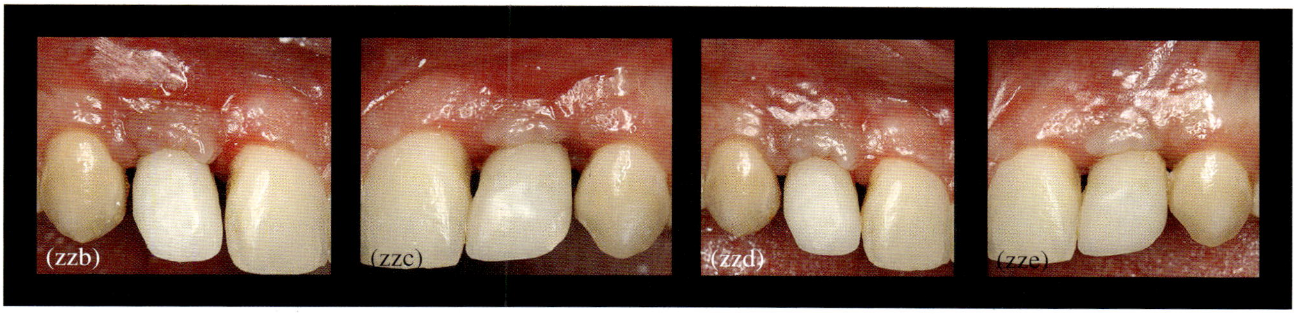

Figure 6.1 (zzb) At eight weeks: Addition of flowable composite on the emergence profile of the temporary crown to condition the soft tissues. (zzc) At eight weeks: Addition of flowable composite on the emergence profile of the temporary crown to condition the soft tissues. (zzd) Soft tissue healing at three months. (zze) Soft tissue healing at three months.

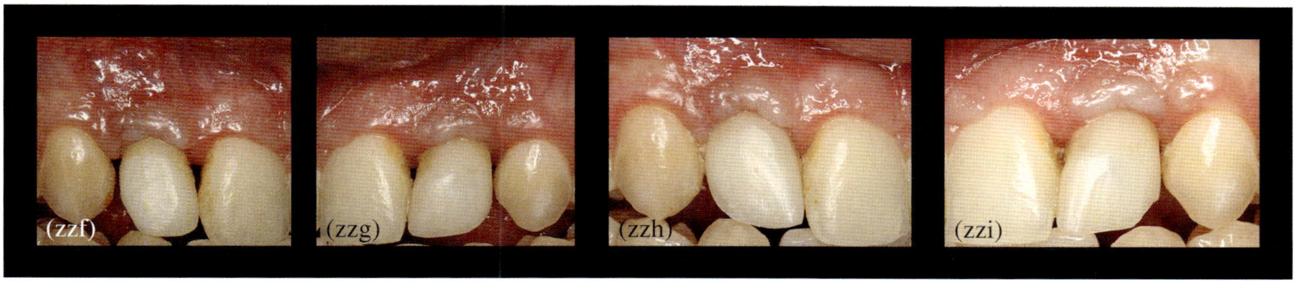

Figure 6.1 (zzf) Soft tissue healing at five months. (zzg) Soft tissue healing at five months. (zzh) Soft tissue healing at nine months. (zzi) Soft tissue healing at nine months.

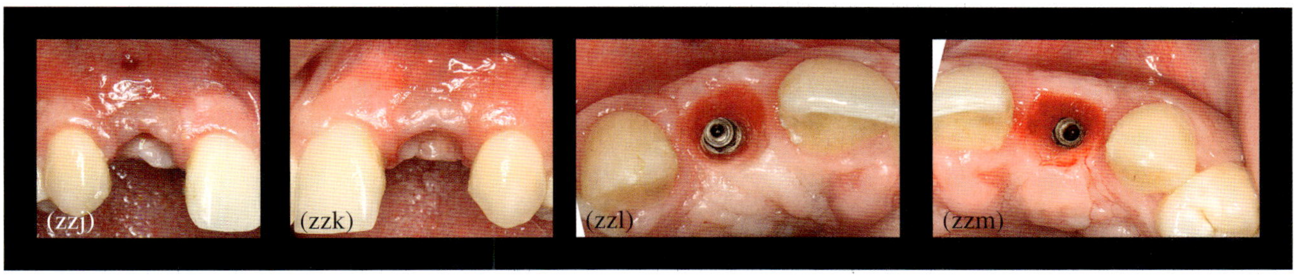

Figure 6.1 (zzj) Conditioned soft tissue ready to receive the final crown. (zzk) Conditioned soft tissue ready to receive the final crown. (zzl) Conditioned soft tissue ready to receive the final crown. (zzm) Conditioned soft tissue ready to receive the final crown.

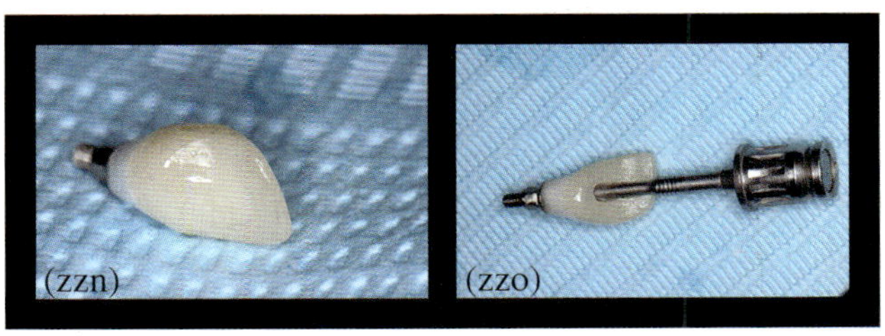

Figure 6.1 (zzn) Lithium disilicate crown cemented extraorally on a customized abutment. (zzo) The crown is perforated extraorally to transform the abutment/crown complex into a screw-retained prosthesis.

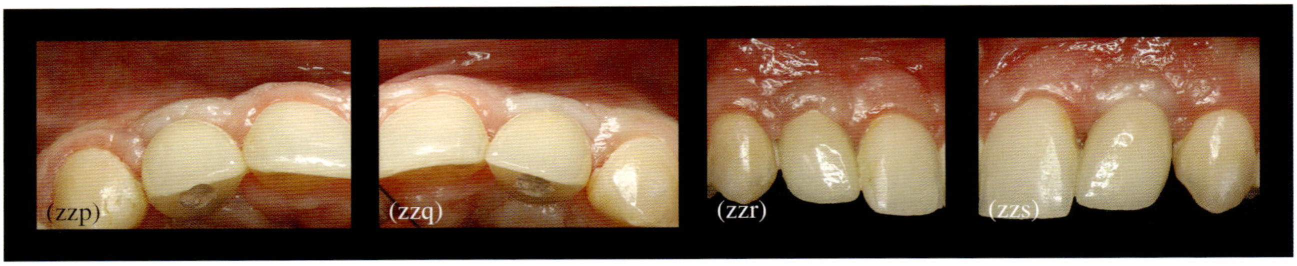

Figure 6.1 (zzp) Insertion of the final crown. (zzq) Insertion of the Final crown. (zzr) Follow-up after crown delivery to monitor the patient's hygiene compliance. (zzs) Follow-up after crown delivery to monitor the patient's hygiene compliance.

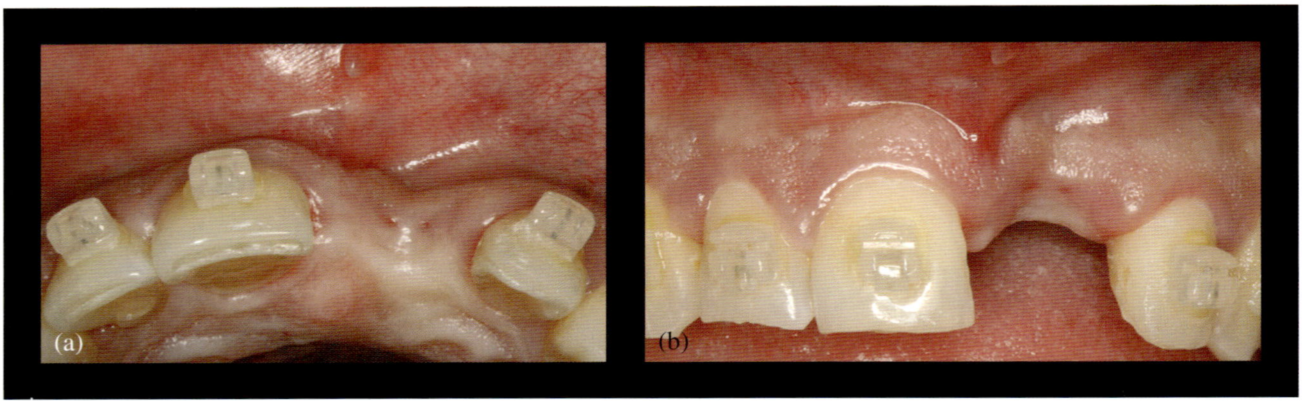

Figure 6.2 (a) Missing left central incisor with obvious buccal ridge defect. (b) Missing left central incisor with obvious buccal ridge defect.

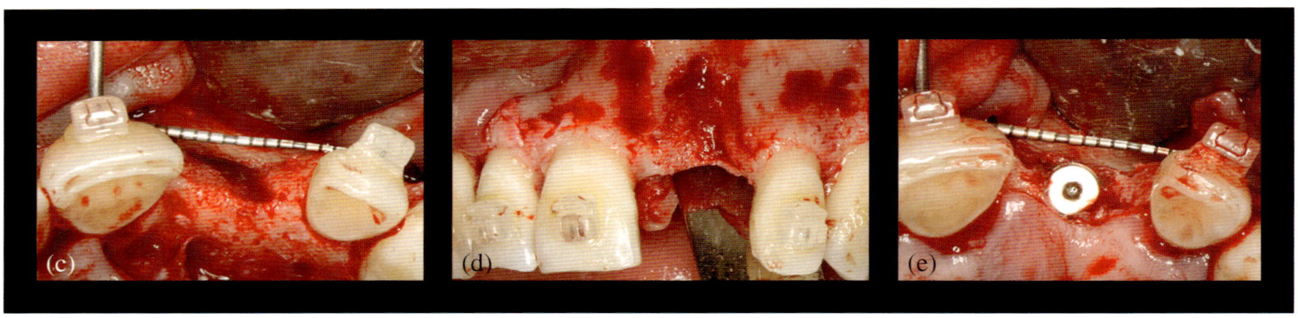

Figure 6.2 (c) Horizontal ridge defect. (d) No defect in the vertical dimension. (e) Implant position in relation to the buccal defect.

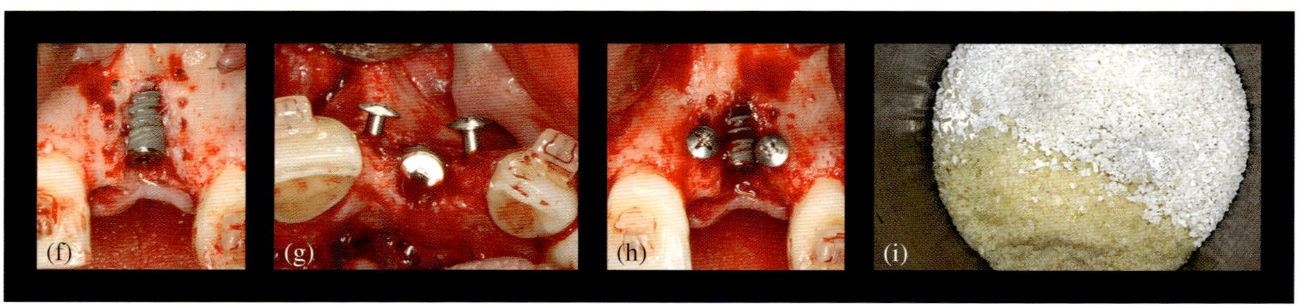

Figure 6.2 (f) Dehiscence-type defect. (g) Placement of two tenting screws, extending in a buccal direction. (h) Placement of two tenting screws, extending in a buccal direction. (i) Preparation of a composite graft consisting of 1 : 1 mixture of an allograft (enCore® combination) and an anorganic bovine bone.

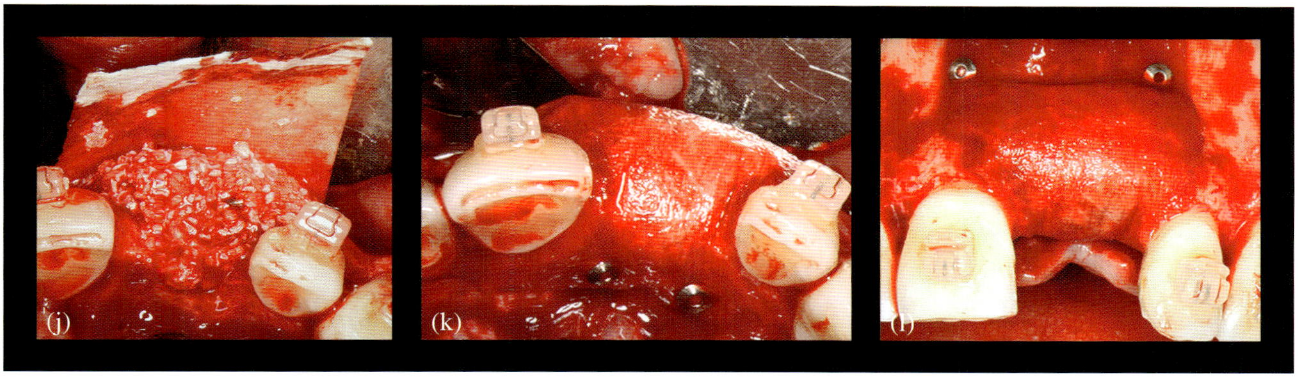

Figure 6.2 (j) Stabilization of a cross-linked collagen membrane (Cytoplast RTM) with two fixation pins placed buccally, creating a pouch-like containment of the particulate graft. (k) Folding of the membrane over the defect and stabilization with additional fixation pins. The presence of the tenting screws will prevent excessive membrane collapse into the defect. (l) Complete immobilization of the membrane/graft complex.

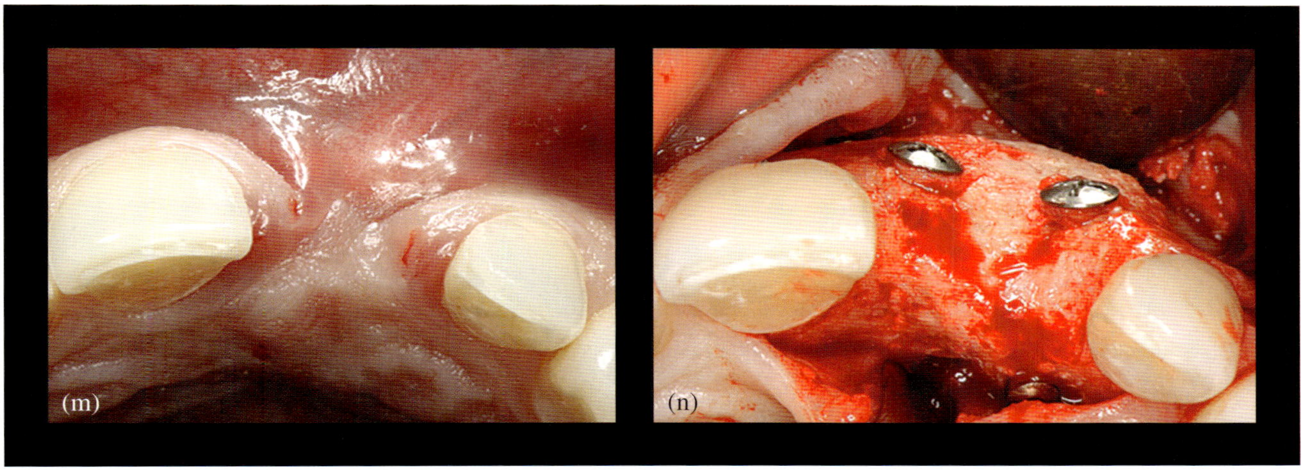

Figure 6.2 (m) Soft tissue aspect after seven months of healing. (n) Second stage surgery at seven months. Regenerated bone completely covering the implant.

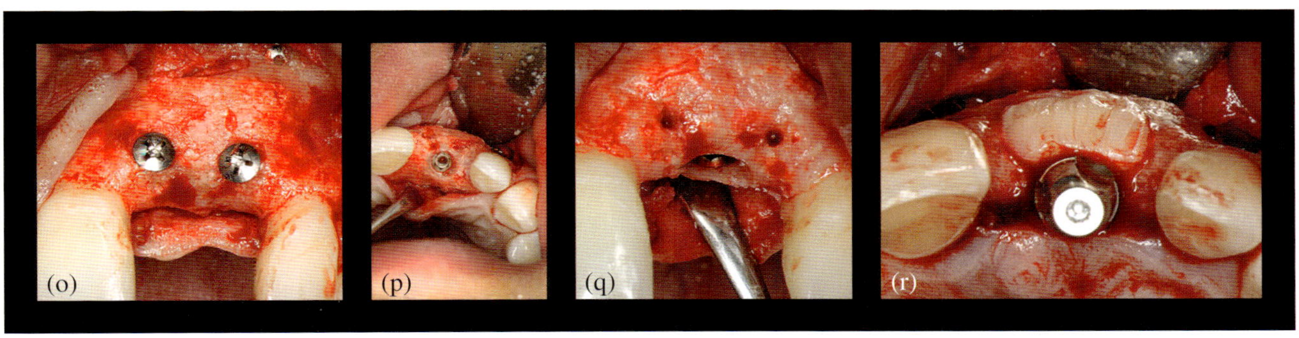

Figure 6.2 (o) Second stage surgery at seven months. Regenerated bone completely covering the implant. (p) Access to the implant platform after osteotomy of the bone covering the implant with a bur. (q) Removal of the tenting screws. (r) Sizing and trimming of a connective tissue graft on the buccal aspect of the ridge. Despite successful regeneration, a small collapse of the membrane occurred between the two tenting screws leading to a small concavity at the coronal aspect of the buccal wall (see (n)). The connective tissue graft aims at filling this residual defect to be able to obtain a natural emergence profile of the prosthesis.

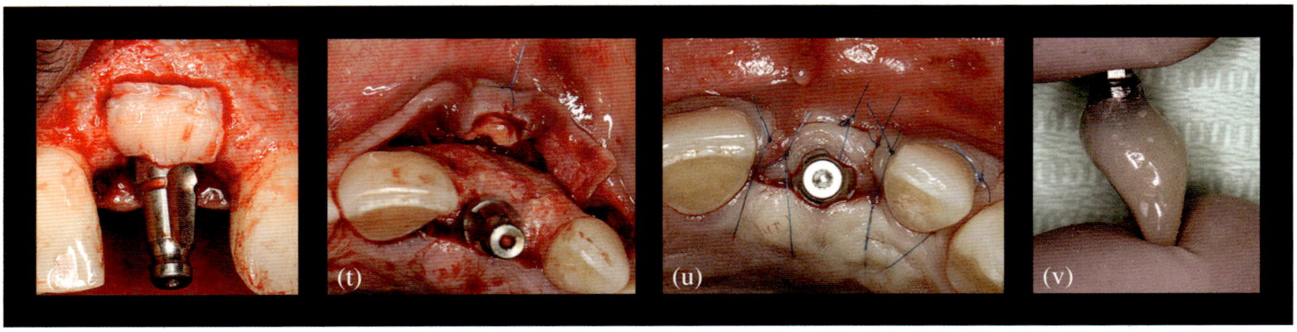

Figure 6.2 (s) Securing of an impression coping onto the implant to prepare for an impression at the end of the surgery. The impression will be used to fabricate a screw-retained temporary prosthesis, to be delivered the following day. (t) Suturing of the connective tissue graft to the internal side of the buccal flap. (u) Wound closure. 6(0) polypropylene sutures. (v) Screw-retained temporary crown delivered the following day. Note the slightly concave buccal emergence profile. The relatively reduced width of the emergence profile is essential at this stage to avoid excessive compression on the wound margins.

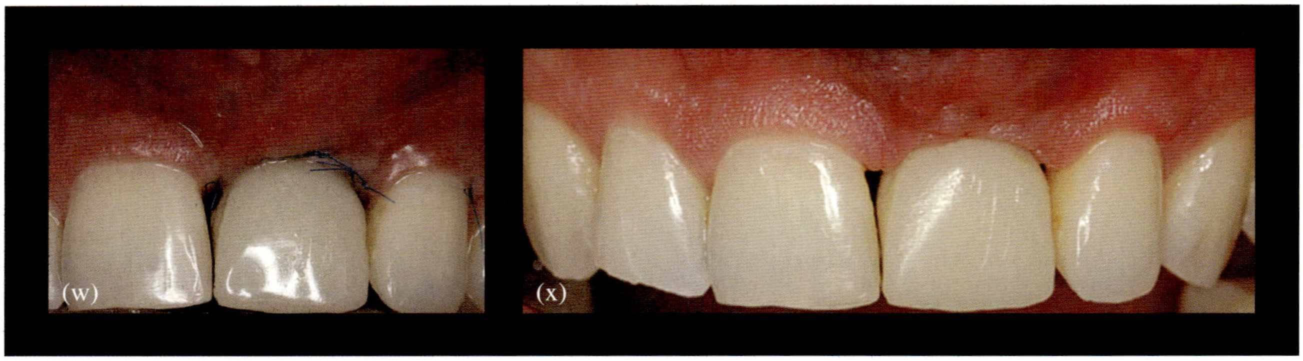

Figure 6.2 (w) Delivery of the temporary crown. (x) One week follow-up. Proper integration of the connective tissue graft. Soft tissue maturation will lead to papillary fill and regularization of the gingival contour.

1999), which is an essential step preceding new bone formation.

6.3.3 Bone Graft and Membrane Placement

Either the bone graft or the membrane could be placed first, depending on the type of membrane used and the configuration of the defect. The implants can be simultaneously inserted (Figures 6.2 and 6.3) or can be placed in a separate surgery after graft maturation (Figures 6.1 and 6.4–6.9).

When non-resorbable membranes are used (Figures 6.1, 6.4 and 6.8–6.10), they should be trimmed and secured on the palatal/lingual aspect with pins or fixation screws on at least two points. The membrane trimming should be carried out in a way that ensures coverage of the entire defect and should extend 2–3 mm beyond the defect borders (Simion et al. 1994). Care should be taken to keep away from adjacent teeth by a minimum distance of 1–1.5 mm (Simion et al. 1994) to prevent bacterial contamination infiltrating the surgical site from the tooth sulcus. The graft is placed taking care to avoid saliva contamination. Then the membrane is folded buccally over the graft and stabilized with pins/screws. The graft should completely fill the space underneath the membrane (Tinti et al. 1996). The graft/membrane complex should be immobile, and the edges of the membrane should be properly fitted to the surrounding bone. When there is no possibility to fit the edges of the membrane onto the bone, the placement of a collagen membrane to cover the exposed areas of the graft has been proposed (Urban et al. 2014).

When a resorbable membrane is used (Figures 6.2, 6.3 and 6.5–6.7), the same approach can be followed. However, the fixation of the membrane can start either buccally (Figures 6.2, 6.3, 6.5 and 6.6) or palatally (Figure 6.7). The placement of a resorbable membrane, and notably a collagen membrane, in contact with the adjacent root should not pose any risk of bacterial infiltration from the tooth sulcus as with non-resorbable membranes. Resorbable membranes are widely used without fixation/stabilization with pins and tacs. However, this practice should be reviewed under the light of two recent studies using bone tacs to stabilize resorbable membranes (Urban et al. 2011, 2013) showing a mean lateral bone gain in ridge width that is considerably higher than what it was achieved with resorbable membrane that are not stabilized with pins. Randomized clinical trials

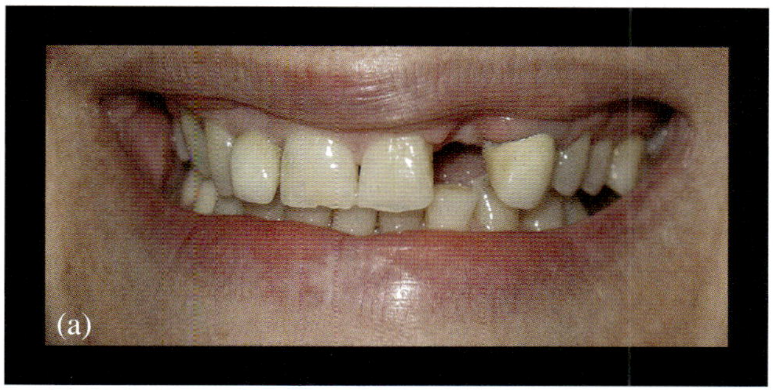

Figure 6.3 (a) Missing left lateral incisor with three-dimensional ridge defect.

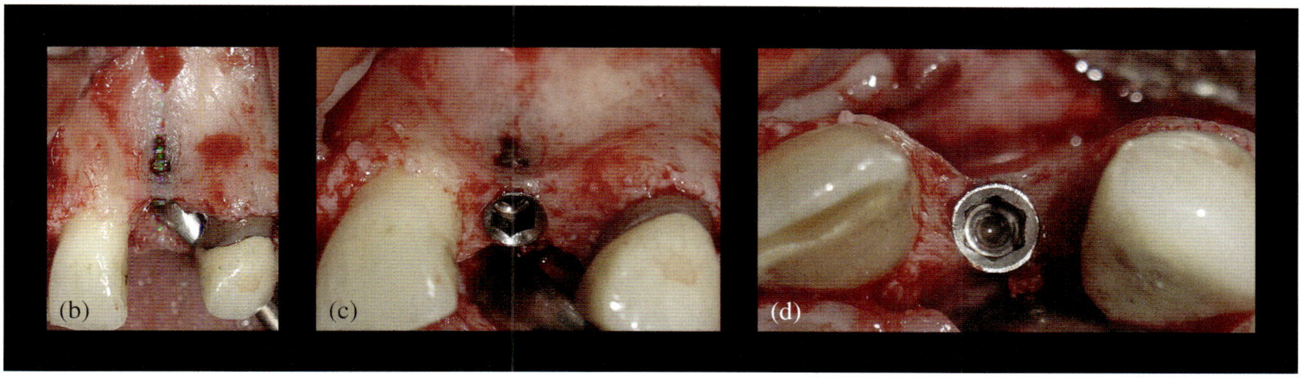

Figure 6.3 (b) Dehiscence-type defect at implant placement. (c) Dehiscence-type defect at implant placement. (d) Dehiscence-type defect at implant placement.

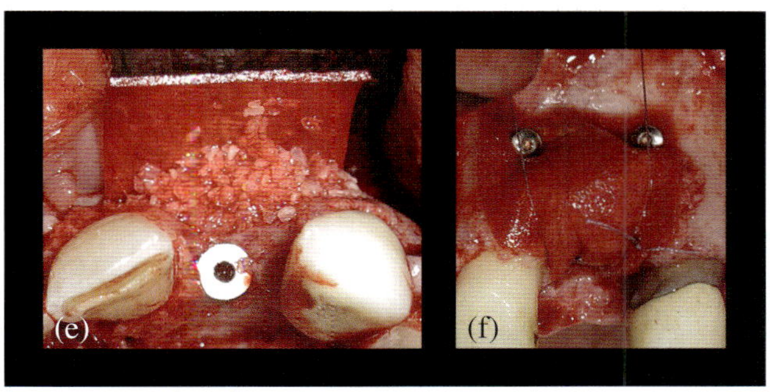

Figure 6.3 (e) Cross-linked collagen membrane (Cytoplast RTM) stabilized buccally with fixation pins creating a pouch that will be filled with the composite graft (1,1 enCore combination allograft and ABB). (f) Adaptation of the membrane onto the defect by using a periosteal mattress suture engaging the buccal periosteum and the palatal flap.

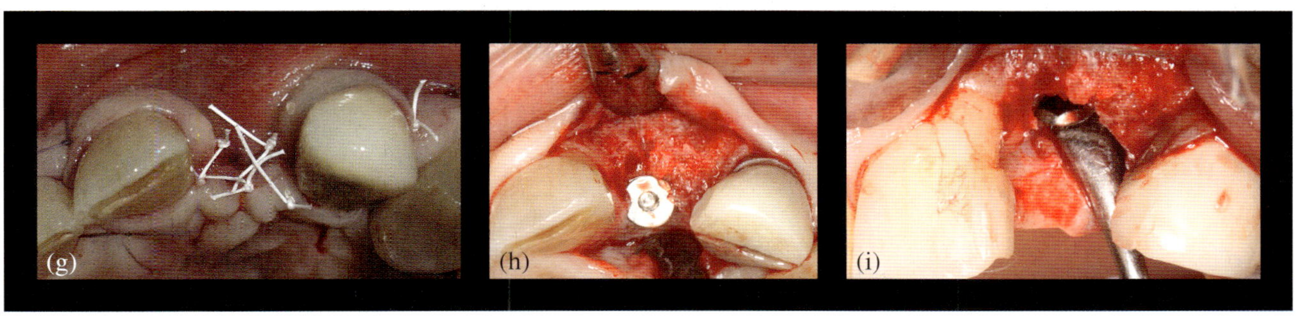

Figure 6.3 (g) Wound closure by means of two lines of sutures on the horizontal incision. (h) Abutment connection surgery at eight months. Complete regeneration of the buccal defect. (i) Abutment connection surgery at eight months. Complete regeneration of the buccal defect.

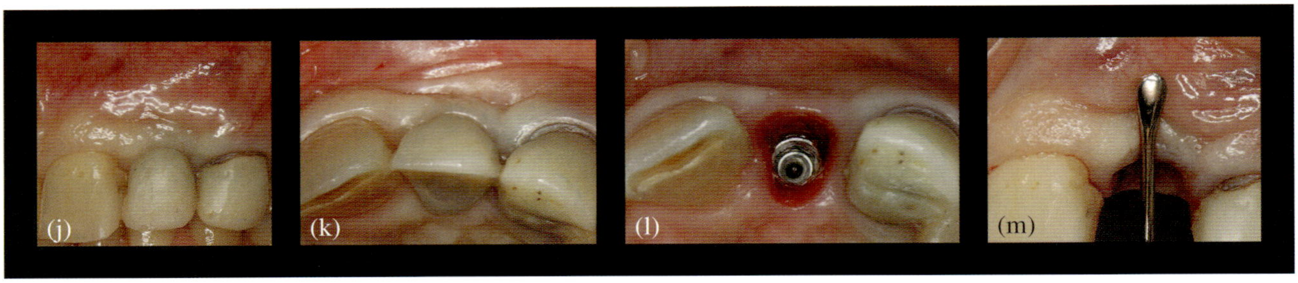

Figure 6.3 (j) Soft tissues after one year of temporization and tissue conditioning. Gingival margin slightly coronal to adjacent teeth. (k) Soft tissues after one year of temporization and tissue conditioning. Slight buccal concavity. (l) Removal of the screw-retained temporary crown to facilitate the creation of a buccal pouch in the soft tissue to accommodate a connective tissue graft. (m) Use of a small tunneling instrument to create a partial thickness buccal pouch.

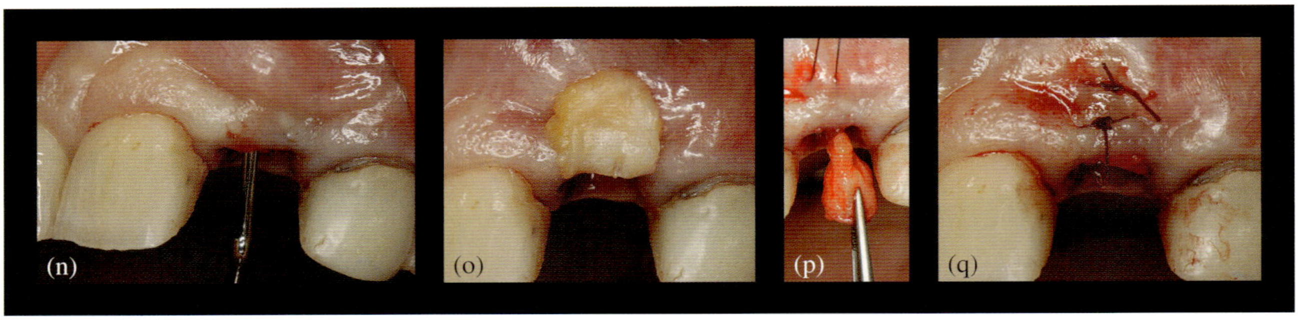

Figure 6.3 (n) Creation of the buccal pouch. (o) Dimensions of the connective tissue graft in relation to the recipient site. (p) Sliding of the connective tissue graft inside the pouch using a mattress suture. (q) Stabilization of the connective tissue graft with an additional mattress suture.

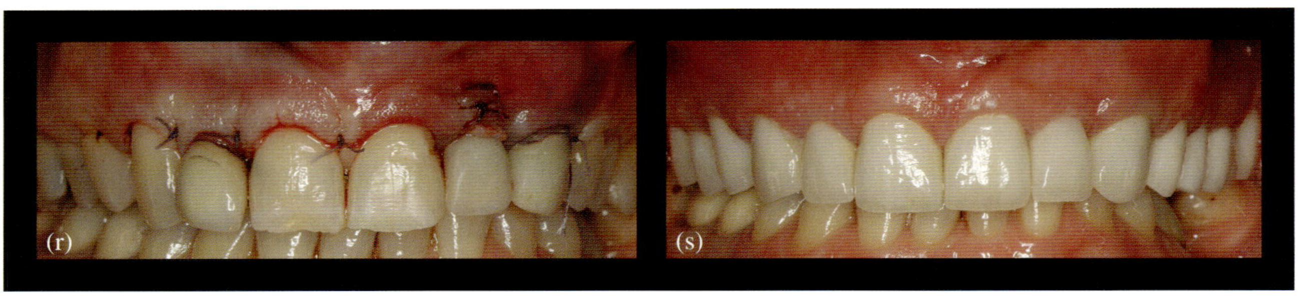

Figure 6.3 (r) A simultaneous crown lengthening on the adjacent teeth is performed to level the gingival margins. (s) Final crowns after one year.

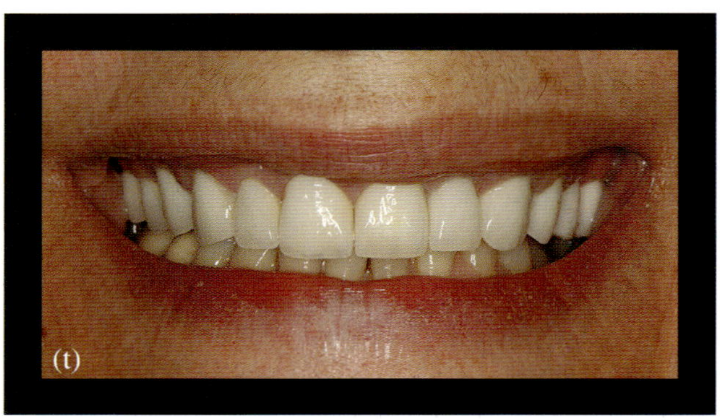

Figure 6.3 (t) Final crowns after one year.

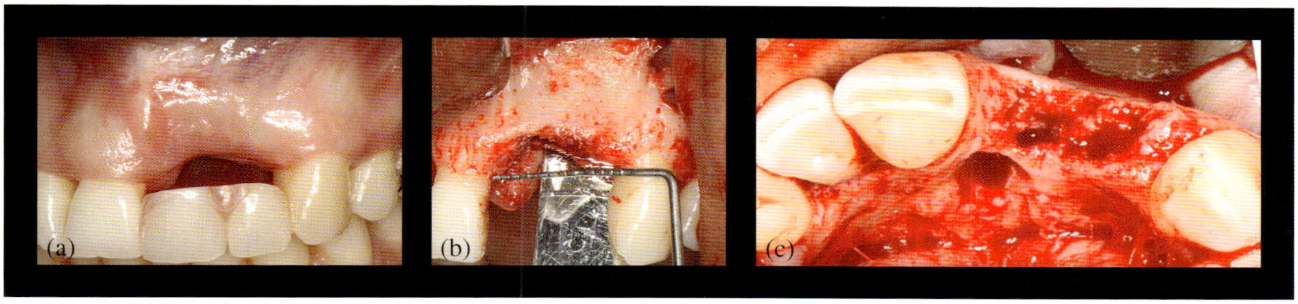

Figure 6.4 (a) Ridge defect on two adjacent sites in the esthetic zone. (b) Vertical component of the ridge defect amounting to more than 5 mm. (c) Occlusal view of the ridge showing the horizontal component of the defect and the presence of the incisive canal that would interfere with proper implant placement. The neuro-vascular bundle on the incisive canal was completely excised to allow bone regeneration in the canal space.

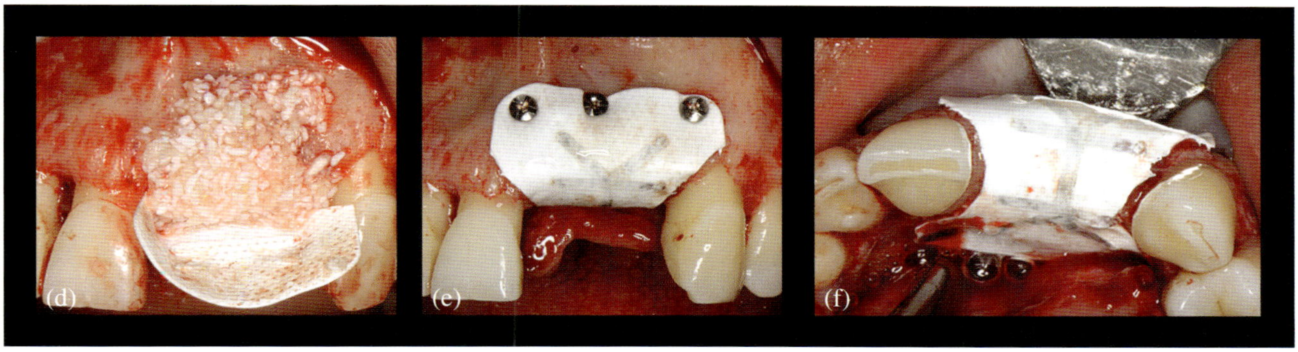

Figure 6.4 (d) Titanium-reinforced d-PTFE (Cytoplast) membrane secured with screws on the palatal aspect of the ridge. Composite bone graft consisting of 1 : 1 mixture of bone allograft (enCore combination) and anorganic bovine bone. (e) Membrane secured buccally with fixation pins. (f) The membrane is kept at a distance of 1–1.5 mm from the adjacent tooth root.

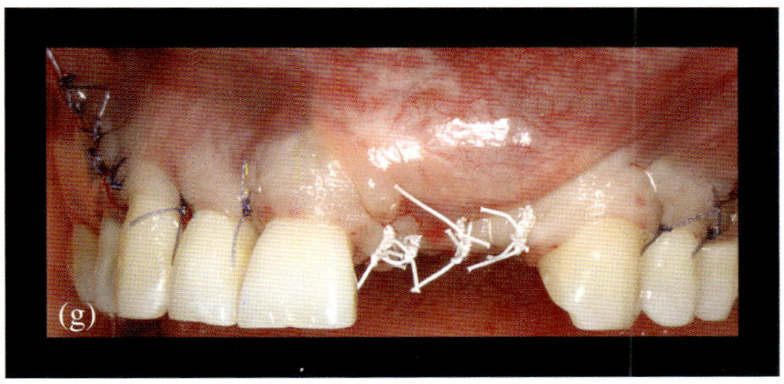

Figure 6.4 (g) Wound closure.

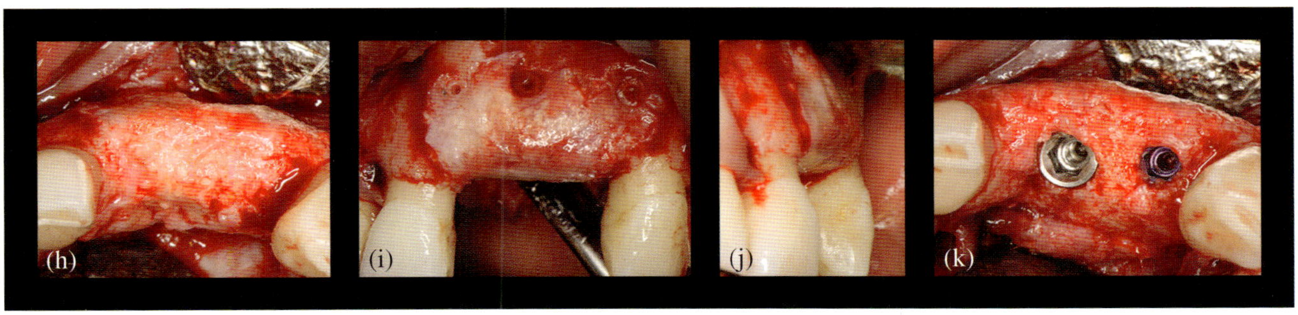

Figure 6.4 (h) Membrane removal at nine months. Occlusal view. Complete regeneration of the ridge defect, including the incisive canal. (i) Membrane removal at nine months. Buccal view. Complete regeneration of the ridge defect. (j) Membrane removal at nine months. Lateral view. Complete regeneration of the ridge defect. (k) Implants placed in a prosthetically driven position.

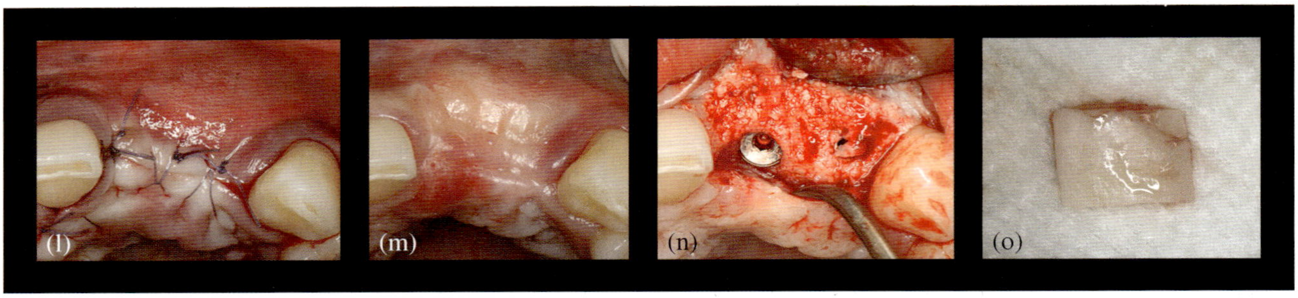

Figure 6.4 (l) Submerged healing. Gottlow sutures using a resorbable thread material. (m) Soft tissue healing after three months. (n) Second stage surgery. Note the overgrowth of bone over the cover screws. (o) Free gingival graft harvested from the tuberosity region. To be de-epithelialized extraorally.

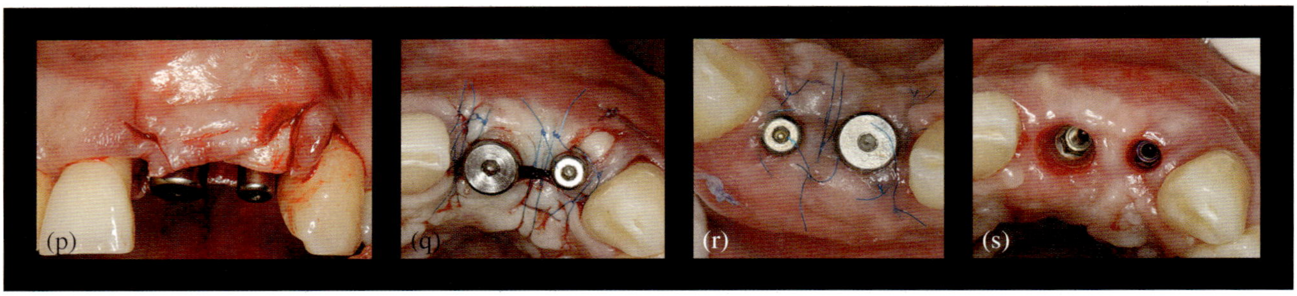

Figure 6.4 (p) The connective tissue graft is grafted buccally. Two small pedicles were separated from the buccal flap laterally to be able to have a primary intention closer at the levels of the papillae. (q) Sutures. 6(0) polypropylene. (r) Soft tissue healing at two weeks. Note the complete integration of the connective tissue graft and the absence of papillary sloughing. (s) Soft tissue maturation after six weeks.

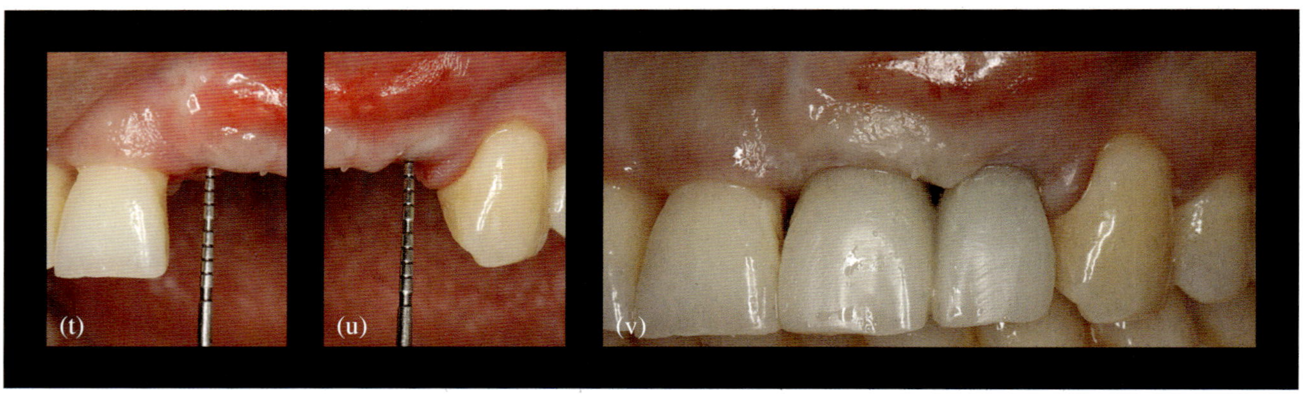

Figure 6.4 (t) Site 21: Presence of 5 mm of soft tissue thickness. (u) Site 22: Presence of 5 mm of soft tissue thickness. (v) Insertion of two temporary screw-retained crowns for the purpose of tissue conditioning.

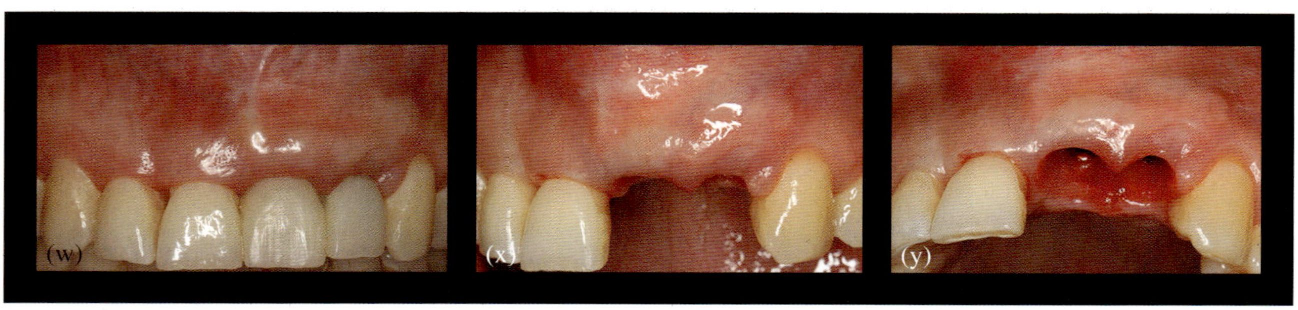

Figure 6.4 (w) After three months. (x) At three months: formation of a pseudo-papilla between 21 and 22. (y) At three months: formation of a pseudo-papilla between 21 and 22.

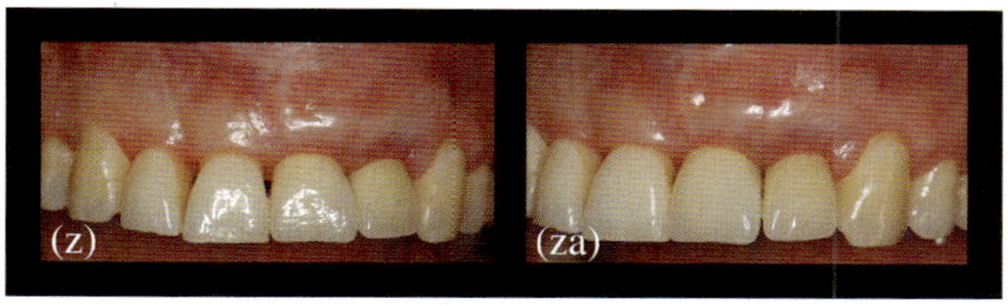

Figure 6.4 (z) Final crowns at seven months post-insertion. (za) Final crowns at seve months post-insertion.

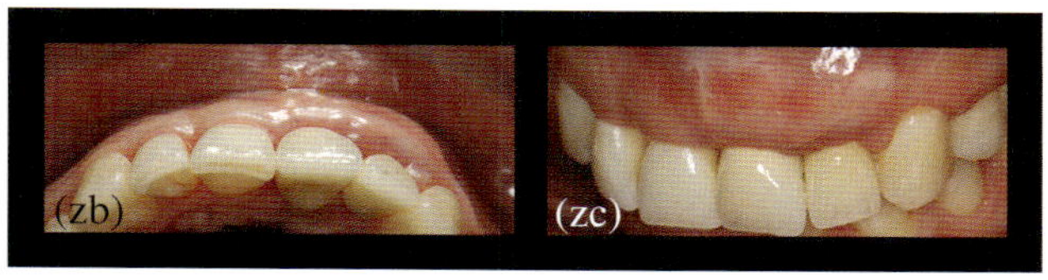

Figure 6.4 (zb) Final crowns at seven months post-insertion. (zc) Final crowns at seven months post-insertion.

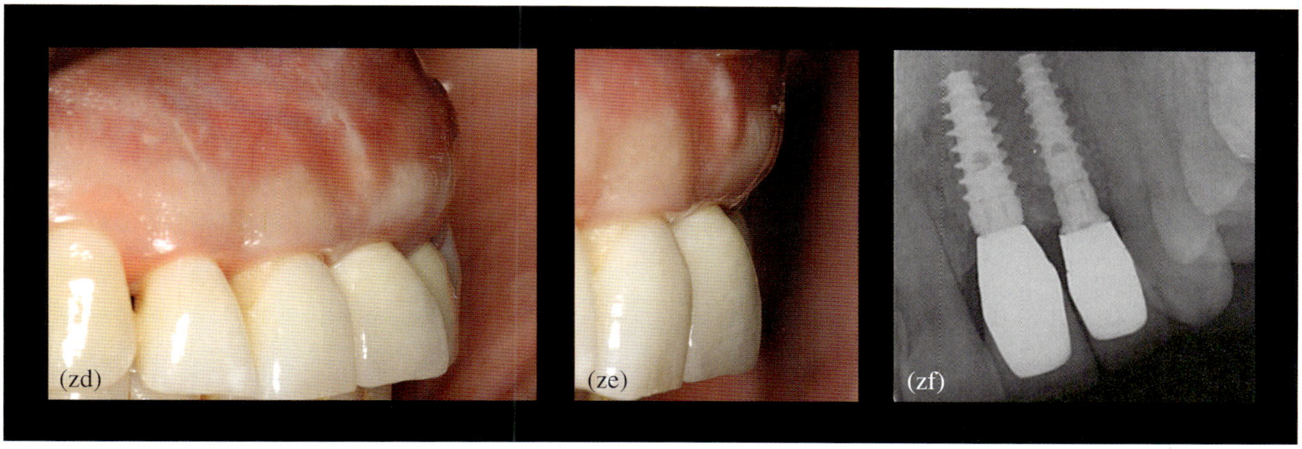

Figure 6.4 (zd) Final crowns at seven months post-insertion. (ze) Final crowns at seven months post-insertion. (zf) Final crowns at seven months post-insertion.

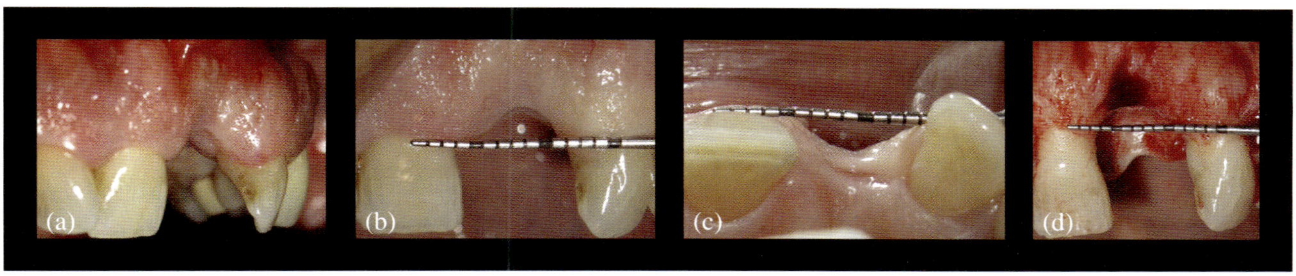

Figure 6.5 (a) Missing left central incisor with three-dimensional ridge defect. (b) Missing left central incisor with three-dimensional ridge defect. (c) Missing left central incisor with three-dimensional ridge defect. (d) Vertical component of the ridge defect.

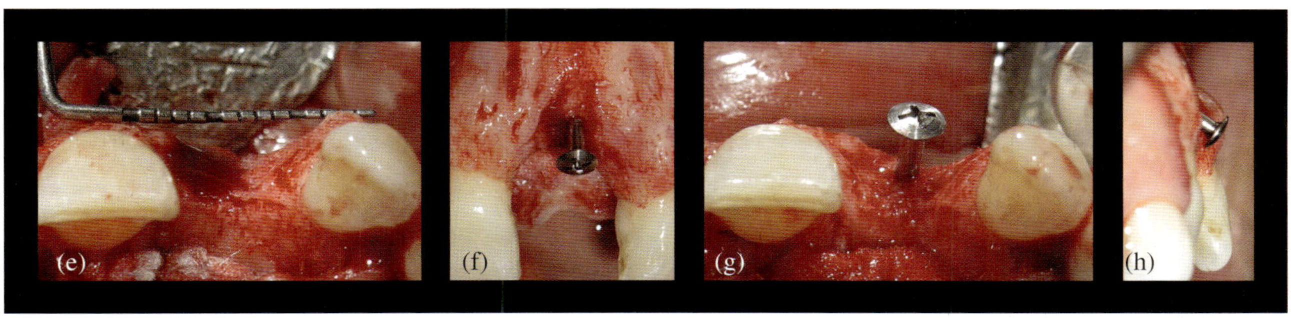

Figure 6.5 (e) Horizontal component of the ridge defect. (f) Placement of one tenting screw in the middle of the defect oriented buccally and coronally. (g) Placement of one tenting screw in the middle of the defect oriented buccally and coronally. (h) Placement of one tenting screw in the middle of the defect oriented buccally and coronally.

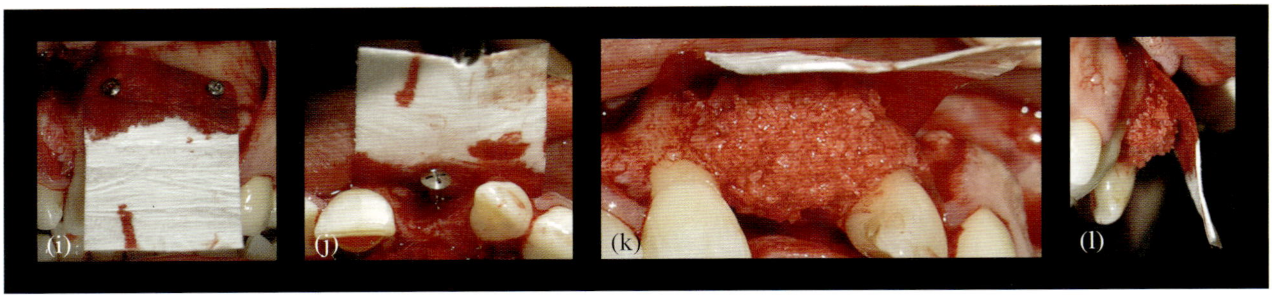

Figure 6.5 (i) Stabilization of a cross-linked collagen membrane (Cytoplast RTM) with two fixation pins placed buccally, creating a pouch-like containment of the particulate graft. (j) Stabilization of a cross-linked collagen membrane (Cytoplast RTM) with two fixation pins placed buccally, creating a pouch-like containment of the particulate graft. (k) Graft placement consisting of an allograft (enCore combination) mixed with autogenous bone collected with a bone scraper. (l) Graft placement consisting of an allograft (enCore combination) mixed with autogenous bone collected with a bone scraper.

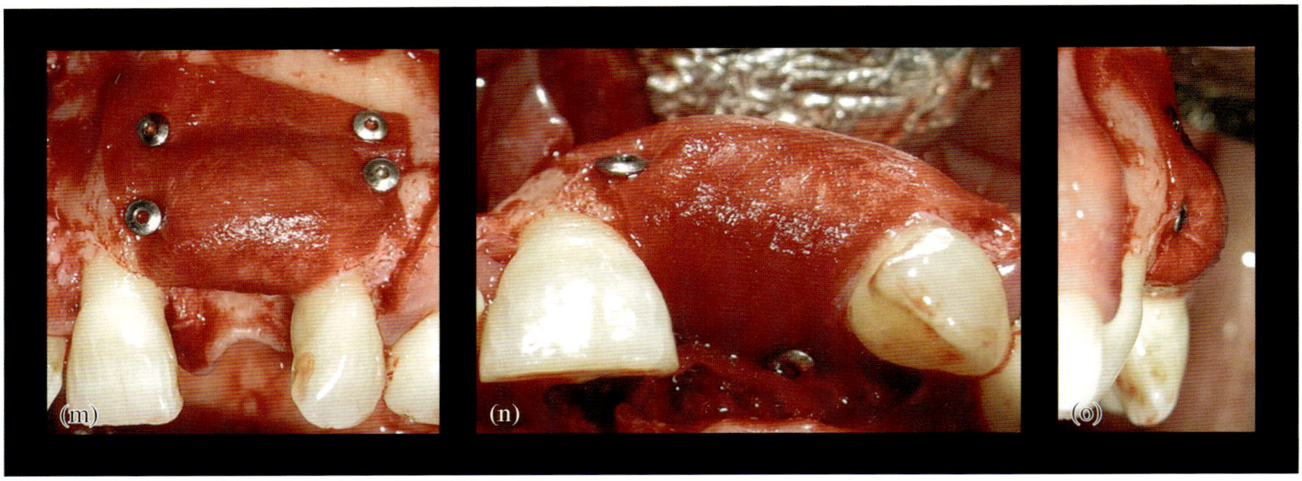

Figure 6.5 (m) Folding of the membrane over the defect and stabilization with additional fixation pins. The presence of the tenting screw will prevent excessive membrane collapse into the defect. (n) Folding of the membrane over the defect and stabilization with additional fixation pins. The presence of the tenting screw will prevent excessive membrane collapse into the defect. (o) Folding of the membrane over the defect and stabilization with additional fixation pins. The presence of the tenting screw will prevent excessive membrane collapse into the defect.

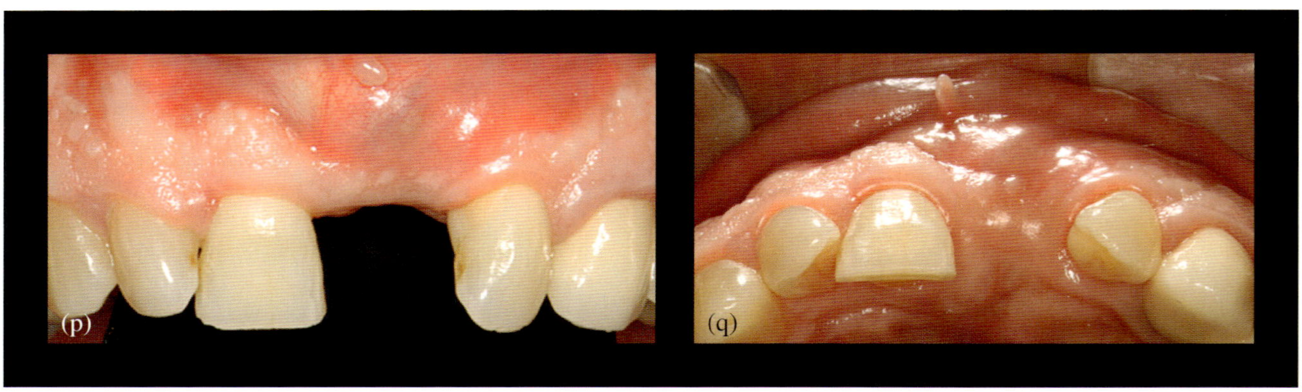

Figure 6.5 (p) Soft tissue healing at six months post-GBR. (q) Soft tissue healing at six months post-GBR.

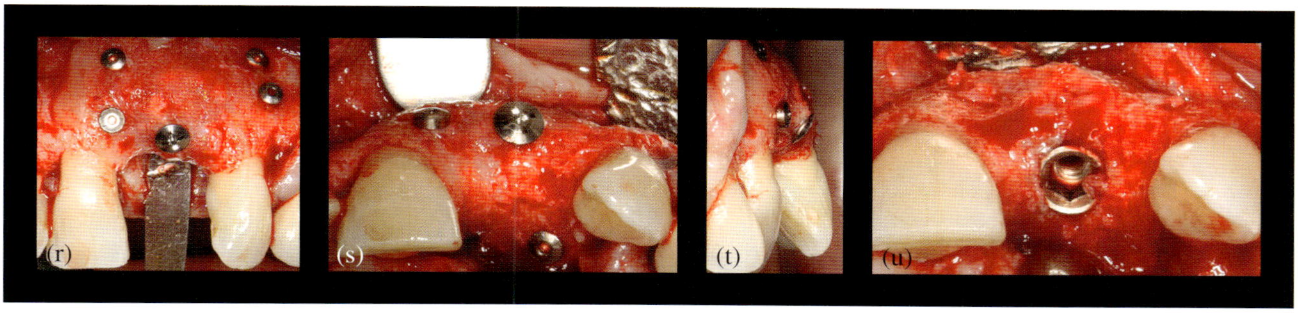

Figure 6.5 (r) Complete three-dimensional regeneration of the defect. (s) Complete three-dimensional regeneration of the defect. (t) Complete three-dimensional regeneration of the defect. Note the presence of regenerated bone around the tenting screw illustrating the importance of space maintenance in GBR. (u) Implant placement.

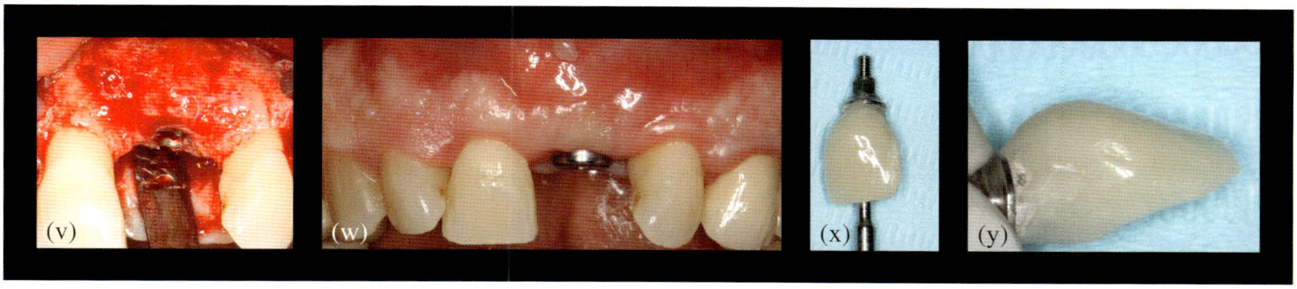

Figure 6.5 (v) Implant placement. (w) Tissue maturation at two months. (x) Fabrication of a screw-retained temporary crown for tissue conditioning. (y) Fabrication of a screw-retained temporary crown for tissue conditioning.

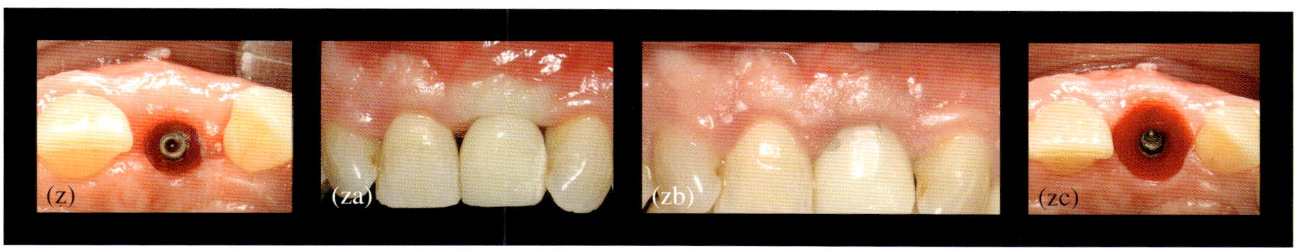

Figure 6.5 (z) Soft tissue emergence profile before the insertion of the temporary crown. (za) Insertion of the temporary crown. (zb) Soft tissue contour five weeks after the insertion of the temporary crown. (zc) Soft tissue emergence profile five weeks after the insertion of the temporary crown.

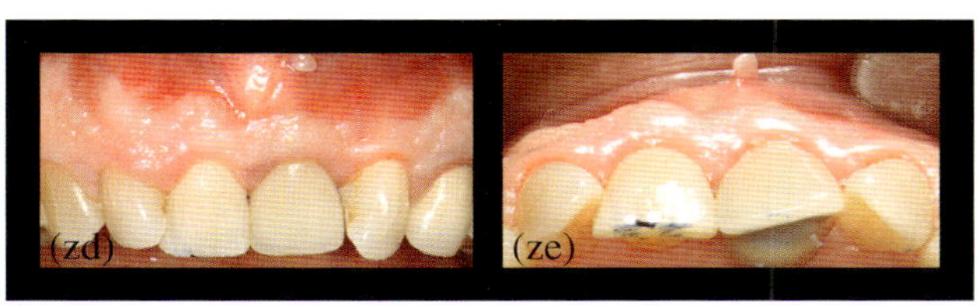

Figure 6.5 (zd) Final crown. Buccal view. (ze) Final crown. Occlusal view.

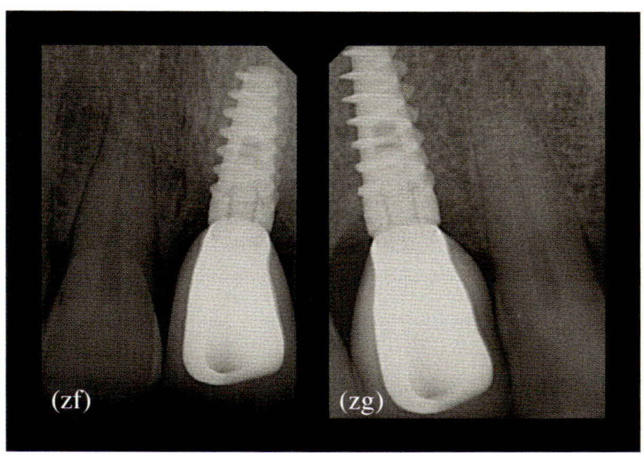

Figure 6.5 (zf) one year radiographic control. (zg) four years radiographic control.

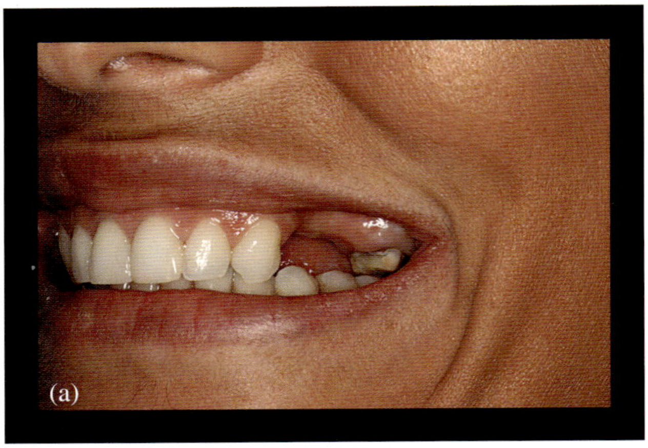

Figure 6.6 (a) Three-dimensional ridge defect on sites 24–25 in a high lip line smile.

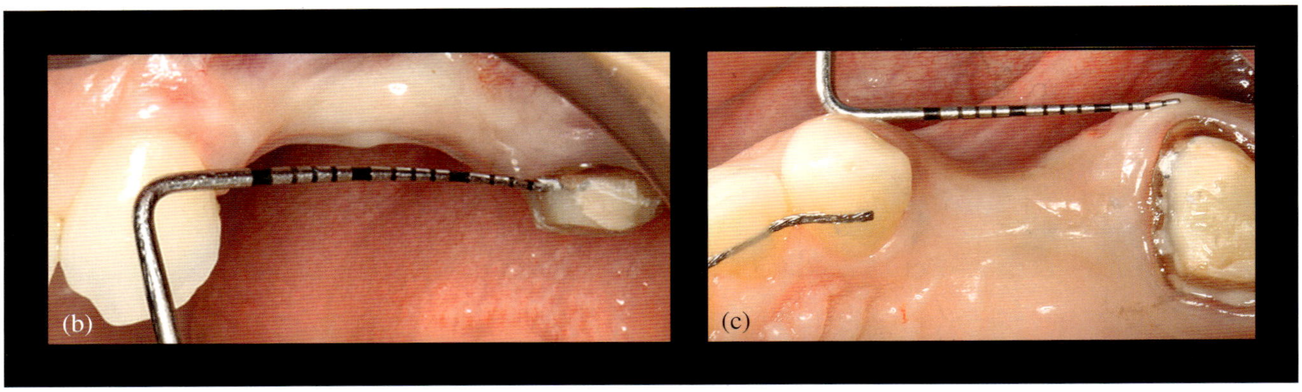

Figure 6.6 (b) Vertical component of the ridge defect. (c) Horizontal component of ridge defect.

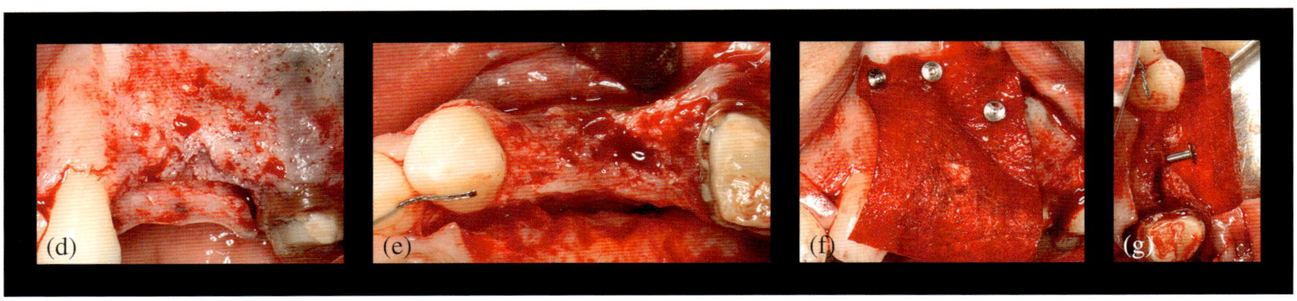

Figure 6.6 (d) Vertical component of the ridge defect. (e) Horizontal component of ridge defect. (f) Stabilization of a cross-linked collagen membrane (Cytoplast RTM) with three fixation pins placed buccally. (g) Occlusal view of the pouch formed by the collagen membrane. Tenting screw is oriented in a lateral and coronal direction.

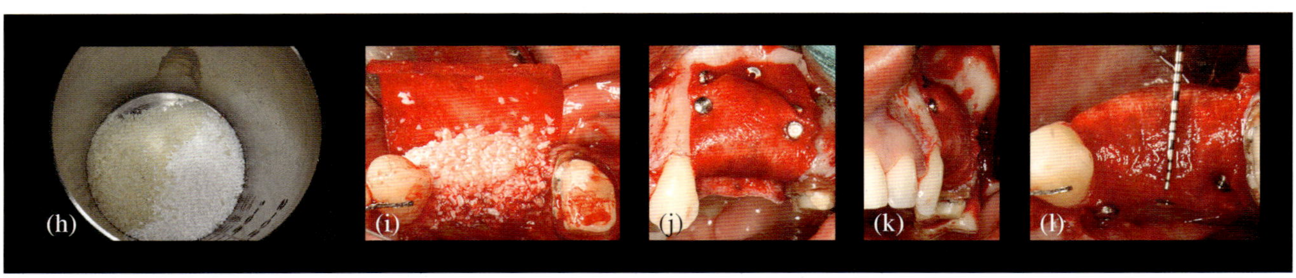

Figure 6.6 (h) Composite graft. 1 : 1 mixture of an allograft (enCore combination) and an anorganic bovine bone. (i) Graft placement in the pouch like space. (j) Folding of the membrane over the defect and stabilization with additional fixation pins. The presence of the tenting screws will prevent excessive membrane collapse into the defect. (k) Lateral view showing a complete fill of the defect with the graft/membrane complex. (l) The presence of the tenting screw will prevent inadvertent reduction in the graft volume during membrane fixation.

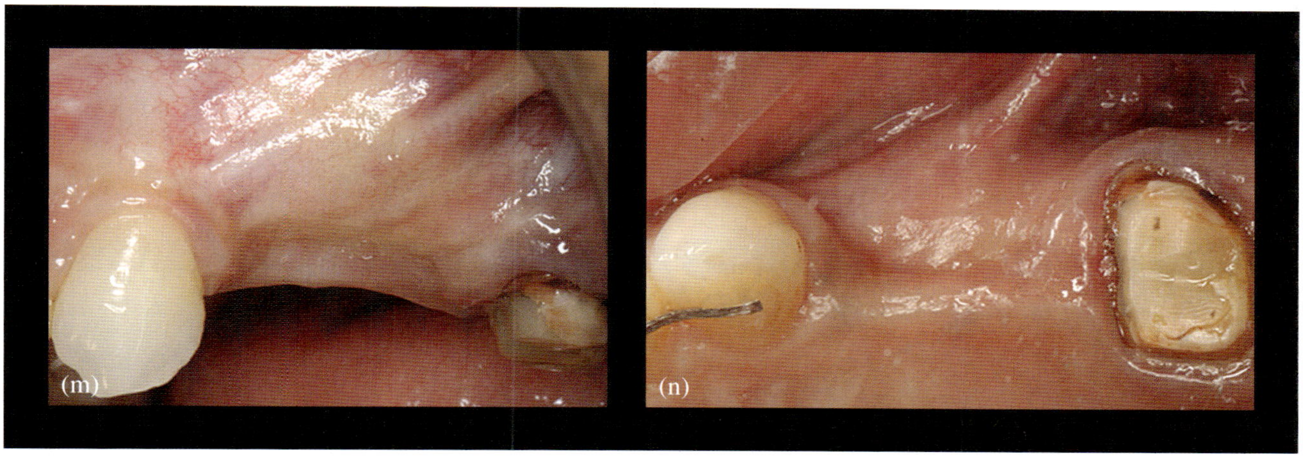

Figure 6.6 (m) Uneventful soft tissue healing. (n) Uneventful soft tissue healing.

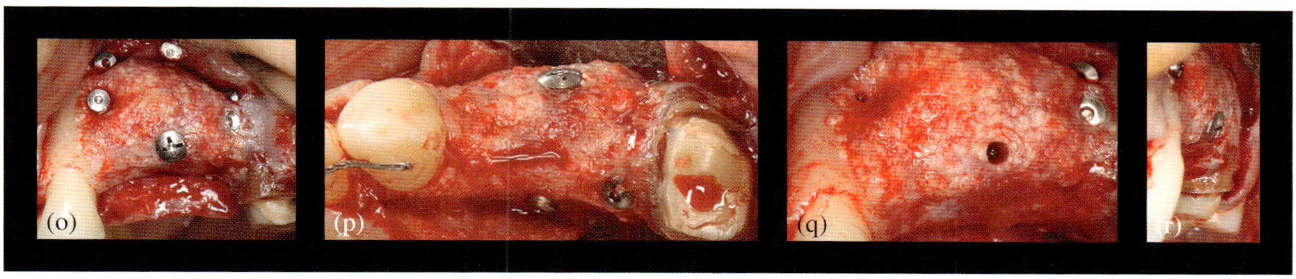

Figure 6.6 (o) Site exposure at seven months for implant placement: All the grafted volume was transformed into a newly regenerated bone. (p) Site exposure at seven months for implant placement: All the grafted volume was transformed into a newly regenerated bone. (q) Close-up view of the regenerated site showing excellent graft integration into the newly formed bone; bleeding at the site of the tenting screw as a sign of graft vitality; bone growth over the fixation pins. (r) Lateral view showing complete three-dimensional regeneration of the defect. Note the presence of regenerated bone around the tenting screw illustrating its importance in preventing membrane collapse into the defect.

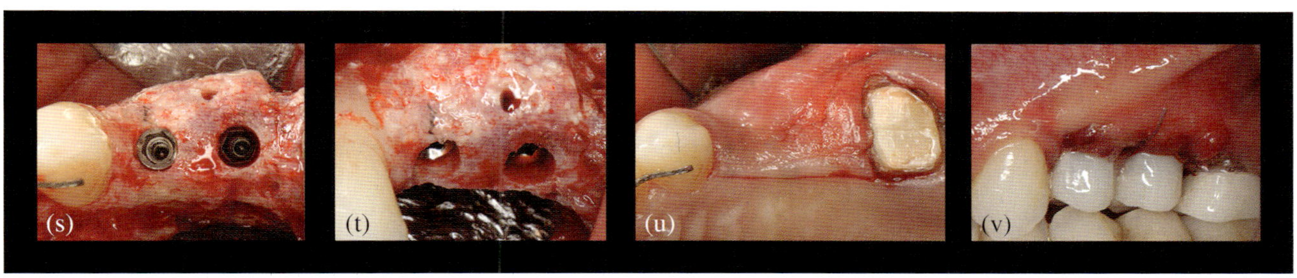

Figure 6.6 (s) Implant placement in a prosthetically driven position. (t) Implant placement in a prosthetically driven position. (u) Second stage surgery after 10 weeks: palatal incision to gain in keratinized tissue buccally to the implants. (v) Second stage surgery after 10 weeks: placement of the temporary crowns (prepared from an index performed at implant placement).

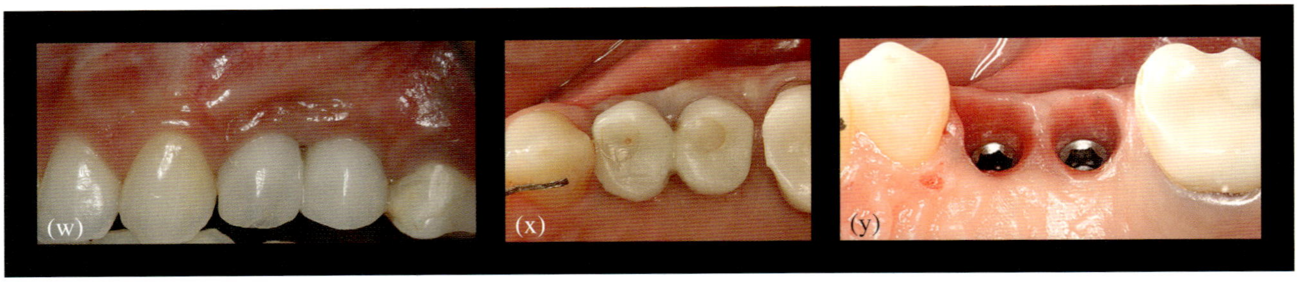

Figure 6.6 (w) Soft tissue maturation after nine months. (x) Soft tissue maturation after nine months. (y) Soft tissue maturation after nine months.

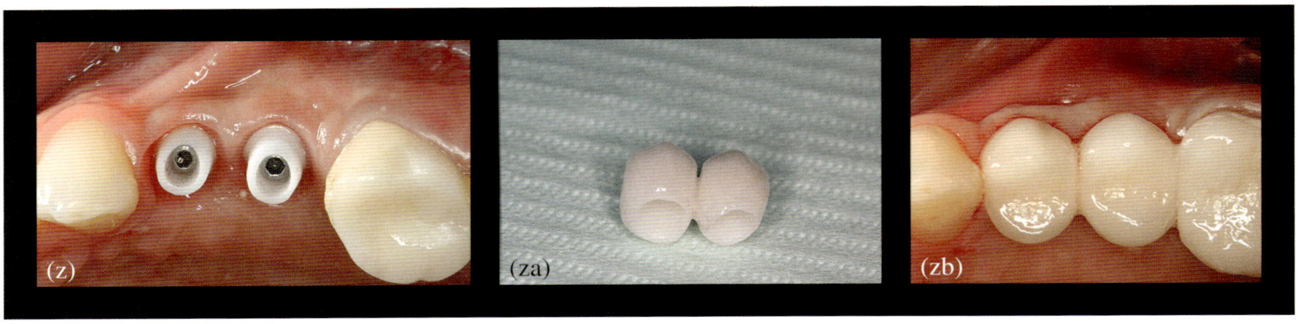

Figure 6.6 (z) Custom made zirconium abutments. (za) Lithium disilicate crowns. (zb) Delivery of the final crowns.

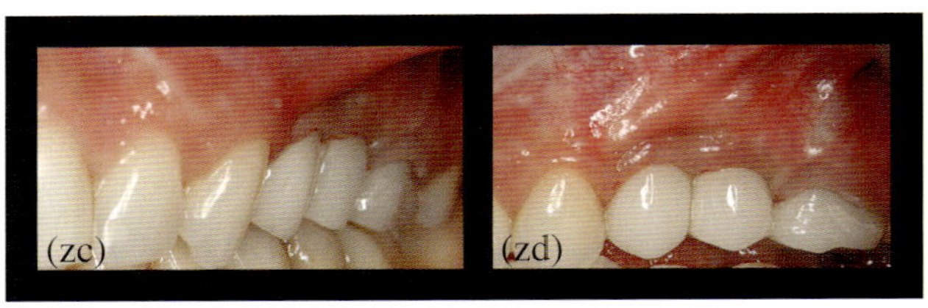

Figure 6.6 (zc) Delivery of the final crowns. (zd) Delivery of the final crowns.

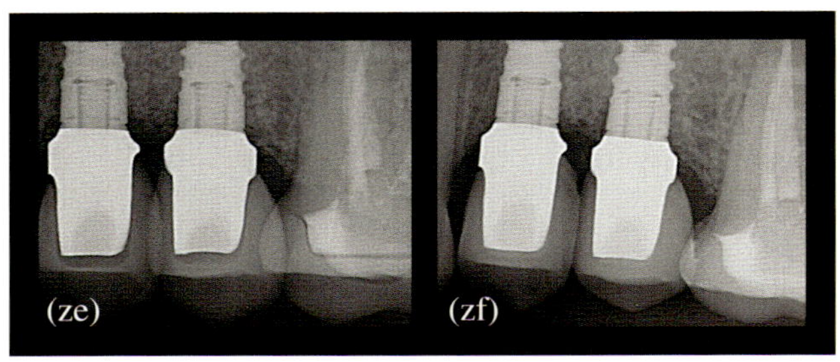

Figure 6.6 (ze) Radiographic control at crown delivery. (zf) Radiographic control at two years.

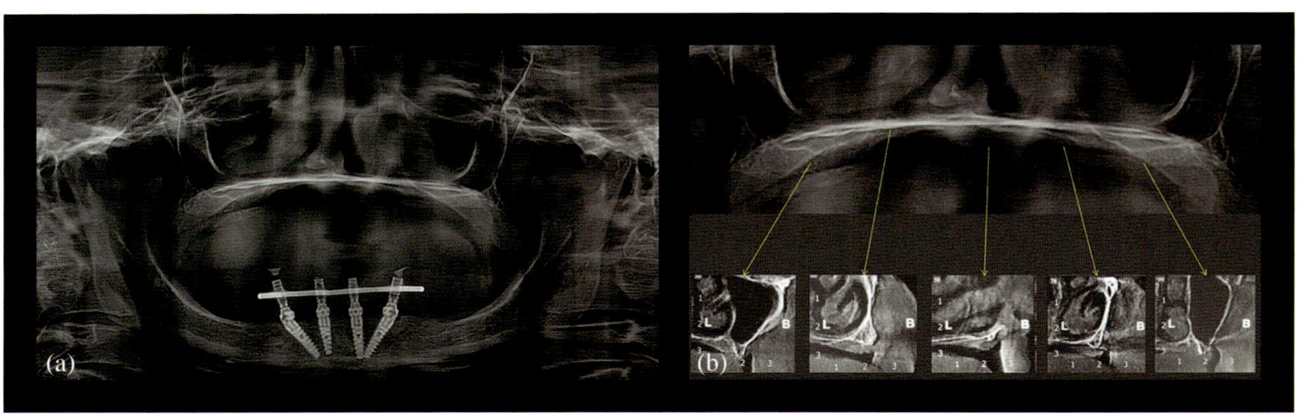

Figure 6.7 (a) Extremely atrophic maxilla in 54 years' old female. (b) Selective axial cuts from a cone beam ct showing the extreme atrophic condition of the maxilla.

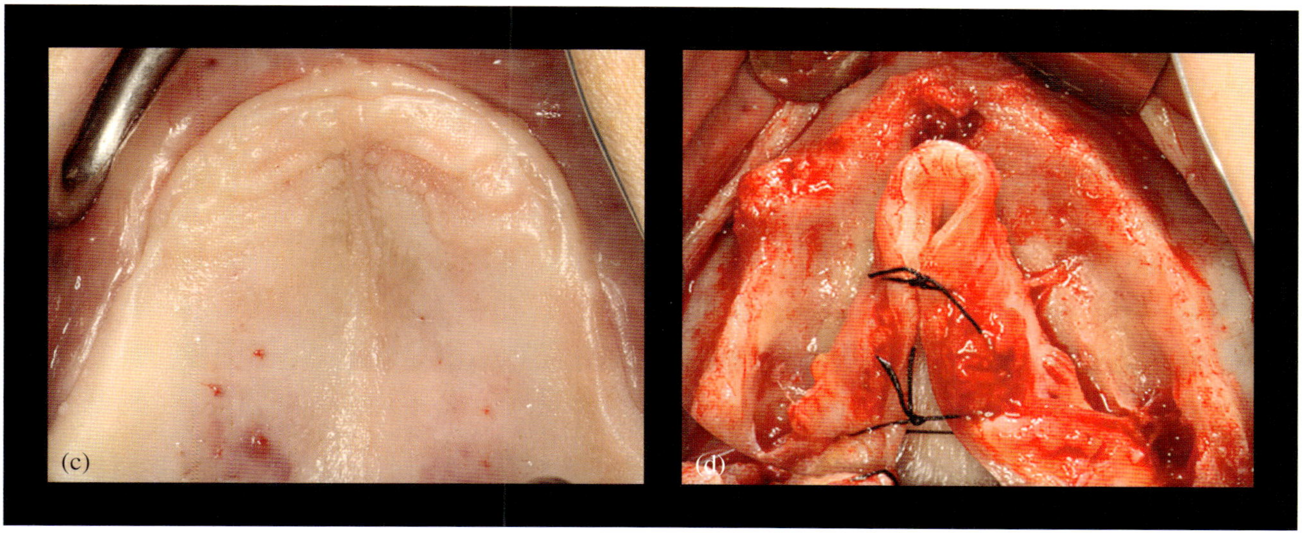

Figure 6.7 (c) Clinical view. (d) Full thickness flap elevation.

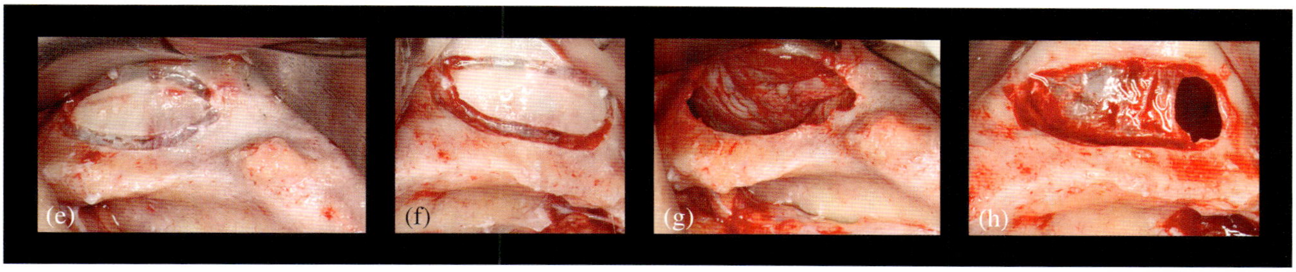

Figure 6.7 (e) Right: Bony window preparation for sinus access. (f) Left: Bony window preparation for sinus access. (g) Right: Elevation of the sinus mucosa. (h) Left: Elevation of the sinus mucosa. Note the occurrence of a mucosal perforation.

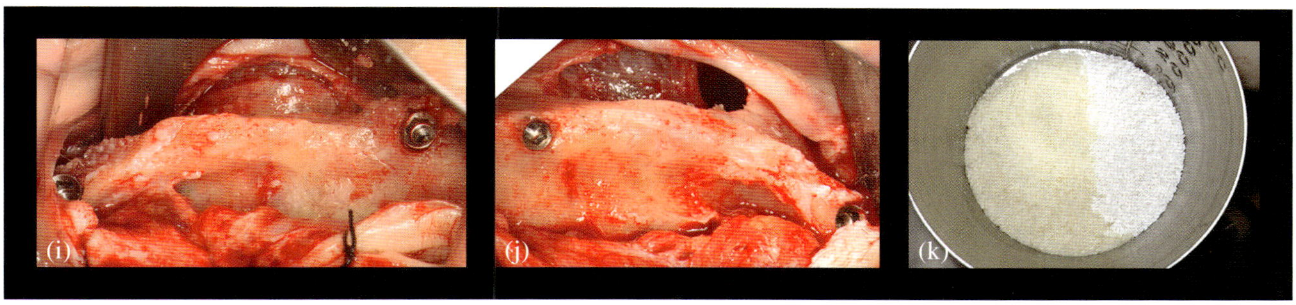

Figure 6.7 (i) Right: Placement of two temporary implants. One in the canine region engaging the nasomaxillary buttress, and one in the tuberosity region engaging the pterygoid bone. (j) Left: Placement of two temporary implants. One in the canine region engaging the nasomaxillary buttress, and one in the tuberosity region engaging the pterygoid bone. (k) Preparation of a composite graft consisting of 1 : 1 mixture of an allograft (enCore combination) and an anorganic bovine bone.

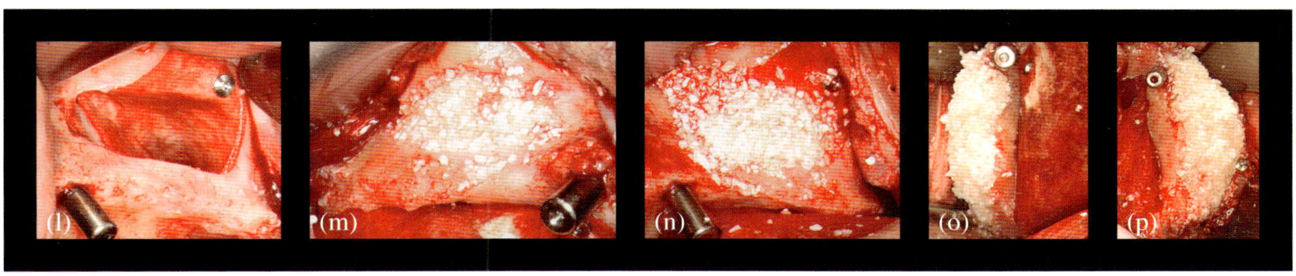

Figure 6.7 (l) Left: patching of the sinus perforation with a cross-linked collagen membrane. The membrane is stabilized with fixation pins. (m) Sinus graft in place. (n) Sinus graft in place. (o) Ridge graft placed laterally, covering the zone of the sinus window. (p) Ridge graft placed laterally, covering the zone of the sinus window.

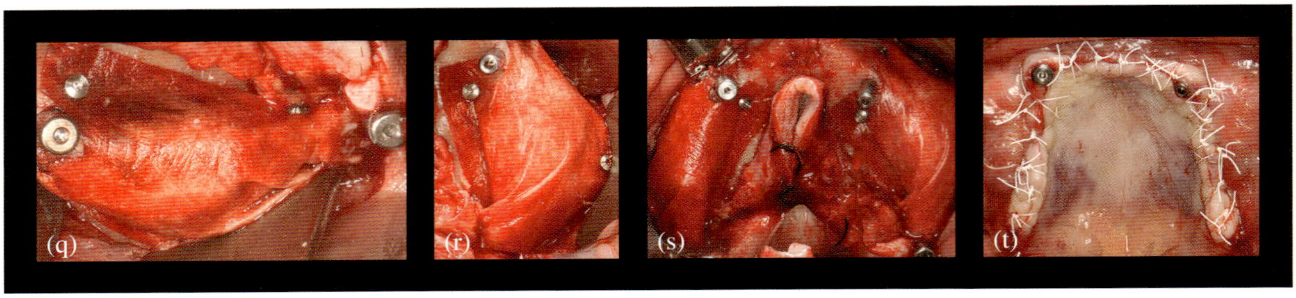

Figure 6.7 (q) Cross-linked collagen membrane (Cytoplast RTM) stabilized with fixation pins consolidating the particulate ridge graft and extending beyond the sinus window. (r) Cross-linked collagen membrane (Cytoplast RTM) stabilized with fixation pins consolidating the particulate ridge graft and extending beyond the sinus window. (s) Occlusal view of the complete maxillary arch showing the combined ridge and sinus augmentation on both sides of the maxilla. In this treatment approach, the anterior part of the maxilla is not grafted. The temporary implants will be immediately loaded with a screw-retained full-arch temporary bridge, providing esthetics and function to the patients during the graft maturation period. (t) Wound closure using two superimposed lines of sutures. Horizontal mattress in the deep layer, and a combination of Gottlow sutures and O sutures in the superficial layer.

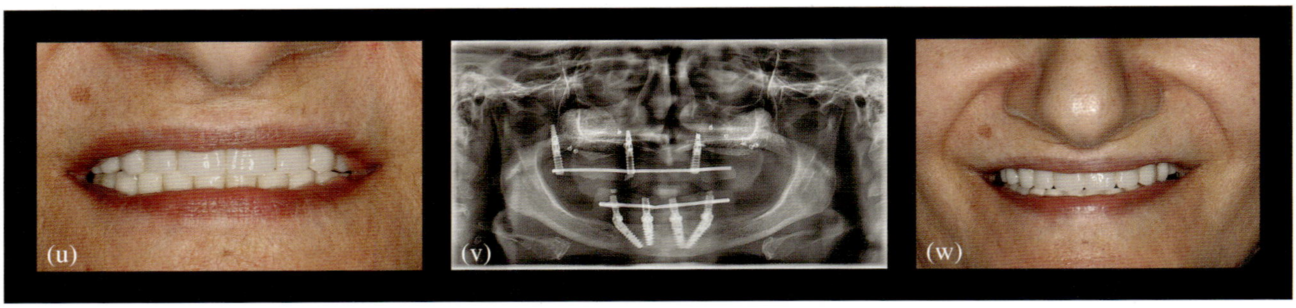

Figure 6.7 (u) Screw-retained temporary fixed prosthesis delivered in the days following the surgery. (v) Radiographic control after the temporary prosthesis delivery. The implant placed in the left tuberosity was mobile and was consequently removed. The prosthesis was attached on the three remaining temporary implants. (w) Temporary prosthesis still in function 14 months after the bone graft surgery.

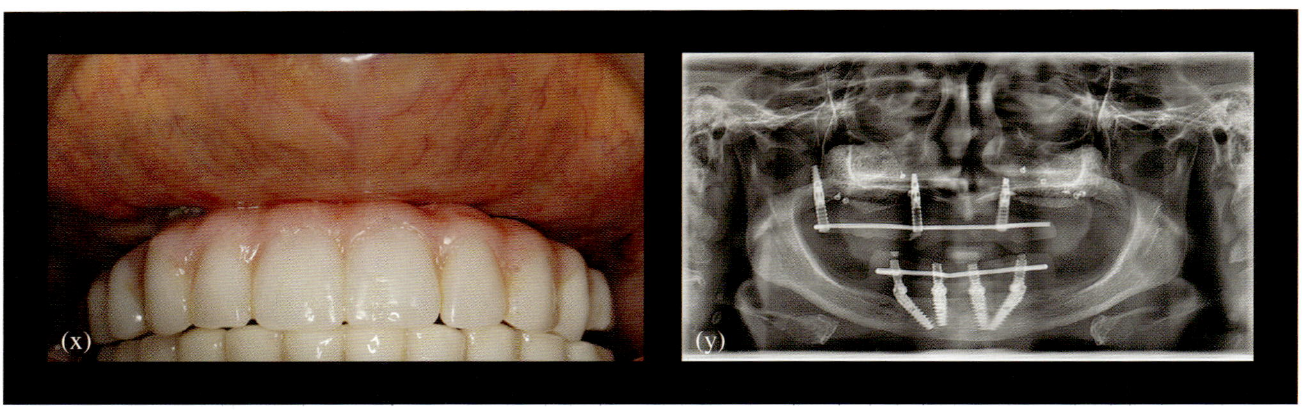

Figure 6.7 (x) Intraoral view of the temporary prosthesis. (y) Radiographic control 14 months after the bone graft surgery.

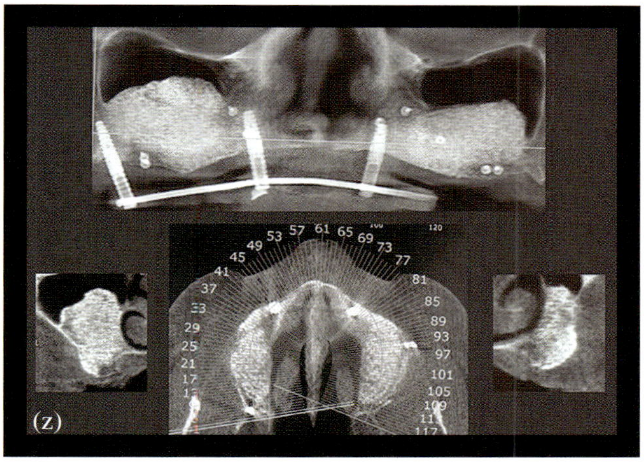

Figure 6.7 (z) Cone beam CT control at 14 months showing the extent of the graft volume in the maxillary sinus and laterally to the alveolar ridge.

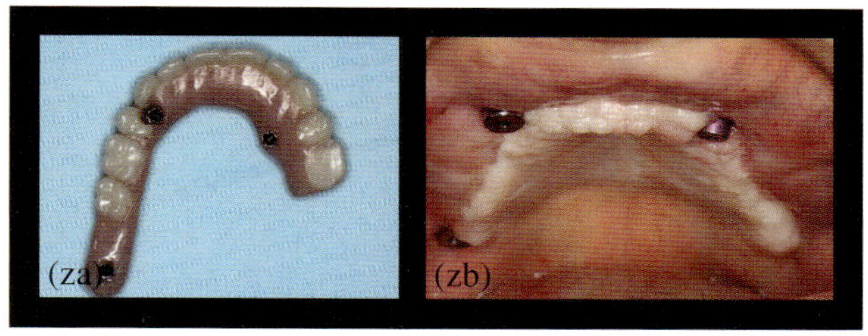

Figure 6.7 (za) Removal of the temporary prosthesis before the implant placement surgery. (zb) Note, laterally, the volume occupied by the ridge graft. Note the reduction in vestibular depth and the absence of keratinized tissue on the occlusal and vestibular aspect of the ridge in the grafted area.

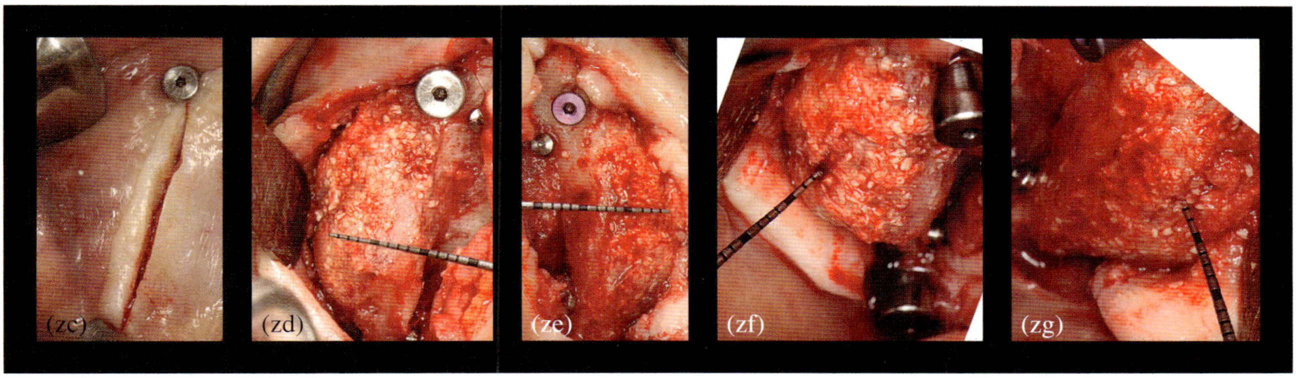

Figure 6.7 (zc) Crestal incision displaced in a palatally to be able to transpose a band of keratinized tissue buccally to the implants. (zd) Substantial increase in ridge width. (ze) Substantial increase in ridge width. (zf) Lateral force probing of the grafted region: only 1 mm of the probe is penetrating the grafted region, showing excellent graft consolidation. (zg) Lateral force probing of the grafted region: only 1 mm of the probe is penetrating the grafted region, showing excellent graft consolidation.

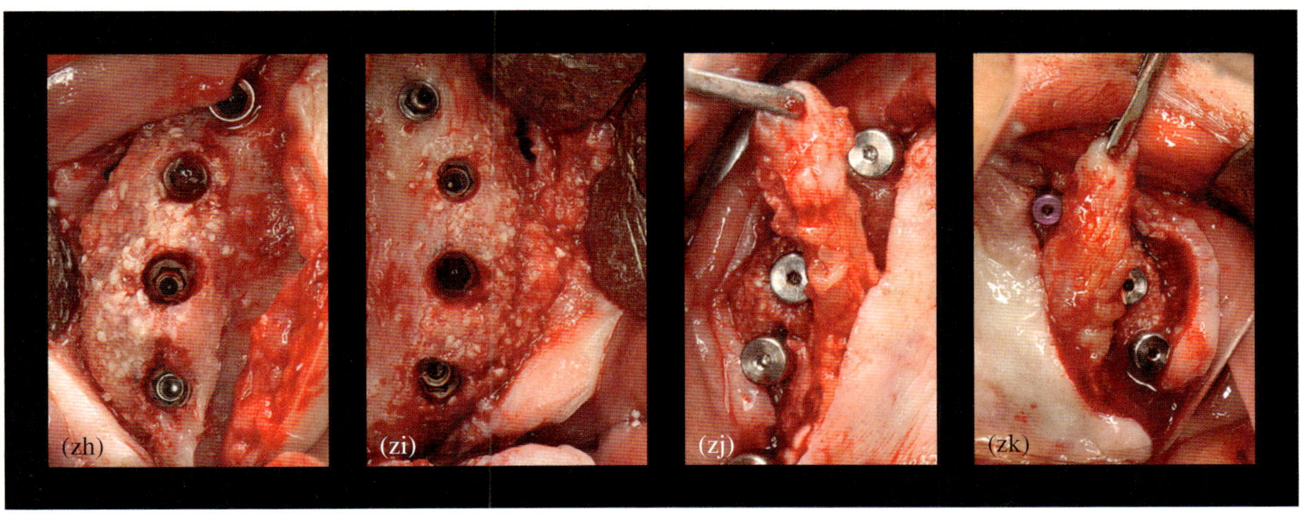

Figure 6.7 (zh) Right: placement of three implants in the grafted area. (zi) Left: placement of three implants in the grafted area. (zj) Palatal pedicle flaps elevated form the thickness of the palatal tissue and rotated laterally to cover the exposed bony area of the alveolar ridge. (zk) Palatal pedicle flaps elevated form the thickness of the palatal tissue and rotated laterally to cover the exposed bony area of the alveolar ridge.

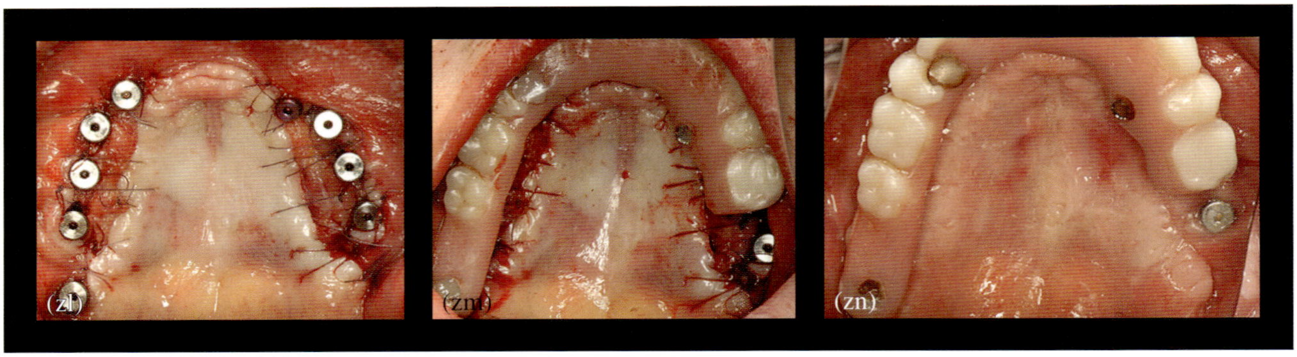

Figure 6.7 (zl) Wound closure. (zm) Temporary prosthesis secured back in place. (zn) Healing of the palatal area after eight weeks.

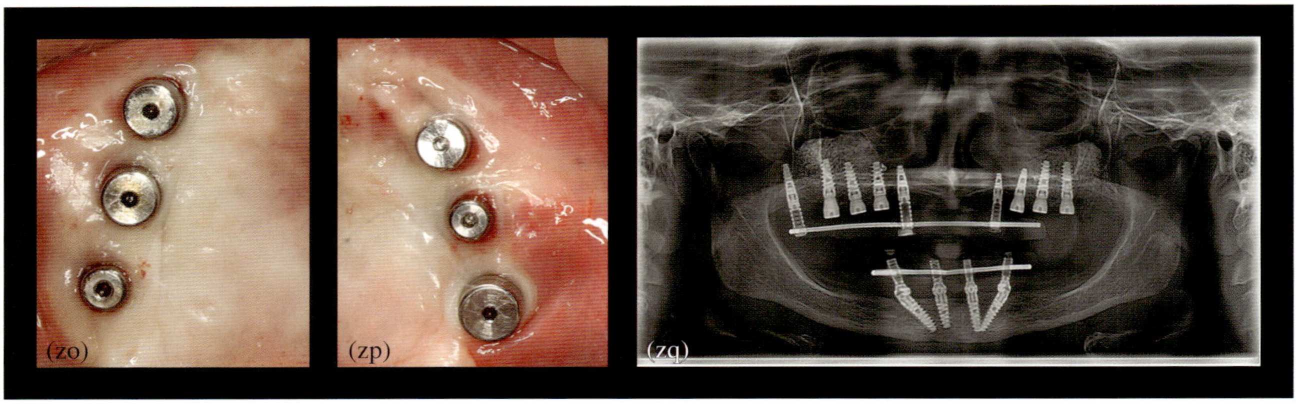

Figure 6.7 (zo) Note the presence of keratinized tissue buccally to the implants. (zp) Note the presence of keratinized tissue buccally to the implants. (zq) Radiographic control four months after implant placement.

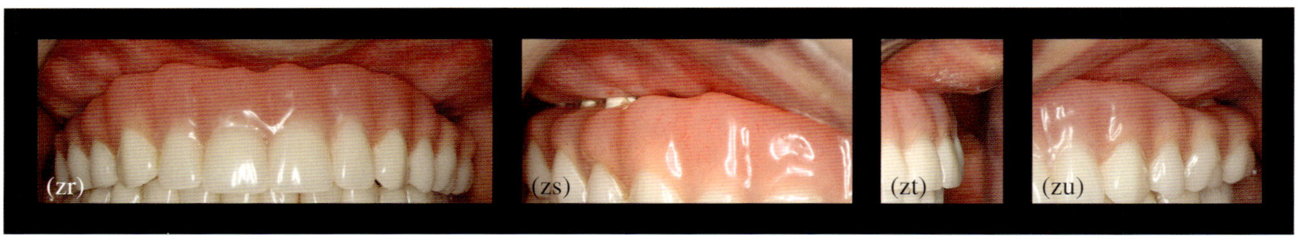

Figure 6.7 (zr) Final prosthesis. (zs) Final prosthesis, right side. Designed to allow hygiene procedures around the implants. (zt) Front part of the prosthesis. The fact that no implants are placed anteriorly allows more freedom in prosthetic construction, notably the creation of a proper lip support. (zu) Final prosthesis, right side. Designed to allow hygiene procedures around the implants.

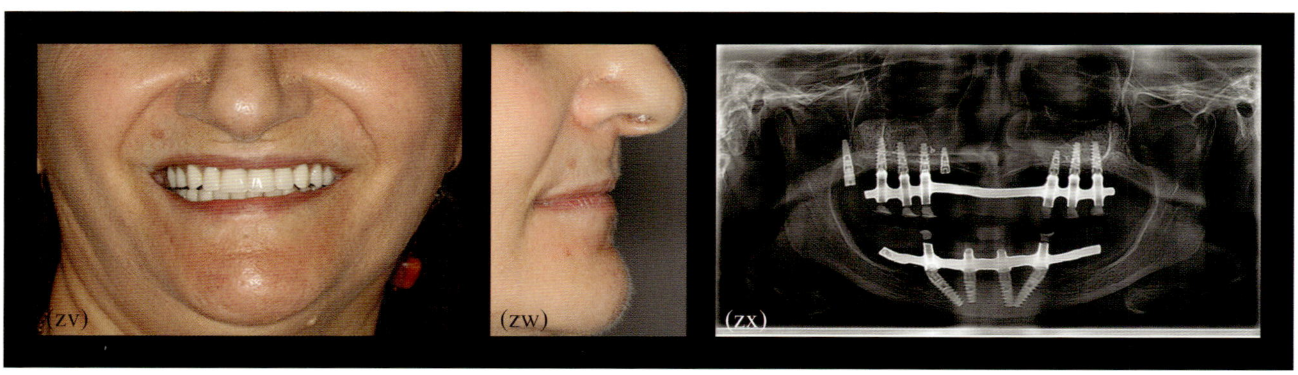

Figure 6.7 (zv) Patient's smile. (zw) Patient's profile. Note the proper lip support. (zx) Two years radiographic control. The right tuberosity implant was not incorporated into the final prosthesis due to access difficulties. The right canine temporary implant was submerged because reverse torqueing was not enough to explant it. The left canine temporary implant was easily explanted with reverse torqueing.

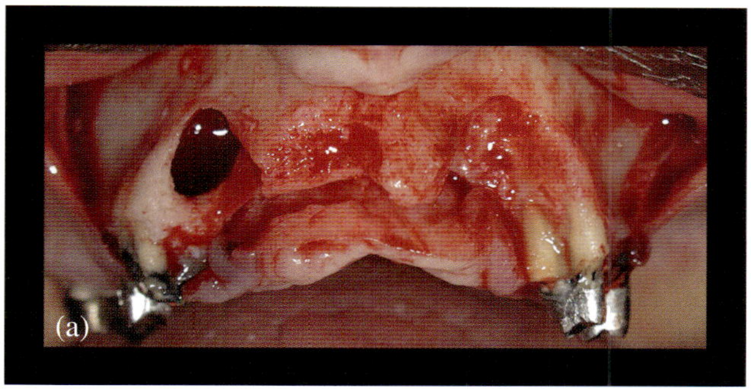

Figure 6.8 (a) Extensive three-dimensional ridge defect in the anterior maxilla and communicating with the right maxillary sinus. Sinus membrane was not perforated.

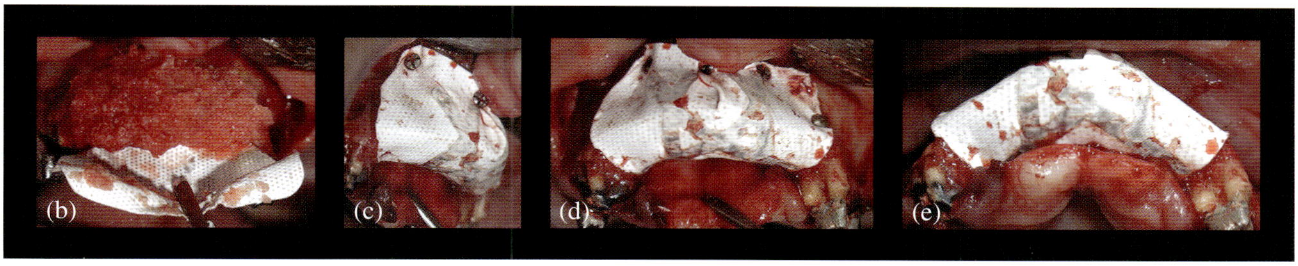

Figure 6.8 (b) Titanium-reinforced d-PTFE (Cytoplast) membrane secured with screws on the palatal aspect of the ridge. Composite bone graft consisting of a mixture of bone allograft (enCore combination) and autogenous bone. (c) Shaping and adaptation of the membrane buccally with miniscrews. The membrane is shaped to allow the re-establishment of the arch curvature. (d) Shaping and adaptation of the membrane buccally with miniscrews. The membrane is shaped to allow the re-establishment of the arch curvature. (e) Shaping and adaptation of the membrane buccally with miniscrews. The membrane is shaped to allow the re-establishment of the arch curvature.

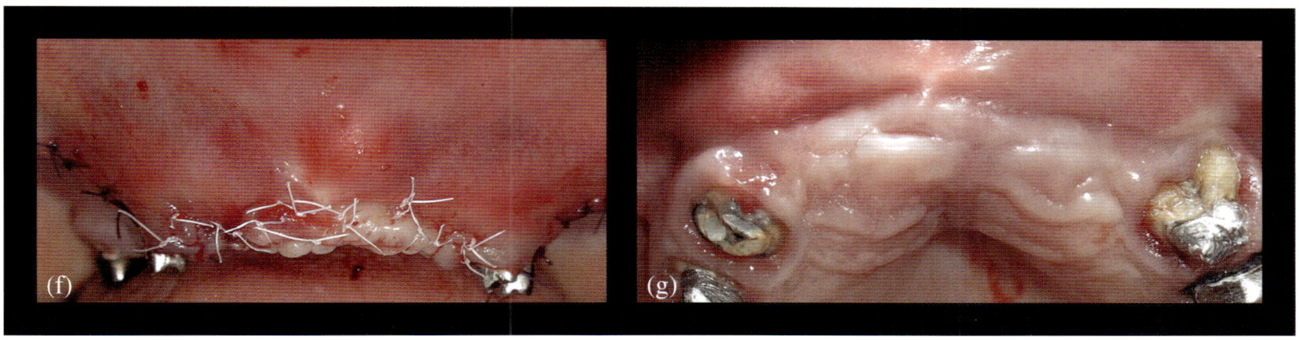

Figure 6.8 (f) Tension free wound closure. (g) Uneventful soft tissue healing.

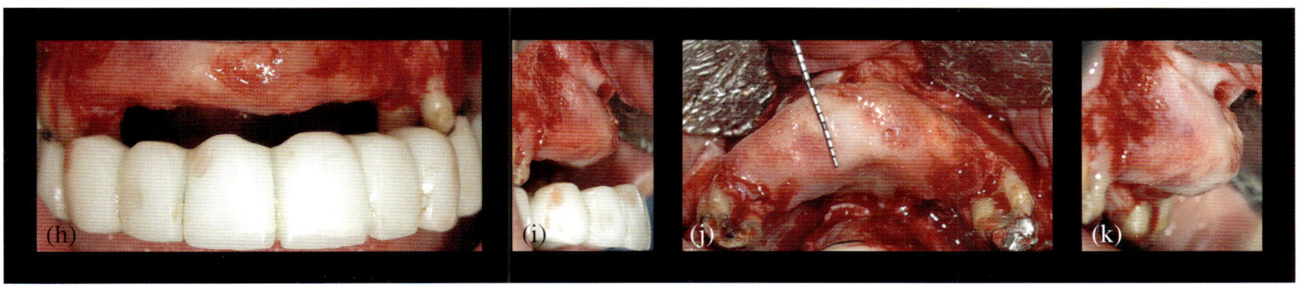

Figure 6.8 (h) Re-entry at nine months: complete regeneration of the space underneath the membrane. Note the presence of the fibrous tissue layer covering the regenerated bone. (i) Re-entry at nine months: complete regeneration of the space underneath the membrane. Note the presence of the fibrous tissue layer covering the regenerated bone. (j) Re-entry at nine months: complete regeneration of the space underneath the membrane. Note the presence of the fibrous tissue layer covering the regenerated bone. (k) Re-entry at nine months: complete regeneration of the space underneath the membrane. Note the presence of the fibrous tissue layer covering the regenerated bone.

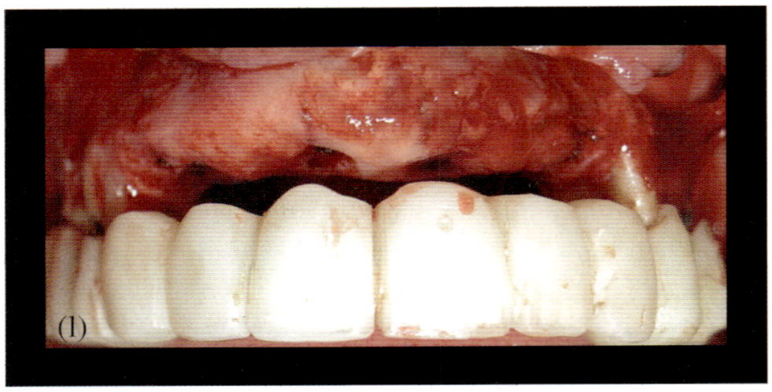

Figure 6.8 (l) Implant placement in a prosthetically driven position.

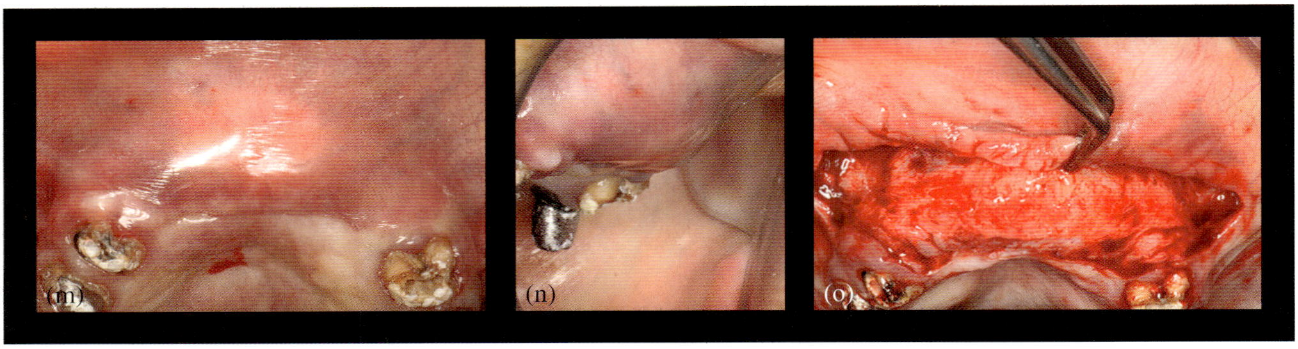

Figure 6.8 (m) Soft tissue healing after implant placement. Note the absence of the vestibule and the absence of keratinized tissue on the crestal and buccal aspect of the ridge. The alveolar mucosa is in contact with palatal gingiva. (n) Soft tissue healing after implant placement. Note the absence of the vestibule and the absence of keratinized tissue on the crestal and buccal aspect of the ridge. The alveolar mucosa is in contact with palatal gingiva. (o) Superficial split thickness incision aiming at repositioning the mucosa at the fornix of the vestibule.

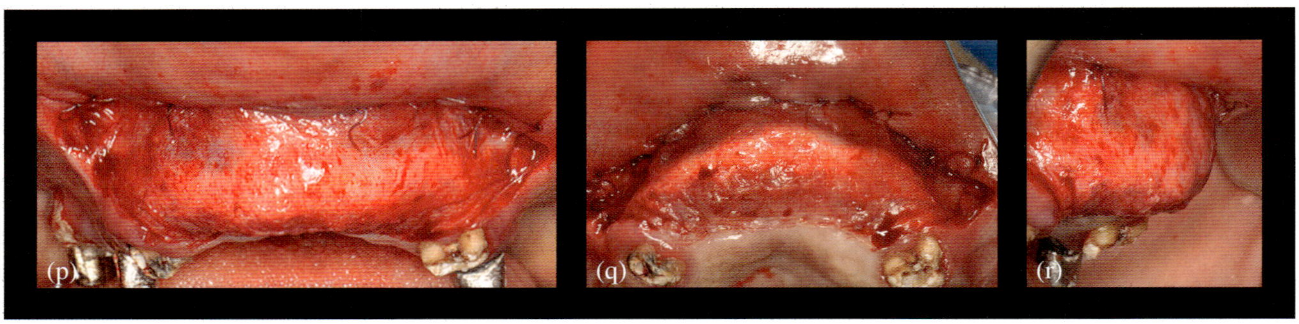

Figure 6.8 (p) Suturing of the partial thickness flap at the fornix of the vestibule. (q) Suturing of the partial thickness flap at the fornix of the vestibule. (r) Suturing of the partial thickness flap at the fornix of the vestibule.

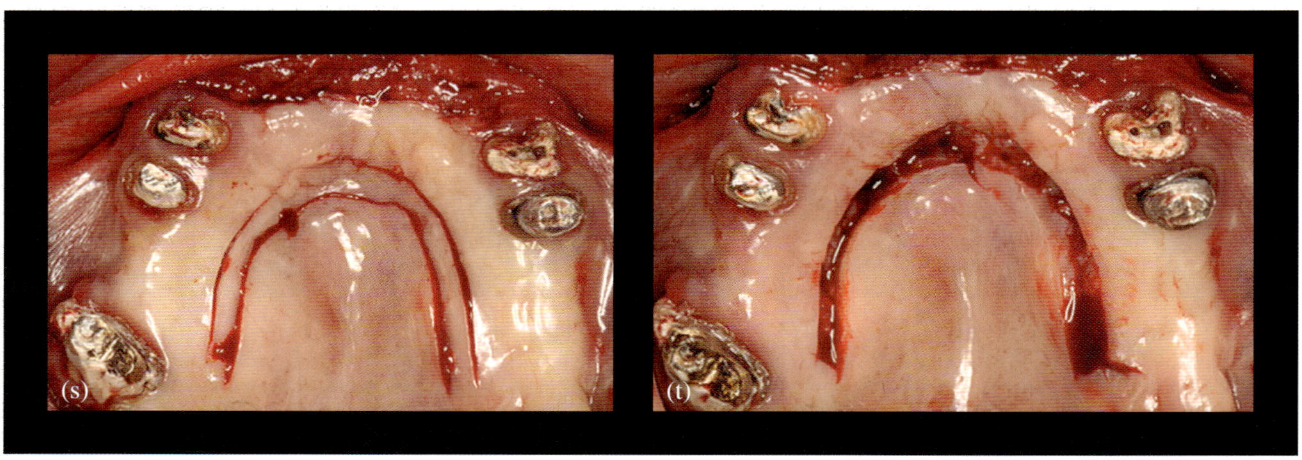

Figure 6.8 (s) Harvesting of a 2–3 mm wide free ging val graft from the palate. (t) Harvesting of a 2–3 mm wide free gingival graft from the palate.

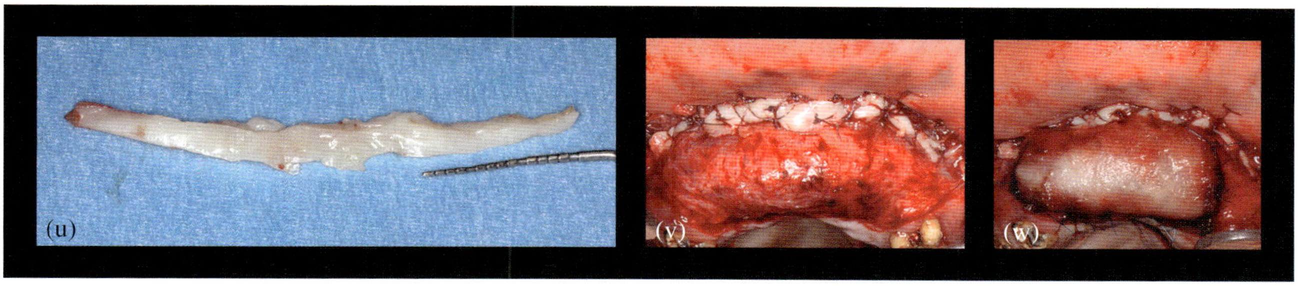

Figure 6.8 (u) Harvesting of a 2–3 mm wide free gingival graft from the palate. (v) Suturing of the gingival graft as apically as possible, preventing re-epithelialization of the wound by epithelial non-keratinized cells migrating from the alveolar mucosa. The only source of epithelial cells would be keratinized palatal tissues. (w) Coverage of the open wound surface by a collagen matrix (Mucograft®) that would help the secondary intention healing.

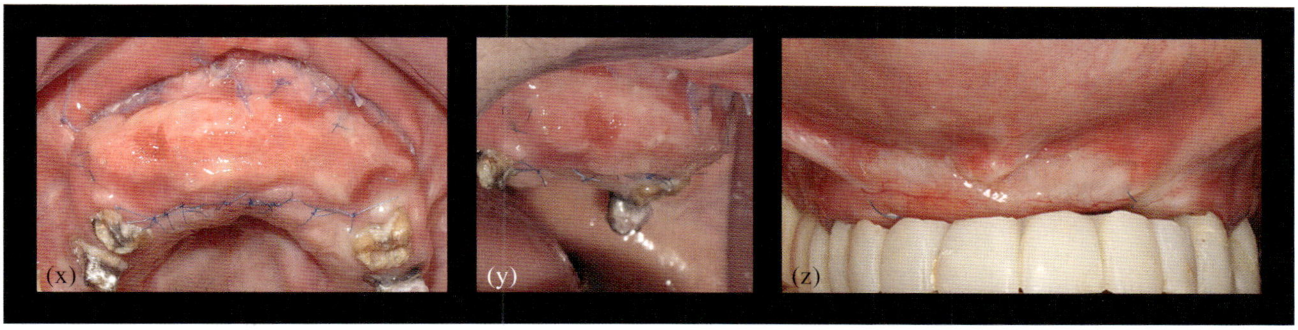

Figure 6.8 (x) Soft tissue healing at two weeks. (y) Soft tissue healing at two weeks. (z) Healing at 2.5 months: re-establishment of the vestibule and the keratinized tissue.

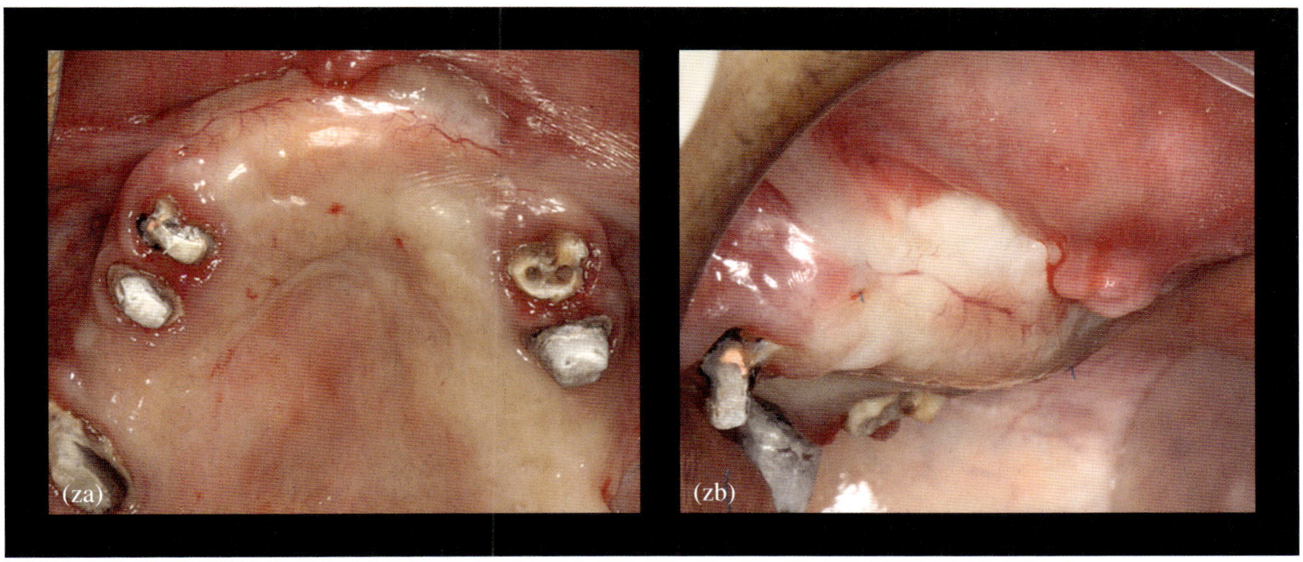

Figure 6.8 (za) Healing at 2.5 months: re-establishment of the vestibule and the keratinized tissue (compare with (m)). (zb) Healing at 2.5 months: re-establishment of the vestibule and the keratinized tissue (compare with (n)).

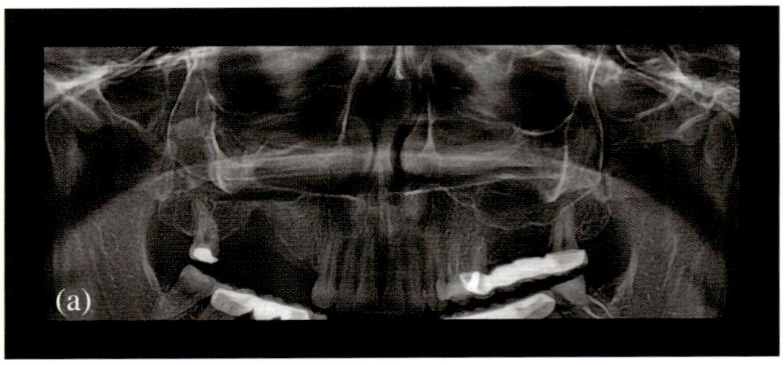

Figure 6.9 (a) 10 mm Vertical defect combined to a narrow ridge in the right maxilla.

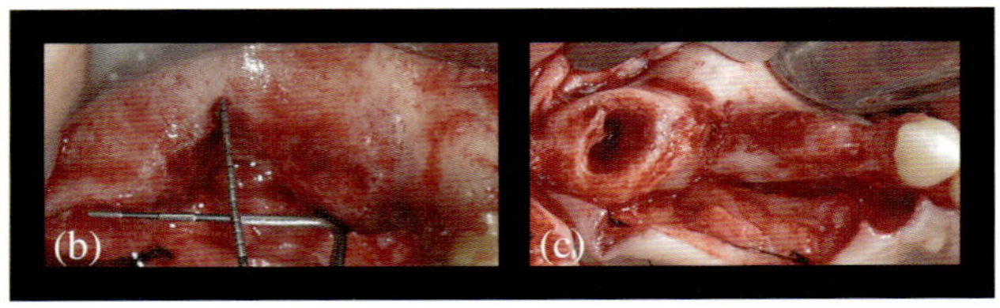

Figure 6.9 (b) 10 mm Vertical defect combined to a narrow ridge in the right maxilla. (c) 10 mm Vertical defect combined to a narrow ridge in the right maxilla.

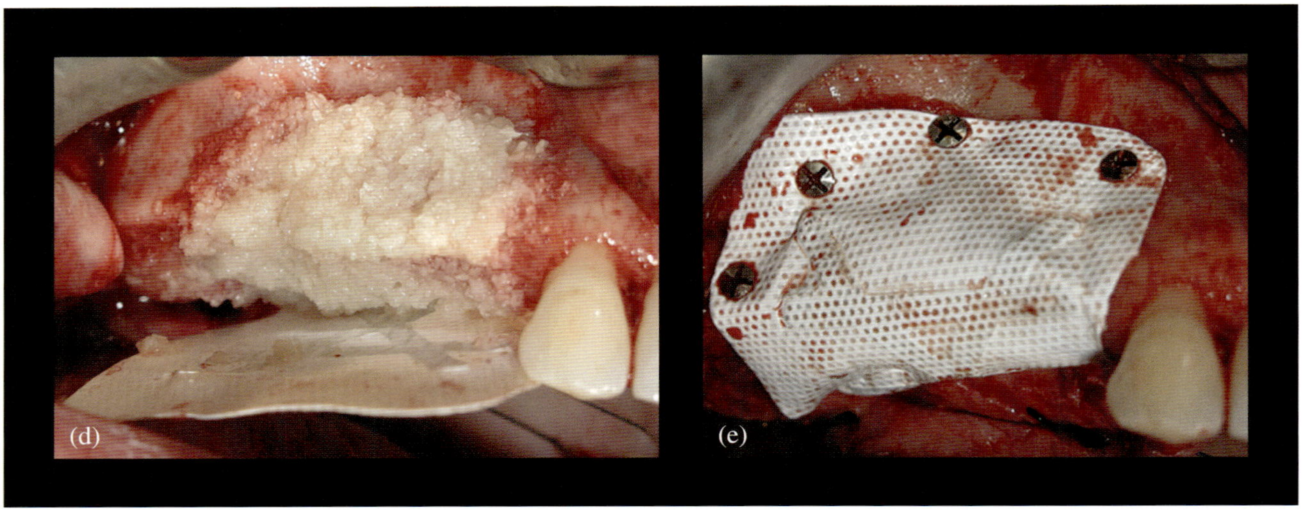

Figure 6.9 (d) Titanium reinforced d-PTFE membrane (Cytoplast) covering a bone allograft (enCore combination). (e) Adaptation of the membrane onto the defect and fixation with miniscrews.

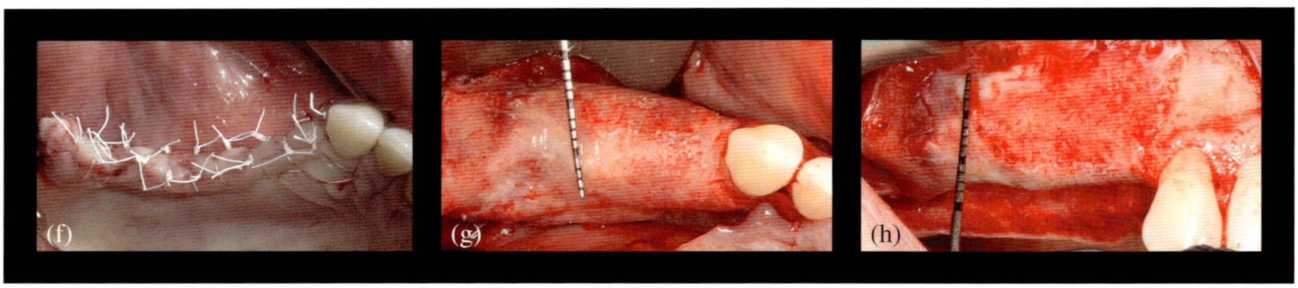

Figure 6.9 (f) Wound closure. Note the displacement of the mucoginigval line in the surgical site. (g) Re-entry at nine months: complete regeneration of the space underneath the membrane. (h) Re-entry at nine months: complete regeneration of the space underneath the membrane.

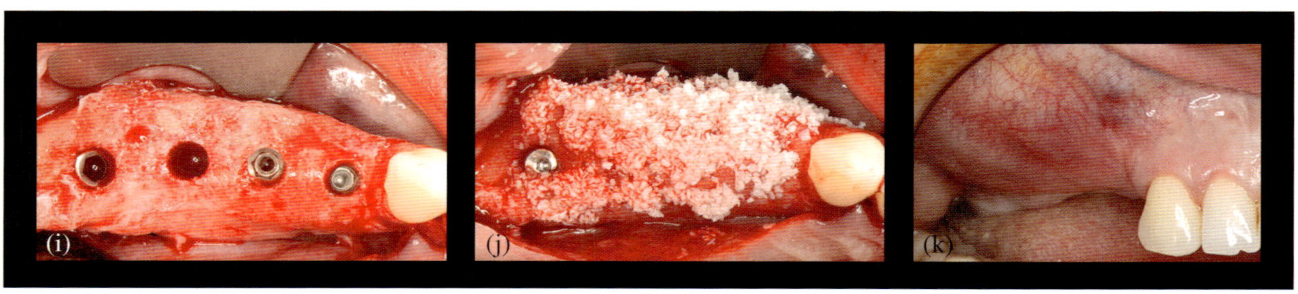

Figure 6.9 (i) Implant placement. (j) Application of a layer of anorganic bovine bone on the outer surface of the regenerated bone in the perspective of limiting graft resorption. (k) Change in the position of the mucoginigval line; absence of keratinized tissue buccally; reduction of vestibular depth.

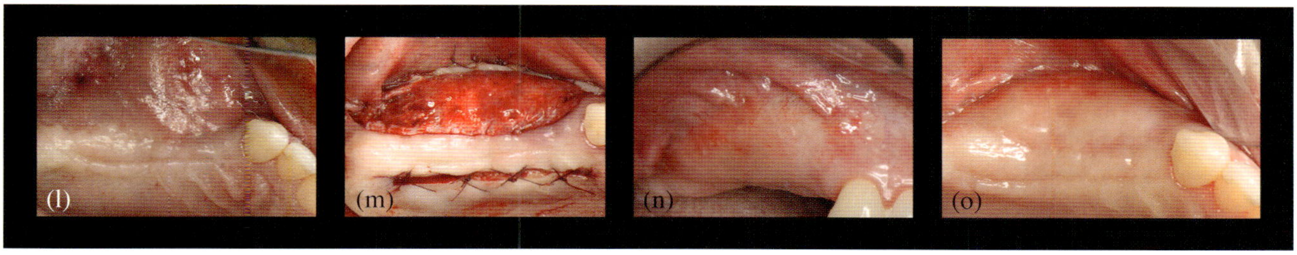

Figure 6.9 (l) Change in the position of the mucoginigval line; absence of keratinized tissue buccally; reduction of vestibular depth. (m) Partial thickness buccal flap repositioned at the vestibular fornix and strip palatal gingival graft (2 mm width) secured as apically as possible. No collagen matrix was applied to the denuded wound. (n) Soft tissue healing at six weeks: re-establishment of the vestibular depth and keratinized tissue buccally. (o) Soft tissue healing at six weeks: re-establishment of the vestibular depth and keratinized tissue buccally.

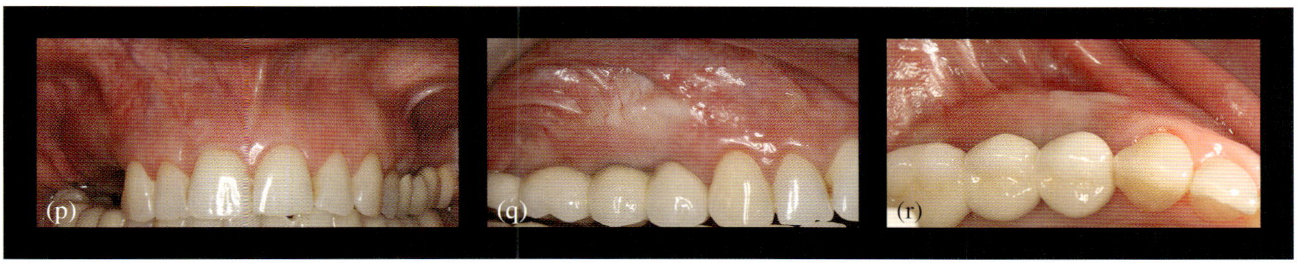

Figure 6.9 (p) Soft tissue healing at six weeks: re-establishment of the vestibular depth and keratinized tissue buccally. (q) Final prosthesis. (r) Final prosthesis.

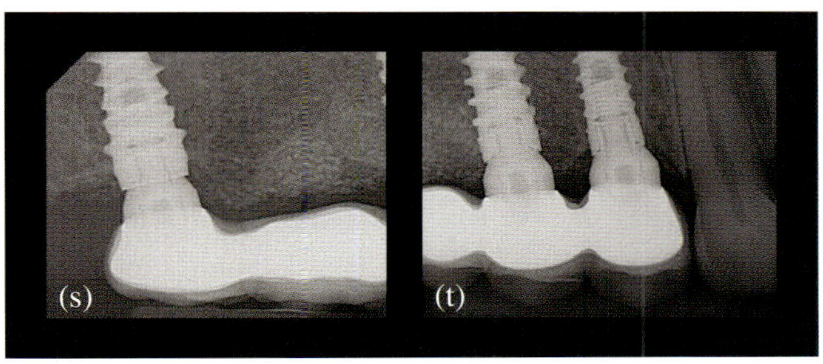

Figure 6.9 (s) Radiographic control at two years. (t) Radiographic control at two years.

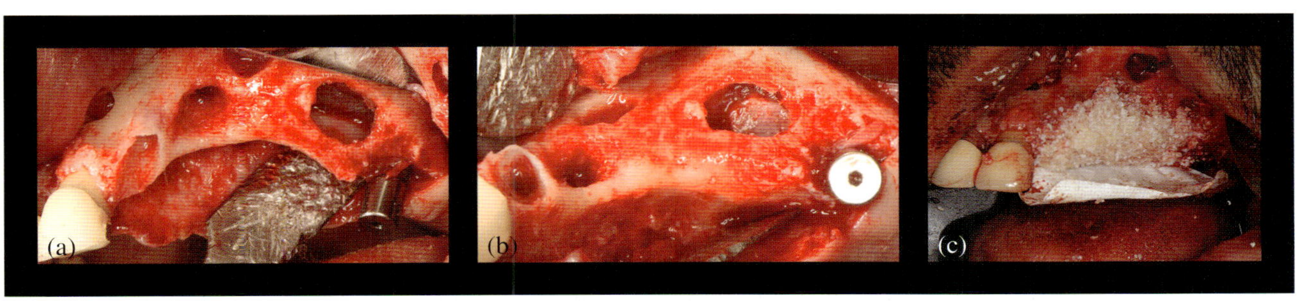

Figure 6.10 (a) Three-dimensional ridge defect combined with a pneumatized left maxillary sinus. (b) Three-dimensional ridge defect combined with a pneumatized left maxillary sinus. (c) Titanium reinforced d-PTFE membrane (Cytoplast) covering a composite graft (1 : 1 allograft and anorganic bovine bone). Sinus grafting was performed simultaneously.

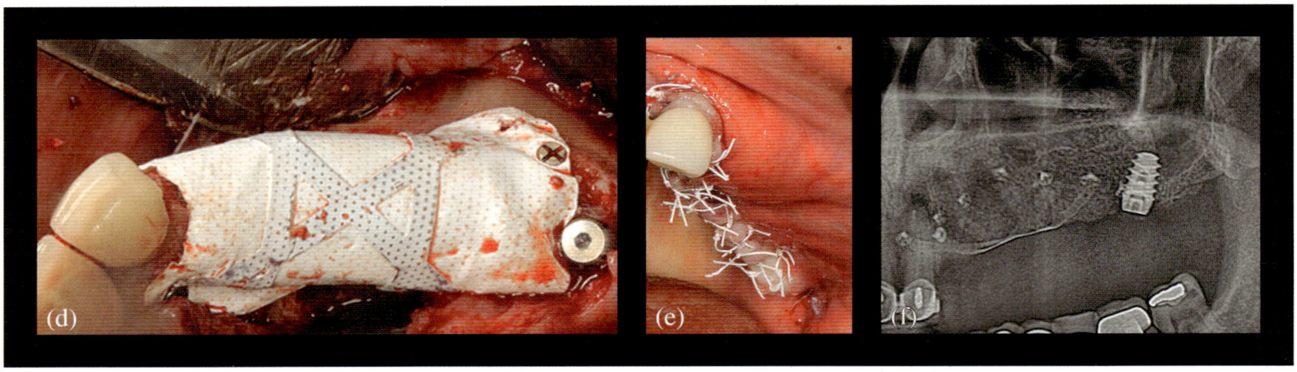

Figure 6.10 (d) Adaptation of the membrane onto the defect and fixation with miniscrews. Note the contact between the membrane and a previously placed dental implant in the distal region. (e) Wound closure. (f) Immediate radiographic control.

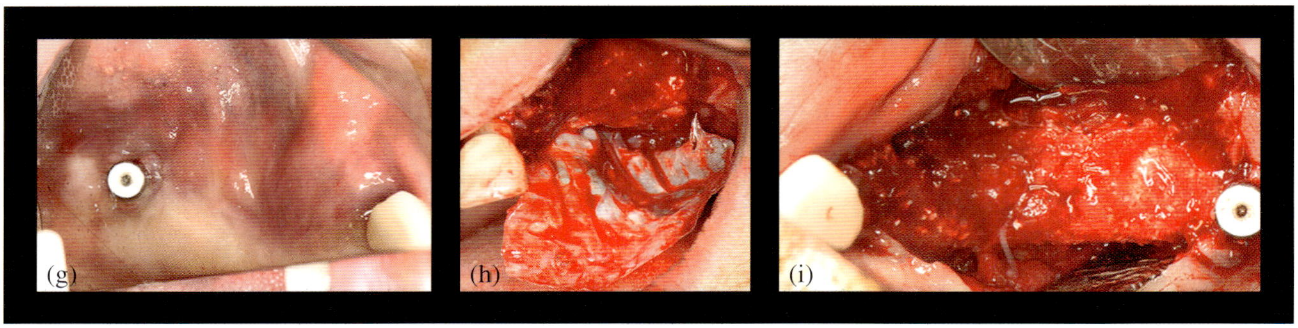

Figure 6.10 (g) Infection with pus formation and swelling that manifested at the seventh week post-operatively. The sinus tract fistula appeared at the level of the previously placed implant. (h) Under antibiotic coverage, the site was surgically accessed, the membrane removed. (i) The site was thoroughly rinsed with saline. No attempt was made to remove the graft. Only loose graft particles were debrided.

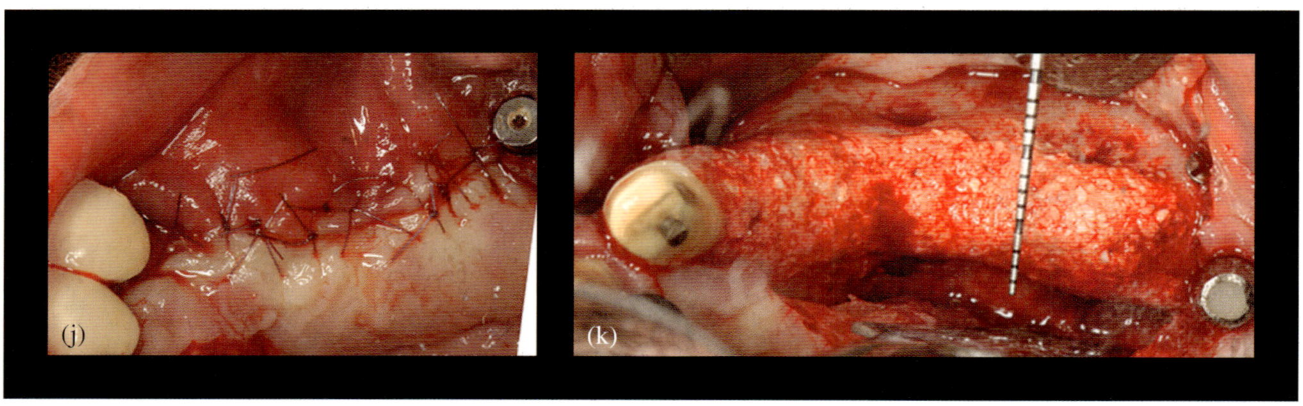

Figure 6.10 (j) Hermetic wound closure using Gottlow sutures. (k) Re-entry after 10 months: Even though a part of the grafted volume was lost, a sufficient bone volume was able to consolidate allowing the placement of dental implants. The sinus graft has consolidated completely.

Table 6.3 Recapitulative table of the most frequently used suture types in the various incision locations.

Incision location	Type of suture	Direction and order	Purpose	Thread type
Horizontal	8-point knot (around the adjacent tooth)	First knot to be performed	Flap positioning	Monofilament: 4(0)
	horizontal mattress (deep horizontal line)	Start on the adjacent tooth and alternate with the closure of the vertical incision	Tissue eversion	Monofilament: 4(0)
	Interrupted sutures and/or Gottlow suture (superficial horizontal line)	Performed after finishing the closure of the deeper horizontal line	Terminal tissue approximation	Monofilament: 4(0) to 6(0)
Vertical	Gottlow suture	Start apically and alternate with the closure of the deep horizontal incision	Tissue eversion and approximation	Monofilament: 4(0) to 6(0)
Adjacent papillae	Simple O suture	Leave to the end	Approximation	Monofilament: 5(0) to 6(0)

with low risk of bias are needed in this respect. In single tooth defect, another way to stabilize the resorbable membrane/bone graft complex beside the use of bone pins is to place a periosteal mattress suture anchored on the palatal flap (Figure 6.3f) (Urban et al. 2016b).

6.3.4 Sutures

Wound closure is a critical step in the GBR procedure. It should evert the flap edges and aim at approximating them on their connective tissue sides. It should provide enough stability to resist the forces generated by the swelling and the muscle pull.

Classically, a tight closure over a grafted site is achieved by placing a first line of horizontal mattress sutures followed by a second line of interrupted sutures along the horizontal incision. The vertical releasing incision is closed with interrupted sutures (Greenstein et al. 2009). We propose the following refinements for the esthetic zone.

After the flaps are liberated they become very mobile and correct flap repositioning is essential to coapt the incised papillary tissues (adjacent to the edentulous site) and avoid major papillary displacement and a subsequent esthetic problem on the adjacent teeth. Instead of starting the suturing at the horizontal incision (over the graft site), we favor a specially designed knot secured around the tooth adjacent to the edentulous site, and having the role of properly positioning the flap around it. This suture pierces the tissues at eight points around the tooth that is adjacent to the edentulous site starting on the side of the tooth that is facing the edentulous site. The needle is inserted from outside the buccal flap at the base of the papilla, about 5 mm from the flap margin. Staying on the same side of the tooth, the internal side of the lingual flap is pierced at the same distance from the flap margin. Then, turning lingually around the tooth and piercing the external side of the lingual flap at the same distance from the flap margin. Now, the needle is brought under the contact point and it pierces the internal side of the buccal flap at the same 5 mm distance from the flap margin. At this stage the suture has entered four points around the tooth and should travel back in the reverse direction at a slightly more coronal level of around 3–4 mm from the flap margins. Coronally to the last exit point, the needle pierces the external aspect of the buccal flap and passes below the contact point to enter the internal side of the lingual flap. Then it turns lingually around the tooth to enter the external side of the lingual flap and finally the internal side of the buccal flap. Now the eight points are completed and the knot is ready to be secured (Table 6.3). After this initial step of flap positioning, we proceed in an alternate fashion in closing the horizontal incision and the vertical incision. The horizontal incision closure should start on the adjacent tooth and move in the direction of the graft. The vertical incision closure should proceed in an apico-coronal direction. The alternate fashion is very important in keeping the flap properly positioned. Otherwise the flaps (notably the buccal flap) will be pulled too much in one direction and will hinder the primary intention closure along the entirety of the incision lines (Table 6.3). Before completing the closure of the horizontal and vertical incisions, the papillae on the adjacent teeth should be coapted with simple knots to secure them in place. The horizontal incision is closed with two lines of sutures. The first line will be using horizontal mattress sutures placed around 4 mm from the flap edge, with 4(0) monofilament material, preferably polytetrafluoroethylene (PTFE). The second using simple knots or preferably a locked horizontal mattress suture called the Gottlow suture (Gottlow et al. 1986) or the Laurell-Gottlow suture (Laurell 1995) with 4(0), 5(0) or even 6(0) monofilament material (Table 6.3) (Figures 6.1s–w, 6.3g, 6.4g, 6.7t, 6.8f, 6.9f and 6.10e). The vertical incision will be closed with a Gottlow suture using 4(0) or 5(0) PTFE material, except the most coronal suture placed in the keratinized tissue, which will be a simple knot. The advantage of using a locked mattress suture over a simple knot in the superficial line of sutures of the horizontal incision is a better tissue coaptation; the advantage of using it in the vertical incision is a reduced risk of tissue laceration and ease of suture removal (Table 6.3).

Sutures should be left in place for two to three weeks.

6.4 Revisiting the Barrier Membranes and the Bone Grafts

During its 25 years of clinical application, the GBR procedure has witnessed the use of several types of membranes and bone graft materials. At the beginnings, only membranes (non-resorbable) were used, and the rationale was centered on the exclusion property of the membrane. After the introduction of bone fillers and resorbable membranes, the rationale shifted towards a synergistic action between the membrane and the bone graft material.

6.4.1 Barrier Membranes

6.4.1.1 Non-resorbable Membranes

Non-resorbable *expanded-polytetrafluoroethylene* (*e-PTFE*) membranes were the first to be introduced. They consist of a bioinert material made in a relatively porous structure. Although the e-PTFE membranes made their mark in GBR and showed excellent results (Aghaloo and Moy 2007), several studies showed reduced outcomes for wound dehiscence (Chiapasco and Zaniboni 2009; Machtei 2001; Simion et al. 1994); especially wound infection that was frequently reported following membrane exposure (Augthun et al. 1995; Nowzari and Slots 1995).

Dense-polytetrafluoroethylene (d-PTFE) was proposed (Bartee and Carr 1995) as a denser structure of PTFE with a pore size not exceeding 3 μm; the aim was to reduce the risk of bacterial colonization when the membrane was intentionally left exposed or following wound dehiscence. These membranes are used in socket grafting surgeries and left intentionally exposed (Fotek, Neiva and Wang 2009). No infectious complications were reported, in contrast to previous reports for e-PTFE membranes, in which membrane exposure usually resulted in infection and impaired bone healing. One study (Ronda et al. 2014) clinically compared e-PTFE to d-PTFE in vertical defects; both membranes showed identical results. In another case series on vertical bone augmentation, d-PTFE membranes were able to support 5.45 mm of vertical bone gain (Urban et al. 2014).

PTFE membranes are also available in *titanium reinforced* form (Figures 6.1k–r, 6.4d–f, 6.8b–e, 6.9d–e and 6.10c–d). The addition of the titanium frame helps maintain the space underneath the membranes in large defects (Dahlin et al. 1988). In the particular case of the esthetic zone, the aim of bone augmentation goes beyond providing sufficient bone volume to accommodate dental implants; it aims at re-establishing ideal three-dimensional ridge shape to support a harmonious soft tissue contour. In this perspective, titanium reinforced-PTFE membranes offer the best available option. The presence of the titanium frame prevents membrane collapse into the defect and favors the re-establishment of optimal ridge contour. This is confirmed by a study using a titanium reinforced e-PTFE membrane to vertically regenerate the bone around titanium miniscrews without the addition of a bone graft. Up to 4 mm of bone was achieved (Simion et al. 1994). The addition of the titanium frame makes this type of membrane the exclusive choice (Table 6.4) in vertical ridge augmentations (Canullo and Malagnino 2008; Rocchietta et al. 2016; Simion et al. 1998, 2001, 2007; Tinti et al. 1996; Todisco 2010; Urban et al. 2009, 2014, 2015). The regenerated bone in the study mentioned previously (Simion et al. 1994) was analyzed histologically; the bone contact with the miniscrews was 42.5%. The newly formed bone was hardly distinguished from the old bone with a pattern of spongious lamellar bone with detectable islands of osteoid tissue in the coronal region. One characteristic of e-PTFE membranes is the occasional presence, at membrane removal, of a soft tissue layer between the membrane and the regenerated bone. This periosteal-like tissue has been extensively described in the literature (Schenk et al. 1994; Simion et al. 1994, 1998; Dahlin et al. 1998) and has been shown to be particularly evident (1–3 mm thick) when the titanium-reinforced membrane for vertical ridge augmentation is used without the association of any graft.

6.4.1.2 Resorbable Membranes

Resorbable membranes were proposed as an alternative to non-resorbable ones, to reduce the risk of complications observed with non-resorbable membranes and to eliminate the need for a second surgery to remove the non-resorbable membrane. Synthetic polymers (polylactic acid and polyglycolic acid) and biopolymers (bovine and porcine collagen) were proposed in the construction of resorbable membranes.

6.4.1.2.1 Collagen Membranes

Nowadays, the majority of the commercially available resorbable membranes developed are type I and type III

Table 6.4 Recapitulative table of the most frequently used membrane types.

Membrane type	Longevity of barrier function	Tissue compatibility	Indication
Titanium reinforced e-PTFE (relatively porous)	Non-resorbable	Maximum	• Vertical defects • Three-dimensional defects
Titanium reinforced d-PTFE (relatively non-porous)	Non-resorbable	Maximum	• Vertical defects • Three-dimensional defects
Native collagen	Relatively short	Maximum	• Lateral defects • Small vertical and small three-dimensional defects
Cross-linked collagen	Longer than native collagen	Suboptimal, but not to the point of affecting outcomes	• Lateral defects • Small vertical and small three-dimensional defects

animal collagen (Figures 6.2j–l, 6.3e–f, 6.5i–o, 6.6f–l and 6.7q–s). The ability of collagen to promote cell adhesion, hemostasis, chemotaxis, along with its low immunogenicity and physiological degradation, make it a suitable material for resorbable membrane construction (Bunyaratavej and Wang 2001). On the other hand, collagen degrades very rapidly, and untreated (native) collagen membranes may lack the stability to maintain barrier function (Rothamel et al. 2005; Zhao et al. 2000). To prolong barrier function, several cross-linking technologies (ultraviolet light, glutaraldehyde, diphenylphosphoryl-azide, hexmethylene diisocyanate, or enzymatic cross-linking using ribose) have been proposed aiming at increasing the number of links between collagen molecules. This leads to stiffer collagen membranes and slows down degradation. The membrane properties vary in terms of the longevity of barrier function and their tissue compatibility.

Longevity of Barrier Function and Tissue Compatibility of Native Collagen Membranes Native collagen membranes were typically described as degrading rapidly. The most documented native collagen membrane is composed of type I and type III porcine dermis collagen. Four weeks after its subcutaneous implantation in rats, a reduction in membrane thickness, transmembrane vascularization, combined with nearly complete biodegradation, was reported (Rothamel et al. 2005; Schwarz et al. 2006). When applied in surgical pouches in the palate of mongrel dogs (Owens and Yukna 2001), moderate to complete degradation was reported one to two months following implantation. In a rat calvarial model, 60% of the membrane material was lost at four weeks, and 80% at nine weeks (Kozlovsky et al. 2009). In contrasting, Ghanaati (2012) have reported a longer barrier function. In a subcutaneous mice model, he reported the absence of membrane degradation and of transmembrane vascularization at 60 days post-implantation. Only mild vascularization was observed on the membrane surface. He described his observation as "membrane integration" in the subcutaneous connective tissue rather than "membrane breakdown." He considered his results as a proof of the efficient barrier function and an explanation of the fact that type I–III native collagen membranes are as successful as e-PTFE membranes in certain clinical scenarios.

In a recent study comparing the degradation profile of type I porcine collagen combined with elastin fibers to a type I–III native collagen membrane (Bozkurt et al. 2014), no or very limited degradation of both membranes was observed at nine weeks. However, the 20 weeks observation period revealed a pronounced thickness loss of 51% for the type I–III collagen membrane and only a slight thickness decrease for the type I collagen-elastin membrane.

Pericardium collagen membranes were also investigated. It is assumed that pericardial collagen, because of its compact properties, shows a certain resistance to degradation (Rothamel et al. 2012). In a dog model, the type I native porcine pericardium collagen membrane resorbed within 8–12 weeks, compared to 4–8 weeks for the type I–III porcine dermis collagen (Rothamel et al. 2012).

Concerning tissue compatibility of native collagen membranes, reports are not consistent. In a subcutaneous rat model, a wide inflammatory zone was noted around a type I–III native collagen membrane at day four. At day 21, a mild inflammation was still present. A strong foreign body reaction was evidenced by the large number of giant cells surrounding the membrane (Zhao et al. 2000). In others animal studies neither inflammatory reaction nor a foreign body reaction were reported for the type I-III native collagen membrane and for type

I native porcine pericardium collagen (Rothamel et al. 2005, 2012). In a rat calvarial defect, only scattered inflammatory cells were observed underneath a type I-III native collagen membrane without the evidence of a foreign body reaction (Kozlovsky et al. 2009). In a subcutaneous mice model, the type I–III native collagen membrane evoked a mononuclear cellular inflammatory response within the membrane thickness, but it did not induce a foreign body reaction (Ghanaati 2012). In a subcutaneous rat model, neither inflammatory reaction nor a foreign body reaction were reported for type I–III native collagen membrane and for type I native collagen-elastin membrane (Bozkurt et al. 2014).

Longevity of Barrier Function and Tissue Compatibility of Cross-linked Collagen Membranes Compared with native collagen membranes, cross-linked membranes have demonstrated a significantly slower degradation associated with decreased vascularization of the membrane body (Paul et al. 1992; Pitaru et al. 1988; Rothamel et al. 2005; Schwarz et al. 2006; von Arx et al. 2005). Cross-linked membranes form a heterogeneous group due to the availability of different cross-linking methods with varying degrees of cross-linking. It was observed that the resorption rate was directly related to the degree of cross-linking (i.e. the higher the degree of cross-linking, the longer the resorption rate). However, when the degree of chemical cross-linking increased, more inflammatory cells seemed to be involved in the process of biodegradation accompanied by a foreign body reaction (Rothamel et al. 2005). Neither inflammatory reaction nor foreign body reactions were reported for a mildly chemically cross-linked collagen prototype membrane nor for an enzymatically cross-linked collagen membrane (Rothamel et al. 2005). A clinical and histologic study in humans evaluating an enzymatically cross-linked collagen membrane reported that collagen layers of the membrane could still be observed seven months following healing. Histologic observation revealed direct apposition of fibrous and bone tissues on the membrane surface (Friedmann et al. 2001). Concerns exist about cellular toxicity of cross-linking agents, such as glutaraldehyde (Speer et al. 1980; Wiebe et al. 1988). Glutaraldehyde is a reference agent for the collagen cross-linking reactions. An in-vitro study showed that cross-linking with glutaraldehyde inhibited the attachment and proliferation of human periodontal ligament fibroblasts and human SaSO-2 osteoblasts (Rothamel et al. 2004). However, in biomaterial research, glutaraldehyde cross-linked collagen is tested for the growth of fibroblasts with high biological efficiency (Chen et al. 2005). In a recent rat calvarial study, glutaraldehyde cross-linked collagen membranes accelerated bone healing of the calvarium defects more than the non-cross linked membranes and did not induce more inflammation as assessed by the concentration of inflammatory cytokines in the tissue surrounding the membrane (Veríssimo et al. 2015).

Although much effort was spent on investigating the degradation profile of collagen membranes, it is obvious that not all aspects have yet been clarified. Some types and degrees of collagen cross-linking are associated with an increased inflammatory reaction coupled with a foreign body reaction. To what extent this tissue reaction may impact osteogenesis is not yet known. Barrier function longevity varies greatly among different types of collagen membranes; the ideal time period that the membrane should retain its barrier function to maximize healing outcomes has still not been determined.

Several studies compared the performance of native and cross-linked membranes in GBR. An animal study (Oh et al. 2003), evaluating native type I–III porcine collagen membrane to glutaraldehyde cross-linked type I bovine collagen membrane for the treatment of dehiscence-type defects, showed no significant difference in bone regeneration, but showed a better bone to implant contact at 16 weeks with the cross-linked membrane. The membrane exposure, when present, generally occurred with both membrane types in a similar frequency and pattern.

In a lateral augmentation model, a randomized clinical trial showed that the ribose cross-linked collagen membrane and the native collagen membrane were comparable in bone augmentation (Friedmann et al. 2011).

In a randomized clinical trial for the treatment of dehiscence peri-implant defects (Annen et al. 2011), significantly more soft tissue dehiscencies and infections were reported for an experimental cross-linked membrane compared with a native one. The linear defect fill values were 44 and 78% respectively. Another randomized clinical trial with a bigger sample size treating the same defect (Becker et al. 2009; Schwarz et al. 2014) and using the same experimental membrane compared to a native one showed that the cross-linked membrane group had better defect fill values (60%) compared to the native collagen membrane group (46%). The difference was not statistically significant, and the authors concluded that both types of membranes resulted in a comparable and clinically important defect fill. The frequencies of soft tissue dehiscences were similar with both membranes. However, for premature exposure, more soft tissue inflammation is observed around the cross-linked membranes. A recent systematic review and a meta-analysis on the treatment of dehiscence peri-implant defects reported that dehiscence complications were more frequent using cross-linked membranes but the odds ratio was not significant (Merli et al. 2016).

Although several studies have been conducted investigating the clinical efficacy of different type of collagen membranes, it is obvious that the comparative performance is not very clear. But owing to their inherent lack of mechanical stability and to their degradation profile, collagen membranes are generally used for dehiscence-type defects (Figures 6.2 and 6.3) and for lateral ridge augmentations (Figure 6.7). At best, they are used for small vertical defects (Figure 6.5) and for small three-dimensional defects (Figure 6.6) (Table 6.4). Well-designed future clinical trials with low risk of bias are needed to test whether the differences in membrane properties are of clinical relevance.

6.4.1.2.2 Synthetic Membranes

Several synthetic polymers were used for the construction of resorbable membranes. The tissue response to the synthetic polymers is usually characterized the presence of an inflammatory infiltrate in and around the membrane coupled with a foreign body reaction (Piattelli et al. 1998; von Arx et al. 2005). A recent systematic review and a meta-analysis (Merli et al. 2016) looked into synthetic poly(lactic-*co*-glycolic acid) membranes compared to e-PTFE membranes. A statistically significant difference was obtained for complete coverage of a dehiscence-type defects in favor of e-PTFE membranes.

6.4.1.2.3 Other Types of Resorbable Membranes/Barriers

Other types of membranes were also proposed.

Acellular dermal matrix (ADM), a bioabsorbable human skin allograft, has been proposed. ADM has several characteristics: it is biocompatible; primary closure may not be critical (Fowler, Breault and Rebitski 2000); no infection occurs upon exposure (Novaes and Souza 2001; Novaes et al. 2002); it enhances gingival thickness by incorporating into the host tissue (Batista et al. 2001; Harris 2002; Henderson et al. 2001); and it provides adequate barrier function lasting longer than two months (Owens and Yukna 2001). In randomized clinical trial treating peri-implant dehiscence-type defect, ADM was equally effective as a chemically cross-linked collagen membrane in regenerating the horizontal and vertical components of the defects (Park et al. 2008).

A xenogenic cortical bone barrier was also proposed (Wachtel et al. 2013; Rossi et al. 2016). Biopsy specimens revealed that the barrier was widely vascularized and integrated with the surrounding soft tissues and the native bone. The presence of osteoclastic lacunae suggested an active remodeling of the particulate graft and a gradual substitution with the newly formed bone.

6.4.2 Bone Grafts

After an initial period where only membranes were used, the addition of bone fillers to the GBR procedure became a standard of practice with the aim of supporting the membrane to avoid volume collapse; acting as a scaffold for bone conduction; acting as an inductor for bone formation; protecting the augmented volume from resorption. Both autografts and bone substitutes in particulate or in block form are used.

6.4.2.1 Autogenous Bone Grafts

With the transplantation of autogenous bone, both osteogenic cells (that are more numerous in the trabecular bone compared to cortical bone) and osteoinductive molecules are brought to the augmented site (Burchardt 1983). Bone morphogenic proteins (BMPs) and other growth factors present in the bone matrix are released during resorption of the autografts (Miron et al. 2016).

Autografts may be harvested from intraoral or extraoral sites. Because of the need to reduce morbidity, most autografts are now collected from intraoral sites in the form of block or particulate grafts.

Block grafts are most frequently collected from the symphysis or the retro-molar region. They offer mechanical stability against pressure from the overlying soft tissue. They may undergo resorption of up to 60% of the initial volume within six months (Johansson et al. 2001; Widmark, Andersson and Ivanoff 1997). To reduce their resorption, a combined approach using onlay black grafting with the GBR procedure was proposed (Chappuis et al. 2017; Maiorana et al. 2005, 2011; von Arx and Buser 2006).

Particulate grafts can be obtained by grinding a bone block with a bone mill (Lundgren et al. 1996; Peleg et al. 1998), can be harvested with a bone scraper (Zaffe and D'Avenia 2007), by means of piezosurgery (Lambrecht 2004) or by collecting the bone slurry during a bone drilling procedure with a filter device (Tinti et al. 1996). A recent study in standardized defects in the mandible of minipigs covered with e-PTFE membranes concluded that all harvesting techniques were equally efficient (Saulacic et al. 2015). However, in a clavarial critical sized defect model, bone slurry/dust was ineffective and performed similarly to the empty control (Clune et al. 2010).

Compared to block grafts, particulate grafts demonstrate a greater osteoinduction and osteoconduction because a much larger area of the graft surface is exposed and due to the faster release of growth factors (Pallesen et al. 2002). Particulate autogenous bone has been shown to be significantly more osteoconductive than any available bone substitute (Buser et al. 1998; Jensen et al. 2006, 2007). Despite their excellent osteoinduction and osteoconduction properties, particulate grafts harvested from intra-oral cortical sites have supposedly neglectable osteogenic potential due to the fact that few osteogenic cells are present in the cortical bone.

Autografts use in GBR is documented in several studies. After an initial period where only membranes were used, clinicians started to use autogenous bone under the membranes. Buser et al. (1996) used croticocancellous blocks combined with bone chips covered by an e-PTFE membrane to treat lateral ridge defects. A mean of 3.5–7.1 mm was achieved. Tinti et al. (1996) used autogenous bone collected from a bone filter covered by an e-PTFE membrane to perform vertical ridge augmentations around protruding implants. After 12 months of healing, an average vertical gain of 4.95 mm was achieved (up to 7 mm). Simion et al. (1998), using autogenous bone chips and an e-PTFE membrane had a mean vertical gain of 5.02 mm. Simion et al. (2001), using an e-PTFE membrane was able to achieve a vertical bone gain of up to 8 mm when particulate autogenous bone grafts were used. When only the blood clot was protected under the membrane or when the demineralized freeze-dried bone allograft (DFDBA) was used, a vertical bone regeneration of more than 4 mm was never achieved. Urban et al. (2009) using particulate autogenous bone combined to an e-PTFE membrane had a mean vertical gain of 5.5 mm. Even though excellent bone forming potential was reported with particulate autogenous bone in GBR, concerns exist about the stability of the augmented bone over time. Simion et al. (2001), in a long-term retrospective study, demonstrated that vertically augmented bone by means of GBR in association with bone chips has a tendency to show a slightly greater amount of marginal bone remodeling than in native bone.

6.4.2.2 Allografts

The grafts of human origin usually used in GBR are freeze-dried bone allograft (FDBA), or DFDBA. Available in block or particulate forms from both cortical and cancellous origins (Block and Degen 2004; Lyford et al. 2003), allografts have been shown to contain osteoinductive growth factors, notably BMPs (Urist and Strates 1971).

DFDBA, being demineralized, have the BMPs exposed with the aim of increasing osteoinductivity. The osteoinductivity of DFDBA was demonstrated by its ability to induce new bone formation when implanted in ectopic non-osseous sites (Miron et al. 2016; Schwartz et al. 1996, 1998). When compared to other bone substitutes (a bovine derived xenograft and a biphasic calcium phosphate graft), DFDBA was the only one to support cell migration as observed with autografts (Miron et al. 2016). Different batches of DFDBA have been shown to contain different concentrations of BMPs with a corresponding variability in osteoinductivity (Schwartz et al. 1996, 1998; Wei et al. 2015). Although allografts contain osteoinductive molecules, there are concerns whether the concentrations of these BMPs are sufficient to clinically induce a relevant osteoinductive effect and whether they are present in an active form (Schwartz et al. 1996). To control the variability in osteoinductivity of DFDBA, some manufacturers are providing presterilization BMP testing and post-sterilization ectopic osteoinductivity testing for every lot.

In critical-size rat calvarial defects, DFDBA and particulate autogenous bone induced a similar bone formation as assessed by histomorphometrical analysis (Chesmel et al. 1998; Mokbel et al. 2008). The DFDBA outperformed anorganic bovine bone (Mokbel et al. 2008) and considerably outperformed biphasic calcium phosphate grafts (Fleckenstein et al. 2006). Only with particulate autogenous bone, some bone formation was noted away from the defects margins (Mokbel et al. 2008).

DFDBA was the first most frequently used bone substitute to replace or to extend particulate autogenous bone grafts used with non-resorbable membranes (Mellonig and Triplett 1993; Rominger and Triplett 1994; Mellonig and Nevins 1995; Nevins et al. 1998; Simion et al. 1998, 2001). In dehiscence-type defects and lateral augmentations, the studies reported favorable outcomes similar to the performance of autogenous bone. Also, in a vertical defect of mean height of 2.68 mm, the DFDBA demonstrated a vertical gain of 3.14 mm with a mean percentage of bone gain of 124% (Simion et al. 1998). In bigger vertical augmentations, however, autografts outperformed DFDBA. In a retrospective clinical study treating vertical defects with titanium reinforced e-PTFE membranes, the sites grafted with DFDBA were not able to achieve a vertical bone regeneration superior to 4 mm, whereas the sites grafted with autogenous bone chips were able to regenerate the bone up to 8 mm (Simion et al. 1998). Some investigators, however, have reported poor histological results with the use of DFDBA compared to autogenous bone in extraction socket defects (Becker et al. 1994, 1995).

Marginal bone remodeling around implant fixtures seemed to be the same when DFDBA or autogenous bone was used under non-resorbable membranes (Simion et al. 2001). However, large scale studies are still lacking to evaluate the stability of the augmented bone.

With the increased use of resorbable membranes, *FDBA* was more frequently used due to its stronger mechanical properties and its better resistance to resorption. Although FDBA has the same BMP content in its organic matrix as in DFDBA, the BMPs are trapped in the mineralized particles. Hence, FDBA are considered less osteoinductive than DFDBA. When FDBA is grafted, osteoclasts break down the mineral content until the FDBA is also demineralized. Osteoinductive proteins then become available to induce new bone formation (Reddi 1994).

According to a human histological study, FDBA may be more osteoconductive than DFDBA (Piattelli et al. 1996). In this study, the FDBA particles that were farthest from the host bone were lined by osteoblasts, actively secreting osteoid matrix and newly formed bone, while in DFDBA only the particles near the host bone were involved in the mineralization processes. However, a recent socket preservation study reported significantly less new bone formation with FDBA (50.63%) compared to DFDBA (80.26%) at 18–20 weeks postoperatively. Both types of graft material were sourced from the same donor, eliminating variables in potential inductivity. DFDBA-treated sites had considerably less residual bone graft material, reflecting the high substitution/biodegradation rate of DFDBA (Wood and Mealey 2012). In a human histological report on allografts use in ridge and sinus augmentations at 6–36 months post-grafting, FDBA and DFDBA produced the same amount of new bone formation, 41.89 and 41.74% respectively (Cammack et al. 2005). While DFDBA may induce bone formation sooner than FDBA, the authors of the previous study supported the possibility that FDBA may "catch up" and provide similar levels of new bone formation.

In a clinical study on ridge augmentation, where FDBA was used alone or combined with autogenous bone chips covered by a cross-linked membrane, the amount of augmentation was not affected by the addition of autogenous bone. With FDBA as a grafting material, the mean lateral bone gain was 5 mm and the mean vertical bone gain was 3.47 mm (Beitlitum, Artzi and Nemcovsky 2010). In a multicenter prospective clinical trial using FDBA of cancellous origin covered by a pericardium collagen membrane, the mean gain in clinical ridge width was only 2.61 mm (Sterio et al. 2013). Remarkably in this study, approximately 50% of the graft material added horizontally was displaced or resorbed during healing, raising concerns about allograft resorption. Histomorphometric analysis revealed a high percentage (58%) of vital bone at re-entry. In a more recent randomized clinical trial, FDBA of cortical and cancellous origin, used alone or in combination with particulate autogenous bone, was placed around lateral tenting screws and covered with an acellular dermal matrix membrane that was stabilized with bone tacs (Caldwell et al. 2015). The amount of augmentation was not affected by the addition of autogenous bone. The mean horizontal bone gain was 3.22 mm. The mean graft resorption between baseline and re-entry was much less than the previous study and amounted to 13.89%. The following factors may account for the reduced graft material resorption/displacement in this study compared to the previous one: the use of tenting screws that may have helped maintain the graft volume; the fixation of the membrane with tacs that may have helped in stabilizing the graft/membrane complex compared to the occasional use of periosteal mattress sutures in the previous study; the use of cortico-cancellous FDBA compared to a cancellous FDBA in the previous study. The performance of cortical FDBA compared to cancellous FDBA was not histologically tested in the human GBR model. However, in a human socket grafting model, new bone formation appeared to be similar with the use of both types of FDBA. Cortical FDBA resisted resorption more than cancellous FDBA as evidenced by a significantly greater percentage of residual graft material in the cortical FDBA group compared to the cancellous one. A better preservation of the ridge contour was also noted in the cortical FDBA group (Eskow and Mealey 2014).

The use of FDBA with a titanium reinforced membrane for lateral ridge augmentation was investigated. The lateral bone gain was in the same range of the previously mentioned studies using resorbable membranes and amounted to 3.2 mm. Histomorphometric analysis revealed a high percentage (47.6%) of new bone formation (Feuille et al. 2003).

A composite DFDBA/FDBA/thermoplastic carrier graft was also tested. In a retrospective case series on the treatment of lateral ridge defects using the composite graft covered by a ribose cross-linked membrane, the mean lateral bone gain was 3.5 mm (Toscano et al. 2010). In a split mouth design clinical trial for the treatment of vertical defects in the posterior mandible using an e-PTFE membrane, the mean vertical bone gain with the composite graft was 4.7 mm compared to 4.1 mm for particulate autogenous bone. Both grafts demonstrated similar histologic characteristics (Fontana et al. 2008).

In all of the studies mentioned above on FDBA use in GBR, neither marginal bone remodeling around the implant fixtures, nor the stability of the regenerated bone volume over time were assessed. Future studies using three-dimensional radiographical assessments of the regenerated volume with long-term follow-ups are needed, especially because there are concerns about the stability of the regenerated bone volume with allografts.

6.4.2.3 Xenografts

Xenografts consist of bone minerals derived from animals or calcifying corals or algae. The organic component has been removed to eliminate the risk of immunogenic reactions and disease transmission. Xenografts of cancellous bovine origin are the most frequently used and extensively documented in GBR. Anorganic Bovine Bone (ABB) possesses osteoconductive properties (Hämmerle et al. 1998; Jensen et al. 2006) and is characterized by its reduced resorption rate. In a mandibular defect model in minipigs, no reduction of ABB volume was observed over one year (Jensen and Terheyden 2009). Human biopsies after sinus grafting documented the continued presence of ABB particles for four years (Piattelli et al. 1999), seven years (Orsini et al. 2007), nine years (Traini et al. 2007) and 10 years (Sartori et al. 2003) postoperatively. They are considered practically close to non-resorbable. ABB is available in particulate form, in a composite form coupled to 10% porcine collagen, and in block from. In ridge augmentations, the ABB was used alone or in combination with autogenous bone to enhance graft healing potential.

Anorganic Bovine Bone Use as the Sole Grafting Material

In Dehiscence-type Defects and Lateral Ridge Augmentations Used as the sole grafting material, ABB covered by either an e-PTFE membrane or a collagen membrane was investigated for the treatment of dehiscence-type defects (Zitzmann, Naef and Schärer 1997). The authors concluded that the treatment was effective. A histological analysis for the same treatment modality performed later (Zitzmann et al. 2001) indicated that ABB can be a suitable material for staged localized ridge augmentation. In a case series, Hämmerle et al. (2008) concluded that ABB covered by a native collagen membrane was able to increase the ridge width by a mean of 3.7 mm. An integration of the ABB particles into the newly formed bone was consistently observed. Merely on the surface of the new bone, some pieces of the grafting material were only partly integrated into bone. However, these were not encapsulated by connective tissue but rather anchored into the newly regenerated bone.

ABB coupled to 10% porcine collagen and covered by an e-PTFE membrane was investigated in a clinical and histological study on the treatment of lateral defects at implants placed in extraction sockets with a missing buccal wall. A horizontal bone gain of 3.75 mm was achieved for an initial defect width of 3.88 mm and a vertical defect fill of 6.5 mm for an initial dehiscence height of 5.88 mm; micro-CT analysis along with histological examination revealed that the ABB particles are embedded in bone; clinically a thin layer of new bone was present along the most external layer of graft particles; histomorphometrically, the amount of new bone formation was in the order of 15.4% (Grunder, Wenz and Schupbach 2011). Implants with dehiscence defects treated with ABB and barrier membranes were followed up for a mean period of 12.5 years (Jung et al. 2013). The survival rate was 91.9% in the collagen membrane group and 92.6% in the e-PTFE membrane group compared to 94.6% for implants entirely surrounded by pristine bone. Differences among the groups were not statistically significant. The mean marginal bone remodeling was similar for the three groups, ranging between 2.36 and 2.53 mm.

In Vertical Ridge Augmentations ABB are seldom used alone in the regeneration of vertical defects. Few studies have documented this application.

Canullo, Trisi and Simion (2006) in a single patient case report using an e-PTFE membrane showed clinical and histological evidence of new bone formation (25.3%) in a vertical defect. The defect height was not mentioned. Canullo and Malagnino (2008), in a retrospective study on 10 cases using an e-PTFE membrane, documented a vertical bone gain of 5.3 mm for an initial mean defect height of 5.1 mm. The healing period was six to eight months. All implants successfully osseointegrated. The histological analysis performed on three biopsies revealed that the surfaces of the graft particles were mostly covered by newly formed bone, even in the most extreme case of a 9 mm vertical defect. A histomorphometry was not performed. Todisco (2010), in a prospective cohort study, have treated 20 patients with a total of 26 sites using ABB with an e-PTFE membrane. After a 12 month healing period, the mean vertical bone gain was 5.2 mm for a mean initial defect height of 5.6 mm. The histomorphometry performed on five samples revealed 52.6% of new bone formation. Marginal bone remodeling amounted to 0.95 mm at one year.

Anorganic Bovine Bone Combined with Autogenous Bone

In Dehiscence-type Defects and Lateral Ridge Augmentations A study with five years of follow-up on implants placed in conjunction with GBR treatment consisting of a combination of ABB (80%) and particulate autogenous bone (20%) covered by an e-PTFE membrane or a native collagen membrane, demonstrated stable marginal bone and soft tissue levels (Dahlin, Simion and Hatano 2010). A more recent study assessed regenerated bone volume stability over a five to nine year period (mean seven years) of a contour augmentation GBR procedure around single implants placed four to eight weeks after tooth extraction. The aim of the procedure was to build a facial bone wall of sufficient height and thickness that would support soft tissue contours over time. ABB and particulate autogenous bone were placed in a sandwich (inner layer of particulate autogenous bone and outer layer of ABB) and covered with a native collagen membrane. The three-dimensional radiographical results showed that the regenerated bone wall was stable over the observation period and had a mean thickness of 2.2 mm. None of the implants developed mucosal recession over time (Buser et al. 2013). The authors concluded that the use of ABB granules seems important for the long-term stability of the regenerated bone because of the low substitution rate of the biomaterial. It can be speculated that ABB granules will not be resorbed during the natural bone remodeling process and thus will help maintain the facial bone wall over time.

The use of ABB with particulated autogenous bone combined with a resorbable membrane stabilized with titanium pins was investigated (Urban et al. 2011, 2013). The average lateral bone gain was 5.56 mm (Urban et al. 2011) and 5.68 mm (Urban et al. 2013), with some sites gaining up to 10 mm. Histologic analysis showed a good integration of ABB particles. Histomorphometry showed an average of autogenous bone (comprising autogenous bone grafts remnants and newly formed bone) of 31% (Urban et al. 2013). The relatively high amount of lateral gain achieved can be attributed to the stabilization of the membrane that immobilizes the graft material, and the use of autogenous bone. A recent study in a pig mandibular defect model shed the light on the importance of stabilizing a collagen membrane with fixation pins (Mir-Mari et al. 2016). It was shown that immediately after wound closure, the group of non-stabilized membranes had 42.8% of the particulate bone graft volume displaced; compared to 22.9% for the group of stabilized membranes. These measurements were for bone graft volume at the coronal level.

In Vertical Ridge Augmentations The combination of ABB and particulate autogenous bone in a 1 : 1 mixture associated with an e-PTFE membrane for vertical ridge augmentation was first tested by Simion et al. (2007) in a prospective case series of seven patients. The healing period was 6–9.5 months (average 27 weeks). Vertical bone gain of up to 5 mm was noted (mean gain was 3.15 mm). The ABB particles demonstrated degrees of integration similar to that of autogenous bone chips. Histomorphometrically, new bone formation was 36.56%. The new bone was more mature towards the apical part. Both the autogenous bone and the ABB particles underwent evident resorption during the healing period. Remodeling of the autogenous bone graft was evidenced by the presence of cutting cones penetration into the bone particles, whereas around the ABB particles osteoclasts were occasionally identified indicating their possible involvement in a visible demineralization process. The latter finding is in agreement with previous reports showing that ABB particles can be resorbed by osteoclasts but seem to undergo a very slow resorption process. The authors concluded that the slow resorption pattern of ABB could be advantageous for the long-term stability of regenerated bone.

In a prospective case series evaluating the use of ABB mixed with autogenous bone in combination with a d-PTFE membrane, the mean vertical bone gain was 5.45 mm, with some sites gaining up to 9 mm (Urban et al. 2014). Histomorphometrically, the autogenous bone (comprising autogenous bone graft remnants and newly formed bone) was 36.6%. None of the cases demonstrated bone resorption throughout the follow-up period, laying more credit to the possible role of ABB in helping the stability of the regenerated bone.

6.4.2.4 Alloplasts

Of the synthetic bone substitutes, calcium phosphate, especially hydroxyapatite (HA), and tricalcium phosphate (β-TCP) are the most investigated. HA is considered osteoconductive but non resorbable, β-TCP is considered more osteoconductive than HA but resorbs rapidly (Buser et al. 1998; Jensen et al. 2006, 2007). A combination of HA and β-TCP, termed biphasic calcium phosphate (BCP), has been proposed to benefit from both the stable space-making properties of HA and the excellent osteoconductive properties of β-TCP (Ellinger, Nery and Lynch 1986). BCPs can be constructed with different HA–TCP ratios. BCPs were investigated in vitro and in vivo with promising results (Chakar et al. 2014; Miron et al. 2016), but clinical documentation in GBR applications is still scarce.

6.4.2.5 Combining Different Bone Substitutes

The only documented combination is for ABB and allografts. This combination was investigated in sinus grafting (Landi et al. 2000) but not in GBR. This combination has the potential of combining the advantages of each biomaterial. The ABB offers its proven osteoconductive potential with a low substitution rate that would eventually help stabilize the regenerated bone volume over time. The allografts, beside their osteoconductive potential, offer the organic component, notably collagen. With DFDBA, the organic component is readily available, while with FDBA it becomes available after the osteoclasts break down their mineral content. Even though their osteoinductive potential can vary considerably, if an allograft that is tested for its osteoinductivity is chosen, a positive effect on bone formation should be anticipated. Moreover, the faster resorption of the allograft would create a more porous architecture allowing revascularization and ingrowth of bone forming cells. The author of this chapter has tested this combination for GBR application (Figures 6.2–6.4, 6.6, 6.7, and 6.10). A clinical and histological report is under preparation.

6.4.2.6 Potential Use of Growth Factors

The two most documented recombinant human growth factors for oral bone regeneration are the platelet derived growth factor (rh-PDGF BB) and the bone morphogenic protein-2 (rh-BMP2). *In vitro* and *in vivo* studies have confirmed that growth factors can enhance the capacity of tissues to regenerate by regulating cell chemoattraction, differentiation and proliferation. While several studies have indicated their effectiveness and their promising potential in enhancing GBR outcomes, clinical documentation is still weak. The discussion of the potential use of growth factors falls outside the scope of this chapter.

6.5 Soft Tissue Corrections after GBR Procedures in the Esthetic Zone

GBR surgery usually results in the translation of the mucoginigval line in a coronal direction. This is due to the advancement of the buccal flap made to achieve a primary intention wound closure. This soft tissue alteration will have three major consequences:

1) Reduction in the width of ***keratinized tissue*** that is usually present on the buccal aspect of the edentulous ridge (Figures 6.7zb, 6.8m–n and 6.9k–l).

2) Reduction in the ***thickness*** of the soft tissues covering the buccal aspect of the ridge (Figures 6.2m and 6.4m).
3) Loss of ***vestibular depth*** (Figures 6.7zb, 6.8m–n and 6.9k–l).

In the esthetic zone, the impact of these soft tissue deformations is more critical than anywhere else in the mouth. Depending on their severity, corrections are sometimes required.

From a functional perspective, the need for keratinized tissue around implants is controversial (Chung et al. 2006). However, from an esthetic perspective the establishment of a keratinized tissue band on the buccal aspect of an implant restoration is important.

When the deformation is minor, usually the abutment connection surgery itself will transpose a band of keratinized tissue buccally to the implant and will increase the buccal soft tissue volume (Figures 6.1zu–zw and 6.6u–v) (Benic et al. 2017). The vestibular depth in this case needs no correction. When the buccal soft tissue volume needs more thickness, a subepithelial connective tissue graft can be applied (Figures 6.2r–u, 6.3l–r and 6.4o–r). To reduce the morbidity of harvesting a connective tissue graft from the palate, an alternative technique utilizing a resorbable collagen matrix soaked in recombinant human PDGF BB was tested (Simion et al. 2012). The results showed a moderate increase in soft tissue volume. In more severe deformations, a severe loss of vestibular depth and keratinized tissue is present (Figures 6.7zb, 6.8m–n and 6.9k–l). In this category of cases, the mucoginigval line is usually located in a palatal position in relation to the submerged implants. Classically, performing a wide free gingival graft will address the vestibular depth problem and the recreation of keratinized tissue in one surgery (Nabers 1966). The drawback of the free gingival graft is the unpleasant color match and its morbidity. To reduce the problem of color matching and to reduce the morbidity of harvesting the graft from the palate, an alternative technique was proposed using a gingival graft of reduced width (strip gingival graft) combined with a xenogenic collagen matrix (Figure 6.8) (Urban et al. 2015). A significant gain in keratinized tissue width (mean of 6.33 mm) at 12 months was achieved (Figure 6.9).

6.6 Complications

6.6.1 Wound Dehiscence and Material Exposure

Wound dehiscence was frequently reported in GBR. Material exposure increases the risk of infection. The risk of exposure was reportedly higher with the use of non-resorbable membranes compared to collagen membranes; but a big heterogeneity exists among reports.

6.6.1.1 PTFE membranes

With PTFE membranes used for vertical augmentations, the range of complications ranged from 0 to 45.5% (Todisco 2010). In a systematic review by Chiapasco and Zaniboni (2009) on the treatment of dehiscence-type defects, the complication rate (expose and/or infection) was reported to be 20% for the e-PTFE membranes. E-PTFE exposure, even if it does not lead to infection, was clinically proven to hinder the effectiveness of the regeneration (Simion et al. 1994). In a meta-analysis by Machtei (2001), the new bone formation in sites without membrane exposure was sixfold greater compared with sites with membrane exposure. Reduced newly formed bone was found in patients where e-PTFE membranes were prematurely exposed during the first three months after implantation compared with those exposed after three to six months or of those that remained unexposed until second stage implant surgery (Mattout and Mattout 2000).

Due to the heterogeneity of reports on membrane exposure with non-resorbable membranes and due to the reduced sample size of the published studies that are usually conducted with a high risk of bias, definitive conclusions cannot be made. Larger scale studies are needed to deliver clear figures. But clinical experience let us assume that a properly managed surgery in an appropriately selected patient should offer no or minimal risk of wound dehiscence with the use of PTFE membranes. Because the classical e-PTFE is no longer available on the market, we consider the use titanium-reinforced d-PTFE membranes as the gold standard in treating vertical defects in the esthetic region, especially because most esthetic defects have at least a small vertical component and are best addressed with a titanium-reinforced membrane. An impeccable soft tissue advancement and closure should offer predictable wound healing.

The d-PTFE membranes, having a pore size of less than 3 μm, are supposedly at a reduced risk of infection when exposed. They are impervious to bacteria. When a d-PTFE membrane is exposed, the patient should be closely monitored to rule out infection. A focused hygiene regimen consisting of 0.2% chlorhexidine gel twice daily to reduce plaque formation and weekly patient follow-up are mandatory (Fontana et al. 2011). In the absence of infection, a d-PTFE membrane can be maintained in place for several weeks, which is the time needed for the bone graft to consolidate. They can then be removed, and graft healing and maturation can proceed on its own. A considerable amount of new bone formation can still be achieved. When infection is suspected or when an obvious purulent exudation is present, the immediate removal of the entirety of the membrane is mandatory, and the underlying infected particles and inflammatory tissue must be curetted (Figure 6.10) (Verardi and Simion 2007; Fontana et al. 2011). The part of the graft that still seems to be consolidated should be kept in place. Chiapasco and Zaniboni (2009) in their previously mentioned systematic review, concluded that although better results (in terms of percentage of bone regeneration) were obtained for uneventful healing with the e-PTFE membranes, an acceptable coverage of the initially exposed implant threads was also achieved for membrane exposure cases (63–100% coverage of the initial defect), with most cases reporting complete or almost complete coverage of the initial defect. Infection and abscess formation can sometimes manifest without membrane exposure. This was correlated with bacterial contamination of the graft and the membrane (Fontana et al. 2011). Membrane removal is required, accompanied by curettage of the infected/loose parts of the graft.

6.6.1.2 Resorbable membranes

With resorbable membranes, and specifically collagen membranes, the risk of exposure is reportedly less than with non-resorbable membranes; 5% of exposure/infection was reported in a systematic review on the treatment of dehiscence-type defects (Chiapasco and Zaniboni 2009). Cross-linked membranes and especially those who are ribose cross-linked have shown a high incidence of exposure compared to native collagen membrane (Friedmann et al. 2011). Interestingly, exposed ribose cross-linked membranes were sometimes able to support secondary intention healing without the exposure of the bone graft material (Moses et al. 2005). With native and chemically cross-linked membranes, the exposure usually heals by secondary intention healing, but more soft tissue inflammation was observed around cross-linked membranes (Becker et al. 2009). Exposure of a collagen membrane should be monitored closely until secondary intention healing has occurred and to exclude any infectious process. Reduced bone quantity and quality should be expected when exposure occurs, but sometimes considerable bone regeneration can still be achieved (Chiapasco and Zaniboni 2009). When infection with purulent discharge happens, removal of the membrane remnants and debridement of the infected graft is indicated.

6.6.2 Neurological Complications

Working in the anterior mandible, lesion to the mental nerve can cause sensory disturbance in the lower lip. Working in the maxillary esthetic zone, lesion to the branches of the infraorbital nerve can cause sensory disturbance to the upper lip and lesion to the buccal branches of the facial nerve can cause reduced upper lip mobility. While the mental nerve and its branches can be surgically localized and isolated, the terminal nerve branches innervating the upper lip run through the thickness of the orbicularis oris muscle and are difficult to visualize. This anatomical characteristic of the upper lip renders it at risk of neurological complications if blind cuts are performed through the muscle. Upper lip neurological complications are likely to be under-reported when major flap advancements are performed in the anterior maxilla. More anatomical research is needed to identify the exact path of the nerve branches of the upper lip.

6.7 Conclusion

Despite lacking an evidence based proof, GBR can be considered today as one of the best techniques to augment the deficient alveolar ridge in an esthetically demanding site. While several other bone augmentation techniques are equally capable of laterally increasing the bone volume, the GBR technique offers the advantage of regenerating the vertical component with a good level of predictability. This capacity in re-establishing the three-dimensional ridge contour is essential for the esthetic outcome.

On the technical level, beside the need for a meticulous flap preparation and an appropriate wound closure, the immobilization of the graft/membrane complex is much needed to optimize the outcome.

The choice of using titanium-reinforced PTFE membranes should be privileged in challenging (especially vertical) defects. The use of collagen membranes, whether native or cross-linked, should be favored in the remainder of defect types.

The choice of the graft material greatly influences the outcome. The bigger the defect, the more important the choice of the graft material. While no graft material alone meets the ideal requirements, composite grafting is favored in certain situations to combine the advantages of different graft types. When using autografts, the biologic potential of the graft is greatly enhanced. ABB, besides being osteoconductive, is valued for its reduced substitution rate and thus for its ability to stabilize the grafted volume against resorption/remodeling. Allografts are favored for their osteoconductive and osteoinductive potential.

In the esthetic zone, GBR procedures are often complemented with soft tissue procedures to thicken the tissues and to re-establish the keratinized mucosa.

References

Aghaloo, T.L. and Moy, P.K. (2007). Which hard tissue augmentation techniques are the most successful in furnishing bony support for implant placement? *Int. J. Oral Maxillofac. Implants* 22 (Suppl): 49–70.

Annen, B.M., Ramel, C.F., Hämmerle, C.H., and Jung, R.E. (2011). Use of a new cross-linked collagen membrane for the treatment of peri-implant dehiscence defects: a randomised controlled double-blinded clinical trial. *Eur. J. Oral Implantol.* 4 (2): 87–100.

von Arx, T. and Buser, D. (2006). Horizontal ridge augmentation using autogenous block grafts and the guided bone regeneration technique with collagen membranes: a clinical study with 42 patients. *Clin. Oral Implants Res.* 17 (4): 359–366.

von Arx, T., Broggini, N., Jensen, S.S. et al. (2005). Membrane durability and tissue response of different bioresorbable barrier membranes: a histologic study in the rabbit calvarium. *Int. J. Oral Maxillofac. Implants* 20 (6): 843–853.

Augthun, M., Yildirim, M., Spiekermann, H., and Biesterfeld, S. (1995). Healing of bone defects in combination with immediate implants using the membrane technique. *Int. J. Oral Maxillofac. Implants* 10 (4): 421–428.

Bartee, B.K. and Carr, J.A. (1995). Evaluation of a high-density polytetrafluoroethylene (n-PTFE) membrane as a barrier material to facilitate guided bone regeneration in the rat mandible. *J. Oral Implantol.* 21 (2): 88–95.

Batista, E.L., Batista, F.C., and Novaes, A.B. (2001). Management of soft tissue ridge deformities with acellular dermal matrix. Clinical approach and outcome after 6 months of treatment. *J. Periodontol.* 72 (2): 265–273.

Becker, J., Al-Nawas, B., Klein, M.O. et al. (2009). Use of a new cross-linked collagen membrane for the treatment of dehiscence-type defects at titanium implants: a prospective, randomized-controlled double-blinded clinical multicenter study. *Clin. Oral Implants Res.* 20 (7): 742–749.

Becker, W. and Becker, B.E. (1990). Guided tissue regeneration for implants placed into extraction sockets and for implant dehiscences: surgical techniques and case report. *Int. J. Periodontics Restorative Dent.* 10 (5): 376–391.

Becker, W., Dahlin, C., Becker, B.E. et al. (1994). The use of e-PTFE barrier membranes for bone promotion aroound titanium implants placed into extraction sockets: A prospective multicenter study. *Int. J. Oral Max. Fac. Imp.* 9: 31–40.

Becker, W., Schenk, R., Higuchi, K. et al. (1995). Variations bone regeneration adjacent to implants augmented with barrier membranes alone or with demineralized freeze-dried bone or autologous grafts: a study in dogs. *Int. J. Oral Max. Fac. Implants.* 10 (2): 143–154.

Beitlitum, I., Artzi, Z., and Nemcovsky, C.E. (2010). Clinical evaluation of particulate allogeneic with and without autogenous bone grafts and resorbable collagen membranes for bone augmentation of atrophic alveolar ridges. *Clin. Oral Implants Res.* 21 (11): 1242–1250.

Benic, G.I. and Hämmerle, C.H.F. (2014). Horizontal bone augmentation by means of guided bone regeneration. *Periodontol.* 66 (1): 13–40.

Benic, G.I., Ge, Y., Gallucci, G.O. et al. (2017). Guided bone regeneration and abutment connection augment the buccal soft tissue contour: 3-year results of a prospective comparative clinical study. *Clin. Oral Implants Res.* 28 (2): 219–225.

Block, M.S. and Degen, M. (2004). Horizontal ridge augmentation using human mineralized particulate bone: preliminary results. *J. Oral Maxillofac. Surg.* 62 (9 Suppl 2): 67–72.

Bozkurt, A., Apel, C., Sellhaus, B. et al. (2014). Differences in degradation behavior of two non-cross-linked collagen barrier membranes: an in vitro and in vivo study. *Clin. Oral Implants Res.* 25 (12): 1403–1411.

Bunyaratavej, P. and Wang, H.L. (2001). Collagen membranes: a review. *J. Periodontol.* 72 (2): 215–229.

Burchardt, H. (1983). The biology of bone graft repair. *Clin. Orthop. Relat. Res.* 174: 28–42.

Buser, D., Dula, K., Belser, U. et al. (1993). Localized ridge augmentation using guided bone regeneration. 1. Surgical procedure in the maxilla. *' Int. J. Periodontics Restorative Dent.* 13 (1): 29–45.

Buser, D., Dula, K., Hirt, H.P., and Schenk, R.K. (1996 Apr). Lateral ridge augmentation using autografts and barrier membranes: a clinical study with 40 partially edentulous patients. *J. Oral Maxillofac. Surg.* 54 (4): 420–432. 432–433.

Buser, D., Hoffmann, B., Bernard, J.P. et al. (1998). Evaluation of filling materials in membrane – protected bone defects. A comparative histomorphometric study in the mandible of miniature pigs. *Clin. Oral Implants Res.* 9 (3): 137–150.

Buser, D., Chappuis, V., Bornstein, M.M. et al. (2013). Long-term stability of contour augmentation with early implant placement following single tooth extraction in the esthetic zone: a prospective, cross-sectional study in 41 patients with a 5- to 9-year follow-up. *J. Periodontol.* 84 (11): 1517–1527.

Caldwell, G.R., Mills, M.P., Finlayson, R., and Mealey, B.L. (2015). Lateral alveolar ridge augmentation using tenting screws, acellular dermal matrix, and freeze-dried bone allograft alone or with particulate autogenous bone. *Int. J. Periodontics Restorative Dent.* 35 (1): 75–83.

Cammack, G.V., Nevins, M., Clem, D.S. et al. (2005). Histologic evaluation of mineralized and demineralized freeze-dried bone allograft for ridge and sinus augmentations. *Int. J. Periodontics Restorative Dent.* 25 (3): 231–237.

Canullo, L. and Malagnino, V.A. (2008). Vertical ridge augmentation around implants by e-PTFE titanium-reinforced membrane and bovine bone matrix: a 24- to 54-month study of 10 consecutive cases. *Int. J. Oral Maxillofac. Implants* 23 (5): 858–866.

Canullo, L., Trisi, P., and Simion, M. (2006). Vertical ridge augmentation around implants using e-PTFE titanium-reinforced membrane and deproteinized bovine bone mineral (Bio-Oss): a case report. *Int. J. Periodontics Restorative Dent.* 26 (4): 355–361.

Casino, A.J., Harrison, P., Tarnow, D.P. et al. (1997). The influence of type of incision on the success rate of implant integration at stage II uncovering surgery. *J. Oral Maxillofac. Surg.* 55 (12 Suppl 5): 31–37.

Chakar, C., Naaman, N., Soffer, E. et al. (2014). Bone formation with deproteinized bovine bone mineral or biphasic calcium phosphate in the presence of autologous platelet lysate: comparative investigation in rabbit. *Int. J. Biomater.* 2014: 367265.

Chappuis, V., Cavusoglu, Y., Buser, D., and von Arx, T. (2017). Lateral ridge augmentation using autogenous block grafts and guided bone regeneration: a 10-year prospective case series study. *Clin. Implant Dent. Relat. Res.* 19 (1): 85–96.

Chen, G., Sato, T., Ohgushi, H. et al. (2005). Culturing of skin fibroblasts in a thin PLGA-collagen hybrid mesh. *Biomaterials* 26 (15): 2559–2566.

Chesmel, K.D., Branger, J., Wertheim, H., and Scarborough, N. (1998). Healing response to various forms of human demineralized bone matrix in athymic rat cranial defects. *J. Oral Maxillofac. Surg.* 56 (7): 857–863. 865.

Chiapasco, M. and Zaniboni, M. (2009). Clinical outcomes of GBR procedures to correct peri-implant dehiscences and fenestrations: a systematic review. *Clin. Oral Implants Res.* 20 (Suppl 4): 113–123.

Chung, D.M., Oh, T.J., Shotwell, J.L. et al. (2006). Significance of keratinized mucosa ini maintenence of dental implants with different surfaces. *J. Periodontal.* 77 (8): 1410–1420.

Clune, J.E., Mulliken, J.B., Glowacki, J. et al. (2010). Inlay cranioplasty: an experimental comparison of particulate graft versus bone dust. *Plast. Reconstr. Surg.* 126 (4): 1311–1319.

Cortellini, P., Prato, G.P., and Tonetti, M.S. (1999). The simplified papilla preservation flap. A novel surgical approach for the management of soft tissues in regenerative procedures. *Int. J. Periodontics Restorative Dent.* 19 (6): 589–599.

Cranin, A.N., Sirakian, A., Russell, D., and Klein, M. (1998). The role of incision design and location in the healing processes of alveolar ridges and implant host sites. *Int. J. Oral Maxillofac. Implants* 13 (4): 483–491.

Dahlin, C., Linde, A., Gottlow, J., and Nyman, S. (1988). Healing of bone defects by guided tissue regeneration. *Plast. Reconstr. Surg.* 81 (5): 672–676.

Dahlin, C., Simion, M., Nanmark, U., and Sennerby, L. (1998). Histological morphology of the e-PTFE/tissue interface in humans subjected to guided bone regeneration in conjunction with oral implant treatment. *Clin. Oral Implants Res.* 9 (2): 100–106.

Dahlin, C., Simion, M., and Hatano, N. (2010). Long-term follow-up on soft and hard tissue levels following guided bone regeneration treatment in combination with a xenogeneic filling material: a 5-year prospective clinical study. *Clin. Implant Dent. Relat. Res.* 12 (4): 263–270.

Ellinger, R.F., Nery, E.B., and Lynch, K.L. (1986). Histological assessment of periodontal osseous defects following implantation of hydroxyapatite and biphasic calcium phosphate ceramics: a case report. *Int. J. Periodontics Restorative Dent.* 6 (3): 22–33.

Eskow, A.J. and Mealey, B.L. (2014). Evaluation of healing following tooth extraction with ridge preservation using cotical versus cancellous freeze dried bone allograft. *J. Periodontol.* 85 (4): 514–524.

Feuille, F., Knapp, C.I., Brunsvold, M.A., and Mellonig, J.T. (2003). Clinical and histologic evaluation of bone-replacement grafts in the treatment of localized alveolar ridge defects. Part 1: mineralized freeze-dried bone allograft. *Int. J. Periodontics Restorative Dent.* 23 (1): 29–35.

Fleckenstein, K.B., Cuenin, M.,.F., Peacock, M.E. et al. (2006). Effect of a hydroxyapatite tricalcium phosphate alloplast on osseous repair in the rat calvarium. *J. Periodontol.* 77 (1): 39–45.

Fontana, F., Santoro, F., Maiorana, C. et al. (2008). Clinical and histologic evaluation of allogeneic bone matrix versus autogenous bone chips associated with titanium-reinforced e-PTFE membrane for vertical ridge augmentation: a prospective pilot study. *Int. J. Oral Maxillofac. Implants* 23 (6): 1003–1012.

Fontana, F., Maschera, E., Rocchietta, I., and Simion, M. (2011). Clinical classification of complications in guided bone regeneration procedures by means of a nonresorbable membrane. *Int. J. Periodontics Restorative Dent.* 31 (3): 265–273.

Fotek, P.D., Neiva, R.F., and Wang, H.-L. (2009). Comparison of dermal matrix and polytetrafluoroethylene membrane for socket bone augmentation: a clinical and histologic study. *J. Periodontol.* 80 (5): 776–785.

Fowler, E.B., Breault, L.G., and Rebitski, G. (2000). Ridge preservation utilizing an acellular dermal allograft and demineralized freeze-dried bone allograft: part II. Immediate endosseous implant placement. *J. Periodontol.* 71 (8): 1360–1364.

Friedmann, A., Strietzel, F.P., Maretzki, B. et al. (2001). Observations on a new collagen barrier membrane in 16 consecutively treated patients. Clinical and histological findings. *J. Periodontol.* 72 (11): 1616–1623.

Friedmann, A., Gissel, K., Soudan, M. et al. (2011). Randomized controlled trial on lateral augmentation using two collagen membranes: morphometric results on mineralized tissue compound. *J. Clin. Periodontol.* 38 (7): 677–685.

Fugazzotto, P.A. (1999). Maintenance of soft tissue closure following guided bone regeneration: technical considerations and report of 723 cases. *J. Periodontol.* 70 (9): 1085–1097.

Ghanaati, S. (2012). Non-cross-linked porcine-based collagen I-III membranes do not require high vascularization rates for their integration within the implantation bed: a paradigm shift. *Acta Biomater.* 8 (8): 3061–3072.

Gottlow, J. (1993). Guided tissue regeneration using bioresorbable and non-resorbable devices: initial healing and long-term results. *J. Periodontol.* 64 (11 Suppl): 1157–1165.

Gottlow, J., Nyman, S., Lindhe, J. et al. (1986). New attachment formation in the human periodontium by guided tissue regeneration. Case reports. *J. Clin. Periodontol.* 13 (6): 604–616.

Greenstein, G., Greenstein, B., Cavallaro, J. et al. (2009). Flap advancement: practical techniques to attain tension-free primary closure. *J. Periodontol.* 80 (1): 4–15.

Grunder, U., Wenz, B., and Schupbach, P. (2011). Guided bone regeneration around single-tooth implants in the esthetic zone: a case series. *Int. J. Periodontics Restorative Dent.* 31 (6): 613–620.

Hämmerle, C.H., Chiantella, G.C., Karring, T., and Lang, N.P. (1998). The effect of a deproteinized bovine bone mineral on bone regeneration around titanium dental implants. *Clin. Oral Implants Res.* 9 (3): 151–162.

Hämmerle, C.H.F., Jung, R.E., Yaman, D., and Lang, N.P. (2008). Ridge augmentation by applying bioresorbable membranes and deproteinized bovine bone mineral: a report of twelve consecutive cases. *Clin. Oral Implants Res.* 19 (1): 19–25.

Harris, R.J. (2002). Cellular dermal matrix used for root coverage: 18-month follow-up observation. *Int. J. Periodontics Restorative Dent.* 22 (2): 156–163.

Henderson, R.D., Greenwell, H., Drisko, C. et al. (2001). Predictable multiple site root coverage using an acellular dermal matrix allograft. *J. Periodontol.* 72 (5): 571–582.

Jensen, S.S. and Terheyden, H. (2009). Bone augmentation procedures in localized defects in the alveolar ridge: clinical results with different bone grafts and bone-substitute materials. *Int. J. Oral Maxillofac. Implants* 24 (Suppl): 218–236.

Jensen, S.S., Broggini, N., Hjørting-Hansen, E. et al. (2006). Bone healing and graft resorption of autograft, anorganic bovine bone and beta-tricalcium phosphate. A histologic and histomorphometric study in the mandibles of minipigs. *Clin. Oral Implants Res.* 17 (3): 237–243.

Jensen, S.S., Yeo, A., Dard, M. et al. (2007). Evaluation of a novel biphasic calcium phosphate in standardized bone defects: a histologic and histomorphometric study in the mandibles of minipigs. *Clin. Oral Implants Res.* 18 (6): 752–760.

Johansson, B., Grepe, A., Wannfors, K., and Hirsch, J.M. (2001). A clinical study of changes in the volume of bone grafts in the atrophic maxilla. *Dentomaxillofac Radiol.* 30 (3): 157–161.

Jovanovic, S.A., Spiekermann, H., and Richter, E.J. (1992). Bone regeneration around titanium dental implants in dehisced defect sites: a clinical study. *Int. J. Oral Maxillofac. Implants* 7 (2): 233–245.

Jung, R.E., Fenner, N., Hämmerle, C.,.H.F., and Zitzmann, N.U. (2013). Long-term outcome of implants placed with guided bone regeneration (GBR) using resorbable and non-resorbable membranes after 12-14 years. *Clin. Oral Implants Res.* 24 (10): 1065–1073.

Kim, Y., Kim, T.K., and Leem, D.H. (2015). Clinical study of a flap advancement technique without vertical incision for guided bone regeneration. *Int. J. Oral Maxillofac. Implants* 30 (5): 1113–1118.

Kleinheinz, J., Büchter, A., Kruse-Lösler, B. et al. (2005). Incision design in implant dentistry based on vascularization of the mucosa. *Clin. Oral Implants Res.* 16 (5): 518–523.

Koymen, R., Karacayli, U., Gocmen-Mas, N. et al. (2009). Flap and incision design in implant surgery: clinical and anatomical study. *Surg. Radiol. Anat.* 31 (4): 301–306.

Kozlovsky, A., Aboodi, G., Moses, O. et al. (2009). Bio-degradation of a resorbable collagen membrane (Bio-Gide) applied in a double-layer technique in rats. *Clin. Oral Implants Res.* 20 (10): 1116–1123.

Lambrecht, J.T. (2004). Intraoral piezo-surgery. *Schweiz. Monatsschr. Zahnmed.* 114 (1): 28–36.

Landi, L., Pretel, R.W., Hakimi, N.M., and Setayesh, R. (2000). Maxillary sinus floor elevation using a combination of DFDBA and bovine-derived porous hydroxyapatite: a preliminary histologic and histomorphometric report. *Int. J. Periodontics Restorative Dent.* 20 (6): 574–583.

Laurell, L. (1995). Guided tissue regeneration in clinical studies: a review. In: *Guided Periodontal Tissue Regeneration* (ed. A. Hugoson, D. Lundgren and B. Lindgren), 68–90. Stockholm: Förlagshuset Gothia.

Lundgren, S., Moy, P., Johansson, C., and Nilsson, H. (1996). Augmentation of the maxillary sinus floor with particulated mandible: a histologic and histomorphometric study. *Int. J. Oral Maxillofac. Implants* 11 (6): 760–766.

Lyford, R.H., Mills, M.P., Knapp, C.I. et al. (2003). Clinical evaluation of freeze-dried block allografts for alveolar ridge augmentation: a case series. *Int. J. Periodontics Restorative Dent.* 23 (5): 417–425.

Machtei, E.E. (2001). The effect of membrane exposure on the outcome of regenerative procedures in humans: a meta-analysis. *J. Periodontol.* 72 (4): 512–516.

Maiorana, C., Beretta, M., Salina, S., and Santoro, F. (2005). Reduction of autogenous bone graft resorption by means of Bio-Oss coverage: a prospective study. *Int. J. Periodontics Restorative Dent.* 25 (1): 19–25.

Maiorana, C., Beretta, M., Battista Grossi, G. et al. (2011). Histomorphometric evaluation of anorganic bovine bone coverage to reduce autogenous grafts resorption: preliminary results. *Open Dent. J.* 5: 71–78.

Majzoub, Z., Berengo, M., Giardino, R. et al. (1999). Role of intramarrow penetration in osseous repair: a pilot study in the rabbit calvaria. *J. Periodontol.* 70 (12): 1501–1510.

Mattout, P. and Mattout, C. (2000). Conditions for success in guided bone regeneration: retrospective study on 376 implant sites. *J. Periodontol.* 71 (12): 1904–1909.

Mellonig, J.T. and Nevins, M. (1995). Guided bone regeneration of bone defects associated with implants: an evidence-based outcome assessment. *Int. J. Periodontics Restorative Dent.* 15 (2): 168–185.

Mellonig, J.T. and Triplett, R.G. (1993). Guided tissue regeneration and endosseous dental implants. *Int. J. Periodontics Restorative Dent.* 13 (2): 108–119.

Merli, M., Merli, I., Raffaelli, E. et al. (2016). Bone augmentation at implant dehiscences and fenestrations. A systematic review of randomised controlled trials. *Eur. J. Oral Implantol.* 9 (1): 11–32.

Mir-Mari, J., Wui, H., Jung, R.E. et al. (2016). Influence of blinded wound closure on the volume stability of different GBR materials: an in vitro cone-beam computed tomographic examination. *Clin. Oral Implants Res.* 27 (2): 258–265.

Miron, R.J., Sculean, A., Shuang, Y. et al. (2016). Osteoinductive potential of a novel biphasic calcium phosphate bone graft in comparison with autographs, xenografts, and DFDBA. *Clin. Oral Implants Res.* 27 (6): 668–675.

Mokbel, N., Bou Serhal, C., Matni, G., and Naaman, N. (2008). Healing patterns of critical size bony defects in rat following bone graft. *Oral Maxillofac. Surg.* 12 (2): 73–78.

Moses, O., Pitaru, S., Artzi, Z., and Nemcovsky, C.E. (2005). Healing of dehiscence-type defects in implants placed together with different barrier membranes: a comparative clinical study. *Clin. Oral Implants Res.* 16 (2): 210–219.

Nabers, J.M. (1966). Extension of the vestibular fornix utilizing a gingival graft – case history. *Periodontics.* 4 (2): 77–79.

Nevins, M., Mellonig, J.T., Clem, D.S. et al. (1998). Implants in regenerated bone: long-term survival. *Int. J. Periodontics Restorative Dent.* 18 (1): 34–45.

Novaes, A.B. and Souza, S.L. (2001). Acellular dermal matrix graft as a membrane for guided bone regeneration: a case report. *Implant Dent.* 10 (3): 192–196.

Novaes, A.B., Papalexiou, V., Luczyszyn, S.M. et al. (2002). Immediate implant in extraction socket with acellular dermal matrix graft and bioactive glass: a case report. *Implant Dent.* 11 (4): 343–348.

Nowzari, H. and Slots, J. (1995). Microbiologic and clinical study of polytetrafluoroethylene membranes for guided bone regeneration around implants. *Int. J. Oral Maxillofac. Implants* 10 (1): 67–73.

Nyman, S., Gottlow, J., Karring, T., and Lindhe, J. (1982). The regenerative potential of the periodontal ligament. An experimental study in the monkey. *J. Clin. Periodontol.* 9 (3): 257–265.

Oh, T.-J., Meraw, S.J., Lee, E.-J. et al. (2003). Comparative analysis of collagen membranes for the treatment of implant dehiscence defects. *Clin. Oral Implants Res.* 14 (1): 80–90.

Orsini, G., Scarano, A., Degidi, M. et al. (2007). Histological and ultrastructural evaluation of bone around Bio-Oss particles in sinus augmentation. *Oral Dis.* 13 (6): 586–593.

Owens, K.W. and Yukna, R.A. (2001). Collagen membrane resorption in dogs: a comparative study. *Implant Dent.* 10 (1): 49–58.

Pallesen, L., Schou, S., Aaboe, M. et al. (2002). Influence of particle size of autogenous bone grafts on the early stages of bone regeneration: a histologic and stereologic study in rabbit calvarium. *Int. J. Oral Maxillofac. Implants* 17 (4): 498–506.

Park, S.-H. and Wang, H.-L. (2007). Clinical significance of incision location on guided bone regeneration: human study. *J. Periodontol.* 78 (1): 47–51.

Park, S.-H., Lee, K., Oh, T.-J. et al. (2008). Effect of absorbable membranes on sandwich bone augmentation. *Clin. Oral Implants Res.* 19 (1): 32–41.

Paul, B.F., Mellonig, J.T., Towle, H.J., and Gray, J.L. (1992). Use of a collagen barrier to enhance healing in human periodontal furcation defects. *Int. J. Periodontics Restorative Dent.* 12 (2): 123–131.

Peleg, M., Mazor, Z., Chaushu, G., and Garg, A.K. (1998). Sinus floor augmentation with simultaneous implant placement in the severely atrophic maxilla. *J. Periodontol.* 69 (12): 1397–1403.

Piattelli, A., Scarano, A., Corigliano, M., and Piattelli, M. (1996). Comparison of bone regeneration with the use of mineralized and demineralized freeze-dried bone allografts: a histological and histochemical study in man. *Biomaterials* 17 (11): 1127–1131.

Piattelli, A., Scarano, A., Coraggio, F., and Matarasso, S. (1998). Early tissue reactions to polylactic acid resorbable membranes: a histological and histochemical study in rabbit. *Biomaterials* 19 (10): 889–896.

Piattelli, M., Favero, G.A., Scarano, A. et al. (1999). Bone reactions to anorganic bovine bone (Bio-Oss) used in sinus augmentation procedures: a histologic long-term report of 20 cases in humans. *Int. J. Oral Maxillofac. Implants* 14 (6): 835–840.

Pitaru, S., Tal, H., Soldinger, M. et al. (1988). Partial regeneration of periodontal tissues using collagen barriers. Initial observations in the canine. *J. Periodontol.* 59 (6): 380–386.

Reddi, A.H. (1994). Symbiosis of biotechnology and biomaterials: applications iin tissue engineering of bone and cartilage. *J. Cell. Biochem.* 56: 192–195.

Rehrmann, A. (1936). Eine Methode zur Schliessung von Kieferhohlen perforationen. *Dtsch. Zahnarztl. Z.* 39: 1136–1139.

Rocchietta, I., Simion, M., Hoffmann, M. et al. (2016). Vertical bone augmentation with an autogenous block or particles in combination with guided bone regeneration: a clinical and histological preliminary study in humans. *Clin. Implant Dent. Relat. Res.* 18 (1): 19–29.

Romanos, G.E. (2010). Periosteal releasing incision for successful coverage of augmented sites. A technical note. *J. Oral Implantol.* 36 (1): 25–30.

Rominger, J.W. and Triplett, R.G. (1994). The use of guided tissue regeneration to improve implant osseointegration. *J. Oral Maxillofac. Surg.* 52 (2): 106–112. 113.

Rompen, E.H., Biewer, R., Vanheusden, A. et al. (1999). The influence of cortical perforations and of space filling with peripheral blood on the kinetics of guided bone generation. A comparative histometric study in the rat. *Clin. Oral Implants Res.* 10 (2): 85–94.

Ronda, M. and Stacchi, C. (2015). A novel approach for the coronal advancement of the buccal flap. *Int. J. Periodontics Restorative Dent.* 35 (6): 795–801.

Ronda, M., Rebaudi, A., Torelli, L., and Stacchi, C. (2014). Expanded vs. dense polytetrafluoroethylene membranes in vertical ridge augmentation around dental implants: a prospective randomized controlled clinical trial. *Clin. Oral Implants Res.* 25 (7): 859–866.

Rossi, R., Rancitelli, D., Poli, P.P. et al. (2016). The use of a collagenated porcine cortical lamina in the reconstruction of alveolar ridge defects. A clinical and histological study. *Minerva Stomatol.* 65 (5): 257–268.

Rothamel, D., Schwarz, F., Sculean, A. et al. (2004). Biocompatibility of various collagen membranes in cultures of human PDL fibroblasts and human osteoblast-like cells. *Clin. Oral Implants Res.* 15 (4): 443–449.

Rothamel, D., Schwarz, F., Sager, M. et al. (2005). Biodegradation of differently cross-linked collagen membranes: an experimental study in the rat *Clin. Oral Implants Res.* 16 (3): 369–378.

Rothamel, D., Schwarz, F., Fienitz, T. et al. (2012). Biocompatibility and biodegradation of a native porcine pericardium membrane: results of in vitro and in vivo examinations. *Int. J. Oral Maxillofac. Implants* 27 (1): 146–154.

Sartori, S., Silvestri, M., Forni, F. et al. (2003). Ten-year follow-up in a maxillary sinus augmentation using anorganic bovine bone (Bio-Oss). A case report with histomorphometric evaluation. *Clin. Oral Implants Res.* 14 (3): 369–372.

Saulacic, N., Bosshardt, D.D., Jensen, S.S. et al. (2015). Impact of bone graft harvesting techniques on bone formation and graft resorption: a histomorphometric study in the mandibles of minipigs. *Clin. Oral Implants Res.* 26 (4): 383–391.

Scharf, D.R. and Tarnow, D.P. (1993). The effect of crestal versus mucobuccal incisions on the success rate of implant osseointegration. *Int. J. Oral Maxillofac. Implants* 8 (2): 187–190.

Schenk, R.K., Buser, D., Hardwick, W.R., and Dahlin, C. (1994). Healing pattern of bone regeneration in membrane-protected defects: a histologic study in the canine mandible. *Int. J. Oral Maxillofac. Implants* 9 (1): 13–29.

Schwartz, Z., Mellonig, J.T., Carnes, D.L. et al. (1996). Ability of commercial demineralized freeze-dried bone allograft to induce new bone formation. *J. Periodontol.* 67 (9): 918–926.

Schwartz, Z., Somers, A., Mellonig, J.T. et al. (1998). Ability of commercial demineralized freeze-dried bone allograft to induce new bone formation is dependent on donor age but not gender. *J. Periodontol.* 69 (4): 470–478.

Schwarz, F., Rothamel, D., Herten, M. et al. (2006). Angiogenesis pattern of native and cross-linked collagen membranes: an immunohistochemical study in the rat. *Clin. Oral Implants Res.* 17 (4): 403–409.

Schwarz, F., Hegewald, A., Sahm, N., and Becker, J. (2014). Long-term follow-up of simultaneous guided bone regeneration using native and cross-linked collagen membranes over 6 years. *Clin. Oral Implants Res.* 25 (9): 1010–1015.

Sclar, A.G. (2003). Surgical techniques for management of peri-implant soft tissues. In: *Soft Tissue Esthetic Considerations in Implant Therapy* (ed. A.G. Sclar), 47–51. Chicago: Quintessnce Books.

Simion, M., Trisi, P., and Piattelli, A. (1994). Vertical ridge augmentation using a membrane technique associated with osseointegrated implants. *Int. J. Periodontics Restorative Dent.* 14 (6): 496–511.

Simion, M., Jovanovic, S.A., Trisi, P. et al. (1998). Vertical ridge augmentation around dental implants using a membrane technique and autogenous bone or allografts in humans. *Int. J. Periodontics Restorative Dent.* 18 (1): 8–23.

Simion, M., Jovanovic, S.A., Tinti, C., and Benfenati, S.P. (2001). Long-term evaluation of osseointegrated implants inserted at the time or after vertical ridge augmentation. A retrospective study on 123 implants with 1-5 year follow-up. *Clin. Oral Implants Res.* 12 (1): 35–45.

Simion, M., Fontana, F., Rasperini, G., and Maiorana, C. (2007). Vertical ridge augmentation by expanded-polytetrafluoroethylene membrane and a combination of intraoral autogenous bone graft and deproteinized anorganic bovine bone (Bio Oss). *Clin. Oral Implants Res.* 18 (5): 620–629.

Simion, M., Rocchietta, I., Fontana, F., and Dellavia, C. (2012). Evaluation of a resorbable collagen matrix infused with rhPDGF-BB in peri-implant soft tissue augmentation: a preliminary report with 3.5 years of observation. *Int. J. Periodontics Restorative Dent.* 32 (3): 273–282.

Speer, D.P., Chvapil, M., Eskelson, C.D., and Ulreich, J. (1980). Biological effects of residual glutaraldehyde in glutaraldehyde-tanned collagen biomaterials. *J. Biomed. Mater. Res.* 14 (6): 753–764.

Sterio, T.W., Katancik, J.A., Blanchard, S.B. et al. (2013). A prospective, multicenter study of bovine pericardium membrane with cancellous particulate allograft for localized alveolar ridge augmentation'. *Int. J. Periodontics Restorative Dent.* 33 (4): 499–507.

Tinti, C. and Parma-Benfenati, S. (1995). Coronally positioned palatal sliding flap. *Int. J. Periodontics Restorative Dent.* 15 (3): 298–310.

Tinti, C., Parma-Benfenati, S., and Polizzi, G. (1996). Vertical ridge augmentation: what is the limit?'. *Int. J. Periodontics Restorative Dent.* 16 (3): 220–229.

Todisco, M. (2010). Early loading of implants in vertically augmented bone with non-resorbable membranes and deproteinised anorganic bovine bone. An uncontrolled prospective cohort study. *Eur. J. Oral Implantol.* 3 (1): 47–58.

Toscano, N., Holtzclaw, D., Mazor, Z. et al. (2010). Horizontal ridge augmentation utilizing a composite graft of demineralized freeze-dried allograft, mineralized cortical cancellous chips, and a biologically degradable thermoplastic carrier combined with a resorbable membrane: a retrospective evaluation of 73 consecutively treated cases from private practices. *J. Oral Implantol.* 36 (6): 467–474.

Traini, T., Valentini, P., Iezzi, G., and Piattelli, A. (2007). A histologic and histomorphometric evaluation of anorganic bovine bone retrieved 9 years after a sinus augmentation procedure. *J. Periodontol.* 78 (5): 955–961.

Triaca, A., Minoretti, R., Merli, M., and Merz, B. (2001). Periosteoplasty for soft tissue closure and augmentation in preprosthetic surgery: a surgical report. *Int. J. Oral Maxillofac. Implants* 16 (6): 851–856.

Urban, I.A., Jovanovic, S.A., and Lozada, J.L. (2009). Vertical ridge augmentation using guided bone regeneration (GBR) in three clinical scenarios prior to implant placement: a retrospective study of 35 patients 12 to 72 months after loading. *Int. J. Oral Maxillofac. Implants* 24 (3): 502–510.

Urban, I.A., Nagursky, H., and Lozada, J.L. (2011). Horizontal ridge augmentation with a resorbable membrane and particulated autogenous bone with or without anorganic bovine bone-derived mineral: a prospective case series in 22 patients. *Int. J. Oral Maxillofac. Implants* 26 (2): 404–414.

Urban, I.A., Nagursky, H., Lozada, J.L., and Nagy, K. (2013). Horizontal ridge augmentation with a collagen membrane and a combination of particulated autogenous bone and anorganic bovine bone-derived mineral: a prospective case series in 25 patients. *Int. J. Periodontics Restorative Dent.* 33 (3): 299–307.

Urban, I.A., Lozada, J.L., Jovanovic, S.A. et al. (2014). Vertical ridge augmentation with titanium-reinforced, dense-PTFE membranes and a combination of particulated autogenous bone and anorganic bovine bone-derived mineral: a prospective case series in 19 patients. *Int. J. Oral Maxillofac. Implants* 29 (1): 185–193.

Urban, I.A., Monje, A., and Wang, H.-L. (2015). Vertical ridge augmentation and soft tissue reconstruction of the anterior atrophic maxillae: a case series. *Int. J. Periodontics Restorative Dent.* 35 (5): 613–623.

Urban, I.A., Monje, A., Nevins, M. et al. (2016a). Surgical management of significant maxillary anterior vertical ridge defects. *Int. J. Periodontics Restorative Dent.* 36 (3): 329–337.

Urban, I.A., Lozada, J.L., Wessing, B. et al. (2016b). Vertical bone grafting and periosteal vertical mattress suture for the fixation of resorbable membranes and stabilization of particulate grafts in horizontal guided bone regeneration to achieve more predictable results: a technical report. *Int. J. Periodontics Restorative Dent.* 36 (2): 153–159.

Urist, M.R. and Strates, B.S. (1971). Bone morphogenetic protein. *J. Dent. Res.* 50 (6): 1392–1406.

Verardi, S. and Simion, M. (2007). Management of the exposure of e-PTFE membranes in guided bone regeneration. *Pract. Proced. Aesthet. Dent.* 19 (2): 111–117.

Veríssimo, D.M., Leitão, R.F.C., Figueiró, S.D. et al. (2015). Guided bone regeneration produced by new mineralized and reticulated collagen membranes in critical-sized rat calvarial defects. *Exp. Biol. Med. (Maywood)* 240 (2): 175–184.

Wachtel, H., Fickl, S., Hinze, M. et al. (2013). The bone lamina technique: a novel approach for lateral ridge augmentation – a case series. *Int. J. Periodontics Restorative Dent.* 33 (4): 491–497.

Wang, H.-L. and Boyapati, L. (2006). "PASS" principles for predictable bone regeneration. *Implant Dent.* 15 (1): 8–17.

Wei, L., Miron, R.J., Shi, B., and Zhang, Y. (2015). Osteoinductive and osteopromotive variability among different demineralized bone allografts. *Clin. Implant Dent. Relat. Res.* 17 (3): 533–542.

Widmark, G., Andersson, B., and Ivanoff, C.J. (1997). Mandibular bone graft in the anterior maxilla for single-tooth implants. Presentation of surgical method. *Int. J. Oral Maxillofac. Surg.* 26 (2): 106–109.

Wiebe, D., Megerman, J., L'Italien, G.J., and Abbott, W.M. (1988). Glutaraldehyde release from vascular prostheses of biologic origin. *Surgery* 104 (1): 26–33.

Wood, R.A. and Mealey, B.L. (2012). Histologic comparison of healing after tooth extraction with ridge preservation using mineralized versus demineralized freeze-dried bone allograft. *J. Periodontol.* 83 (3): 329–336.

Zaffe, D. and D'Avenia, F. (2007). A novel bone scraper for intraoral harvesting: a device for filling small bone defects. *Clin. Oral Implants Res.* 18 (4): 525–533.

Zhao, S., Pinholt, E.M., Madsen, J.E., and Donath, K. (2000). Histological evaluation of different biodegradable and non-biodegradable membranes implanted subcutaneously in rats. *J. Craniomaxillofac. Surg.* 28 (2): 116–122.

Zitzmann, N.U., Naef, R., and Schärer, P. (1997). Resorbable versus nonresorbable membranes in combination with Bio-Oss for guided bone regeneration. *Int. J. Oral Maxillofac. Implants* 12 (6): 844–852.

Zitzmann, N.U., Schärer, P., Marinello, C.P. et al. (2001). Alveolar ridge augmentation with Bio-Oss: a histologic study in humans. *Int. J. Periodontics Restorative Dent.* 21 (3): 288–295.

7

Perfecting Implant Related Esthetic via Using Optimum Surgical Guides

Giampiero Ciabattoni[1], Alessandro Acocella[2], and Roberto Sacco[3, 4, 5]

[1] Faenza, Italy
[2] Prato, Italy
[3] Barts and The London School of Medicine and Dentistry, London, UK
[4] Eastman Dental Institute, London, UK
[5] King's College Hospital, London, UK

7.1 Introduction

The use of osseointegrated dental implants for treating patients was first outlined in 1969 (Brånemark et al. 1969). The word 'osseointegration' was defined as a direct contact between the surface of an implant and the bone tissue (Brånemark et al. 1977). Schroeder et al. used the term "functional ankylosis" for the same condition (Schroeder et al. 1981). Later, osseointegration was defined as: "a clinical process where a rigid fixation of alloplastic materials is achieved and maintained, in bone tissue during functional loading" (Albrektsson and Zarb 1993).

Dental implant rehabilitation is now widely considered as a predictable treatment option for replacing missing dentition.

A systematic review has shown that the survival rate of a single tooth dental implant restoration is comparable to a three-unit fixed partial restoration at 10-years of follow up (Pjetursson et al. 2007).

Therefore, the request and use of dental implants in the replacement of anterior missing teeth has increased recently.

A major element influencing the functional, biologic, and esthetic achievement of implant rehabilitation is the quantity of residual hard and soft tissue. It has been confirmed that tooth loss results in constant and progressive bone tissue resorption and remodeling of the edentulous areas (Devlin and Ferguson 1991; Sobolik 1960).

In the esthetic zone, clinical success is highly dependent on achieving long-term soft tissue and hard tissue results (Belser et al. 2004; Kan et al. 2003).

Clinicians have to carefully consider the present tissue architecture, and they must be aware of the surgical implant positioning and subsequent bone remodeling process (Cardaropoli, Lekholm and Wennstrom 2006).

An increasing understanding and awareness of the nature of soft tissue and biological width have simplified the practitioners' ability to utilize dental implant rehabilitations in esthetic regions in a more predictable way (Martegani et al. 2007; Tarnow et al. 1992; Zetu and Wang 2005).

Grunder (2000) considered an intact buccal plate as a substantial factor in esthetic success outcome (Grunder 2000). In relation to the mesial-distal dimension, researches have highlighted the differences of implants positioned adjacent to natural teeth and implants positioned adjacent to an other implant fixture. It has been suggested that implants should be placed at least 1.5 mm away from an adjacent tooth and there should not be less than 3 mm between two implants to reduce crestal bone loss (Buser, Martin and Belser 2004). Single implant cases benefit from the hard and soft tissue of adjacent dentition. It has been determined that the interproximal bone of a tooth-bound dental implant is dependent on the level of bone at the adjacent tooth (Avivi-Arber and Zarb 1996; Grunder 2000). Thus, it has been agreed that the presence of papillae are mainly influenced by the interproximal bone level of the adjacent teeth (Cardaropoli et al. 2006; Kan et al. 2003).

Advances in Esthetic Implant Dentistry, First Edition. Abdelsalam Elaskary.

Companion website: www.wiley.com/go/elaskary/esthetic

Proper dental implant planning, positioning, and consequently exact transfer on the model cast should be considered as the most important factors for long-term success of prosthetic restorations with dental implants (Mischkowski et al. 2006; Wismeijer, Casentini and Chiapasco 2010). Since poor implant placement compromises esthetics and function, as well as increasing the risk of implant failure due to biomechanical overload, computer-guided surgical systems are the latest tools that can achieve ideal results with a potential long-term success rate (Ruppin et al. 2008). Based on conventional model casts or digital imaging systems, surgical templates have been developed to create continuity between diagnosis, prosthetic planning, and surgical phases, to guide the dental surgeon to improved precision and safety during dental implant placement (Brief et al. 2005).

In this chapter we analyze the utility of guided implant surgery and its value in the context of the esthetic implant dentistry.

7.2 Conventional Guided Implant Placement: Clinical and Surgical Planning

Prosthetic rehabilitation in esthetic areas in the maxilla using dental implants represents a challenge for any clinician. Factors that are potential sources of complication are bone resorption including bone quality, soft tissue management, and anatomical variables.

To have a long-term outcome and benefit for the patient, the treatment plan should consider all these difficulties and variables.

With the introduction of three-dimensional (3D) diagnostic imaging and treatment planning technologies in implant dentistry, the preparation and placement of dental implants has become the norm in quality patient care (Casselman et al. 1991; Rothman et al. 1988).

In any surgical implant therapy and especially in immediate loading techniques, prosthetic-dental implant plans are essential to succeed.

Guided implant surgery has helped facilitate, simplify, and overcome the most common challenges in dental implant therapy.

In the early 1990s, a group of software was presented that allowed the extra feature of placing graphic dental implants on the cross-sectional images (ImageMaster-101). The first type of Sim/Plant was presented by CSI in 1993, allowing the positioning of virtual implants on CT images. At the end of the 1990s, Simplant 6.0 was presented. This new software added the creation of a 3D reformatted image. Materialize (Leuven, Belgium) introduced the technology for performing osteotomies to specific depth and direction through a surgical stent. Thereafter, Nobel-Biocare (Zurich, Switzerland) introduced the NobelProcera/NobelGuide technology. The NobelGuide technology was introduced as an implant planning and placement system for both straight and tapered Nobel Biocare dental implants. In 2011, a completely redesigned upgrade of the NobelGuide software, NobelClinician, was introduced to complement the previous software.

Currently there are many software products from other manufacturers, such as Easy-Guide (Keystone Dental, Burlington, MA, USA), Straumann coDiagnostiX (Straumann, Basel, Switzerland), VIP Software (BioHorizons, Birmingham, AL, USA), Implant Master (IDent, Foster City, CA, USA), which are now available as well (Jung et al. 2009).

Modern implant software can reconstruct anatomical areas in 3D, allowing clinicians to virtually plan implant placement from a CT or cone beam computed tomography (CBCT) scan.

This type of approach enables any clinician to operate on difficult cases with a minimally invasive approach, providing a prosthetic restoration that has a predictable success rate (Table 7.1) (Balshi, Wolfinger and Balshi 2006; Moraschini et al. 2015; Parel and Triplett 2004).

7.2.1 Pre-surgical and Virtual Planning

Clinical examination before any type of surgery is extremely important. The clinical investigation before guided surgery includes a full patient medical history, preliminary radiographic (intra-oral and/or panoramic radiographs) digital photographs, mounted dental models, and the degree of mouth opening. Following the prelaminar examination each patient should be prepared for high-resolution spiral CT (Figures 7.1–7.4a).

Study casts should be obtained from well-extended impressions of the patient alveolar ridge/ridges; further, the model casts should be mounted in an articulator with all anatomic landmarks.

The patient must be able to open their mouth sufficiently to accommodate at least additional 10 mm length of the burs used with the surgical template to prepare the implant sites.

The technician then fabricates dentures/wax-up with the teeth in an ideal centric occlusion and in the appropriate position for phonetics, esthetics, and vertical dimension. The position of the teeth will be duplicated in the final fixed restoration.

The prosthesis created should have exceptional soft tissue adaptation with an exact fit to the underlying mucosa. The flanges should be a minimum of 3 mm thick and overextended into the buccal and labial vestibules. For this purpose, understanding the different mucosa

Table 7.1 Overview of the implant and prosthesis cumulative survival rates in selected studies (Moraschini et al. 2015).

	Number of implant inserted			Number of implants failed			Failure type				
Study	Maxilla	Mandible	Total	Maxilla	Mandible	Total	Early	Delay	Late	Implant Survival rate %	Prosthesis survival rate %
van Steenberghe et al. (2005)	184	0	184	0	0	0	0	0	0	100	100
Malo et al. (2007)	72	20	92	2	0	2	0	2	0	97.8	100
Komiyama et al. (2012)	124	52	176	10	9	19	8	11	0	89.2	83.9
Johansson et al. (2009)	312	0	312	2	0	2	0	2	0	99.4	96.2
Puig (2010)	128	67	195	2	2	4	4	0	0	97.9	100
Gillot et al. (2010)	211	0	211	4	0	4	1	2	1	98.1	100
Meloni et al. (2010)	90	0	90	2	0	2	0	2	0	97.8	Non reported
D'haese et al. (2012a)	78	0	78	1	0	1	1	0	0	98.7	Non reported
Di Giacomo et al. (2012)	22	38	60	1	0	1	1	0	0	98.3	91.6
Komiyama et al. (2008)	Non reported	Non reported	165	3	0	3	1	2	0	98.2	100
Landazuri-Del Barrio et al. (2013)	0	64	64	0	6	6	0	6	0	90.6	Non reported
Marra et al. (2013)	177	135	312	6	1	7	3	3	1	97.8	100
Browaeys et al. (2014)	36	44	80	0	0	0	0	0	0	100	100

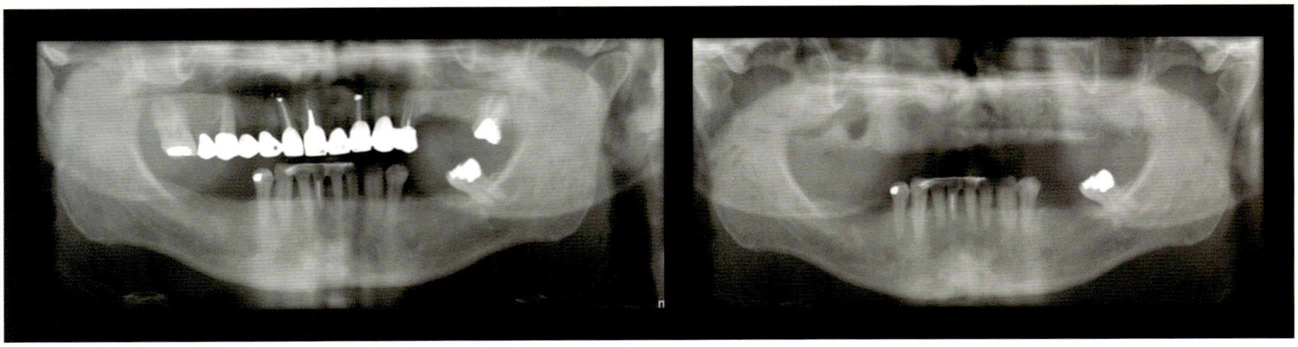

Figure 7.1 Preliminary orthopantomography (OPG): before removing the failed dentition and after six months of healing time.

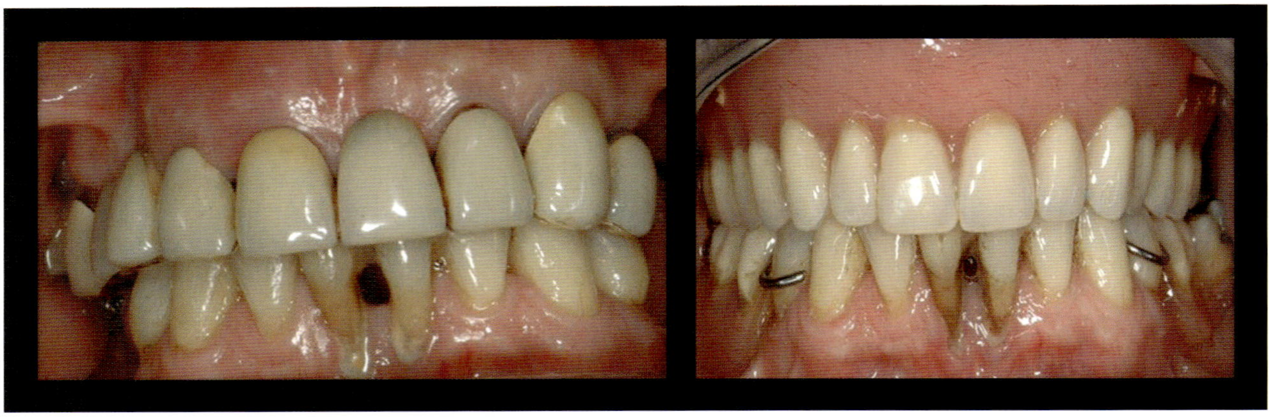

Figure 7.2 Intra-oral clinical picture: before removing the failed dentition and after six months from the extraction.

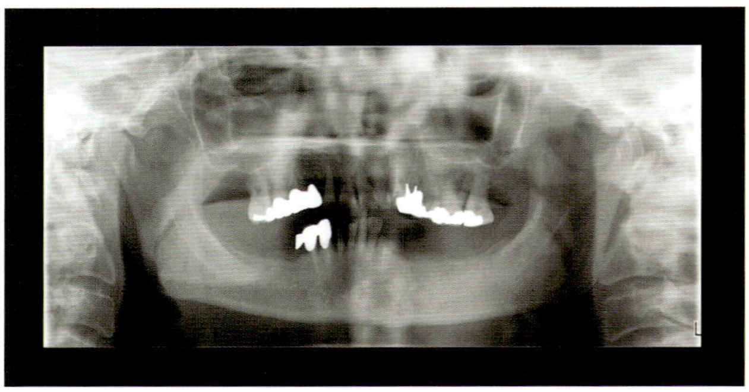

Figure 7.3 Preoperative X-ray showing failed dentition.

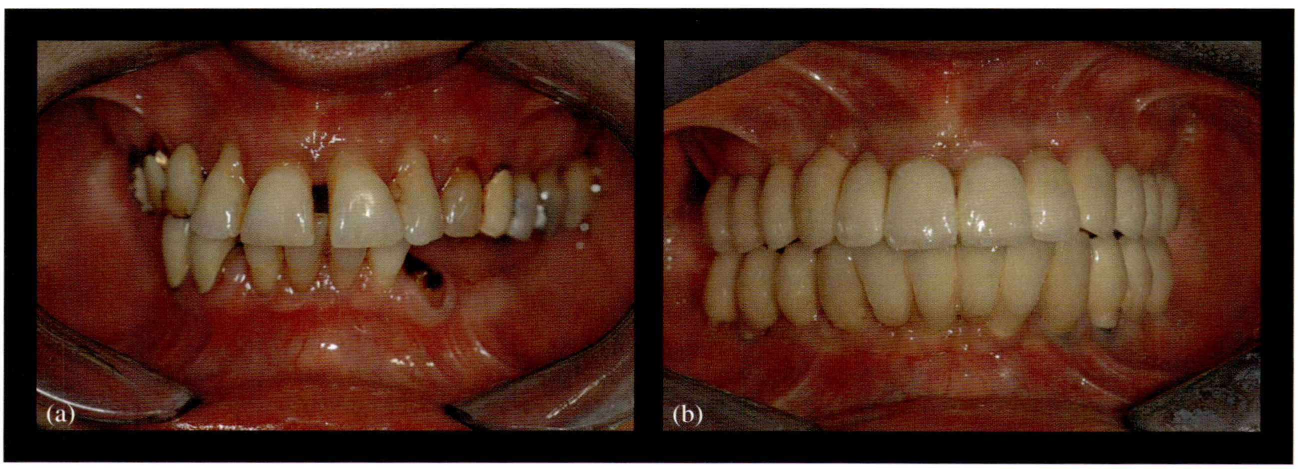

Figure 7.4 (a) Before guided surgery; (b) After guided surgery and final prosthetic result.

thickness and resilience in both the maxilla and the mandibular alveolar ridge is important, this can increase the chances of a vertical surgical stent malposition, which can lead to errors in implant positioning.

Vasak et al. (2011) observed that the deviation of the implant placement in the maxilla is proportional to the thickness of the mucosa. Therefore, to minimize the risks of this error, before any surgery it is fundamental to aim for the perfect fit of the surgical stent in the maxilla. Moreover, to decrease the chances of a surgical stent fracture, with an increased mucosa thickness in the maxilla it is always advisable to have the surgical stent with 3–4 mm thickness (uniformly) (Schneider et al. 2009; Yong and Moy 2008).

In partially edentulous cases, once the ideal occlusion is reached, an additional 3 mm thickness of acrylic is added to cover the occlusal surfaces of the existing teeth, and inspection windows are placed. The palate is also covered with acrylic, which helps stabilize the surgical stent during surgery. In mandibular cases, the denture is extended to cover the retromolar area. All these features need to be reproduced in the surgical stent.

The denture, or an exact duplicate, is then prepared as the radiological guide. Ten to twelve fiducial markers (notch) are placed in an alternate pattern at different levels to the occlusal plane on the buccal flanges, and the palatal and lingual surfaces. Each site is prepared with a 2 mm wide round bur and filled with gutta percha.

A rigid vinyl polysiloxane bite registration (silicon or surgical registration index), taken in centric occlusion, is used to stabilize the radiographic guide during the CT scanning procedure.

Checking the correct relationship between the registration index and the opposite dentition before the CT scan and the surgical procedure minimizes any potential implant placement errors. Several studies have shown that malposition or absence of the registration index are a source of in accuracy during implant placement (Block and Chandler 2009; D'haese et al. 2012a).

Subsequently, two CBCT scans are made with acquisition slices of 0.4 mm: the first, of the patient wearing the radiographic guide while occluding into the bite registration, and the second, of the radiographic guide alone, positioned in approximately the same orientation as in the first scan. These two Digital Imaging and Communication in Medicine (DICOM) formatted files are then transferred into the surgical planning software and the data of the patient's alveolar bone and radiological guide are then converted into 3D images (Figures 7.5a and 7.6). The clinician can identify any anatomical limits and therefore plan the surgery. According to current literature, it is advisable to perform flapless surgery and/or computer implant surgery with not less than 4 mm (width) and 12 mm residual alveolar bone height (Becker et al. 2009; de Almeida et al. 2010).

Most of the guided implant software uses a 3D screen and a 2D panel. The radiological markers (gutta percha fiducial marks) allow for the fusion/matching of these two scans, thus showing the association of the denture teeth to the underlying bone.

The virtual placement of the implants can then be carried out according to the anatomical limits identified.

Using 3D and cross-sectional views of the alveolar bone, along with an image of the overlying virtual prosthesis in exact relationship to the underlying bone, the implants can be virtually placed in the bone in relation to the position of the teeth in the final prosthesis (Figures 7.5b and 7.7a, b).

The 3D image can be rotated in all spatial planes to evaluate the bony anatomy. The implant abutment and guide sleeve of the surgical template can be positioned with each implant.

In some cases, due to a thin or in adequate alveolar ridge, guided surgery can still be used. Literature describes alveolar bone expansion or trans-alveolar mini-sinus lift using osteotomes rather than drills with a guided surgical approach (Pozzi and Moy 2014). Small bone defects can be corrected during guided surgery.

In contrast, in cases where regenerative surgery (large bone defects) is required, it is always advisable to approach the case in stages (Komiyama et al. 2008).

Nowadays many software programs are able to analyze bone quality, which is essential when immediate loading is planned. Using computer-guided surgery, clinicians can identify areas with better bone quality.

Once the virtual implant planning is completed, the position of the anchor pins (surgical stent stabilization pins) can be planned. Normally there is a minimum of one horizontal stabilization pin in partially edentulous cases and up to four in edentulous cases (mainly buccal) (Figure 7.5a, b and 7.6). However, in a recent study the authors have suggested the need to plan for the positioning of at least two anchor pins buccally and two palatally or posteriorly to avoid any movement of the surgical stent (D'haese et al. 2012b).

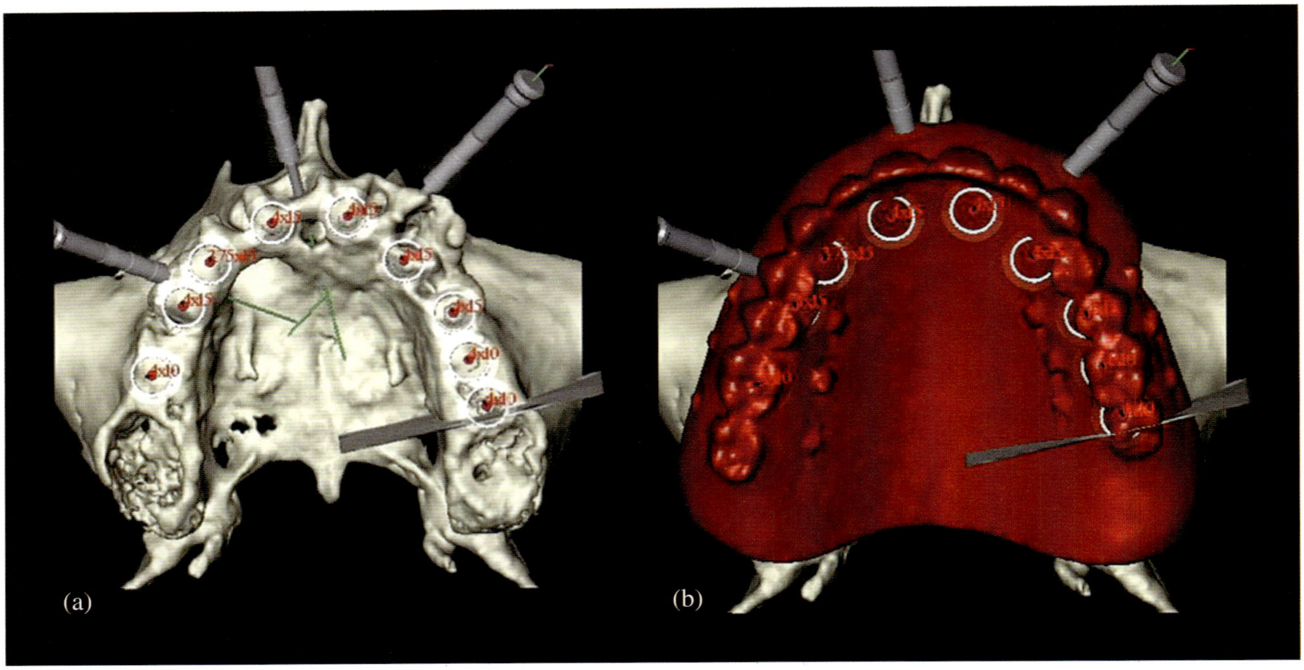

Figure 7.5 (a) Maxilla virtual planning; (b) Implant Virtual Planned in relation with the future prosthesis.

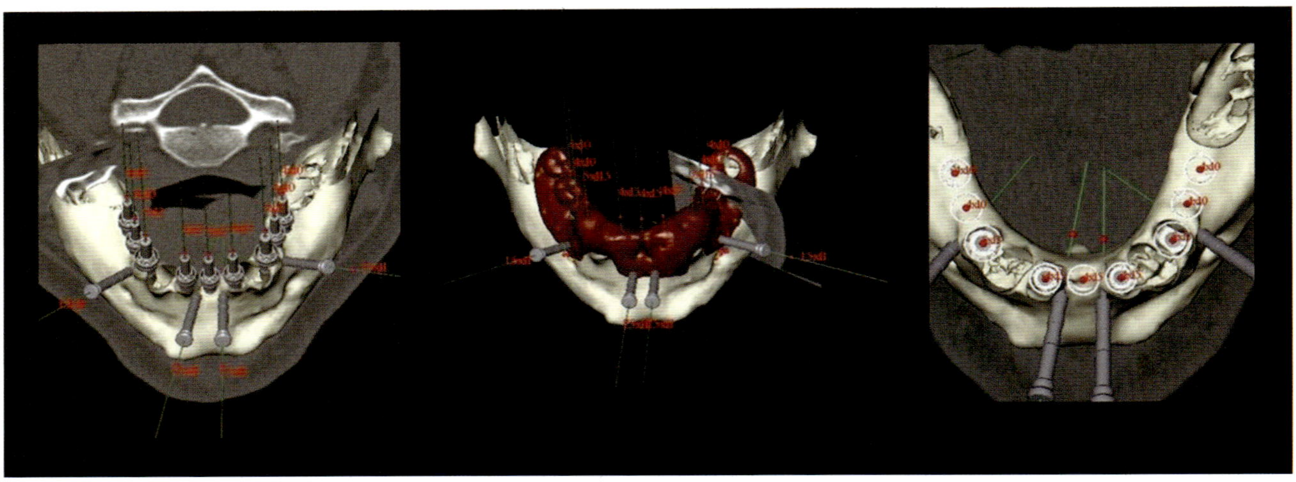

Figure 7.6 Mandible virtual planning.

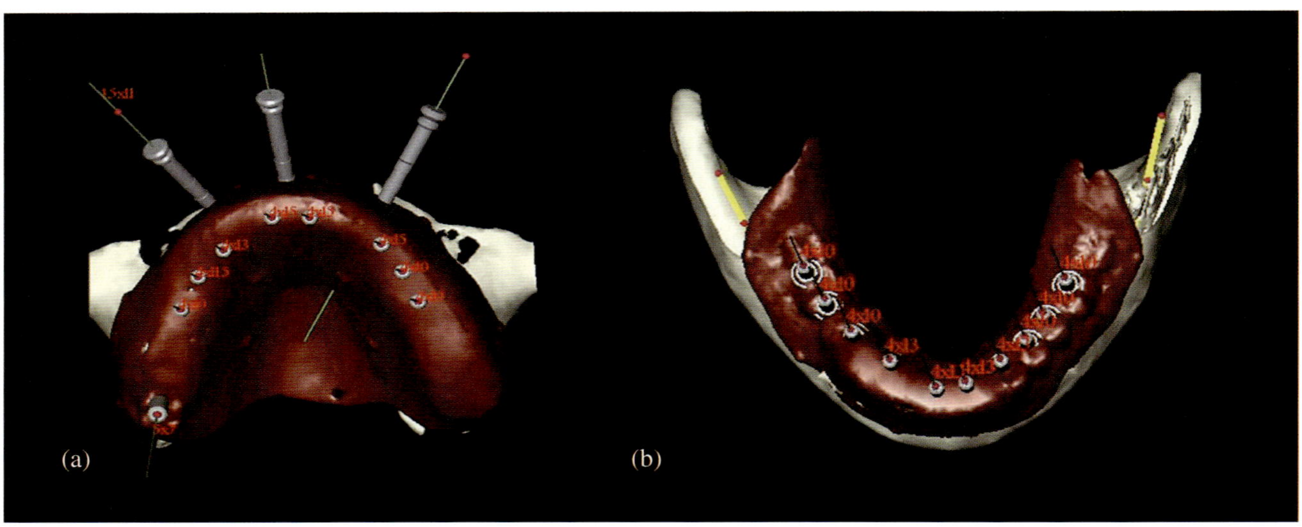

Figure 7.7 Virtual planning; (a) Maxilla; (b) Mandible.

Moreover, during the planning phase of the anchor pins, inclining the longitudinal axis to avoid soft tissue interferences (perioral soft tissue) is always recommended.

After the clinician has approved the virtual treatment plan, the digital planning file is emailed to the manufacturing facility for fabrication of the stereolithically-constructed surgical template/stent. The surgical template is delivered to the dental practice and a try-in is scheduled to confirm the accuracy of its fit.

For those cases in which an immediate provisional prosthesis will be inserted at the time of surgery or soon thereafter, the surgical template is sent to the dental laboratory for the provisional restoration. At this stage the dental technician can use the precision of the surgical template/stent for the presurgical construction of the master cast. According to our clinical experience, to achieve better accuracy it is advisable to take an accurate impression with a special tray from which a master cast is constructed. The master cast is adjusted/drilled/cut according to the position of the connected implant replicas to the surgical template/stent. The use of this technique reduces technical errors and allows a better reading of the soft tissue details.

At this stage the provisional restoration is constructed according to the information provided by the clinician.

7.2.2 Surgical Procedure

Once the patient is prepared, local anesthesia is administered, and the surgical template is placed with the surgical index. A slow local anesthetic injection technique is always recommended to minimize any soft tissue swelling. As an alternative, the patient can be asked to bite on the registration index for 10 minutes to dissipate local anesthesia. Before starting any surgery it is important to make sure that the surgical template is exactly seated on the underlying mucosa. Once the patient bites into the surgical index, and no discrepancy is observed, a 1.5 mm twist drill is used to prepare the anchor pin sites. Once the pins are placed, the surgical index is removed.

Some computer-guided surgical system use osteosynthesis screws in order to anchor the surgical stem; however, this may create macro-displacements of the surgical template. It is always advisable to start inserting the more distal anchor pins. Once the surgical template is fixed, it is good practice to always check that the surgical guide template is not under pressure.

A tissue punch is used to remove the core of gingiva from the alveolar bone, from each guide sleeve. The initial implant preparation begins with the counterbore starter drill.

The use of the counterbore starter drill is important for remove the initial cortical bone from the alveolar ridge; this is very useful in the anterior maxilla; however, this phase cannot be performed when the cortical bone is extremely thin. Moreover, it is always advisable to start preparing the distal surgical site for a better stabilization of the surgical stent.

Successive-sized twist drills with drill-stops are used with corresponding twist drill sleeves to prepare each implant site to the exact position and depth as determined in the virtual plan. The preparation is undersized in diameter in soft bone, and in dense bone; a bone tap is used after the final width of the implant site is prepared. All burs are irrigated with copious amounts of cold saline, and the burs are used in a 'pumping' manner to allow the irrigant to flow to the apex of the preparation to prevent the bone from overheating. The implant is connected to a guided implant mount and inserted into the prepared osteotomy site with the torque wrench or implant drill. The implant is inserted to the depth at which the implant mount contacts the drill guide sleeve in the surgical template. Overtightening the implant can displace, and sometimes fracture, the surgical template. In softer bone, overtightening can cause the implant threads to strip the preparation, and the implant will 'spin,' losing its initial stability in bone.

The optimal insertion torque should aim between 30 and 35 N cm (Figure 7.8).

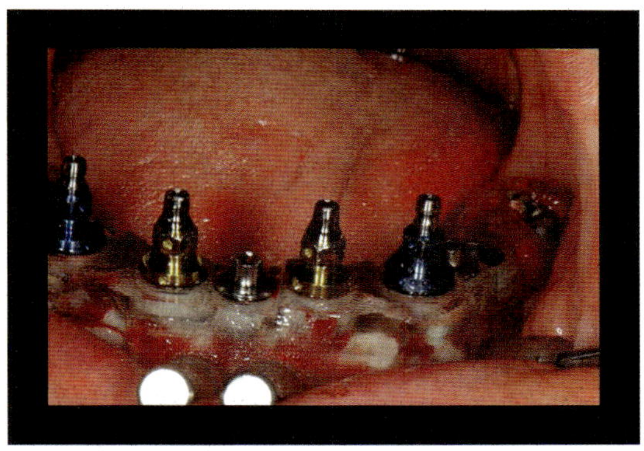

Figure 7.8 Implant positioned at their final height.

Following the placement of the implants, the guided implant mounts, template abutments, and stabilization pins as well as the surgical template are removed. The implant sites are inspected and any residual overlying soft tissue is eliminated. The provisional restoration is connected to the implants. Postoperative diagnostic images show the precise position of the implant abutments on the implants. Usually, minimal occlusal adjustments are needed. Fully edentulous cases are normally immediately loaded. Partially edentulous cases are either kept out of occlusion or placed with light occlusal contacts with delayed loading (Figures 7.9 and 7.10). After the osteointegration the dental implants, the patient can receive a final and permanent prosthetic rehabilitation (Figures 7.4b and 7.11–7.14).

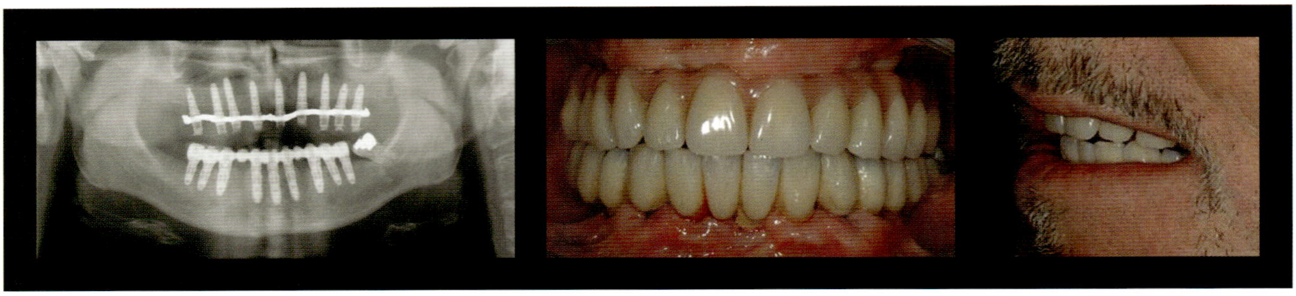

Figure 7.9 Temporary restoration placed immediately after surgery.

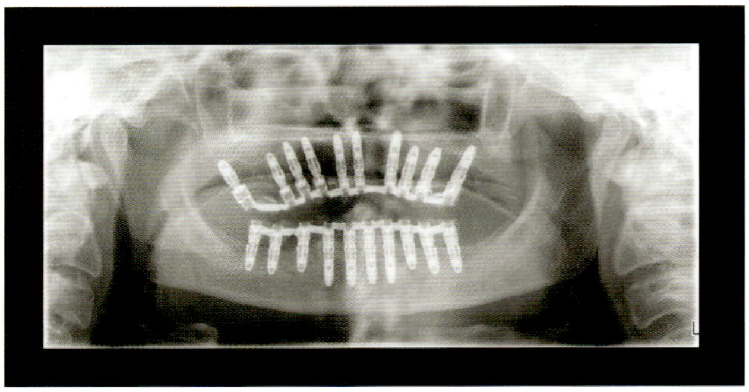

Figure 7.10 Panoramic X-ray after surgery, showing temporary full mouth rehabilitation immediately loaded.

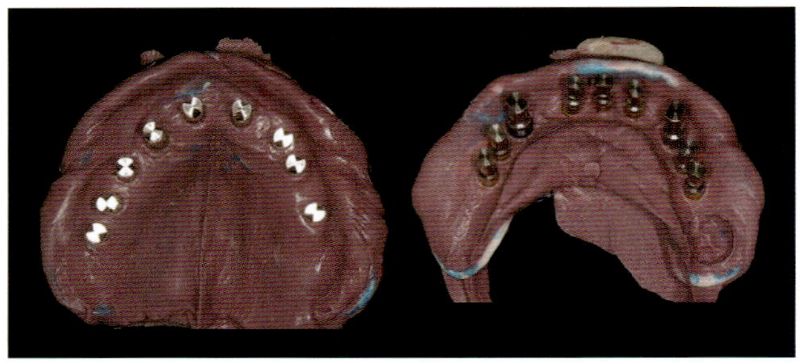

Figure 7.11 Precision impression after six months for final restoration.

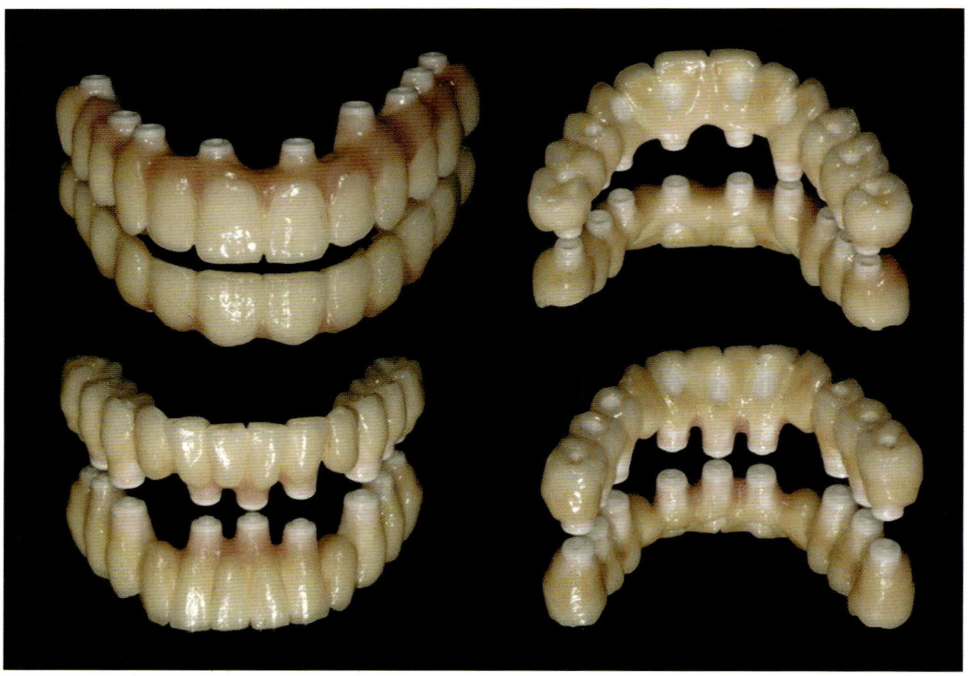

Figure 7.12 Procera implant bridge rehabilitation in zirconia.

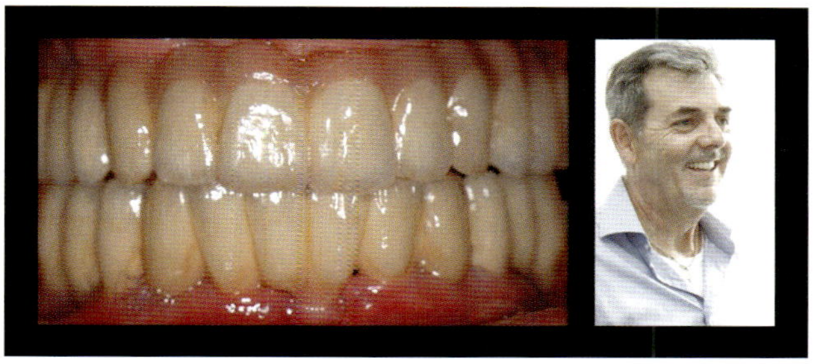

Figure 7.13 Clinical result of the procera implant bridge.

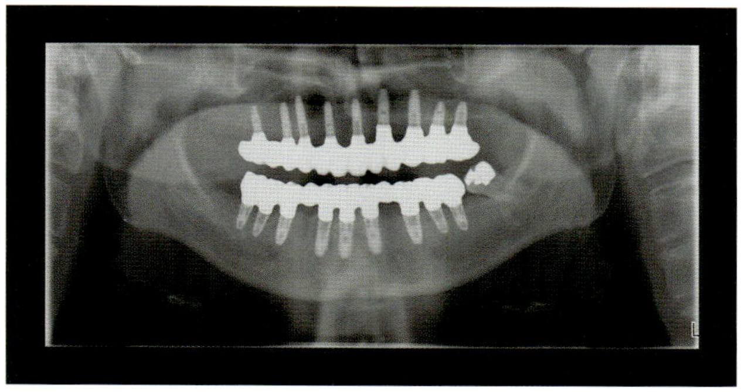

Figure 7.14 X-ray at five-year follow-up.

7.3 Post-extractive Guided Implant Placement: Clinical and Surgical Procedure

Immediate dental implant positioning in fresh extraction sites was introduced about 40 years ago (Schulte and Heimke 1976). Several researches have demonstrated successful clinical outcomes using this procedure with a high cumulative survival rate and stable crestal bone levels, similar to delay implant placement (Becker et al. 1998; Chen, Darby and Reynolds 2007; Sanz et al. 2013).

Initially, researchers showed that immediate implant placement could maintain alveolar bone dimensions (Paolantonio et al. 2001; Watzek et al. 1995). However, more recent clinical trials do not support this theory, indicating significant changes in the ridge dimensions after the positioning of an immediate implant (Botticelli et al. 2004, 2006).

Immediate implant placement is normally used due to esthetic needs.

This kind of dental implant surgery represents a challenge for clinicians and is rated either as an advanced or a complex difficulty level according to the straightforward, advanced, complex (SAC) classification established by the International Team of Implantology (ITI) (Dawson and Chen 2009).

According the ITI Consensus Conferences in 2003 and 2008, clinicians can choose from different implant placement timing options (Chen et al. 2009; Hammerle, Chen and Wilson 2004):

1) Immediate implant placement (type 1) on the day of extraction;
2) Early implant placement after four to eight weeks of soft tissue healing (type 2);
3) Early implant placement after 12–16 weeks of partial bone healing (type 3);
4) Late implant placement after complete bone healing of at least six months (type 4).

Each treatment approach has indications that depend on the clinical situation and clinician's experience (Buser and Chen 2009).

A literature review published in 2009 concluded that immediate implant placement in the anterior maxilla is associated with a significant risk of esthetic complications, mainly recession of the facial mucosa (Chen and Buser 2009). Several studies have proved that 20–30% of immediate implants generated mucosal recession of ≥1 mm (Cordaro, Torsello and Roccuzzo 2009; Kan et al. 2007;). Such soft tissue recession is produced either by the absence of a facial bone wall to support the facial mucosa, or a facial malposition of the implant, or by a combination of the two (Chen and Buser 2010). Other studies have observed marginal mucosal recession ranging from 0.06 to 1 mm, with most of the recession occurring within the first three months following delivery of the implant restoration (Bengazi, Wennstrom and Lekholm 1996; Oates et al. 2002; Priest 2003).

Moreover, it has been suggested that gingival biotype may affect soft tissue esthetic outcomes with dental implants (Kois 2001).

According to Kois (2001), a thick biotype alone does not confer resistance to marginal tissue recession. However, sites with a thin tissue biotype had a higher frequency of recession of 1 mm or greater compared with thick sites (45.8 vs. 33.3%, respectively) with a mean recession of 1.8 ± 0.82 mm (range 1–3 mm) and 1.3 ± 0.52 mm (range 1–2 mm), respectively. Sites with a thin tissue should thus be considered as having a greater risk of marginal tissue recession when compared with thick sites, particularly if the implants are buccally positioned (85.7% for thin vs. 66.7%) (Kois 2001).

The ideal positioning of an implant in all three dimensions, regardless of the implant system used, has been well described in the dental literature. Several guidelines have been indicated as key to obtain the best possible esthetic results in implant placement. First, the position of the implant depends on the planned restoration that the implant will support. Second, the implant platform should be placed 3 mm apical to the zeniths of the predetermined facial-gingival margins of the planned restorations. Third, the center of the implant should be placed at least 3 mm palatal to the anticipated facial margins. The objective is to avoid poor facial bone thickness and gingival recession (Hänggi et al. 2005; Kois 2001).

Guided implant surgery using CBCT, virtual treatment planning software, and stereolithographic surgical templates has certainly been a major accomplishment to provide optimal three-dimensional implant positioning for both anatomical as well as prosthetic factors (Jung et al. 2009). Mucosa-supported templates offer the potential for higher predictability and less invasive flapless implant surgery together with reduced intraoperative discomfort and postoperative patient morbidity (Nkenke et al. 2007). Operative time and surgical error are also reduced (Scotti et al. 2010). The potential advantages of flapless implant placement in the esthetic zone may include reduced mucosal recession and maximum preservation of peri-implant papillae due to avoidance of mucoperiosteal flap elevation (Koutrach and Nimmo 2010).

Nevertheless, guided surgery aimed at improving implant esthetics has so far not been explored in scientific literature.

In the next section we discuss the most difficult challenges in guided surgery in the esthetic area and the use of a new technique to overcome them: the double-template technique (DTT).

7.3.1 Pre-surgical and Virtual Planning

Guided surgery can be useful in placing implants in a post-extraction site. A correct placement is crucial in this type of therapy.

From a clinical standpoint, the necessary examinations include a full medical history, preliminary X-ray digital photographs, mounted dental models, and the degree of mouth opening (Figure 7.15). Following these clinical exams, each patient should have a high-resolution spiral CT. Study casts should be obtained from well-extended impressions of the patient alveolar ridge/ridges, model casts should be mounted in an articulator with all anatomic landmarks.

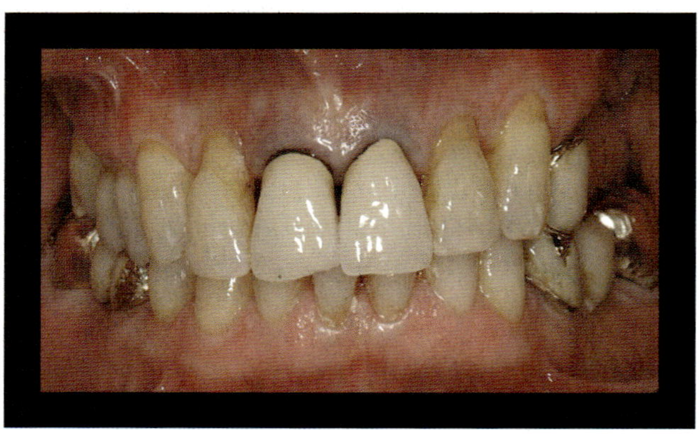

Figure 7.15 Intra-oral clinical picture of failed dentition.

The technician then fabricates a prosthetic acrylic replica with the teeth in the ideal centric occlusion and in the appropriate position for phonetics, esthetics, and vertical dimension.

Six to eight small (1, 5 mm) gutta-percha markers are randomly inserted in the prosthetic acrylic replica, acting as radio-opaque markers according to the double scanning technique. A silicone radiographic index is prepared and double-CT scan procedure is carried out: in one scan the patient wears the prosthesis and the radiographic index, and in the other one the prosthesis alone.

The master cast is duplicated and the teeth to be extracted are removed from the cast at the gingival level.

Particular care has to be taken to leave the gingival margin intact around them. Diagnostic probing to the alveolar crest of the unrestorable teeth at the interproximal, buccal, and palatal aspects are performed and accurately reported on the cast.

A wax-up of the teeth in the corrected final position is then done. This provides valuable information to the clinicians when planning the depth level of the implant shoulder. If the teeth that need to be extracted are misaligned, wax-up of the ideal final prosthetic position is performed and serves as guide for modification of the double-piece radiographic guide before the CT scan, as reported by Cantoni and Polizzi (2009).

The ideal profile of the prosthetic restoration is visualized in the software during the virtual planning suggesting the correct implant angulation.

The buccal borders of the surgical guided stent have to be extended up to the fornix, bypassing the undercuts determined by the flared teeth. These hyperextended borders support a sufficient number of pins and a sufficient amount of resin to support the metal cylinder in alignment with the post-extraction sites.

Based on the standard protocol, the patient will then undergo a CT scan before the extraction of the unrestorable teeth, wearing the radiographic guide.

The DICOM files obtained from the CT scan will include data regarding the anatomy of the patient's jaw and the ideally planned teeth positions and buccal emergency profile in relation with the correct prosthetic plan.

The two resulting sets of axial CT slices are processed with a software planning program and fused on the basis of radio-opaque markers. In this way the surgeon is able to perform a virtual planning with an ideal implant insertion and can have a clear vision of the prosthetic result to be achieved.

In the healed sites, implants are virtually placed in a standard mode while in the planned extraction sites, implants are always planned to be inserted in a palatal position because of the highly predictable buccal plate resorption in order to gain good primary stability. Furthermore, the fixture is always virtually planned to be placed at 2.5–3 mm below the coronal aspect of the buccal plate (Chen et al. 2007; Kan et al. 2003). Sometimes, in maxillary areas and especially in complex restorations (all-on-four and/or full arch), implants are virtually planned to engage the sinus or nasal cortical plate to achieve an optimum primary stability. Another advantage of software-guided implants in post-extractive sites is the possibility of choosing an optimal implant diameter, thus reducing the potential gap from the implant surfaces and the buccal plate. A gap less than 2 mm allows the clinician to avoid using grafting materials, while preserving a good esthetic outcome.

In clinical practice, if the gap between the implant and the buccal cortical plate is more than 2 mm, the use of graft material should be considered.

All implants are usually planned the right direction across the arch and in a sufficient number to allow an immediate loading protocol. In addition, implants are planned to be parallel to each other both on the front and the sagittal plane to facilitate the adaptation of the prosthesis at the end of procedure.

A minimum of three to four anchor pins and one or two anchor pins are always planned on the palatal/lingual aspect aiming to achieve excellent surgical template stability, and to prevent any movement, which may lead to inaccurate implant placement.

The authors of this chapter normally perform guided surgery in post-extractive cases, always obtaining data for two virtual software implant plans. Each patient receives two guided surgical stents, one for the implant placed in both healed and post-extraction sites and one with the implants inserted only in the healed sites.

The two digital plans are sent to the manufacturing facility for fabrication of the stereolithic surgical template/stent. The manufacturing facility fabricates two surgical guides, having the same shape, number, and position of the anchor pins as well as the same sleeves corresponding to the implants inserted in healed sites for the patient (Figure 7.16a, b).

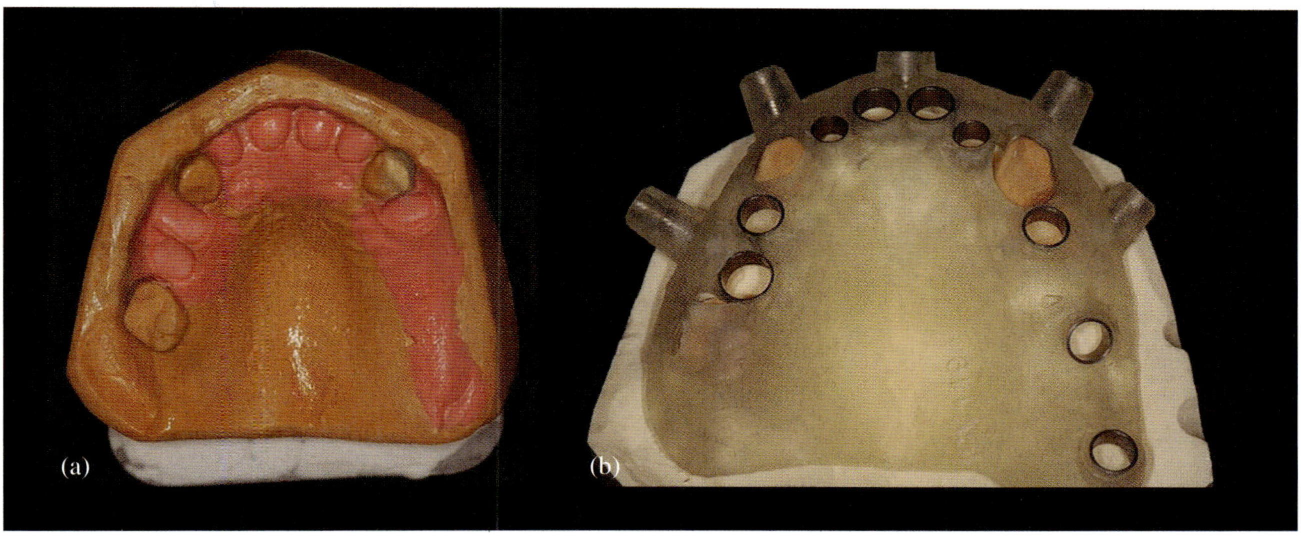

Figure 7.16 (a) Model cast where teeth were removed according to the virtual surgical plan; (b) Surgical stent included the post-extractive sites, positioned and checked before the surgical procedure.

The template with the sleeves only for the healed sites is used first as a pre-extractive template. This kind of template is very stable because is supported by the residual teeth, anchor pins, and the implant positioned in healed sites. The implants inserted in non-post-extractive sites during the surgical procedure are used as *reference implants* for re-positioning the second template, after the extraction of the unrestorable teeth.

Subsequently, the second post-extractive surgical guide template, with the same anchor pin positions, is accurately repositioned and stabilized using the reference implants.

Once the two surgical templates are delivered, the first pre-extractive template is checked and any interference is removed and then tried in the patient's mouth. The second surgical template (post-extractive template) is checked on the model cast where the technician simulated the extraction. At this stage any interferences between the guide and the model cast are assessed. The surgical sleeves and the surrounding resin often interfere with the soft or hard tissues. This interference is removed, when possible, from the template by removing part of resin and avoiding touching the metallic cylinders. Any damage to the metallic sleeves must be avoided. Interference to soft or hard tissue is removed from the cast and accurately communicated to the clinician. If some parts of the model cast require removal, it is duplicated before any removals to avoid losing any important information about the shape of the soft tissue. Once all the interferences are removed from the guide and/or the cast and the second guide fits perfectly on the model cast, the implant analogues are secured to the surgical guide, the master cast is adjusted/drilled/cut according to the position of the connected implant replicas to the surgical template/stent.

A titanium-acrylic resin full provisional prosthesis is pre-fabricated to the base of the post-extractive surgical template and the master cast.

7.3.2 Surgical Procedure

Once the patient is draped and prepared, local anesthesia is administered, and the first surgical template (pre-extractive surgical template) is placed and positioned with the surgical index.

Before starting any surgery it is important to make sure that the surgical template is sits precisely on the underlying mucosa. Once checked that no discrepancy exists, with the patient biting into the surgical index, the surgical template is fixed to the bone structure using the anchor pins.

A tissue punch is used to remove the mucosa from the alveolar bone, and each guide sleeve (pre-extractive surgical template) ensuring the soft tissue is carefully removed from each surgical site. The initial implant preparation begins with the counterbore starter drill. Subsequently, drills with increasing diameter are used to prepare the implant osteotomies in the conventional manner.

Once all planned fixtures in non-extractive surgical sites are placed, the first surgical template (pre-extractive surgical template) is removed and all the scheduled extractions are performed in a non-traumatic way to preserve integrity of the alveolus walls. An accurate alveolar bone curettage is performed to remove all granulation tissue and soft tissue remnants. Moreover, a periodontal probe is recommended to evaluate the integrity of the buccal plate of the post-extraction sockets.

The second surgical template (post-extractive template) is then inserted and fixed with the anchor pins in the same position as the first guide and with the expansible template-abutments screwed onto the fixture previously inserted in the healed sites.

This technique allowed the surgeon to re-place and stabilize the second drilling template in the same position as the previous one and perfectly according to the virtual planning.

Implant sites are prepared in the fresh extraction sockets using sleeves and drills of different diameters as previously described and according to the implant virtual planning. To secure primary stability, the drilling protocol might include under preparation according to the bone density in different sites.

Screw-tapping is performed for very dense bone and countersinking is sometimes carried out to eliminate crestal bone interferences that may compromise a good seating of the pre-fabricated prosthesis.

All implants should be inserted using a torque controller wrench aiming to an insertion torque of 35 N cm (Figure 7.17a, b). Excessive insertion torque can produce unwanted implant deviations with a consequent loss of accuracy and may compromise the result of the procedure.

Once the surgical template (post-extractive template) is removed, the implant sites are inspected and any residual

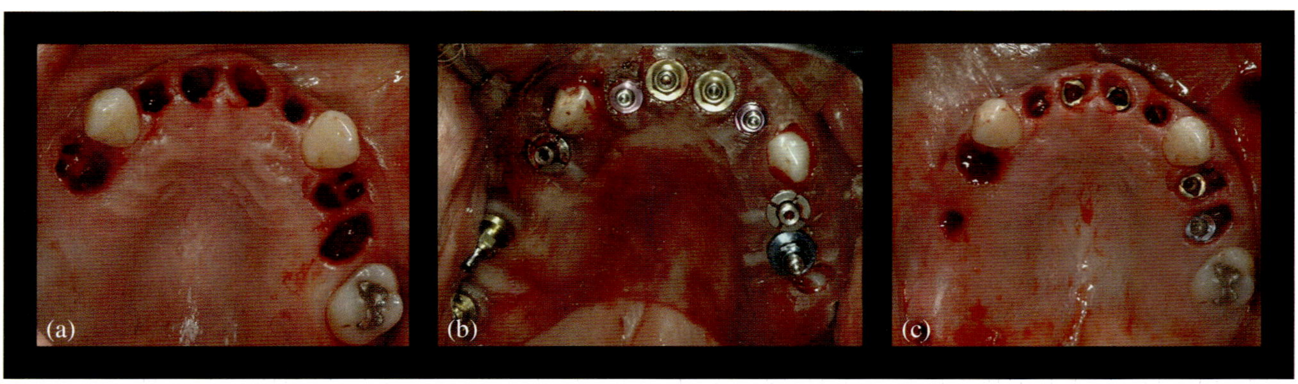

Figure 7.17 (a) Intra-oral picture at the time of the dental extractions; (b) Implant surgical placement using the virtual planned surgical stent; (c) Intra-oral picture of implant positioned in the empty alveolar sockets using the guided surgical stent.

overlying soft tissue is removed (Figure 7.17c). The temporary restoration is connected to the implants. Postoperative diagnostic images confirm the precise seating of the implant abutments on the implants. Usually, minimal occlusal adjustments are needed. Normally, after the osteointegration of the dental implants, the patient receives a final and permanent prosthetic rehabilitation (Figures 7.18a, b and 7.19a, b).

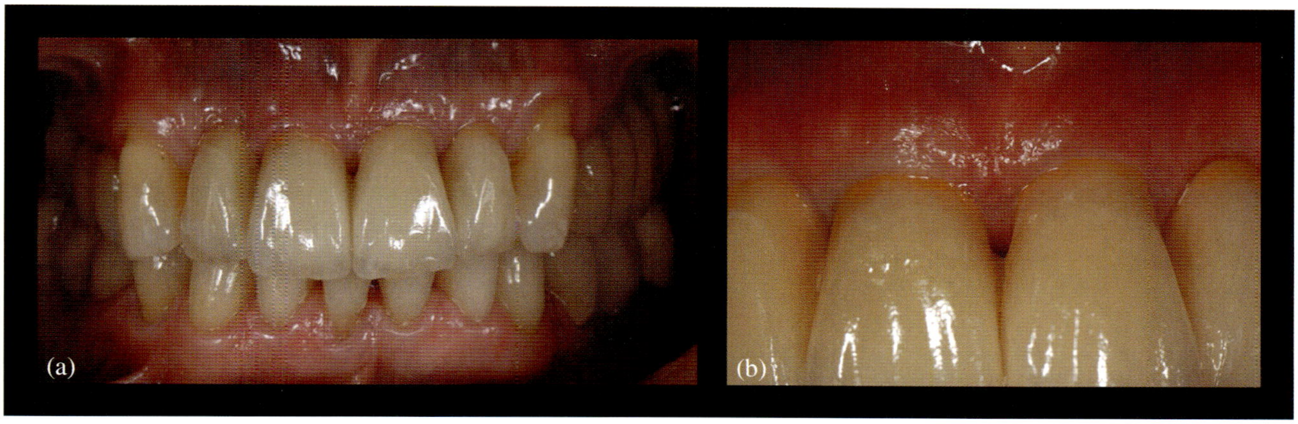

Figure 7.18 (a) Clinical image of the final restoration; (b) Higher magnification of the papilla between the post-extractive implants.

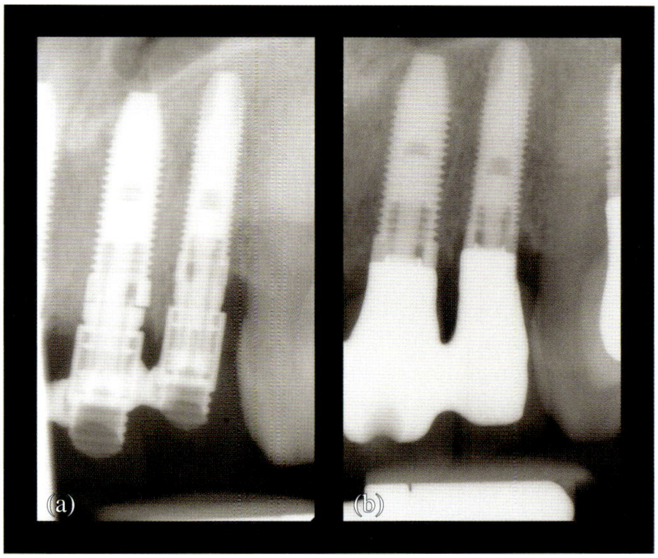

Figure 7.19 (a) Periapical X-ray of the temporary restoration soon after the implant placement; (b) Periapical X-ray at five years of follow-up.

References

Albrektsson, T. and Zarb, G.A. (1993). Current interpretations of the osseointegrated response: clinical significance. *Int. J. Prosthodont.* 6: 95–105.

Avivi-Arber, L. and Zarb, G.A. (1996). Clinical effectiveness of implant-supported single-tooth replacement: the Toronto study. *Int. J. Oral Maxillofac. Implants* 11 (3): 311–321.

Balshi, S.F., Wolfinger, G.J., and Balshi, T.J. (2006). Surgical planning and prosthesis construction using computed tomography, CAD/CAM technology, and the Internet for immediate loading of dental implants. *J. Esthet. Restor. Dent.* 18: 312–323.

Becker, B.E., Becker, W., Ricci, A., and Geurs, N. (1998). A prospective clinical trial of endosseous screw-shaped implants placed at the time of tooth extraction without augmentation. *J. Periodontol.* 69: 920–926.

Becker, W., Goldstein, M., Becker, B.E. et al. (2009). Minimally invasive flapless implant placement: follow-up results from a multicenter study. *J. Periodontol.* 80 (2): 347–352.

Belser, U.C., Schmid, B., Higginbottom, F., and Buser, D. (2004). Outcome analysis of implant restorations located in the anterior maxilla: a review of the recent literature. *Int. J. Oral Maxillofac. Implants* 19 (Suppl): 30–42.

Bengazi, F., Wennstrom, J.L., and Lekholm, U. (1996). Recession of the soft tissue margin at oral implants. A 2-year longitudinal prospective study. *Clin. Oral Implants Res.* 7: 303–310.

Block, M.S. and Chandler, C. (2009). 'Computed tomography–guided surgery: complications associated with scanning, processing, surgery, and prosthetics. *J. Oral Maxillofac. Surg.* 67 (11 Suppl): 13–22.

Botticelli, D., Berglundh, T., and Lindhe, J. (2004). Hard-tissue alterations following immediate implant placement in extraction sites. *J. Clin. Periodontol.* 31: 820–828.

Botticelli, D., Persson, L.G., Lindhe, J., and Berglundh, T. (2006). Bone tissue formation adjacent to implants placed in fresh extraction sockets: an experimental study in dogs. *Clin. Oral Implants Res.* 17: 351–358.

Brånemark, P.-I., Adell, R., Breine, U. et al. (1969). Intraosseous anchorage of dental prostheses. I. Experimental studies. *Scand. J. Plast. Reconstr. Surg.* 3: 81–100.

Brånemark, P.-I., Hansson, B.O., Adell, R. et al. (1977). Osseointegrated implants in the treatment of the edentulous jaw. Experience from a 10-year period. *Scand. J. Plast. Reconstr. Surg.* 16: 1–32.

Brief, J., Edinger, D., Hassfeld, S., and Eggers, G. (2005). Accuracy of image-guided implantology. *Clin. Oral Implants Res.* 16 (4): 495–501.

Browaeys, H., Dierens, M., Ruyffelaert, C. et al. (2014). Ongoing crestal bone loss around implants subjected to computer-guided flapless surgery and immediate loading using the all-on-4 concept. *Clin. Implant Dent. Relat. Res.* 17 (5): 831–843.

Buser, D. and Chen, S.T. (2009). Implant placement in postextraction sites. In: *20 Years of Guided Bone Regeneration in Implant Dentistry*, 2e (ed. D. Buser), 153–194. Chicago: Quintessence Publishing.

Buser, D., Martin, W., and Belser, U.C. (2004). Optimizing esthetics for implant restorations in anterior maxilla: anatomic and surgical consideration. *Int. J. Oral Maxillofac. Implants* 19 (suppl): 43–61.

Cantoni, T. and Polizzi, G. (2009). Implant treatment planning in fresh extraction sockets: use of a novel radiographic guide and CAD/CAM technology. *Quintessence Int.* 40: 773–781.

Cardaropoli, G., Lekholm, U., and Wennstrom, J.L. (2006). Tissue alterations at implant-supported single-tooth replacements: a 1-year prospective clinical study. *Clin. Oral Implants Res.* 17 (2): 165–171.

Casselman, J.W., Deryckere, F., Hermans, R. et al. (1991). Denta Scan: CT software program used in the anatomic evaluation of the mandible and maxilla in the perspective of endosseous implant surgery. *Rofo* 155 (1): 4–10.

Chen, S.T. and Buser, D. (2009). Clinical and esthetic outcomes of implants placed in postextraction sites. *Int. J. Oral Maxillofac. Implants* 24 (Suppl): 186–217.

Chen, S.T. and Buser, D. (2010). Esthetic complications due to implant malpositions: etiology, prevention, and treatment. In: *Dental Implant Complications Etiology, Prevention, and Treatment* (ed. J.T. Froum), 134–155. Hoboken, NJ: Wiley-Blackwell.

Chen, S.T., Darby, I.B., and Reynolds, E.C. (2007). A prospective clinical study of non-submerged immediate implants: clinical outcomes and esthetic results. *Clin. Oral Implants Res.* 18 (5): 552–562.

Chen, S.T., Beagle, J., Jensen, S.S. et al. (2009). Consensus statements and recommended clinical procedures regarding surgical techniques. *Int. J. Oral Maxillofac. Implants* 24 (Suppl): 272–278.

Cordaro, L., Torsello, F., and Roccuzzo, M. (2009). Clinical outcome of submerged vs. non-submerged implants placed in fresh extraction sockets. *Clin. Oral Implants Res.* 20: 1307–1313.

Dawson, T. and Chen, S.T. (2009). *The SAC Classification in Implant Dentistry*. Berlin: Quintessence Publishing.

de Almeida, E.O., Pellizzer, E.P., Goiatto, M.C. et al. (2010). Computer-guided surgery in implantology: review of basic concepts. *J. Craniofac. Surg.* 21 (6): 1917–1921.

Devlin, H. and Ferguson, M.W. (1991). Alveolar ridge resorption and mandibular athrophy. A review of the local and systemic factors. *Br. Dent. J.* 170: 101–104.

D'haese, J., Van De Velde, T., Komiyama, A. et al. (2012a). Accuracy and complications using computer-designed stereolithographic surgical guides for oral rehabilitation by means of dental implants: a review of the literature. *Clin. Implant Dent. Relat. Res.* 14 (3): 321–335.

D'haese, J., Van De Velde, T., Elaut, L., and De Bruyn, H. (2012b). A prospective study on the accuracy of mucosally supported stereolithographic surgical guides in fully edentulous maxillae. *Clin. Implant Dent. Relat. Res.* 14 (2): 293–303.

Di Giacomo, G.A., da Silva, J.V., da Silva, A.M. et al. (2012). Accuracy and complications of computer-designed selective laser sintering surgical guides for flapless dental implant placement and immediate definitive prosthesis installation. *J. Periodontol.* 83: 410–419.

Gillot, L., Noharet, R., and Cannas, B. (2010). Guided surgery and presurgical prosthesis: preliminary results of 33 fully edentulous maxillae treated in accordance with the NobelGuide protocol. *Clin. Implant Dent. Relat. Res.* 12 (Suppl 1): 104–113.

Grunder, U. (2000). Stability of the mucosal topography around single-tooth implants and adjacent teeth: 1-year results. *Int. J. Periodontics Restorative Dent.* 20: 11–17.

Hammerle, C.H., Chen, S.T., and Wilson, T.G. Jr. (2004). Consensus statements and recommended clinical procedures regarding the placement of implants in extraction sockets. *Int. J. Oral Maxillofac. Implants* 19 (Suppl): 26–28.

Hänggi, M.P., Hänggi, D.C., Schoolfield, J.D. et al. (2005). Crestal bone changes around titanium implants. Part I: a retrospective radiographic evaluation in humans comparing two non-submerged implant designs with different machined collar lengths. *J. Periodontol.* 76 (5): 791–802.

Johansson, B., Friberg, B., and Nilson, H. (2009). Digitally planned, immediately loaded dental implants with prefabricated prostheses in the reconstruction of edentulous maxillae: a 1-year prospective, multicenter study. *Clin. Implant Dent. Relat. Res.* 11: 194–200.

Jung, R.E., Schneider, D., Ganeles, J. et al. (2009). Computer technology applications in surgical implant dentistry: a systematic review. *Int. J. Oral Maxillofac. Implants* 24: 92–109.

Kan, J.Y., Rungcharassaeng, K., Umezu, K., and Kois, J.C. (2003). Dimensions of peri-implant mucosa: an evaluation of maxillary anterior single implants in humans. *J. Periodontol.* 74 (4): 557–562.

Kan, J.Y.K., Rungcharassaeng, K., Sclar, A., and Lozada, J.L. (2007). Effects of the facial osseous defect morphology on gingival dynamics after immediate tooth replacement and guided bone regeneration: 1-year results. *J. Oral Maxillofac. Surg.* 65 (7 Suppl.1): 13–19.

Kois, J.C. (2001). Predictable single tooth peri-implant esthetics: five diagnostic keys. *Compend. Contin. Educ. Dent.* 22: 199–206. quiz 208.

Komiyama, A., Klinge, B., and Hultin, M. (2008). Treatment outcome of immediately loaded implants installed in edentulous jaws following computer-assisted virtual treatment planning and flapless surgery. *Clin. Oral Implants Res.* 19 (7): 677–685.

Komiyama, A., Hultin, M., Nasstrom, K. et al. (2012). Soft tissue conditions and marginal bone changes around immediately loaded implants inserted in edentate jaws following computer guided treatment planning and flapless surgery: a 1-year clinical follow-up study. *Clin. Implant Dent. Relat. Res.* 14: 157–169.

Koutrach, M. and Nimmo, A. (2010). Preservation of existing soft-tissue contours in the transition from a tooth to an implant restoration in the esthetic zone using a flapless approach: a clinical report. *J. Prosthodont.* 19: 391–396.

Landazuri-Del Barrio, R.A., Cosyn, J., De Paula, W.N. et al. (2013). A prospective study on implants installed with flapless-guided surgery using the all-on-four concept in the mandible. *Clin. Oral Implants Res.* 24: 428–433.

Malo, P., de Araujo Nobre, M., and Lopes, A. (2007). The use of computer-guided flapless implant surgery and four implants placed in immediate function to support a fixed denture: preliminary results after a mean follow-up period of thirteen months. *J. Prosthet. Dent.* 97: 26–34.

Marra, R., Acocella, A., Rispoli, A. et al. (2013). Full-mouth rehabilitation with immediate loading of implants inserted with computer-guided flap-less surgery: a 3-year multicenter clinical evaluation with oral health impact profile. *Implant Dent.* 22: 444–452.

Martegani, P., Silvestri, M., Mascarello, F. et al. (2007). Morphometric study of the interproximal unit in the esthetic region to correlate anatomic variables affecting the aspect of soft tissue embrasure space. *J. Periodontol.* 78 (12): 2260–2265.

Meloni, S.M., De Riu, G., Pisano, M., and Cattina Tullio, A. (2010). Implant treatment software planning and guided flapless surgery with immediate provisional prosthesis delivery in the fully edentulous maxilla. A retrospective analysis of 15 consecutively treated patients. *Eur. J. Oral Implantol.* 3: 245–251.

Mischkowski, R.A., Zinser, M.J., Neugebauer, J. et al. (2006). Comparison of static and dynamic computer-assisted guidance methods in implantology. *Int. J. Comput. Dent.* 9 (1): 23–35.

Moraschini, V., Velloso, G., Luz, D., and Barboza, E.P. (2015). Implant survival rates, marginal bone level changes, and complications in full-mouth rehabilitation with flapless computer-guided surgery: a systematic review and meta-analysis. *Int. J. Oral Maxillofac. Surg.* 44 (7): 892–901.

Nkenke, E., Eitner, S., Radespiel-Tröger, M. et al. (2007). Patient-centred outcomes comparing transmucosal implant placement with an open approach in the maxilla: a prospective, non-randomized pilot study. *Clin. Oral Implants Res.* 18: 197–203.

Oates, T.W., West, J., Jones, J. et al. (2002). Long-term changes in soft tissue height on the facial surface of dental implants. *Implant Dent.* 11: 272–279.

Paolantonio, M., Dolci, M., Scarano, A. et al. (2001). Immediate implantation in fresh extraction sockets. A controlled clinical and histological study in man. *J. Periodontol.* 72: 1560–1571.

Parel, S.M. and Triplett, R.G. (2004). Interactive imaging for implant planning, placement, and prosthesis construction. *J. Oral Maxillofac. Surg.* 9: 41–47.

Pjetursson, B.E., Bragger, U., Lang, N.P., and Zwahlen, M. (2007). Comparison of survival and complication rates of tooth supported fixed partial dentures and implant supported fixed partial dentures and single crowns. *Clin. Oral Implants Res.* 18 (Suppl.3): 97–113.

Pozzi, A. and Moy, P.K. (2014). Minimally invasive transcrestal guided sinus lift (TGSL): a clinical prospective proof-of-concept cohort study up to 52 months. *Clin. Implant Dent. Relat. Res.* 16 (4): 582–593.

Priest, G. (2003). Predictability of soft tissue form around single-tooth implant restorations. *Int. J. Periodontics Restorative Dent.* 13: 19–27.

Puig, C.P. (2010). A retrospective study of edentulous patients rehabilitated according to the 'all-on-four' or the 'all-on-six' immediate function concept using flapless computer-guided implant surgery. *Eur. J. Oral Implantol.* 3: 155–163.

Rothman, S.L., Chaftez, N., Rhodes, M.L. et al. (1988). CT in the preoperative assessment of the maxilla and mandible for endosseous implant surgery. *Radiology* 169 (2): 581.

Ruppin, J., Popovic, A., Strauss, M. et al. (2008). Evaluation of the accuracy of three different computer-aided surgery systems in dental implantology: optical tracking vs. stereolithographic splint systems. *Clin. Oral Implants Res.* 19 (7): 709–716.

Sanz, M., Cecchinato, D., Ferrus, J. et al. (2013). Implants placed in fresh extraction sockets in the maxilla: clinical and radiographic outcomes from a 3-year follow-up examination. *Clin. Oral Implants Res.* 25: 321–327.

Schneider, D., Marquardt, P., Zwahlen, M., and Jung, R.E. (2009). A systematic review on the accuracy and the clinical outcome of computer-guided template-based implant dentistry. *Clin. Oral Implants Res.* 20 (Suppl 4): 73–86.

Schroeder, A., van den Zypen, E., Stich, H., and Sutter, F. (1981). The reaction of bone, connective tissue and epithelium to endosteal implants with titanium-sprayed surfaces. *J. Maxillofac. Surg.* 9: 15–25.

Schulte, W. and Heimke, G. (1976). The Tubinger immediate implant. *Quintessenz.* 27: 17–23.

Scotti, R., Pellegrino, G., Marchetti, C. et al. (2010). Diagnostic value of NobelGuide to minimize the need for reconstructive surgery of jaws before implant placement: a review. *Quintessence Int.* 41: 809–814.

Sobolik, C.F. (1960). Alveolar bone resorption. *J. Prosthet. Dent.* 10: 612–619.

van Steenberghe, D., Glauser, R., Blomback, U. et al. (2005). A computed tomographic scan-derived customized surgical template and fixed prosthesis for flapless surgery and immediate loading of implants in fully edentulous maxillae: a prospective multicenter study. *Clin. Implant Dent. Relat. Res.* 7 (Suppl 1): 111–120.

Tarnow, D.P., Magner, A.W., and Fletcher, P. (1992). The effect of the distance from the contact point to the crest of bone on the presence or absence of the interproximal dental papilla. *J. Periodontol.* 63 (12): 995–996.

Vasak, C., Watzak, G., Gahleitner, A. et al. (2011). Computed tomography-based evaluation of template (NobelGuide™)-guided implant positions: a pro-spective radiological study. *Clin. Oral Implants Res.* 22 (10): 1157–1163.

Watzek, G., Haider, R., Mensdorff-Pouilly, N., and Haas, R. (1995). Immediate and delayed implantation for complete restoration of the jaw following extraction of all residual teeth: a retrospective study comparing different types of serial immediate implantation. *Int. J. Oral Maxillofac. Implants* 10: 561–567.

Wismeijer, D., Casentini, P., and Chiapasco, M. (2010). Pre-operative assessment and prosthetic planning: the edentulous patient. In: *ITI Treatment Guide* (ed. D. Wismeijer, D. Buser and U. Belser), 13–34. Berlin, Germany: Quintessence Publishing.

Yong, L.T. and Moy, P.K. (2008). Complications of computer-aided-design/computer-aided-machining-guided (NobelGuide) surgical implant placement: an evaluation of early clinical results. *Clin. Implant Dent. Relat. Res.* 10 (3): 123–127.

Zetu, L. and Wang, H.L. (2005). Management of inter-dental/inter-implant papilla. *J. Clin. Periodontol.* 32 (7): 831–839.

8

Restorative Space & Implant Position Optimization

8.1 Restorative Space Management

Restorative space assessment at the pre-operative phase is an important step in providing a predictable esthetic implant-supported restoration. It is common to find many clinicians faced with a restorative dilemma as a result of the failure to or overlooking of the assessment of the restorative space prior to implant fixture placement. The restorative dentist is sometimes faced with insufficient restorative space, and is then left with few options for correction. The available space after tooth extraction is called the *restorative space*; its boundaries are the mesiodistal, buccolingual, and vertical axes. The amount of restorative space is usually governed by many factors including teeth drift, tooth overeruption, bone resorption, and malocclusion. The available restorative space that will host the implant fixtures and their related restorative components, should be carefully assessed and is vital for the esthetic and functional outcome. Insufficient restorative space often leads to many unsatisfactory clinical situations, including improper masticatory function and poor occlusal curve orientation. Fortunately, modern dentistry offers an array of techniques that can enable the correction of a deficient restorative space to an acceptable level.

Implant positioning in the posterior alveolar ridge is governed by factors such as occlusion, biting loads (English 1993), opposing dentition, parafunctional habits, quality and quantity of the available bone, and the existing location of the anatomical landmarks, while the esthetic zone is governed by other factors such as smile line, lip support, facial symmetry, quantity and quality of soft tissues, periodontal phenotype, emergence profile, type of prosthetic components to be used, and the future contour of the desired final restoration. Abiding by these factors not only ensures success but also the long-term esthetic and functional outcome, with a special emphasis on the value of three-dimensional dental implant fixture positioning in addition to using a relatively atraumatic surgical techniques, accurate osteotomy sizing, exerting no pressure on the alveolar bone, minimizing heat generation to the bone, and achieving primary implant stability (Burger and Klein-Nulend 1999; Buser et al. 1999; Herrmann 2000), and it is advisable to avoid direct biting loads at the bone–implant interface during a sufficient healing period when there is no plan has been implemented for immediate load protocol (Block, Kent, Guerra 1997; Brunski, Puleo and Nanci 2000; Szmukler-Moncler et al. 1998).

Clinicians should exercise extra care so they do not compromise sulcular depth or gingival biological health in an attempt to achieve optimal implant placement (Misch 1995) to reduce the risks of morbidity and implant failure (Elaskary et al. 1999a, b). Implant failure is not only limited to the breakdown of the integration between the implant and investing bone but also encompasses the failure to achieve esthetic and phonetic goals, and to offer the patient satisfaction (Meffert 1992).

The introduction of more predictable therapeutic modalities, restorative materials, surgical, and restorative techniques have significantly expanded available treatment options and offered a better outcome. Mastering these modalities offers a maximum benefit for the patient. In other words, when many treatment options are available, the skill lies in how to select the best option, which involves careful patient selection and achieving a comprehensive treatment plan (Karthik, Sivakumar and Thangaswamy 2013).

8.2 Loss of Restorative Space

The distance from the occlusal plane of any of the arches to the crest of the alveolar ridge of the opposing arch is referred to as the available restorative space. The available restorative space will dictate the prosthetic design choices. The implant position should satisfy all

Advances in Esthetic Implant Dentistry, First Edition. Abdelsalam Elaskary.

Companion website: www.wiley.com/go/elaskary/esthetic

biologic parameters, thus, reducing the tendency for a poor occlusal scheme (Boyd 2009; Evans and Chen 2008; Spalding and Cohen 1992). Over time, edentulous areas that are not promptly restored may lead to drifting, tipping, rotation, and super-eruption of neighboring and/or opposing teeth (Geckili et al. 2011), thus leading to space reduction. Intrusion, extrusion, correction of tipped teeth, and reduction of crowding or excessive spacing are treatments that an orthodontist can provide (Goodacre et al. 1997). Regaining the lost inter-occlusal space can often can be achieved by using all the disciplines of modern dentistry (see Figure 8.1a and b).

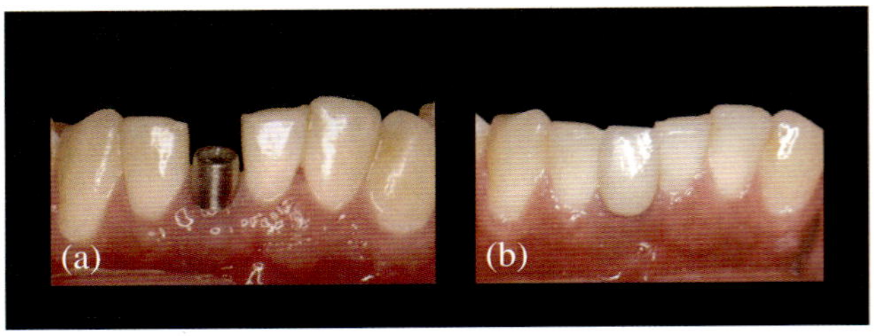

Figure 8.1 (a) and (b) Insufficient horizontal space that lead to faulty implant supported restoration.

Lost intermaxillary space must be regained prior to implant placement and restoring the biological occlusal contours can be accomplished by periodontal, orthodontic, conservative restorative, and surgical procedures, either individually or combined (Geckili et al. 2011). The procedures used depend on the clinician's choice, and the available mastered knowledge, such as intrusion of the extruded natural teeth, posterior maxillary alveoloplasty, or enameloplasty of the extruded natural teeth to minor adjustments as well as endodontic treatment and periodontal surgical skills (Chen et al. 2004). Preprosthetic surgical procedures should be performed before the insertion of the implants to restore lost interarch space. The use of screw-retained restoration is yet another predictable option for solving a deficient interarch space, because of the low profile of the screw-retained abutments when compared to cement-retained ones.

8.3 Magnitude of Restorative Space

8.3.1 Horizontal Space Component

Adequate mesiodistal (horizontal) restorative space must be present to provide a restoration that simulates natural tooth contours, as this space allows the proper spreading of the implant supported restorations within the arch. It allows the placement of the optimal number of implants replacing lost teeth, correlated with the available buccolingual width of the bone, proposed location, and angulation of the adjacent teeth roots (Shenoy 2012) (see Figure 8.2a and b).

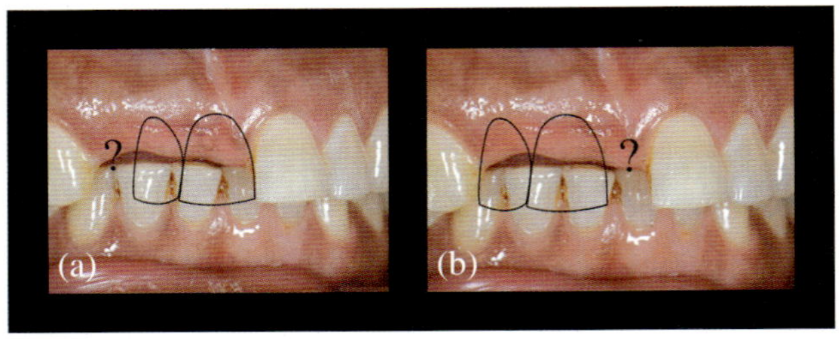

Figure 8.2 (a) and (b) Imaginary situations to provide a mesial or distal diastema.

The optimal distribution of dental implants, (spreading) within the available horizontal space respect (1) the adjacent biologic natural teeth space, (2) an adjacent implant biologic space, and (3) the high occlusal loads in relation to the surface area of the implants used (Shenoy 2012). This in turn will offer (1) the development of a healthy papilla, (2) the development of proper prosthetic contours, (3) healthy peri-implant tissue status, (4) hygienic implant-supported restorations, and (5) and the development of harmonious occlusion (Shenoy 2012) (see Figure 8.3a and b).

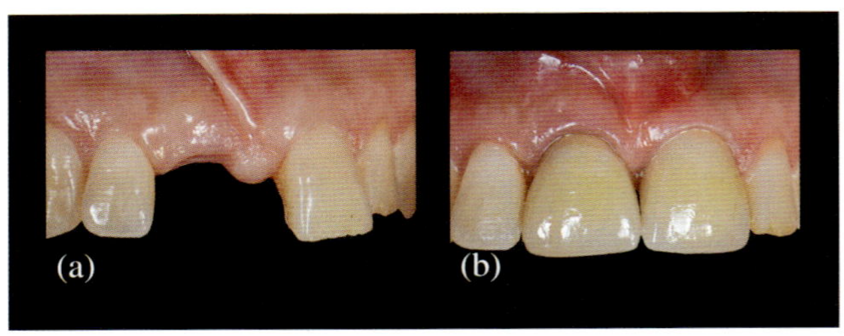

Figure 8.3 (a) Excessive mesiodistal space due to the pre- existing median diastema, (b) The case finally restored closing the median diastema as pair patient request.

The mesiodistal space shows the size of the future implant-supported restoration to be used (molar or premolar) and the number of teeth being replaced. The natural maxillary first and second premolars and the first molar have an average mesiodistal size of 7.1, 6.6, and 10.4 mm, respectively. The dimensions of these teeth at the cementoenamel junction (CEJ) are 4.8, 4.7, and 7.9 mm. At a distance 2 mm from the CEJ, the teeth measure 4.2, 4.1, and 7.0 mm. Decisions need to be made about the implant size to be used. The following guidelines should be considered when selecting implant size and evaluating mesiodistal space for implant placement: (1) the implant should be at least 1.5 mm away from the adjacent teeth, (2) the implant should be at least 3 mm away from an adjacent implant, and (3) a wider diameter implant should be selected for molar teeth (Danza et al. 2011).

8.3.2 Vertical Space Component

The vertical space may be rendered deficient due to overeruption of the natural teeth when the opposing dentition is lost for a long time or may be excessive due to alveolar bone resorption due to long-term tooth loss. Posterior mandibular fixtures should be placed so that the exit hole of the screw access should point to the middle of the occlusal surface (Figure 8.4a and b). Posterior maxillary implants should be placed so that the exit angle of the screw access points toward the inner incline of the buccal cusp. Placing dental implants in off-angle positions always complicates the restorative outcome. On examination, the space between the residual ridge and the opposing occlusal plane should be evaluated. Replacing premolar and molar teeth requires ample space between the residual ridge and the opposing occlusion; 7 mm would be considered the bare minimum (Jivraj and Chee 2006) (see Figure 8.5a and b).

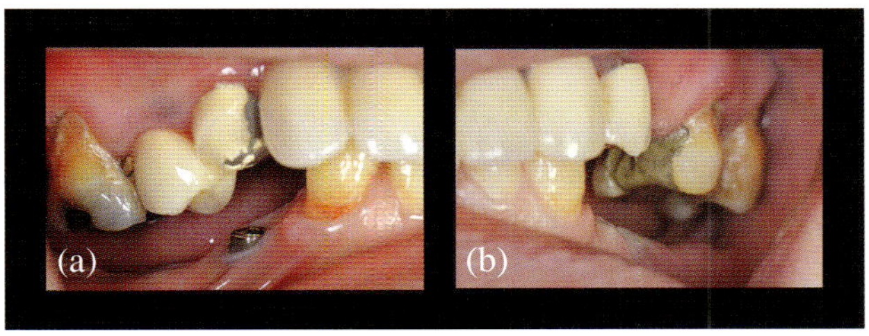

Figure 8.4 (a) and (b) Deficient vertical space due to over eruption.

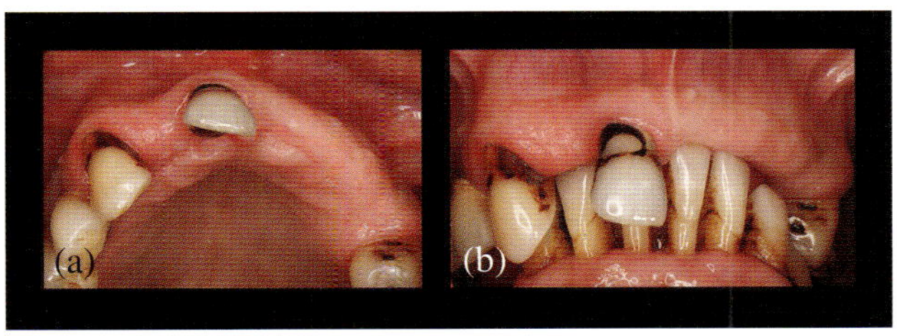

Figure 8.5 (a) Missing maxillary dentition. (b) The patient in occlusion showing over erupting lower teeth that hinders implant placement (Deficient vertical enter arch space).

8.4 Methods to Optimize Deficient Horizontal Space

The degree of horizontal space deficiency dictates the suitable method for space optimization. Minor clinical interventions can be selected for minor space discrepancies; however, other surgical interventions that involve further aggressive maneuvers could be undertaken to correct larger space insufficiencies.

8.4.1 Enameloplasty/Coronoplasty

Enameloplasty, or tooth recontouring, or stripping, is a procedure in which small amounts of tooth enamel are removed by modifying length, shape, or surface. It is indicated when there is a minimal degree of deficient mesiodistal space and can offer an effective and minimally invasive treatment approach. Approximately 0.5 mm of the enamel surface can be removed, the degree of reduction is limited to prevent dentin hypersensitivity (Stewart and Prescott 1976). Intentional root canal treatment of the tooth with perfectly vital pulp may be necessary in some patients with pre-existing hypersensitivity (Ingle and Bakland 2002).

Coronoplasty is the selective reduction of occlusal areas with the primary purpose of influencing mechanical contact to establish an ideal occlusion, relieving premature contacts and eliminating occlusal disharmonies. It is believed that ideal occlusal adjustment is not only responsible for eliminating injurious occlusal forces, but is also equally important in providing the functional stimulation necessary for the preservation of periodontal health (Malathi et al. 2014).

The correction of the occlusal supracontacts, is facilitated by: (1) grooving (correcting the grooves and fissures), (2) spherodizing (restoring the buccolingual width of the occlusal surface to normal dimensions), and (3) pointing (restoring the cusp point contours) (Carranza and Jolkovsky 1991). In coronoplasty elimination of tipped molars through selective reshaping of the occlusal surfaces of teeth results in more favorable distribution of the occlusal forces. The practice of enamel stripping, coil springs, and power chains are also important in optimizing the space requirements of an implant surgical site presented with insufficient horizontal space. Enamel stripping is a frequent technique used to gain additional restorative space and the practitioner should be comfortable performing this procedure, either with diamond strips, burrs, or discs (Livas, Jongsma and Ren 2013) (see Figure 8.6a–h).

For minor vertical space insufficiency, occlusal reduction could be performed to offer more restorative space (Rosenstiel 1998). The steps of coronoplasty might involve:

1) Removal of any excessive enamel in various cuspal positions.
2) Open or adjust any disturbing proximal contacts.
3) Removal of the gross occlusal disharmonies.
4) Polishing of the rough surfaces. (Carranza and Jolkovsky 1991).

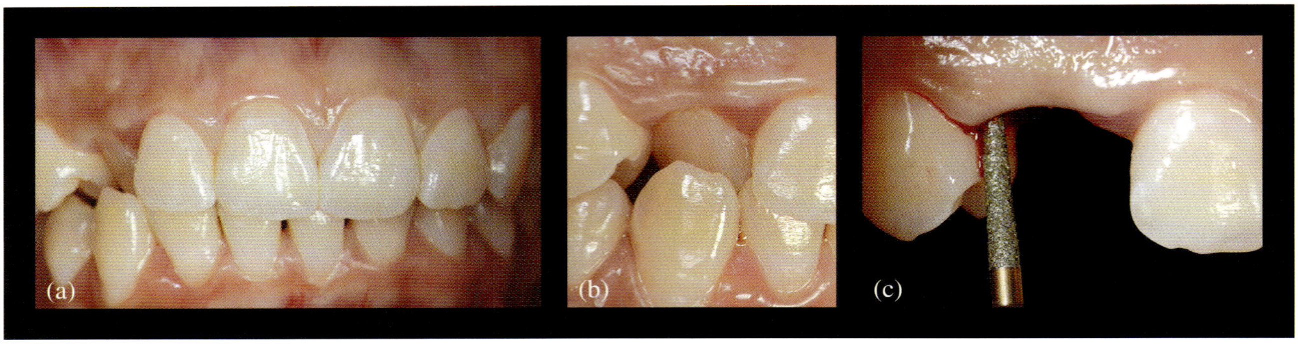

Figure 8.6 (a) and (b) Palataly inclined right canine, (c) Enameloplasty done around the adjacent tooth to compensate for the mesiodistal space.

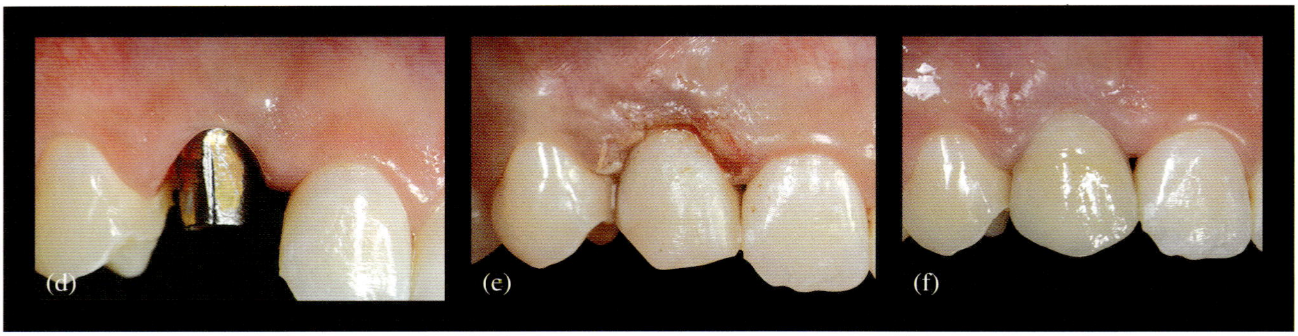

Figure 8.6 (d) Abutment in place, (e) Soft tissue optimization, (f) Final case restored.

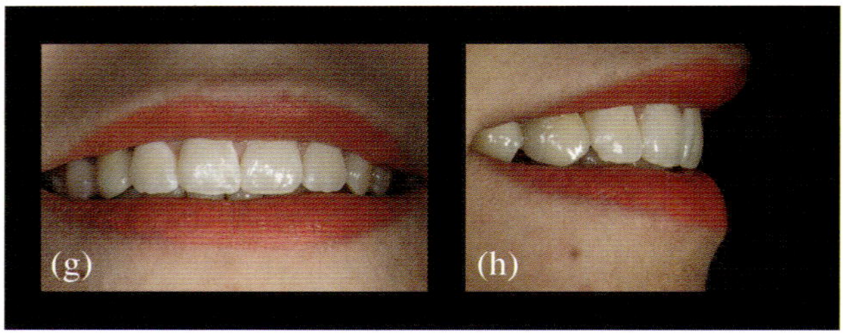

Figure 8.6 (g) and (h) Buccal and lateral view.

8.4.2 The Use of Narrow Diameter Implants

Narrow diameter implants (NDIs) are designed for placement in locations where placement of the regular diameter implants is not possible due to the reduction of the available horizonal space or the narrow diameter of the missing tooth to be replaced. Narrow diameter implants may be utilized in areas with limited spaces between adjacent teeth, between convergent tooth roots, or in narrow ridge situations. Additionally, narrow diameter implants can be used to replace narrow diameter teeth including the lateral maxillary and mandibular incisors. Because of the anterior placement of NDIs, esthetic considerations are also crucial for prosthetic fabrication. Several studies have assessed the effectiveness of narrow diameter implants. For instance, an evaluation of 316 NDIs followed over a 10-year period demonstrated a cumulative survival rate of 92.3% without any implant fractures (Buser et al. 1997). Similarly, another study examined 510 implants with diameters ranging from 3.0 to 3.5 mm from multiple implant systems (Lee et al. 2005). Only three of the implants were lost, demonstrating a survival rate of 99.4%. In general, these long-term studies have shown that small diameter implants can exhibit survival rates comparable to regular platform ones, suggesting that narrow diameter implants can be a predictable treatment option for situations in which large diameter implants cannot be placed. However, unfortunately those NDIs cannot be considered as the load becomes magnified as we go posteriorly (see Figure 8.7a–i).

8.4.3 Orthodontic Movement

Most horizontal space insufficiency can be treated by orthodontic teeth movement, but the restorative dentist will occasionally be confronted with complex treatment planning decisions resulting from (Miller 1995): (1) a non-esthetic position of the anterior dentition caused by overcrowding or excessive spacing, (2) a poor position of posterior abutments due to malocclusion, (3) supraeruption and occlusal plane discrepancies, (4) mesial drift into edentulous areas, and (5) collapse of the occlusal vertical

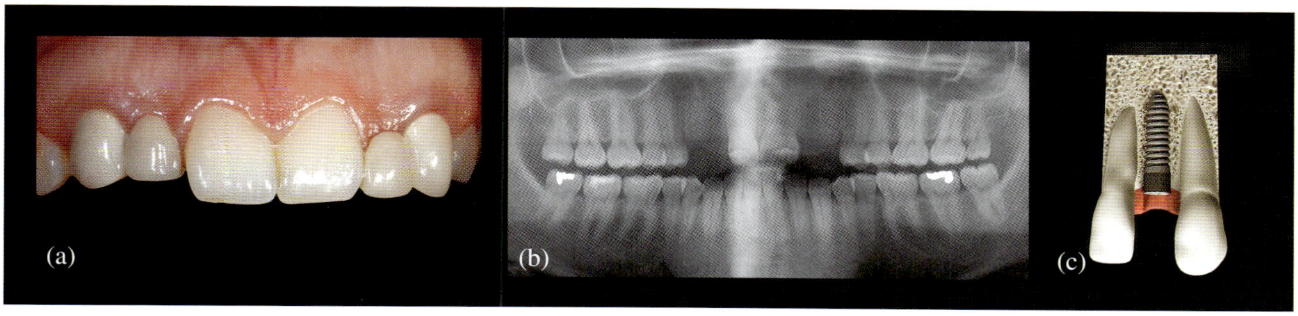

Figure 8.7 (a) Poor restorative outcome as a result of deficient mesiodistal space, (b) Radiographic panoramic view showing the available restorative space, (c) Sketch for the use of narrow implant in limited mesiodistal spaces.

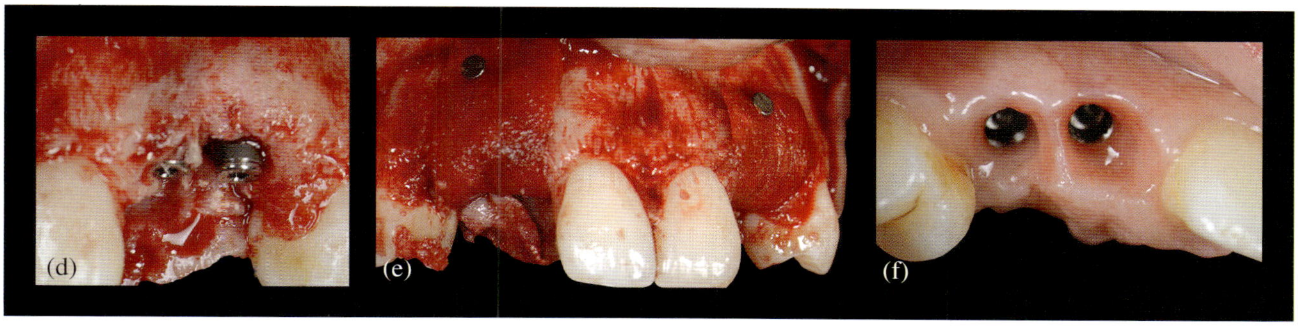

Figure 8.7 (d) Two narrow implants (3 mm diameter) were placed and the bone defect was grafted, (e) Collagen membranes where tacked in place, (f) Soft tissue contour is finalized.

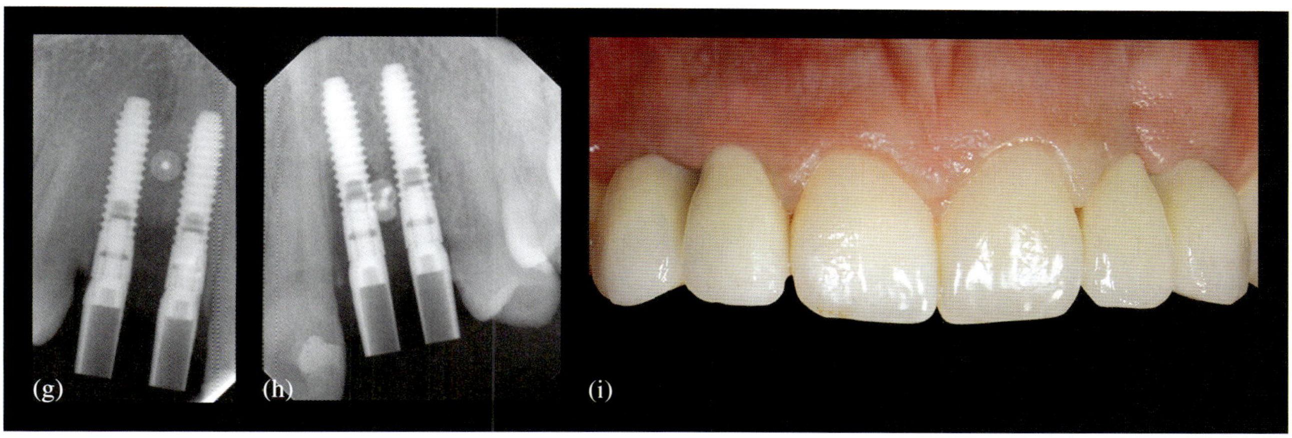

Figure 8.7 (g) and (h) Periapical radiographic view showing implants in position, (i) Case finally restored.

dimension due to loss of posterior teeth. An interactive collaborative approach between orthodontists and restorative dentists is deemed necessary for effective management of these problems (see Figure 8.8a–f). Natural teeth intrusion, extrusion, uprighting of tipped teeth, and reduction of crowding or excessive spacing are treatments that an orthodontist can provide routinely. Implants can also be used for orthodontic anchorage to improve treatment outcomes (Goodacre et al. 1997).

The orthodontic profession is undergoing a rapid and enormous growth phase with expansion in its approach toward interactive care. The more progressive specialists recognize that if treatment with optimal long-term prognoses is to be provided a collaborative approach provides a better result in the future. There are many areas where orthodontists are in close collaboration with prosthodontic specialists, such as prior to the replacement of missing teeth, closure/consolidation of spaces for esthetic and periodontal improvement, intrusion or extrusion of certain teeth, correction of axial inclination of teeth, and space maintenance and management of impacted teeth.

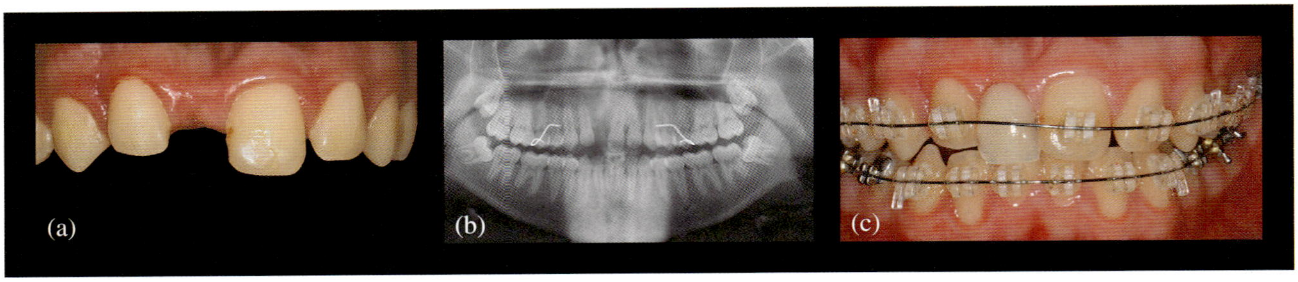

Figure 8.8 (a) Deficient horizontal mesiodistal space that hinders proper implant restorative space, (b) Panoramic radiographic view showing the defective space, (c) Orthodontic treatment for natural teeth distalization.

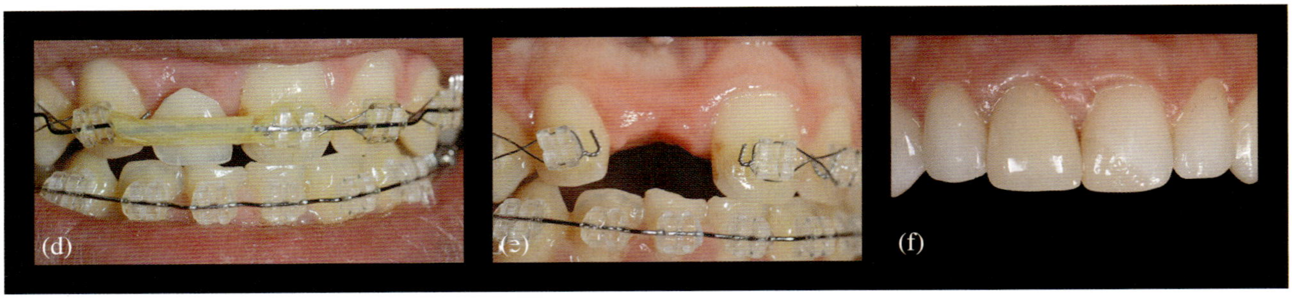

Figure 8.8 (d) and (e) Space optimization achieved post orthodontic treatment, (f) Final prosthesis in place.

The clinician makes an assessment about the mesiodistal space required for an optimal anatomically contoured restoration. Contralateral teeth can be used as a reference to communicate spatial requirements (see Figure 8.9a–c). If the tooth to be replaced has not yet been removed, several decisions should be made prior to the extraction. If bone deficiencies are present, orthodontic tooth eruption of the tooth prior to extraction can help to increase the amount of hard and soft tissue in the future implant site.

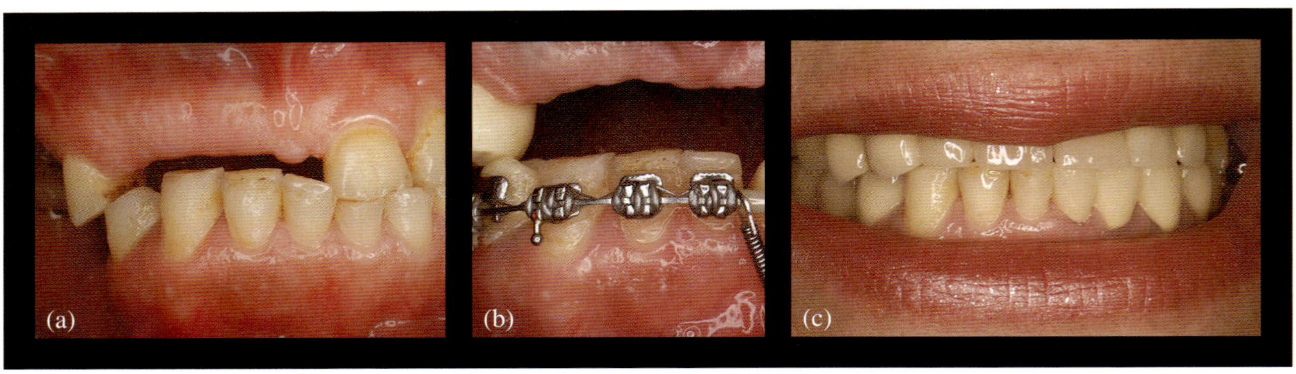

Figure 8.9 (a) Deficient vertical space, (b) Orthodontic teeth intrusion, (c) Final case restored.

A diagnostic wax-up as shown in Figure 8.10a–c acts as a visual aid for the orthodontist so that an appropriate space can be created. When lateral incisors are congenitally missing it is not uncommon to find that the adjacent roots have drifted into the space, making placement of implants difficult. Often orthodontic therapy is required to create space for implant placement and also for the prosthetic restoration by uprighting natural teeth roots. Ideally the maxillary lateral incisor should be two-thirds the width of the central incisor. Most central incisors are 8–10 mm wide. If the central incisor is 8 mm wide then the lateral should be 5.5 mm, if the central is 9 mm then the lateral should be 6 mm, and if it is 10 mm then the lateral should be 6.7 mm. The range of most lateral incisors varies from 5.5 to 6.7 mm. In some situations the orthodontist may create less than an ideal width for the lateral incisor.

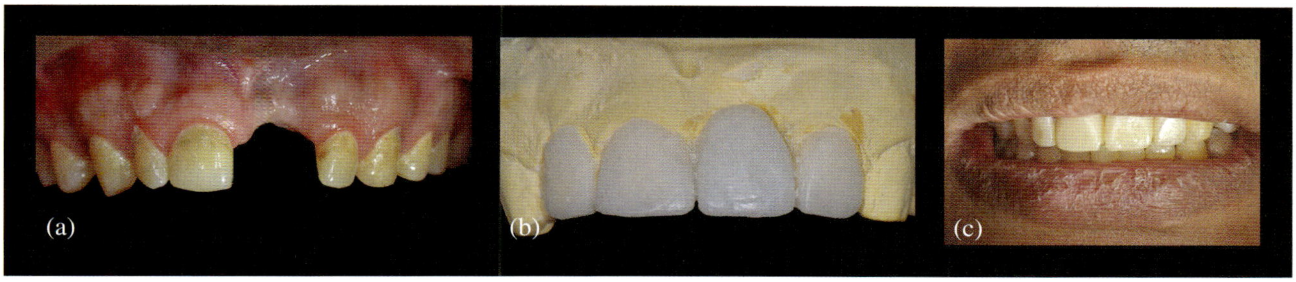

Figure 8.10 (a) Excessive horizontal restorative space, (b) Wax up made, (c) Mockup try in.

If space is not available the orthodontist should consider enamel stripping interproximally from the central incisors and the canines to provide additional width for the central incisor crown (teeth stripping or enameloplasty).

The use of orthodontic techniques may help to avoid the need for invasive procedures, such as mucogingival surgeries (Seibert and Salama 1996), distraction osteogenesis (Chin and Toth 1996), guided tissue repair (Hämmerle and Jung 2003), or bone graft applications (van Steenberghe et al. 1997). The discomfort caused by the use of orthodontic devices such as wires, braces, or other appliances for orthodontic treatment can be a disadvantage from the esthetic and hygienic perspectives. Similarly, there may be a need for conservative periodontal surgery, such as gingivoplasty, for correction of the cervical levels between adjacent teeth (see Figure 8.11a–g).

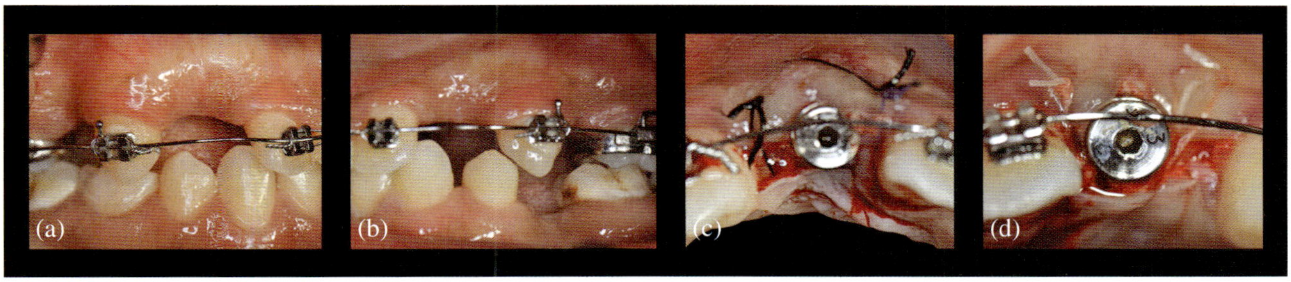

Figure 8.11 (a) and (b) Excessive horizontal space for the maxillary right and left side, (c) and (d) The most mesial implants being placed while orthodontic movement being in process.

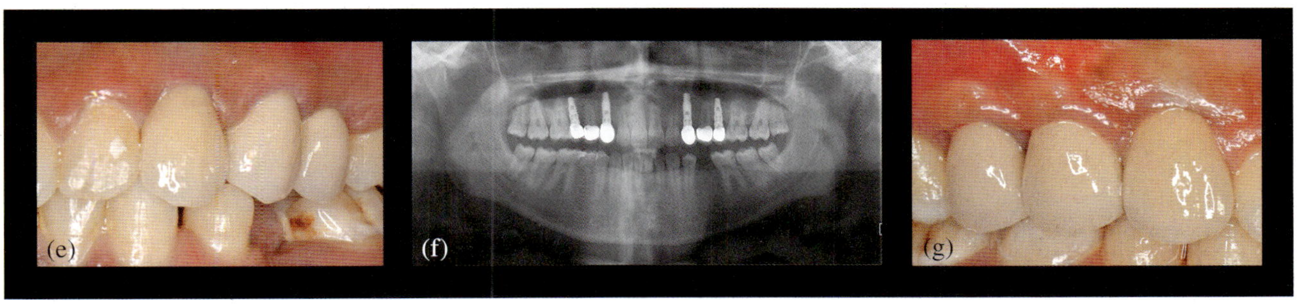

Figure 8.11 (e) Close up (left side), (f) Full mouth O.P.G. radiograph, (g) Close up (Right side).

8.5 Methods to Optimize Vertical Space Insufficiency

8.5.1 Orthodontic Management

8.5.1.1 Excessive Space

Forced orthodontic eruption might be an alternative approach to surgery for increasing and improving the hard and soft tissue contours. Initially described by Heithersay and Hirsch (1993) and Ingber (1974), this technique has been used to correct isolated bone defects, reposition the gingival margin, and lengthen the natural tooth crown (Ingber 1974; Johnson and Sivers 1986; Potashnick and Rosenberg 1982). Forced orthodontic eruption, also known as orthodontic extrusive remodeling, forced eruption, or orthodontic extraction (Korayem et al. 2008; Salama and Salama 1993), is an osteophysiologic- and orthodontic-based technique. In 1993, Salama and Salama (1993) applied this technique to lengthen the alveolar bone crest and replace the gingival tissue, improving the soft, and hard tissue profiles at the sites of implant placement. They performed orthodontic extrusion in hopeless teeth with periodontal involvement.

Some authors (Mantzikos and Shamus 1997, 1999; O'Neal and Butler 2002; Salama and Salama 1993) have reported that teeth with periodontal involvement and without periapical lesions can be extruded to develop bone and gingival tissues in a coronal direction before implant placement. Lengthening of the vertical buccal bone plate and the alveolar bone crest allows good implant placement, providing a more natural emergence profile of the prosthesis relative to the adjacent teeth and enhancing the cervical gingival levels. The increase in keratinized gingival and bone tissues allows a more esthetically pleasing final restoration (Mantzikos and Shamus 1999; O'Neal and Butler 2002).

The extrusion movement of a tooth involves the application of tension forces in all regions of the periodontal ligament to stimulate bone apposition. The entire alveolar bone connected to the root of the periodontal ligament exhibits this movement, as does the gingival tissue (Bach, Baylard and Voyer 2004; Cuoghi et al. 2010). Usually, this movement produces forces that might cause rapid extrusion and smaller crown migration of the supporting tissues, presumably because the rapid movement exceeds the tissues' physiological capacity for adaptation (Cuoghi et al. 2010; Sabri 1989). The rapid extrusion movement is associated with risks of ankylosis (Oesterle and Wood 1991) and root resorption (Minsk 2000) of the tooth, phenomena that can be limited by controlling the extrusion forces (Malmgren, Malmgren and Frykholm 1991).

Korayem et al. (2008) published a systematic review of the literature on the development of the alveolar region through orthodontic extrusion for later implant placement. They found 19 case reports that showed clinically significant gains in bone and gingival tissues, which improved the quality and quantity at the implant site. In all of the clinical cases cited, the extrusion movement was performed in the anterior region of the dental arch. The most common indication for extrusion and extraction of the teeth was poor prognosis of the tooth due to periodontal disease, with severe horizontal bone loss, interproximal or circumferential to the teeth (Korayem et al. 2008). The extrusion time of the teeth varied from 4 to 28 weeks. The retention period of the teeth for tissue adaptation ranged from immediate extraction to up to six months after the final active extrusion treatment.

Korayem et al. (2008) also found no consensus concerning a standard clinical protocol for orthodontic extrusion, but they recommended certain behaviors based on the literature. They indicated forces of 15 and 50 N cm for the anterior and posterior teeth, respectively, and a slow and steady extrusion rate of $\leq$2.0 mm month^{-1}. A retention and stabilization period of $\geq$1 month for each month of active extrusion was recommended prior to extraction. Overlay wires were recommended to reinforce anchorage and to avoid the tipping of adjacent teeth toward the tooth undergoing active extrusion. They also indicated that a buccal root torque component may be applied concomitantly to increase the buccolingual bulk of the alveolar bone. Nevertheless, of the many orthodontic extrusion methods that are available in the literature, it is the responsibility of the orthodontist to implement and monitor the effects caused by force application (Bach et al. 2004; Cuoghi et al. 2010). The orthodontist must seek to avoid detrimental effects, such as ankylosis (Oesterle and Wood 1991) and root resorption (Minsk 2000), as well as excessive forces that could make vertical bone gain impracticable (Erkut et al. 2007; Holst et al. 2007; Malmgren et al. 1991) (see Figure 8.12).

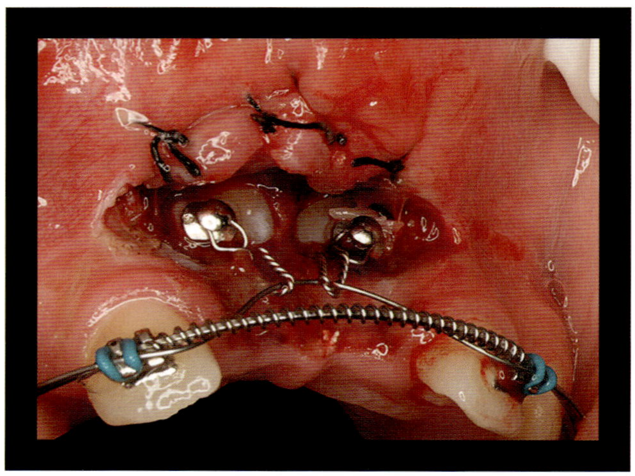

Figure 8.12 Orthodontic extrusions of two retained central incisors to develop natural contours.

Orthodontic brackets may be used to control the application of forces in a desired direction. This control is very important when bone must be gained in any non-axial direction (Tondelli, Kay and Kuabara 2014). By bonding brackets to the facial tooth surface (with a more cervical position in the tooth to be extruded), extrusion can be performed at low-magnitude forces, allowing new tissues to form (Salama and Salama 1993). The action line of the extrusion force passes buccally to the resistant center of the tooth and creates a moment (i.e. tendency to incline) on the tooth, which moves the root apex and leads to bone formation in the buccal direction (Korayem et al. 2008). Inclination and torque control must be performed later in the extrusion process and with a rectangular wire. The orthodontist must avoid loss of mechanical control, which can lead to excessive root apex tipping.

Orthodontic extrusion allows a tooth that has suffered bone loss to be restored by repairing the crown root ratio. It avoids the need for implant placement or the mutilation of adjacent teeth through the installation of a fixed prosthesis. In the case of a hopeless tooth, the technique enables the implant to be fixed at a better angle and position, resulting in better function and esthetics (Salama and Salama 1993). Orthodontic extrusion allows the restorative dentist to create a more harmonious gingival level and esthetically pleasing effect by providing the patient with a restoration that mimics the contralateral side. Extrusion is performed at a rate of 1 mm week^{-1} and a stabilization period of one month for each millimeter extruded. Extrusion is the most predictable method of vertical bone development (Rose, Jivraj and Chee 2006). It is likely that patients requiring dental implants to replace multiple missing teeth will need horizontal bone augmentation in addition to extrusion (Chen et al. 2004). Extrusion allows the clinician to develop the peri-implant site vertically to give the patient esthetically proportionate restorations (see Figure 8.13a–c).

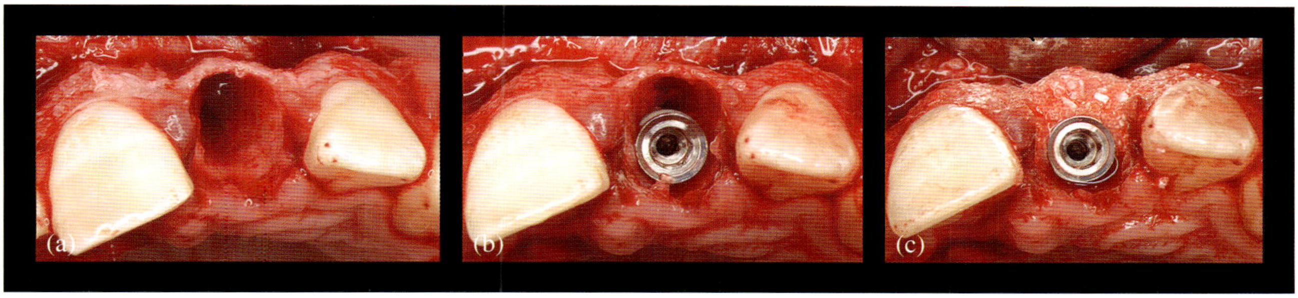

Figure 8.13 (a) An extraction socket condition, (b) The implant head is placed in the optimal buccolingual position. Note the space left for natural emergence between the implant and the crest of the bone, (c) The space is filled with bone-grafting material.

Orthodontic teeth extrusion promotes the development of a better area for implant installation at sites of moderate or severe periodontal involvement, thereby increasing the amount and quality of bone, which directly influences implant stability (Buskin, Castellon and Hochstedler 2000). Other treatment modalities, such as allogeneic or autologous bone grafts, guided tissue regeneration, and distraction osteogenesis, may contribute to the same goal (Chen et al. 2004; Hämmerle and Jung 2003; van Steenberghe et al. 1997). The use of forced extrusive orthodontic movers can be used only for minor deficiencies, the regular routine bone grafting.

8.5.1.2 Management of Deficient Vertical Restorative Space

Orthodontic intrusion of the overerupted antagonistic tooth to facilitate implant rehabilitation is a predictable treatment strategy and a routine orthodontic procedure. However, it is usually limited to one tooth only and so the task is formidable with routine orthodontic mechanics while control of the anchorage is difficult. Recently, the introduction of miniscrew implants to the orthodontic armamentarium has widened the scope of intervention (Kanomi 1997; Kravitz et al. 2007a; Park et al. 2001). Preprosthodontic intrusion of an over-erupted tooth with the aid of miniscrew implants is simple and less invasive (Kravitz et al. 2007a; Sohn, Lee and An 2008). Use of miniscrew implants in preprosthodontic management has drawn great interest in recent years among researchers and clinicians. It is a predictable option with fewer side effects (Kravitz et al. 2007a; Sohn et al. 2008). Recent studies have revealed that the average intrusion of maxillary molars is between 3 and 4 mm and a combination of a single miniscrew implant and a fixed appliance (partial) is a predictable and effective procedure to achieve maxillary molar intrusion (Kravitz et al. 2007b; Yao et al. 2005). No definite consensus exists on where exactly the miniscrew implant should be placed when a single screw is used for maxillary first molar intrusion. The placement of the screw in D4 bone quality revealed an associated failure rate (35–50%) (Jaffin and Berman 1991). A miniscrew can be placed in the buccal dentoalveolus between the second premolar and the first molar at the mucogingival junction, while a raised transpalatal arch will effectively counter the buccal tipping of the molar and help in intrusion (Kravitz et al. 2007b). A miniscrew implant in the midpalatal area can also provide an effective intrusive force, but it should be combined with a rigid transpalatal bar to prevent the horizontal component of the force tipping the teeth. When tipping occurs the roots invariably move buccally (Park et al. 2005); however, use of two screws on both buccal and palatal sides will effectively produce true intrusion to direct a force through the center of resistance of a molar, and simultaneous buccal and palatal forces should be applied (Sivakumar and Sivakumar 2014). Still the most critical factor for molar intrusion was the point of application of the intrusive force (Chun et al. 2000; Park et al. 2005). Nevertheless, the anatomic constraints that often exist hinder the optimal positioning of miniscrew implants (see Figure 8.14a–i).

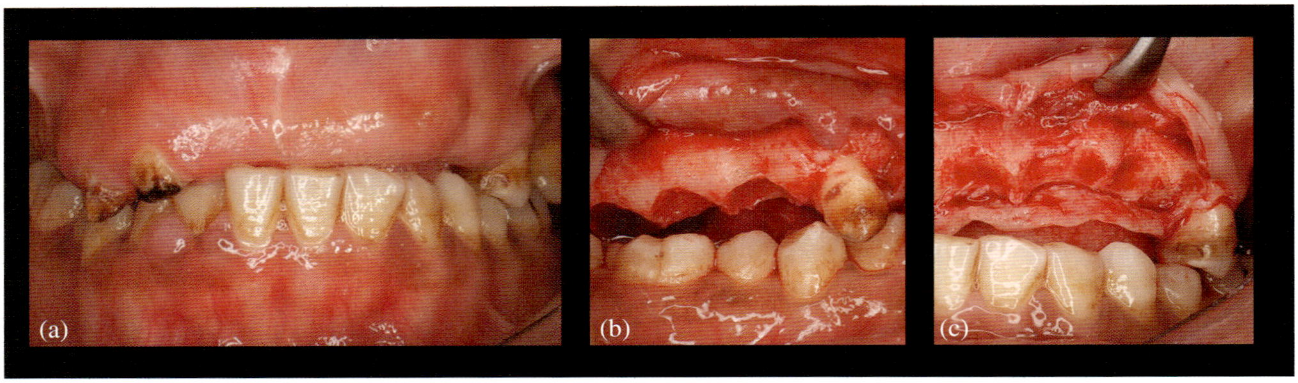

Figure 8.14 (a) Insufficient vertical space (complete collapse), (b) and (c) Osseous re-contouring (resection) ample of bone height allowed such procedure.

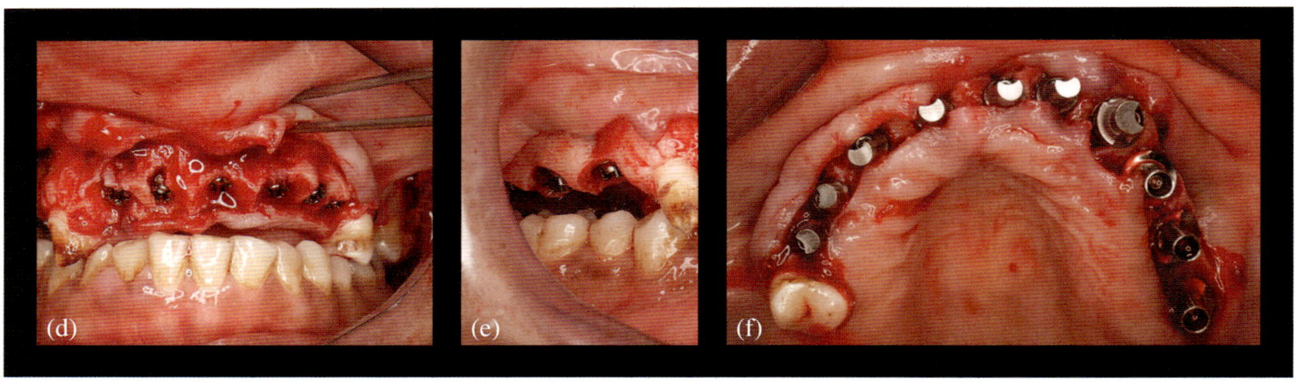

Figure 8.14 (d) and (e) Implants placed revealing sufficient vertical restorative space, (f) Final abutments connected for immediate loading.

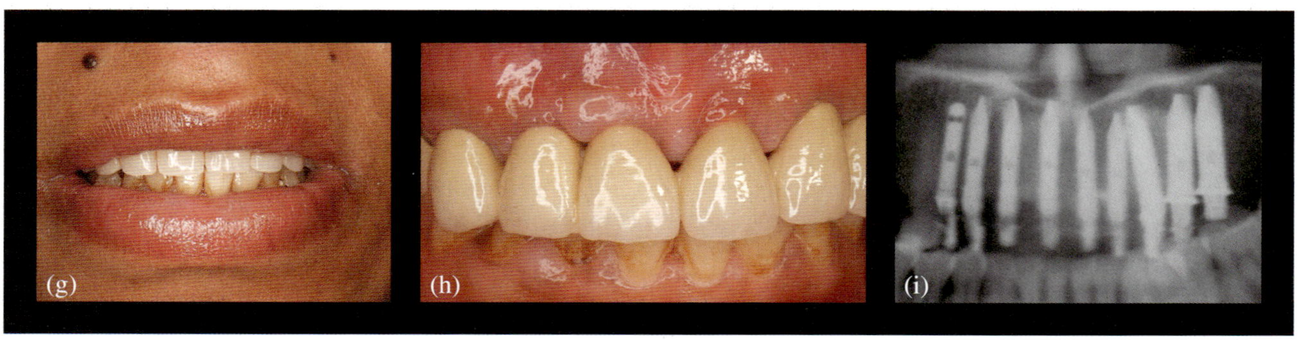

Figure 8.14 (g) and (h) Final case restored, (i) Panoramic radiographic view showing sufficient implant height inserted.

8.5.1.3 Screw-retained Abutments

The size and contours of the planned prosthesis require an optimal restorative space (see Figure 8.15a–c). A single-unit, screw-retained restoration has the benefit of using fewer components, as it is directly connected to the implant fixture. It also provides a more predictable retention of the restoration unlike the cement-retained abutments, which require sufficient height to offer retention to the above restoration (Berglundh and Lindhe 1996; Misch et al. 2005). Screw-retained abutments can help solve the problem of limited interarch space to a great extent. They also provide better provisional options as there is the ability to remove and replace the restoration easily at consecutive appointments, they often offer a predictable solution in implant dentistry.

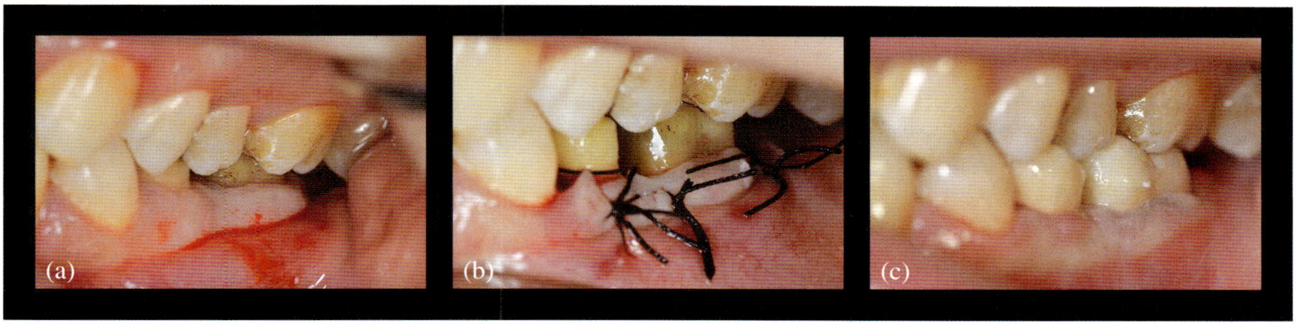

Figure 8.15 (a) Insufficient vertical space, (b) Crown lengthening procedure, (c) Final case restored.

A screw-retained restoration screws directly on to the implant body and requires an even smaller crown height space than cement-retained restorations; however, it exhibits weaker porcelain strength at the screw–hole interface (Kendrick and Wong 2009), and presents a greater incidence of screw loosening (Jemt 1991; Kline et al. 2002). If at least 2 mm of occlusal clearance is planned, then, just like natural teeth, there will be enough room for occlusal porcelain to be used (Blair et al. 2002).

Screw-retained abutments offer superior esthetic outcomes, and can even solve faulty implant angulations. The modern evolution of milling devices offer a versatile option of milling the screw-retained abutments along with the restoration that is attached to it to give a superior precision and perfect fit. The custom fabricated abutments offer a harmonious scalloped contour that matches the gingival curvatures.

8.5.2 Crown Lengthening

Tooth crown lengthening is employed when there is overeruption of the opposing tooth within the arch that needs to be repositioned apically, without the need to perform orthodontic tooth intrusion. The basic need for such procedure (in this clinical application) is to offer more tooth structure for the retention of the future crown. As with any procedure, the patient needs to be informed of any potential complications such root sensitivity, root resorption, and transient mobility of the teeth. Usually when crown lengthening is performed, it is accompanied by root canal treatment to restore the harmony of the occlusal curves (Narayan, Narayan and Jacob 2011). Pre-operative restorative assessment includes tooth location within the arch, periodontal considerations, crown-to-root ratio, and the potential space to be gained (see Figure 8.16a–d).

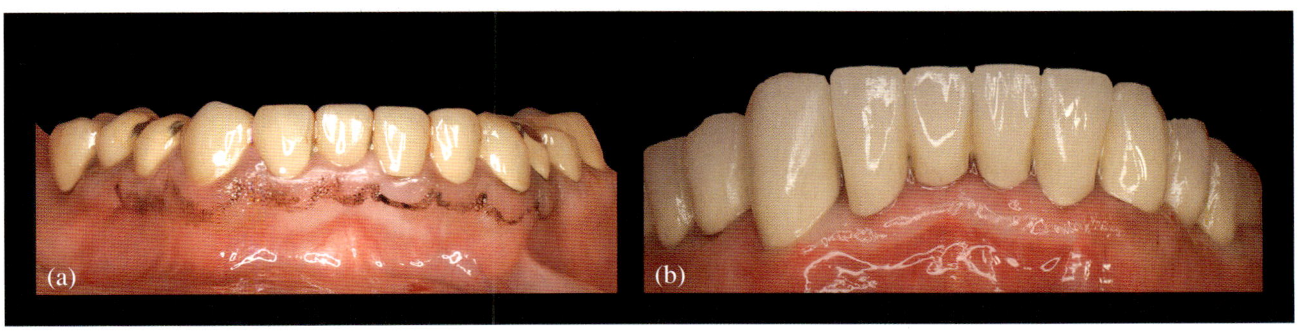

Figure 8.16 (a) and (b) Apical repositioning flap.

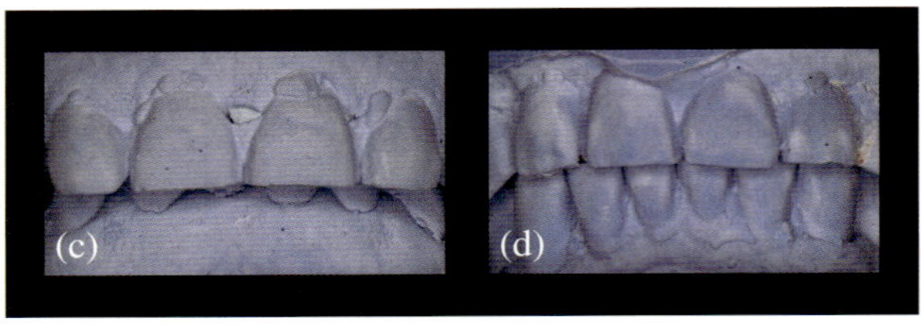

Figure 8.16 (c) and (d) Study cast showing the change of the inter-maxillary teeth relationship.

A classification system for esthetic crown lengthening procedures has been proposed by Lee (2004). Type I – involves sufficient soft tissue present allowing gingival exposure of the alveolar crest or violation of the biologic width (Narayan et al. 2011). Type II – sufficient soft tissue allows gingival excision without exposure of the alveolar crest, Type III – gingival excision to the desired clinical crown length will expose the alveolar crest. Type IV – gingival excision will result in inadequate band of attached gingiva. Maynard and Wilson (1979) recommended a minimum of 3 mm of attached gingiva in the presence of subgingival restorative therapy. Only an apically repositioned flap without osseous resection is done when there is no adequate width of attached gingiva and there is a biologic width of more than 3 mm on multiple teeth (Nugala et al. 2012) (see Figure 8.17).

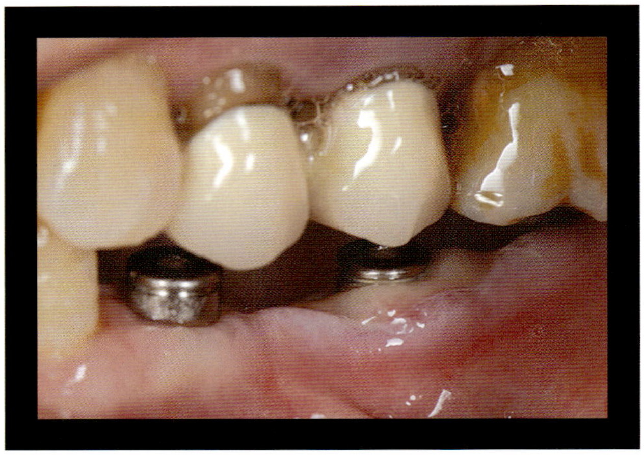

Figure 8.17 Insufficient vertical space due to over eruption of the maxillary teeth.

The alveolar bone is reduced by ostectomy and osteoplasty to expose the required tooth length in a scalloped fashion and to follow the desired contour of the overlying gingiva (see Figure 8.18a–f). As a general rule, at least 4 mm of sound tooth structure must be exposed, so that the soft tissue will proliferate coronally to cover 2–3 mm of the root, thereby leaving only 1–2 mm of a supragingivally located sound tooth structure (Nugala et al. 2012) (see Figure 8.19a–c).

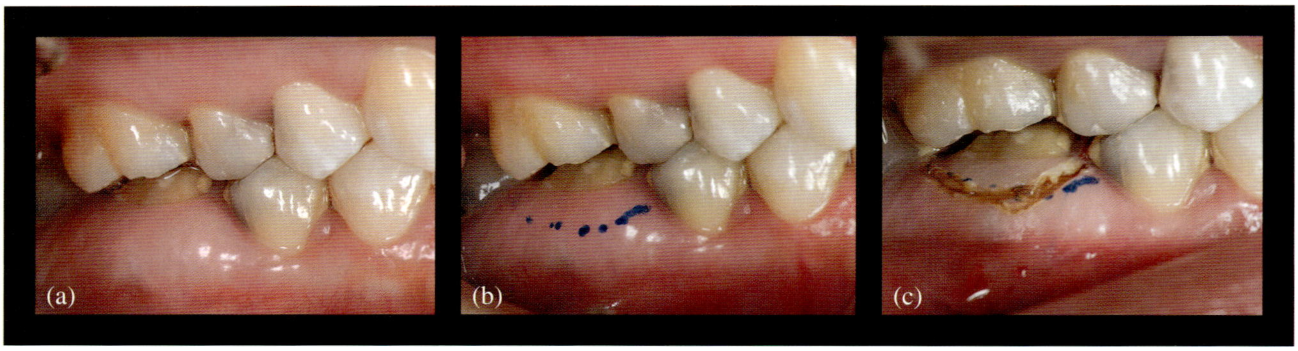

Figure 8.18 (a) Insufficient vertical space, (b) Blue marker is used to mark the future gingival margins, (c) Laser gingivectomy and osseous contouring to the marked lines.

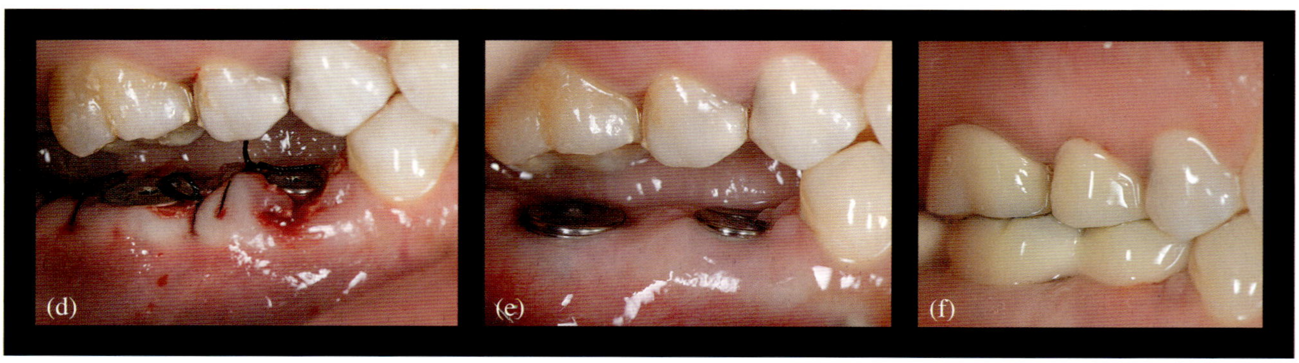

Figure 8.18 (d) Two implants positioned allowing a better vertical restorative space, (e) Two months post healing, (f) Final screw retained restoration in place.

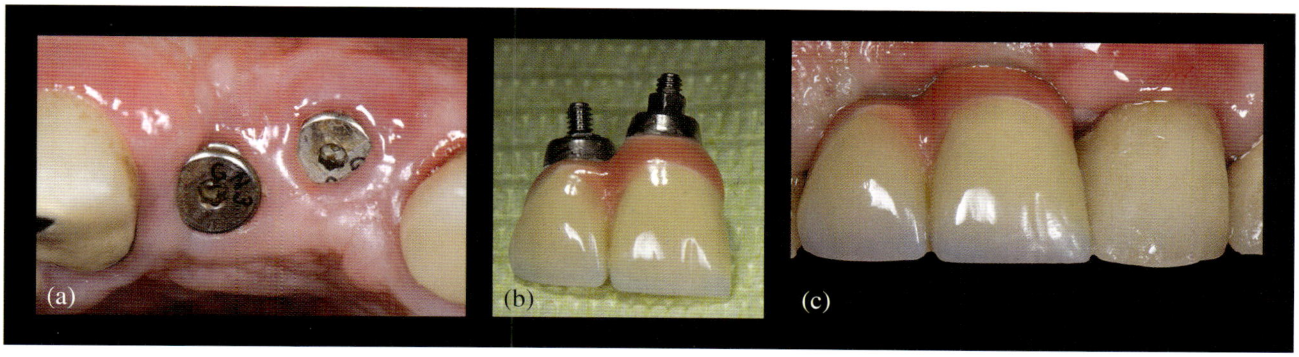

Figure 8.19 (a) Poor labially placed implants, (b) and (c) Corrected by screw retained implant supported prosthesis.

In the prosthetic phase, after healing is completed, extension of the preparations subgingivally to attain better retention form may have adverse reactions in the periodontium. As chamfer preparations are necessary to provide the room for the ceramic material of a restoration, there is usually no apparent reason for more than minimal or no extension below the gingival crest (Sharma et al. 2012).

8.5.3 Osseous Crest Management

Preprosthetic surgery is defined as surgical procedures designed to facilitate fabrication of a prosthesis or to improve the prognosis of prosthodontic outcome (Chari and Shaik 2016). The procedures may include alveoloplasty, maxillary tuberosity reduction, exostoses and tori removal, and reduction of genial tubercles.

Alveolectomy, which is the surgical removal or trimming of the alveolar process, can be used to trim the excessive bone tissues to facilitate prosthetic rehabilitation whenever there is excessive interdental, interseptal, or buccal alveolar crest after extraction. They might be trimmed with forceps or a round bur and then smoothed with a bone file. Another procedure is alveoloplasty, which sometimes refers to a surgical recontouring of the alveolar process. This procedure might involve simple alveoloplasty, interseptal alveoloplasty, Dean's alveoloplasty, Obwegeser's modification and post-extraction alveoloplasty (Obwegeser 1966). The principles of osseous resective surgery, as it is conceived today, dates back to Schluger (1949) and Friedman (1955). They aimed to eliminate osseous defects so that a consistency between osseous topography and gingival tissue could be re-established, but at a more apical level. The need for an optimal prosthetic rehabilitation often dictates this procedure (Hempton and Dominici 2010). Osseous ressective surgery is the combined use of both osteoplasty and ostectomy to re-establish harmonious marginal bone morphology around the teeth.

When ressective osseous surgery is performed to eliminate osseous deformities or to reshape healthy bone for exposure of tooth structure, the final contours of the underlying osseous structure influence the overlying gingival tissues (Hempton and Dominici 2010). Wound healing should result in a scalloped gingival architecture with a minimized sulcus depth.

The decision on the amount of osseous structure removal will depend on the use of a prefabricated surgical stent to verify the accurate amount of bone to be removed (see Figure 8.20a and b).

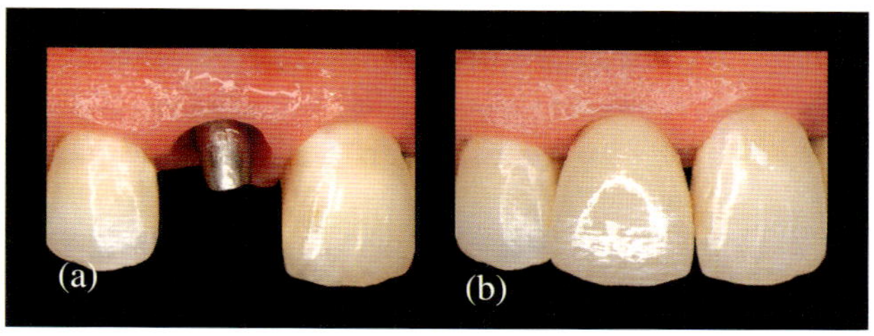

Figure 8.20 (a) and (b) Optimum implant positioning that provides optimum emerges profile and soft tissue related prosthetic margins.

8.5.4 Distraction Osteogenesis (for Optimization Excessive Vertical Space)

Insufficient alveolar height would most likely result in an improper crown–implant height ratio (Garcia et al. 2002). When excessive restorative interarch space exists, the clinician is often faced with two main issues: (1) the poor esthetic shape of the restorations, and (2) the minimal bone height for placing dental implants. Decreased alveolus size in the vertical dimension is a common finding in patients going for prosthetic rehabilitation as a result of long-term edentulism, failed bone graft technique, orofacial pathology, or injury.

The introduction of distraction osteogeneses dates back to 1905 when Ilizarov and Deviatov (1969) applied it on the facial region for animals and 20 years later in human beings. The principle involved an intentional osteotomy of the proposed area followed by a traction force applied to the callus. The process has been used in the maxilla and mandible. The recent availability of miniature distraction devices allowed even better treatment outcome from bone distraction. Alveolar distraction can be divided into two categories, (vertical distraction) and (horizontal distraction). The process of distraction avoids bone grafting procedures using other body parts and their associated complications. Complications associated with the procedure might include the malposed distracted segment, formation of bone defects, fracture of the transport segment, and infections leading to failure of the overall procedure (Jonsson and Siemssen 1998).

Distraction osteogenesis of the edentulous alveolar ridges may be considered an alternative to many other surgical techniques, such as alloplastic graft augmentation, autogenous onlay bone grafting, and guided bone regeneration (Urbani 2001). Alveolar distraction is now widely used for treating severe forms of alveolar ridge insufficiency (Gaggl, Schultes and Kärcher 2000; Keller, Tolman and Eckert 1998).

Distraction osteogenesis allows alveolar bone gain without requiring the inclusion of foreign materials. There is no need for a donor site and a clinically controlled bone gain is obtained (Urbani 2001). As the bone segment is transported, soft tissue advancement is also achieved (Uckan et al. 2002).

Histologic studies show that a satisfactory bone callus is obtained after two months. Urbani (2001) and Consolo et al. (2000) state that after three months implants can be positioned correctly. They believe that distractor removal times may range from 30 to 60 days. However early removal of the device might lead to serious consequences. Urbani (2001) reported a mean time of 87 days before implant insertion. It is also important to place the distraction device according to the correct distraction vector to avoid a labial deficiency of the distracted segment. Orientation of the distraction rod should be made toward the middle of the adjacent teeth in the buccolingual axis.

One of the main problems in alveolar distraction is accurate control of the direction. When the transport segment is relatively long (more than about 2 cm), it may be difficult to achieve accurately controlled osteogenesis using only one distraction device. There is a possibility of tilting in the longitudinal axis of the distraction. In such cases, one solution is to use two distractors for each transport segment.

8.6 Factors Influencing Implant Positioning

Several factors contribute to accurate implant positioning. These factors are not so much technical as they are treatment-related, and they help ensure predictable esthetic results (see Figure 8.21a and b). These factors are given in the following sections (Elaskary 2008).

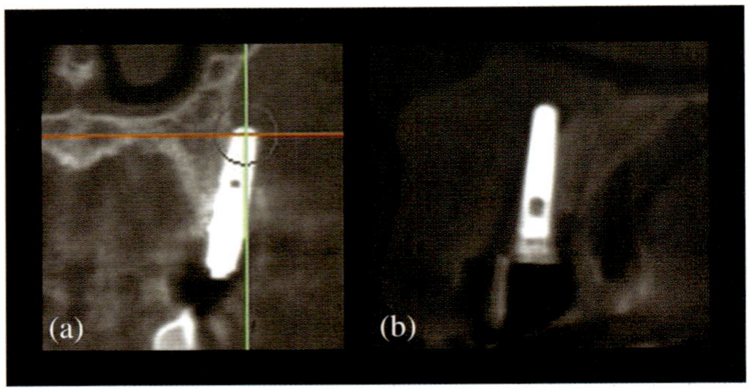

Figure 8.21 (a) and (b) Improper implant positioning (poor angulation) as a result of not using accurate positioning device.

8.6.1 The Grip

During the drilling procedure, the grip of the handpiece influences the implant's optimal position to a great extent. The control of the clinician's hand while drilling, using either a palm grip or pen-grasping grip, optimizes the positioning procedure. The palm grip sometimes provides better control over other grips, especially in maxillary premolar locations. It is the author's personal opinion that the palm grip offers greater control of the drilling procedure in the maxillary posterior areas. This preference is due to the nature of the drilling procedure, which differs from the regular turbine handpiece grip that is used for cavity preparation. The nature of the slow speed and high torque during dental implantology procedures, as well as the bone resistance, allows the palm grip to assist in achieving better positioning control (Elaskary 2008).

8.6.2 Accuracy of the Surgical Guide

The more accurate the surgical template, the more accurate the implant positioning. New types of templates are being fabricated with computer-aided design/computer-aided manufacturing (CAD/CAM) technology that offers precise positioning in terms of locating the axial location of the implant head within the alveolar ridge. These precise surgical templates are being used with a computed tomography (CT) scan-based planning system (Tardieu, Vrielinck and Escolano 2003) that allows the surgeon to select the optimal location for implant placement, taking into account specific anatomic characteristics of the patient and thus using optimal bone densities. The precision of the perpendicular reconstruction images along the axis of the arch (orthogonal frontal oblique sections) is almost 95%. Thus, the precision of these reconstruction sections is amply sufficient for clinical application in implant therapy (see Figure 8.22a and b).

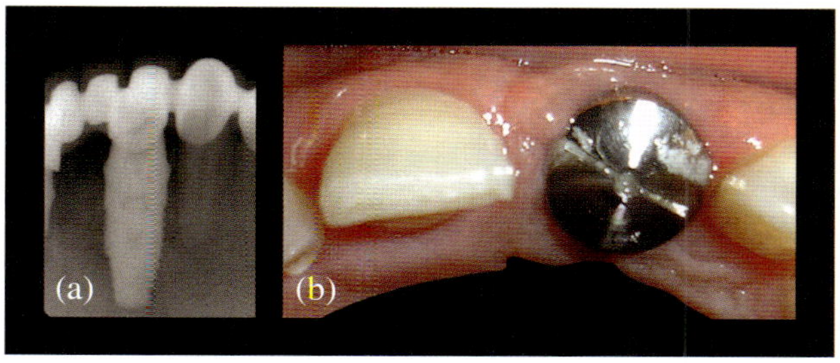

Figure 8.22 (a) Wrong implant size selection, (b) Faulty implant size selection.

The goal of this technology is to allow the clinician to use an individualized drill guide that fits exactly on the bone crest of the patient. A CAD/CAM program uses the shape of the scanning template and the 3D information of the plan. A stereolithographic drill guide allows a physical transfer of the implant planning to the patient's mouth. The scannographic template is designed so that it can be transformed into a temporary fixed or final prosthesis for immediate loading (Elaskary 2008).

An available planning software system, NobelGuide® (Nobel Biocare AB, Göteborg, Sweden), was introduced to maximize the implant positioning from the three dimensions. It also makes it possible to measure soft tissue height, which is considered an outstanding advantage, and the axial position of the dental implant. This subsequently transfers most of the surgical and prosthetic planning and fabrication outside the patient's mouth and allows the planning to be done prior to implant installation. This revolutionary treatment planning and surgical implementation system transfers extraoral planning into the mouth with accuracy and ease. Therefore, placing implants, abutments, and restorative components is simultaneous by using either conventional modeling or a computer-aided 3D design. This system gives the exact position and depth of the implants prior to surgery. The laboratory can then produce a surgical template that guides the surgical procedure from the start to a completely successful placement. The case is planned in a computer based on CT scan data, which offers a more precise picture of anatomy, compared to model-based planning. A customized surgical template and the required implant-related components then can be ordered and used according to the preplanned case.

8.6.3 Sharpness of the Cutting Flutes of the Drills

Because drills become blunt with use, each implant manufacturer states the number of times a set of drills should be used, after which they should be discarded. The sharpness of the drill prevents it from wobbling in the surgical site and the subsequent deviation from the intended angulation or position. In fact, the sharpness of the rosette or the pilot drill that is used for the pilot osteotomy is the most valuable because it guides the primary path for the other drill to follow (Elaskary 2008).

8.6.4 The Use of Positioning Devices

Many implant positioning devices are now available in the market, and some positioning devices are now available to help keep an optimized distance between the implant and the natural teeth. A novel implant positioning system called the IPS set (Storz am Markt GMBH, Emmingen-Liptingen, Germany) was introduced to assist in maintaining the proper implant position and angulation during the preparation of the surgical site. It consists of a series of sleeves and spreaders that maintain the proper interproximal dimensions and help determine the proper apical level of the implant head during surgery (Elaskary 2008). The system facilitates selection of the implant diameter and axis, maintains exact spacing between the adjacent tooth and the implant or between adjacent implants, is compatible with any implant system, is useful for orthodontists in determining prospective implant positions in cases in which teeth are missing as a result of a congenital defect, and is suitable for use as seating tips in spacing templates (Iglhaut 2003).

8.6.5 The Use of Computerized Navigation Surgery

Computerized navigation surgery is a developing technology for intraoperative tracking and guidance of surgical instruments to enhance minimally invasive procedures. It is considered to be a new era in perfecting implant positioning within the alveolar ridge and has evolved to facilitate minimally invasive procedures (Casap et al. 2005). This surgery, also called *image guided implantology*, can be used with flapless or flapped implant placement protocols for flapless implant placement where the surgery may be perceived as a blind procedure that includes a risk of cortical plate perforation. The computerized navigation system provides real-time imaging of the drill and transforms flapless implant surgery into a fully monitored procedure. The surgeon can rely on the computerized navigation to adjust the position and angulation of the drill in absolute coordination with the presurgical digital implant plan. The highly accurate intraoperative navigation enables precise transfer of the detailed presurgical implant plan to the patient (Elaskary 2008). Intraoperative computerized navigation in implant dentistry mandates that an interfacing template be firmly attached to the operated jaw throughout the surgery. In the partially edentulous patient, this template may be an acrylic resin splint that is mounted over the existing natural teeth, while in fully edentulous jaws, stabilizing bone screws might be used (Casap et al. 2005).

8.6.6 Implant Morphology and Design

Modern implant dentistry has versatile research dimensions, such as the implant design. The modern implant design has several additional morphological modifications that differ from the original standard classic designs and was originally made to simulate the original tooth morphology in most of the designs. Unfortunately, all missing teeth in the same dental arch cannot be restored with the same implant design due to the unique and versatile nature of human tooth roots. Some roots possess antirotational characters, some have stronger anchorage characters, and still others have a greater load-bearing capacity. Therefore, the comparison between natural teeth and dental implants is unfair and dental implants should not be called third dentition (Elaskary 2008).

When restoring natural dentition with conventional prostheses, the anatomy of the existing natural teeth and periodontium serve as guides for replicating the original natural form and contours. Unfortunately, dental implants do not provide the same valuable guides that are available when restoring natural dentition, especially when multiple teeth are missing. Consequently, before inserting dental implants, the clinician should develop an imaginary picture that will act as a guide or reference during the treatment plan. This is accomplished by properly assessing the original shape of the osseous bed and the biological dimensions of the missing dentition and relating them to the restorative components that will be used. Understanding the basic morphology of the missing tooth in relation to the implant fixture design along with its related components becomes an absolute necessity for achieving successful esthetic results (see Figure 8.23).

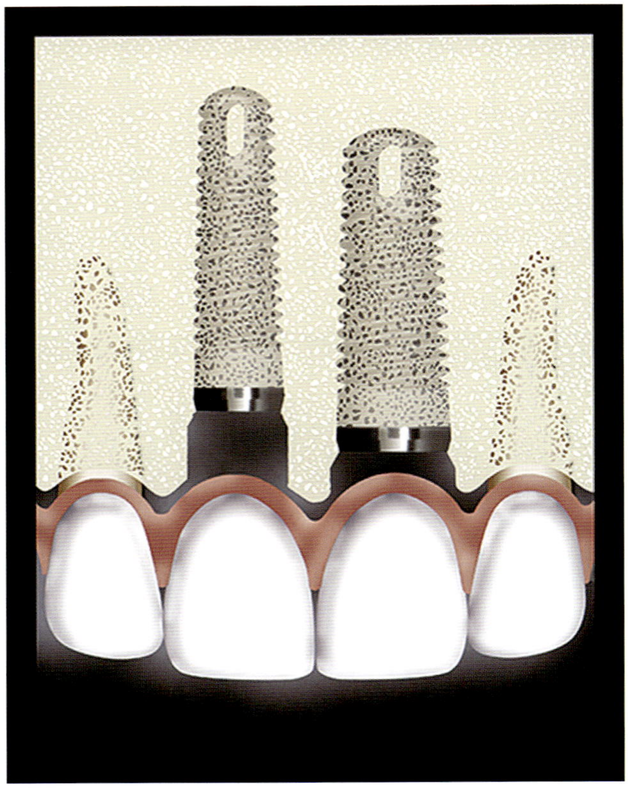

Figure 8.23 A drawing showing the effect of using different implant diameters in relation to apical sinking.

Many scholars study the technical advancements in implant designs. As a result, a better understanding of bone behavior and cellular activities has led to the invention of new designs. The changes involved include implant surface treatments, predictable interface connections, versatile unique implant sizes, and new implant-related prosthetic components. The newly introduced dental implant designs have led many clinicians to dramatically improve the clinical outcome of dental implants from both esthetic and functional standpoints and to take implant-supported restorations to new levels. Thus, selection of the optimum implant design and size is now an integral part of every treatment plan that seeks a superior esthetic outcome (Elaskary 2008).

The elements of implant design are:

1) The implant surface topography (micro characters).
2) The overall physical geometry (macro characters), such as length, diameter, and macroscopic threads, vents, and grooves.
3) The implant material composition.

These factors contribute to the implant's overall design. The question inevitably arises regarding which design features best stabilize the implant in the receptor site, assist the implant mechanical anchorage in the bone, best distribute occlusal loads, and provide the maximum esthetic outcome (Elaskary 2000).

Root form implant design should focus on several aspects when it is being used for the new modern loading modalities. For example, cylinder implants and finned implants press against the walls of the receptor site when the implant is tapped into place via a friction fit. These two particular designs cannot be used predictably for modern loading concepts due to the diminished initial bone–implant contact. In addition, they do not offer initial cortical bone engagement because they are not simply screwed in place; they are tapped in place. Therefore, the initial amount of bone that comes into direct contact with screw-type implants becomes important for the long-term survival of the implant (Johansson and Albrektsson 1987).

However, Sennerby and others (1992) observed that the removal torque of screw-type implants depends on the amount of available compact bone, rather than on the total amount of surrounding bone. Therefore, an ideal implant design should focus on achieving a maximum number of threads that should engage dense cortical bone for maximum stability. Also, the number of threads increases the amount of area available to bear loading; hence, the greater the number of threads, the greater is the functional surface area. Some threaded implants have a 1.5 mm distance between the threads, whereas others have a 0.4 mm distance. The smaller the distance between the threads, the greater is the thread number, and corresponding surface area (Misch et al. 2004).

The thread depth also influences the implant design; the greater the thread depth, the greater is the functional surface area and mechanical anchorage. The thread depth can range from 0.2 to 0.42 mm (Misch et al. 2004). Thread geometry may affect the strength of early osseointegration and the bone implant interface. Osseointegrated implants either have a V thread or a reverse buttress thread, or a square thread design. The V-shaped thread design offers 10 times greater shear force applied to bone when compared with other thread shapes. The V thread and reverse buttress thread geometries are similar in terms of bone maintenance around them, while the square thread demonstrates statistically significantly higher values of bone support (Misch et al. 2004). A tapered form for a root-shaped implant design presents unique physical characteristics:

1) It reduces the tendency for apical perforation when an immediate placement method is selected, as compared with those that are parallel-walled.
2) It might avoid damaging the adjacent roots.
3) It offers greater initial stability.
4) It compresses bone against its walls.

In addition to threads, many root-form implants contain vents for bone anchorage to enhance post-healing mechanical fixation. Most of the screw-type implants have one or more vents in their apical regions (Gores, Hayes and Unni 1989). In addition, connecting screws are an integral part of any designed implant-retained prosthetic system. Fatigue, loosening, and breaking of the screws are expected throughout the loading cycles intraorally (Elaskary 2008).

A study by Yousef and others (2005) was designed to understand the parameters of screw loosening, using an *in vitro* model, which included torque, screw head rotation, changes in screw dimension, and distortion of the implant–abutment joint. Implants (4 × 10 mm) were potted in autopolymerizing blocks. Abutments were placed with screws tightened with a 35 Newton centimeter (N cm) torque and standardized crowns were fabricated. Three implant systems were used: Nobel Biocare USA, Inc. (Yorba Linda, CA, USA), 3i Implant Innovations, Inc. (Palm Beach Gardens, FL, USA), and Bio-Lok International, Inc. (Deerfield Beach, FL, USA). Seven samples were tested for each system. The samples were loaded with 300 N loads for 50 000 cycles at 1 Hz. Torque turn audits were performed at 10 000, 25 000, and 50 000 cycles. At the conclusion of the loading, counterclockwise rotation of the abutment screw was measured. The screws were retrieved and measurements were made and compared with the controls. Finally, one sample from each group was embedded in resin, sectioned longitudinally, and examined under the standard error of the mean (Elaskary 2008).

The Nobel Biocare system showed a 9.4 N cm loss of torque from the loading protocol. This result was accompanied by a counterclockwise rotation of 7° and a 200 μm elongation of the screw. Compression and distortion of the longitudinally sectioned joint architecture was observed with the standard error of the mean. No loss of torque, counterclockwise rotation, or lengthening of the screws was observed in the 3i and BioLok International systems. Intimate adaptation of the joint without distortion was seen in the longitudinal sections. Screw loosening appears to follow specific parameters that include counterclockwise rotation, lengthening of the screw, and distortion of the screw joint. This process is likely to be associated with both the physical properties of the screw as well as its configuration. This observation suggested that each implant screw joint "adapts" to its environment based upon its design and material characteristics.

The surface topography of the implant can range from relatively smooth, machined, rough, plasma sprayed, sand blasted, and acid etched to a porous form of hydroxyapatite (HA). There is a positive correlation between the degree of primary mechanical fixation of the implant and increasing roughness of the implant surface (Carlsson et al. 1988). This work was supported by Carlsson et al., who found that rough-surfaced titanium screws demonstrated a higher removal torque in comparison to smooth-surfaced duplicates after six weeks in rabbits (Carlsson et al. 1988).

The implant–abutment connection becomes an important element in implant design. It predicts the stability and fixation of the restorative components and helps minimize the marginal bone loss upon loading. It also resists rotation and future connecting screw loosening. Most implant connections consist of internal threads to both retain and facilitate the removal of the abutments. The main geometrical form of the common interlocking elements can be a hexagon or octagon, which mates with a complementary abutment to prevent rotation. The ideal abutment connection is internal with interlocking geometry to prevent rotation and for better load bearing (Elaskary 2008).

A root form implant design is used to restore missing teeth. The standard root form screw-type implant body is 3.75 mm in diameter, and the diameter of its platform might flare up to 4.1 mm. The cylinder design of endosseous implants usually has a 4 mm body diameter and the same platform dimensions as the screw type (Jansen and Weisgold 1995). The abutments for the cylindrical and screw-type implants start with the same diameter as the implant's platform and then flare out to 4.5 or 5 mm. While these dimensions might vary somewhat among implant manufacturers or be due to laboratory modifications of the abutment, most of the standard implant diameters require a crown with a minimum diameter of 5.5 mm at the CEJ level and 7 mm at the level of the contact points when a missing central incisor is being restored, for instance.

The clinician should compensate for the difference in the diameter of the implant and the cervical dimension of the missing tooth to obtain natural biological contours of implant-supported restorations. This is accomplished by soft tissue expansion procedures through the provisional prosthesis to allow a smooth transition from the implant head diameter to that of the natural diameter. Selecting an implant diameter that is wider than or similar to the tooth to be replaced results in an incorrectly sized crown that does not biologically fit with the surrounding tissues (Elaskary 2008).

A recent study by Nebot et al. (2006) evaluated the implant platform modification, shifting the implant–abutment interface medially to minimize invasion of the biologic width. The study assessed 30 control cases and 30 study cases using the platform-modification technique. Interproximal bone resorption on the medial and distal of each implant was assessed using digital radiography at one, four, and six months. The mean value of bone resorption observed in the mesial measurement for the control group was 2.53 mm, whereas it was 0.76 mm for those patients in the study group. The mean value of bone resorption observed in the distal measurement for patients in the control group was 2.56 mm, whereas it was 0.77 mm for those in the study group. The study group had a significant reduction of bone loss in comparison to the control group ($P < 0.0005$), which indicated the clinical usefulness of the platform switching technique.

The implant diameter is directly related to the root diameter at the crest of the alveolar ridge. For example, if a missing maxillary central incisor to be replaced with a dental implant has a diameter that ranges between 7 and 8.5 mm at the CEJ level and between 5 and 6 mm at the bone level, the diameter of the implant to be used may vary from 4 to 6 mm, and so forth (Wheeler 1950). Therefore, the diameter of the implant should be related to the diameter of the root at the bone emergence level and not the CEJ level, because if the diameter of the implant exceeds the diameter of the root at the bone level, it will eventually cause crestal bone resorption. The diameter of the missing tooth can be verified by measuring the dimensions of the same tooth on the contralateral side or by verifying it on a study cast. The width of the implant dictates its position within the alveolar ridge; wider implants are less apically positioned while narrow diameter implants are more apically placed to allow for "running room" to stack the prosthetic components in it (Elaskary 2008).

The use of a specific formula for selecting a particular implant diameter for a specific tooth might not be ideal because there are many other variables that must be considered in the implant diameter selection process. Some of these include variations in the tissue phenotype, differences in the size of the same tooth's diameter among different individuals, changes that occur to the remaining bone after extraction, the altered soft tissue contours, and the variation in implant diameters. Thus, the clinician's personal evaluation is the best method for selecting the proper implant size and an individualized treatment approach is better than applying a generalized rule to different clinical situations (Elaskary 2008).

8.6.7 Implant Positioning Rationale

Placing an implant in the esthetic zone requires accurate attention to all treatment details, not only to achieve clinically accepted results but also to preserve the existing natural details. An optimum osseous dimension and restorative dimension should be key in any accurate 3D positioning procedure. The natural balance between these two dimensions should be preserved in implant therapy as it contributes to the complete biological integration of the dental implant within its housing (Jansen and Weisgold 1995). Certain guidelines assist in placing the implant in a 3D fashion – the interproximal dimension, which represents the relationship anteroposteriorly between the implant and the natural teeth mesiodistally, and the labiopalatal dimension, which relates to the mediolateral axis, and the sagittal dimensional axis, which is the apicoincisal dimension (Elaskary 2008).

8.6.7.1 Mesiodistal Position

The mesiodistal position of the implant in relation to the adjacent teeth or between adjacent implants has a direct impact on the esthetic outcome and the interproximal marginal integrity of the future restorative contours. It directly affects hygiene maintenance around implant-supported restorations and adjacent natural components. In ideal soft and hard tissue conditions, the implant should be positioned midway in the center of the available mesiodistal space to obtain a centrally positioned prosthesis. The potential risk of improper mesiodistal positioning of the implant is the approximation to the interdental papilla or, worse, impinging on it. This can cause blunting of the papilla and possible damage to the periodontium of the adjacent tooth to the implant site by compromising the blood supply, which could lead to external root resorption. External root resorption highlights the importance of not using parallel walled roots for dental implants. The use of a tapered implant design may reduce the chance of adjacent root approximation, especially when restoring areas with limited mesiodistal space or with curved roots.

Grunder et al. (2005) noted that the optimal distance between an implant and a natural tooth should not be less than 1.5 mm. The tooth attachment will be in jeopardy if this minimum distance is not maintained; in turn, this will cause a reduction or loss of the interproximal papilla. If the distance between two implants is less than 3 mm, the interproximal bone level is expected to be more apical to the implant shoulder and therefore exhibit a reduced or absent papilla. This situation is even more critical in thin-scalloped tissue phenotypes because, in these cases, the implant head is usually positioned more apical than the bone attachment of the adjacent teeth. Only if the implant-to-implant distance is greater than 3 mm can the interproximal bone peak be maintained above the implant head. In cases where the interimplant distance cannot be optimized, the future restoration will show many clinical discrepancies (see Figure 8.24a–c).

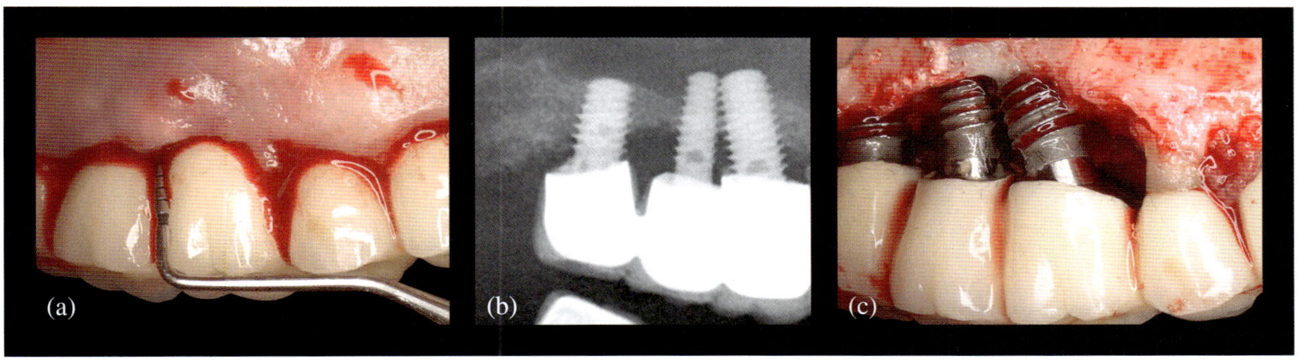

Figure 8.24 (a) Soft tissue inflammation with deep pocketing related to an implant supported bridge, (b) Radiographic view showing two close implants mesiodistally as well as impinging prosthetic margins, (c) Note the proximity of the two implants that hinders any hygiene measures.

The presence of diastemas demands more careful mesiodistal positioning of dental implants. With diastemas, the available interproximal space is larger than the original missing tooth size. In these cases, precise surgical templates ensure optimal implant positioning (Kennedy, Collins and Kline 1998) to determine the exact position of the missing tooth and at the same time to preserve the original size of the diastema prior to tooth loss (see see Figure 8.25a–c).

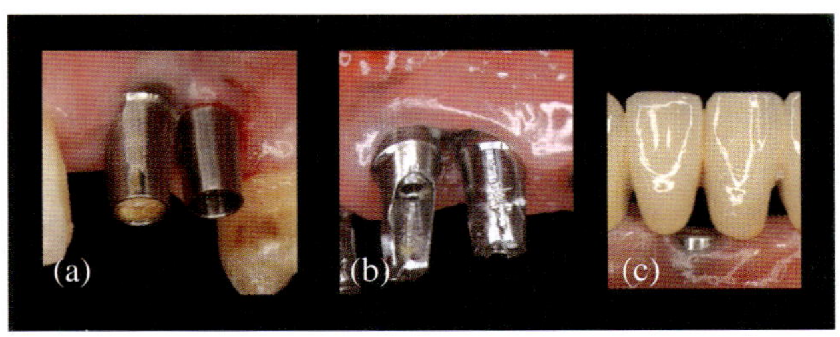

Figure 8.25 (a–c) Three examples of faulty mesiodistal implant positioning.

For multiple missing teeth within a larger space, the clinician has the freedom to design the shape of the diastema according to some guiding factors such as the preplanned teeth size, the patient's desire, and the midline position. Optimized clinical results can be obtained via a thorough fabrication of a wax-up and careful pre-surgical planning. For single-tooth replacements, the method for calculating the minimum space required for the optimal mesiodistal positioning of the implant should include the width of the periodontal ligament (average 0.25 mm) and a minimum of 1 mm of sound bone should be kept between the implant and the periodontal ligament of the adjacent natural tooth (Ohenell et al. 1992). The measurements accounting for the periodontal ligament and sound bone should be doubled to calculate both the mesial and distal aspects of the implant. Simply stated, the required distance for placing a 4 mm diameter implant between two teeth would be calculated by adding 1 mm + 0.25 mm + 4 mm + 0.25 mm + 1 mm. The resulting sum of 6.5 mm is the minimum space needed to position the implant mesiodistally. When multiple implants are used, the previous equation may be used by adding a distance of 2–3 mm between each implant (Elaskary et al. 1999a).

These measurements are only a guideline; every case should be approached on an individual basis. The mesiodistal position of an implant depends on the mesiodistal dimension of the available edentulous space, the presence or absence of diastemas, the size of the missing teeth (if a record exists), the type of the abutment to be used, and the adjacent root proximity (Elaskary 2008).

8.6.7.2 Implant Angulation Rationale

The labiopalatal position of the implant within the alveolar ridge influences the emergence point of the implant-supported restoration as well as its contagious marginal contours and the profile of the final restoration (see Figures 8.26a–c, 8.27a–c, and 8.28a–c). Generally, a proper emergence profile is desirable, for both esthetic and hygienic reasons. Therefore, the labial contour of the implant head has to emerge, as do adjacent natural teeth (see Figure 8.29).

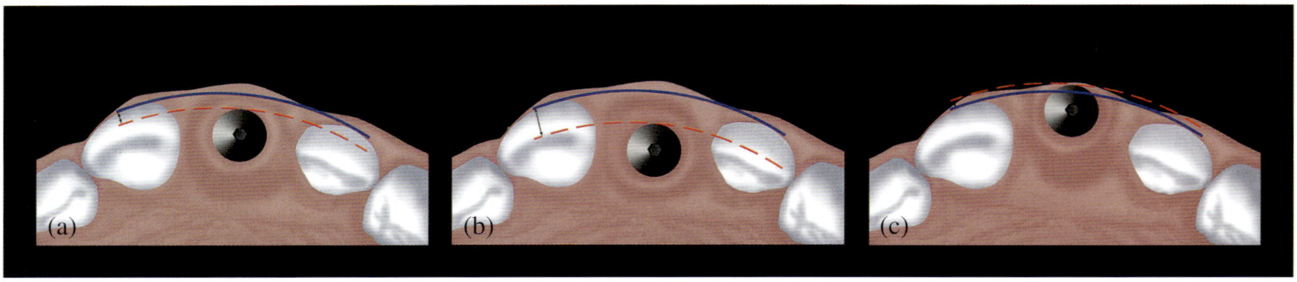

Figure 8.26 (a–c) An illustration showing the different situations of the buccolingual levels of the implant placement. The red line represents the implant head level, and the blue line represents the natural teeth natural buccal contour. In (a) an optimal space between the implant head and the natural teeth buccal contours, while in (b) the distance is too far from the natural buccal contour, and in (c) the implant head is placed at a very close distance from the natural buccal contour, which makes it difficult to restore.

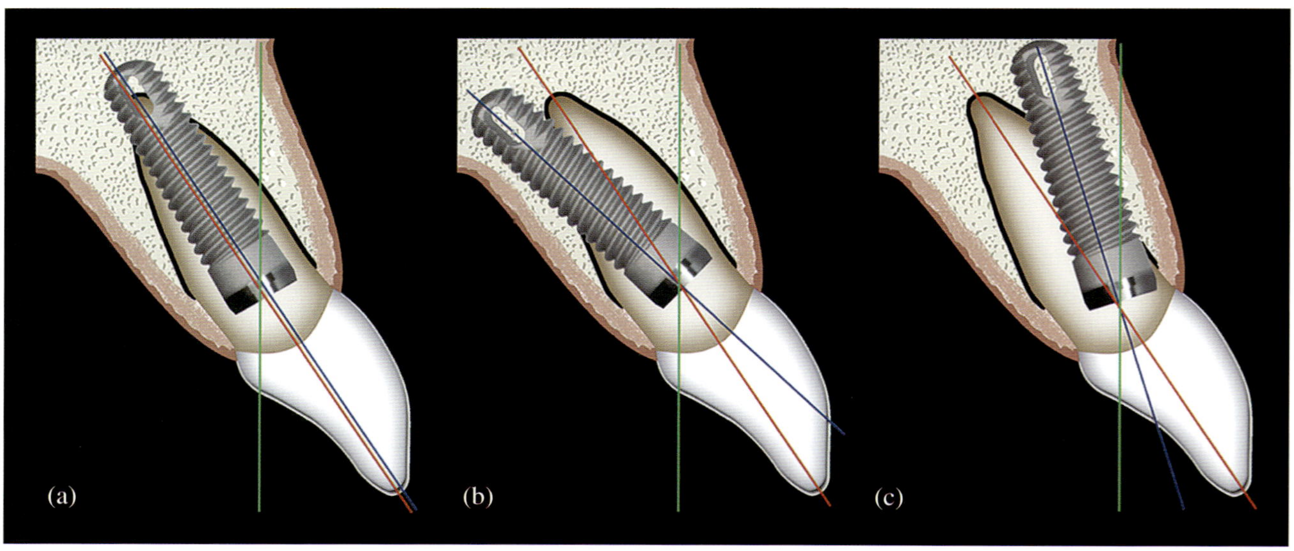

Figure 8.27 (a–c) The red line represents the original natural tooth axis, the blue line represents the implant fixture axis, and the green line represents the sagittal axis of the patient. In (a) the implant fixture is coinciding with the natural tooth position. In (b) the implant is slightly palatal to the sagittal plane. In (c) the implant is placed in a labial position at a 45° angle to the sagittal axis.

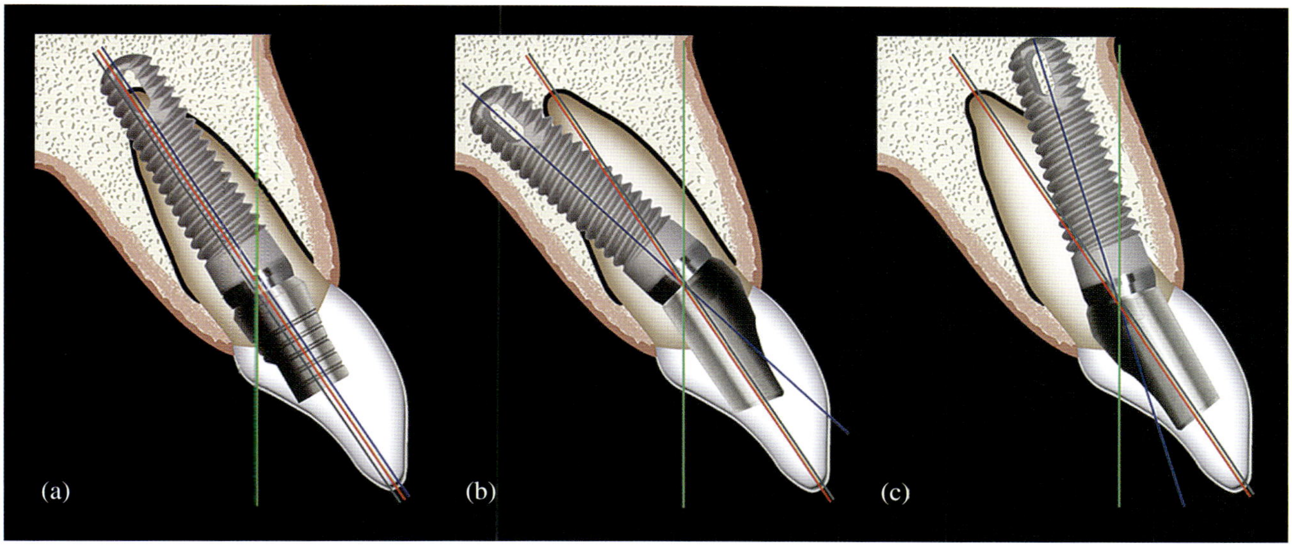

Figure 8.28 (a) When the implant fixture is placed in the same tooth position, the abutment used at the same plane of the implant fixture, (b) and (c) The slight implant fixture angulation to the labial or the lingual form natural tooth axis dictated the use of angulated abutments.

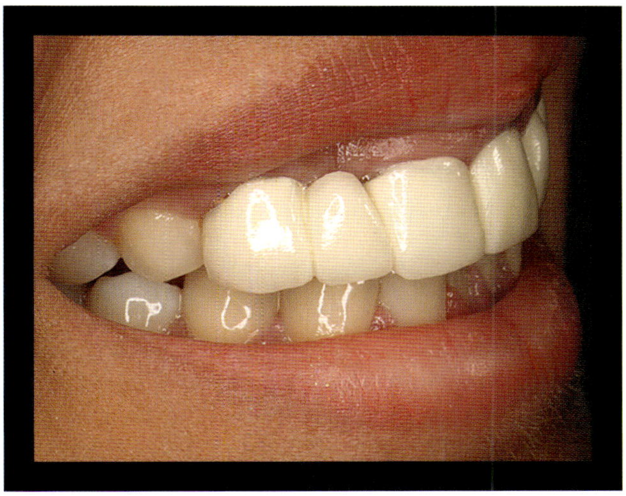

Figure 8.29 Poor prosthetic outcome due to poor implant positioning (mesiodistal).

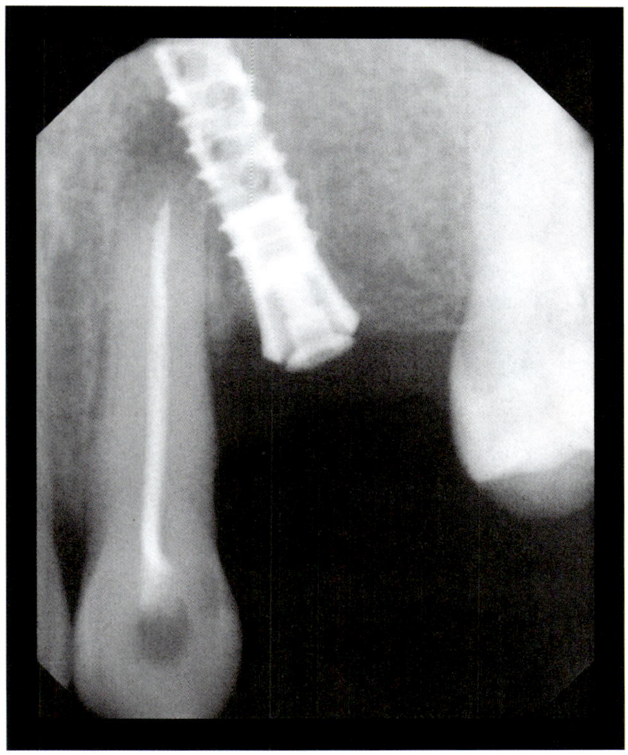

Figure 8.30 Poor mesiodistal implant positioning that injured the root apex of the adjacent tooth.

The labiopalatal position of the implant body within the alveolar ridge depends to a great extent on the accuracy of the surgical template and the clinician's stable grasp of the handpiece. Accurate labiopalatal placement can be achieved by leaving 1 mm of intact labial bone covering the implant surface (Grunder et al. 2005). The bone on top of the implant should be almost equal to that of the adjacent natural component (in cases of a single missing tooth) (see Figure 8.30).

In perfect bone situations, the implant should be placed as close to the buccal contour as the volume of the available bone permits, leaving 1.5 mm from the buccal edge of the bone (Potashnick 1998). For example, in 6 mm of bone width, a 3.75-mm diameter implant should be placed labiopalatally to leave sufficient bone on the labial aspect of the implant body to maintain an optimal osseointegration. If the labiopalatal dimension of bone is less than 6 mm, a smaller diameter implant may be used.

Several methods can treat a deficient bone width; bone dilators and bone splitting methods can be used to increase or expand the amount of available bone accordingly (Jansen and Weisgold 1995).

The placement of the implant in this dimension is critical. A misplaced implant can violate the integrity of the labial plate of bone with subsequent bone fenestration or dehiscence, leading to a final implant-supported restoration with bulky, over-contoured margins. This situation is clinically impossible to correct, even with the use of angulated abutments. In fact, angulated abutments might further complicate the situation because their metallic gingival collar can potentially displace the soft tissue in a more labial direction, resulting in soft tissue recession or grayish, discolored gingiva at the emergence level.

There is a direct relationship between the labial edge of the implant interface and the highest point of the future crown contour. When the distance of the labial edge of the implant interface and the highest point of the future crown contour at the emergence level increases, there are more restorative complications in the implant-supported prosthesis. In the worst cases, when the distance is too large, the final restoration will appear to be severely 'ditched-in' when viewed sagittally. Consequently, fabrication of a restoration with a ridge-lap design at its labial margin to be aligned with the adjacent natural teeth might be the only solution. A ridge-lap design hinders hygiene maintenance around the restoration labial contour, thereby facilitating plaque accumulation and leading to possible inflammation and apical migration of the gingival margin. This may be a potential threat to the implant's very existence, because pocket formation may ensue, resulting in implant failure. As a result of the modified ridge-lap design, there will be an increased strain on the implant surface due to an off-axis loading (Parel and Sullivan 1989).

Many factors control the implant angulation: the available alveolar process angulation, the existing occlusion, the precision of the surgical template, and the mode of implant placement protocol, whether immediate or delayed. Some authors classify implant angulation according to its relation to the occlusal plane (Daftary 1995). The implant may be inserted perpendicular to the occlusal plane, which provides a far more palatal positioning of the final restoration, resulting in a ridge-lap design of the restoration. An angulation of approximately 65°, or 45° to the occlusal plane, results in the most labial positioning of the implant head with optimal esthetic results. This placement often requires using an angulated abutment (see Figure 8.31a and b).

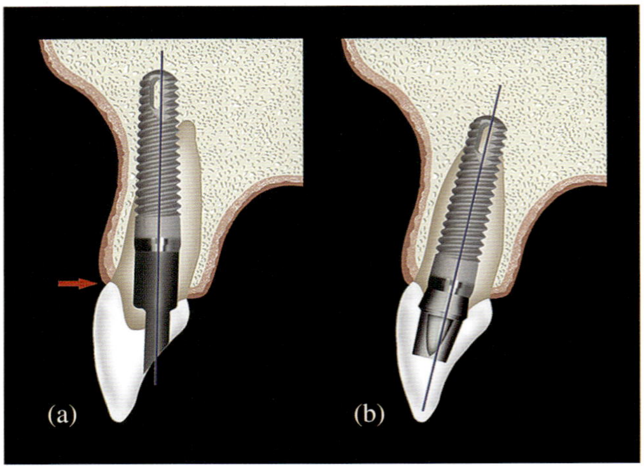

Figure 8.31 (a) Illustration showing the long-axis positioning of the implant fixture when using a cement-retained abutment, (b) Illustration showing the long-axis positioning of the implant when using a screw-retained abutment.

Usually when an immediate implant is placed, the use of angulated abutments in both scenarios does not affect the implant survival. The angulation of the implant within the alveolar ridge is not restricted only to the labiopalatal dimension but can also be in a mesiodistal direction (see Figure 8.32a–l).

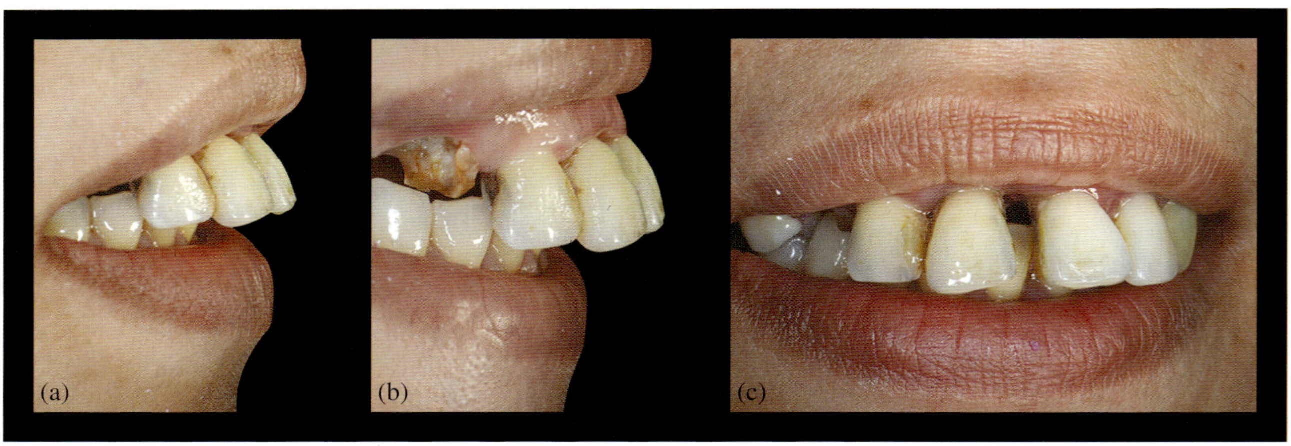

Figure 8.32 (a–c) Clinical picture showing excessive gingival display, severe hopeless teeth with labial protrusion along with undesired diastema.

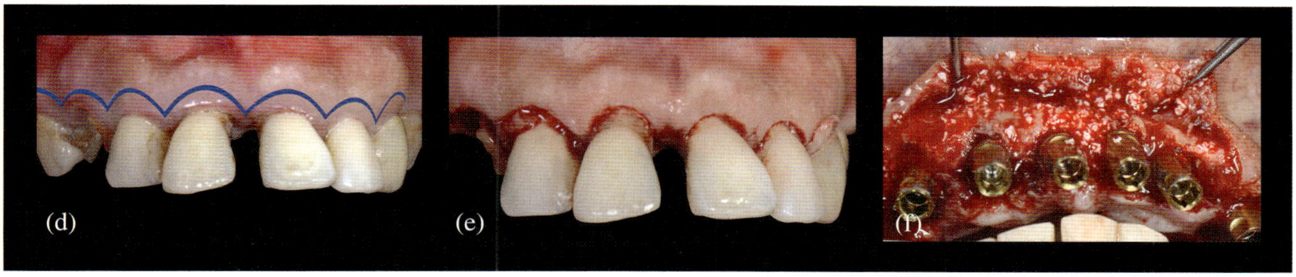

Figure 8.32 (d) Planning of the incision design and gingival re-contouring, (e) Laser re-contouring of the gingiva, (f) Flap elevated, hopeless teeth removed, implants placed, one-time abutment connected, bone voids filled with particulate allograft.

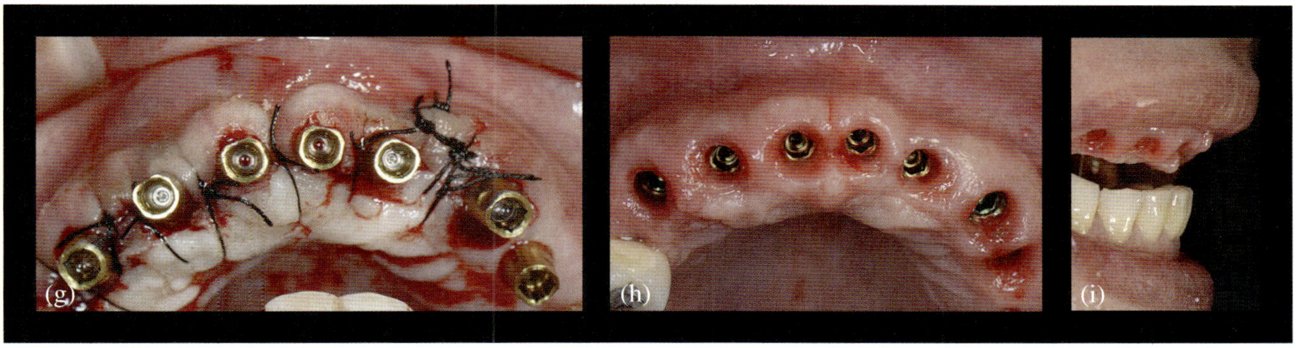

Figure 8.32 (g) Flap sutured, (h) Two months post implant insertion showing favorable soft tissue condition, (i) Profile view showing the enhancement of excessive gingival display as well as the labial profile.

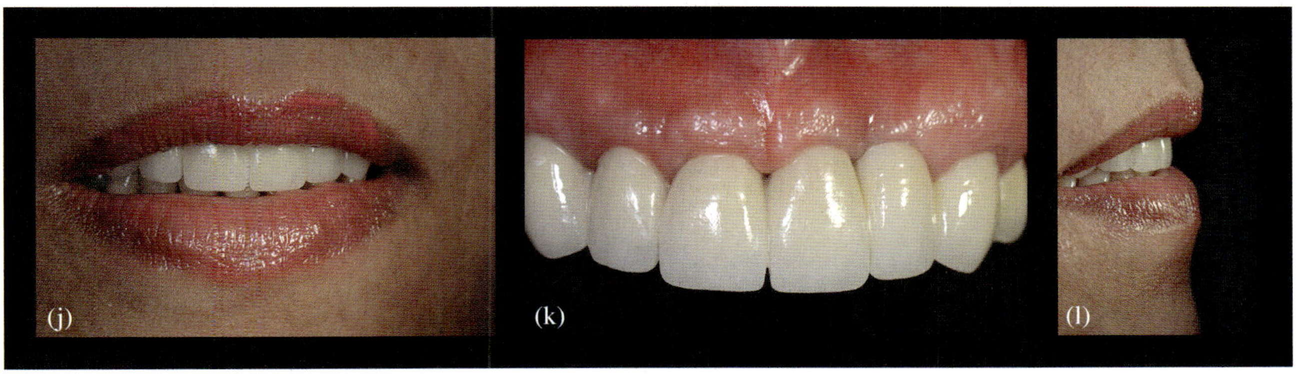

Figure 8.32 (j–l) Final case restored showing an enhanced gingival display, tissue profile and lip support.

A recently developed technique (Koyanagi 2002) to optimize the implant angulation within the alveolar ridge guides the head of the contra-angle handpiece with the surgical guide rather than guiding the drill itself through a guide hole or tube placed into a surgical template. This method is designed to prevent the drill from contacting the template, tube, or other material. The surgical guide should enable the operator, equipped with all of the information gained from preoperative examinations, to prepare the surgical site in the predetermined direction without being influenced by the clinician's visual or tactile senses. Preparation of the planned implant bed is thereby facilitated and the implant angulation is optimized. The described technique allows objective assessment and determination of implant location, inclination, and depth for individual treatment situations.

The final abutment might influence the labiopalatal positioning of the implant as well as its angulation. The final abutment and the final restoration should be determined before starting implant placement. There are two main types of final abutments – screw-retained abutments and cement-retained abutments. The choice of positioning of the implant fixture will depend on the space needed to gain accessibility to the abutment. For example, when cement-retained abutments are used, the implant is positioned exactly in the center of the long axis of the future implant-supported crown. On the other hand, when screw-retained abutments are used, the implant should be placed slightly palatal to the long axis of the crown to access the connecting screw from the palatal side (Davidoff 1996).

8.6.7.3 Axial Positioning Rationale

Implant positioning in relation to its axial level influences the amount of exposure the final restoration will receive, which in turn dramatically affects the esthetic outcome of the restoration (Jansen and Weisgold 1995). Apicoincisal positioning is no less important than the mesiodistal and labiopalatal positioning aspects of the implant. Unfortunately, surgical templates that offer apicoincisal positioning guidance for functional or esthetic implant placement are few. They are often difficult to fabricate and they are not cost-effective. Most of the recent computer-generated templates have a metallic stop to control the apical extent of the drill. The optimal axial positioning of the implant head allows the final restoration to emerge naturally through the marginal gingival tissues with no violation to the gingival sulcus (Wheeler 1974), allowing the contours of the restoration to develop in a progressive manner within the peri-implant soft tissue housing. As a result, the final prosthetic result appears as if it emerges naturally (see Figure 8.33a–c).

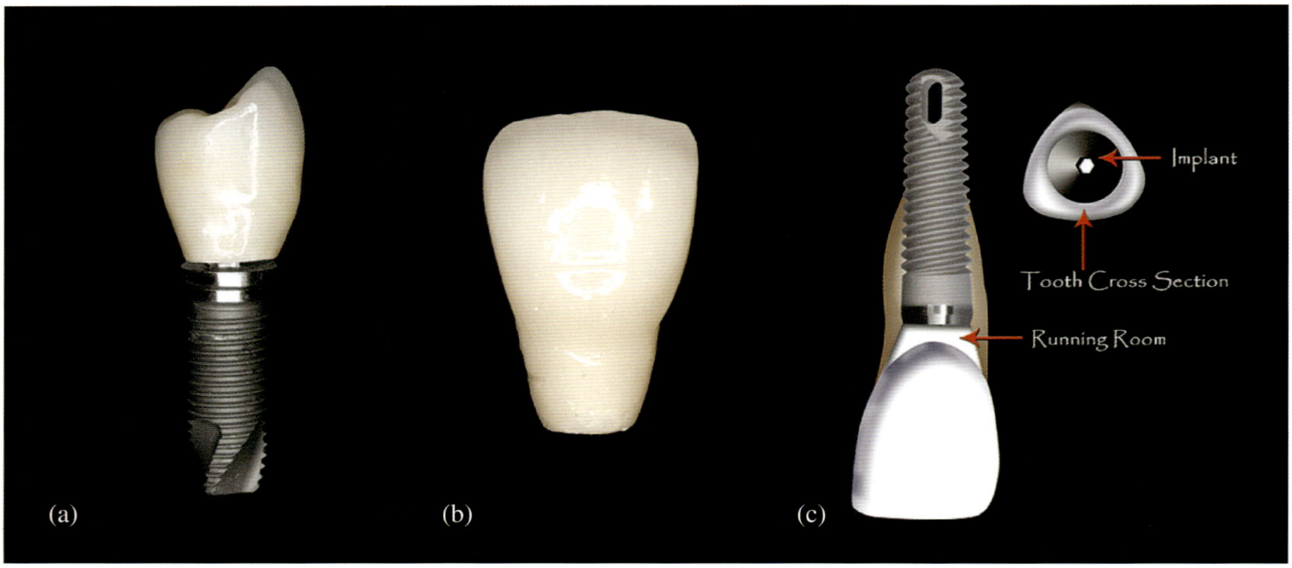

Figure 8.33 (a) An implant with its prosthetic component. Note the difference between the size of the final crown and the cervical implant dimension, (b) An implant-supported restoration that has the transition from the cross section of the implant diameter to the original natural crown size diameter, (c) An illustration showing the difference in cross section between implant and natural tooth and the running room.

Several factors control the location of the implant head in an axial dimension, including (1) the amount of space available for restoration, (2) the topography of the remaining bone, (3) the marginal gingival location of the adjacent natural teeth, and (4) the selected implant diameter. The optimal axial location of the implant head is necessary due to the anatomical difference between the fixture morphology and that of the natural tooth at the cervical level. A morphological transition from the narrow circular implant neck of the implant head to that of the natural tooth form is naturally required (Elaskary 2008).

The reference location of all axial implant positioning is an imaginary line connecting the gingival zeniths of the adjacent natural teeth. There is a greater urgency for restoring natural gingival contours surrounding the new restorations when a natural tooth reference is missing and multiple adjacent implants are to be used. These implants should be placed at the alveolar crest within the circumference of the missing teeth to be restored. This enables the clinician to develop appropriate natural embrasures on both sides adjoining the restorations and duplicate a natural gingival profile (Potashnick 1998). The ideal apicoincisal implant positioning places the implant head 2–3 mm apical to the line connecting the gingival zeniths of the adjacent natural teeth. This subsequently allows 'running room' throughout the biological width of the implant when it is correctly positioned in an apicoincisal plane (Parel and Sullivan 1989) (see Figure 8.34a–c).

The 'running room' is a space of 2–3 mm in depth and surrounds the implant head circumferentially. This room allows for stacking or building up of prosthetic components to create the natural gingival emergence of

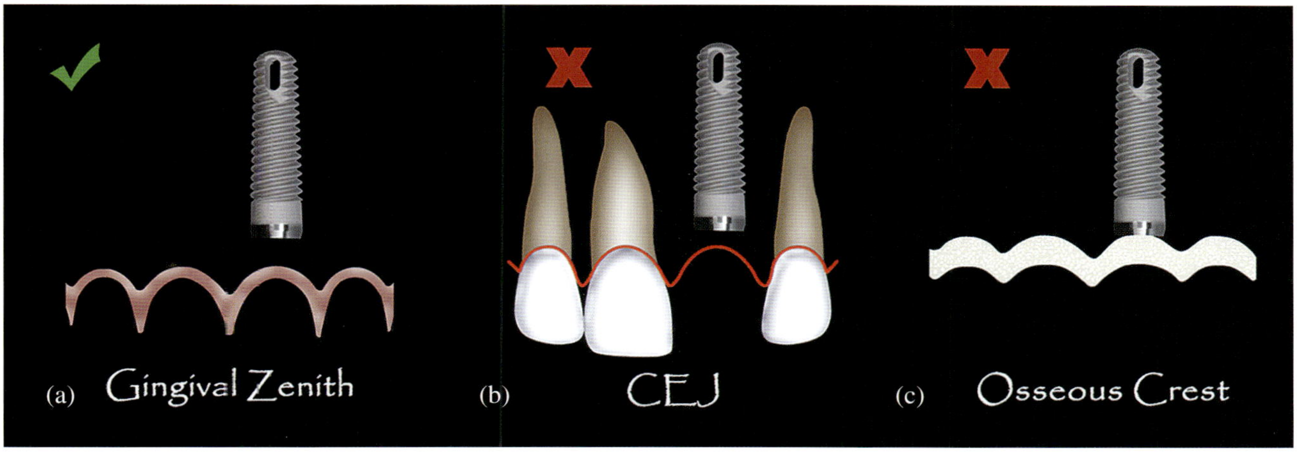

Figure 8.34 (a–c) An illustration showing the three different positioning possibilities.

the final restoration. If any modification or expansion of the gingival tissues to match the original crown size takes place in this particular space, the progressive use of the provisional restoration will develop the original cross-sectional shape of the missing natural tooth. The use of anatomical abutments has not proven to be more effective than the progressive use of the provisional restoration. Because the gingival tissue does not have a memory to keep its original dimensions without existing support, the peri-implant soft tissue tends to collapse and regain its original circular shape (due to the pressure from the circular collagen fibers surrounding the biological seal) upon its removal from the gingival sulcus. Clinically speaking, natural biological contours could be replicated without the need for anatomical abutments. Provisional prostheses have proven to give an optimal gingival influence with great clinical predictability (see Figure 8.35a–d).

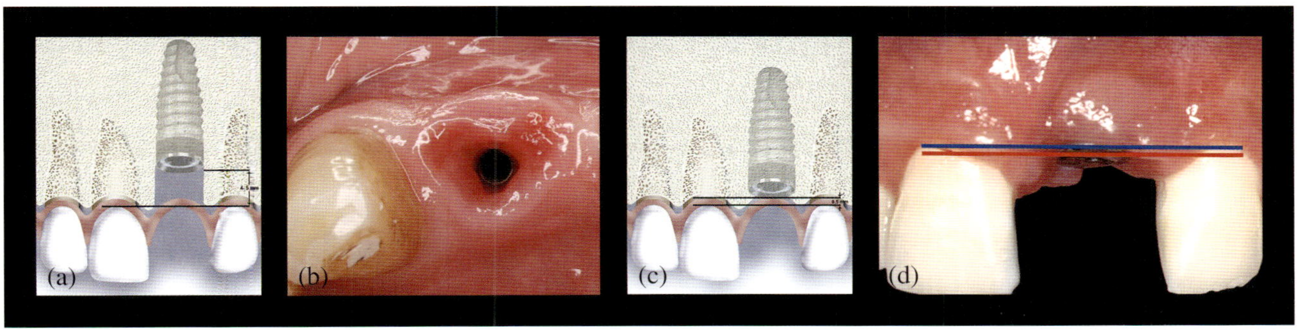

Figure 8.35 (a) Diagram showing too far apical placement of an implant fixture, (b) Tissue hyperplasia and irritation as a result of the too far apical implant placement due to the long pocketing in the trans mucosal area, (c) Diagram showing too far incisal placement of an implant fixture, (d) Clinical picture of too far incisally placed implant that hinders esthetic restorative result (bulky crown).

The implant diameter has an inverse relationship to the amount of subgingival sinking. It influences the amount of axial sinking of the implant head, because implants with wide diameters eventually require less space for making the transition into a natural tooth form than narrow-diameter implants. Bear in mind that not all the biological concepts are violated. The screw design implant ranks first to allow a more precise axial placement than the cylindrical designs. Its mechanical characters allow control of the depth while threading the fixture in the bone. The cylinder design, on the other hand, requires the use of an implant retrieval tool to adjust the implant's optimal vertical position, which makes the procedure difficult to control (Elaskary 2008).

Gingival zenith of the adjacent natural teeth is considered to be the landmark or the reference in apicoincisal implant positioning. Therefore, for several reasons, it is recommended that the location of the implant head be related to a line connecting the gingival zenith of the adjacent remaining natural dentition rather than to a line connecting the CEJ or the crest of the ridge. For instance, the gingival zenith is not a static landmark; it sometimes moves apically, such as in the case of gingival recession, because it represents the actual clinical marginal level of the soft tissue at the time of implant placement. In contrast, the CEJ is a constantly static landmark. It follows a uniformly fixed scalloped path along the root surface. It also pursues a wavy course that has a rise and fall on both buccolingual and interproximal margins. This scalloped line does not move when gingival recession occurs; thus, it does not allow for optimal apicoincisal positioning in the case of gingival recession and in cases of placing an implant in unbalanced soft tissue margins. Also, the wavy course of the CEJ does not give a stable reference with which to measure. The use of the deepest part of the gingival zenith allows the final implant-supported restoration to attain the same marginal level as that existing around natural dentition.

The crest of the ridge is a less than ideal reference point for making a measurement to relate the implant head because the nature of bone resorption sometimes makes it variable in its levels. In other words, in many instances the osseous housing is not the optimal landmark. Soft tissue thickness on top of it can be variable as well, which might lead to unpredictable variable measurements. For example, when the alveolar ridge has undergone a process of vertical osseous resorption, the implant head will eventually be situated above the bone level. Therefore, the osseous crest should not be taken as a reference measuring point (Elaskary 2008).

8.7 Treatment of Malposed Implants

Implant osseointegration is not the only factor that affects the success of implant-supported restorations; the position and angulation of the implant strongly influence the treatment esthetics, and function outcome. Precise preoperative assessment of the surgical site is required for providing an optimal implant position and restoratively driven treatment planning (Park et al. 2001) (see Figure 8.36a–e).

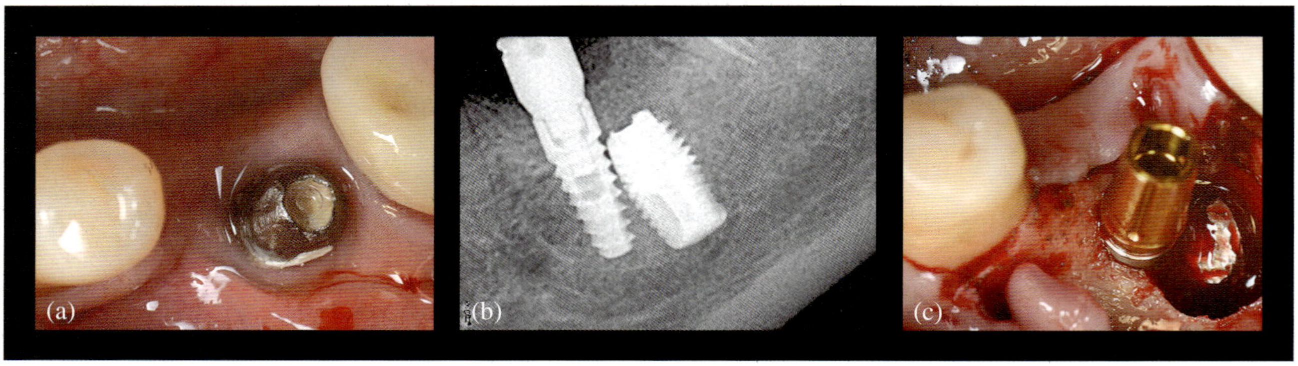

Figure 8.36 (a) Pre-operative view of implant placed in poor mesiodistal position, (b) Radiographic view showing poor implant positioning, (c) Reduction of poorly positioned implant and placement of a new one.

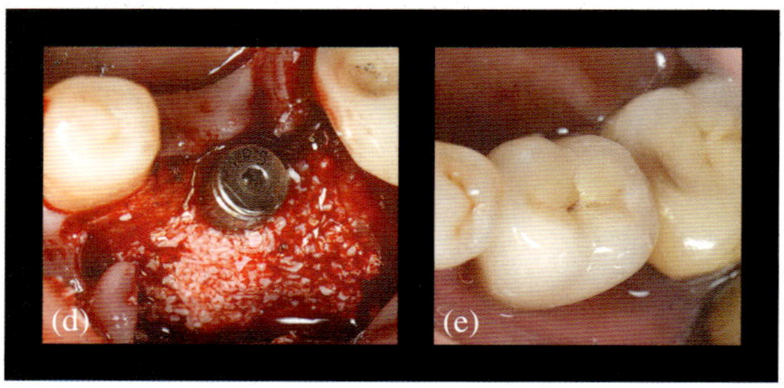

Figure 8.36 (d) The defect is grafted, (e) Case finally restored.

Most of the poor treatment outcome consequences arise when implants are not optimally placed in one or more geometric planes (e.g. mesiodistally, buccolingually, and apicocoronally) according to the previously mentioned guidelines. Placing the implant before deciding on a future restorative plan can often lead to irreversible errors. Using a surgical guide helps to provide an accurate guidance for implant placement in the ideal position, provided that the guide is fabricated according to the correct artificial teeth setting in the diagnostic model or on the virtual planning software. Malpositioned implants are less amenable to modification or corrections. In the esthetic zone, malposed implants can be problematic and may have to be removed and new implants placed (Froum et al. 2011). In fact out of clinical experience, the majority of poorly positioned dental implant fixtures in the esthetic zone would be deemed for removal (see Figure 8.37a–e).

The implant position should be in line with some of the landmarks for adjacent teeth and centered in relation to the opposing occlusion to avoid a malocclusion situation or overload on the prosthesis (Misch and Resnik 2012). Using a surgical guide helps to provide

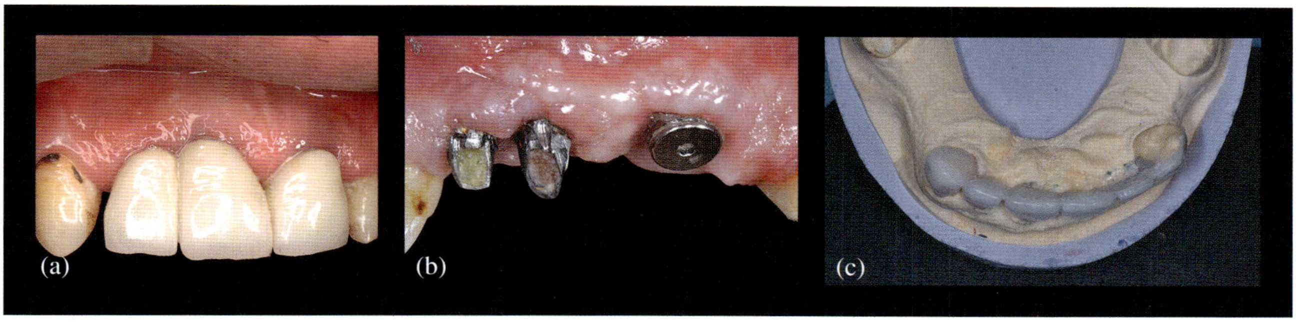

Figure 8.37 (a) Too close placed implants (improper mesiodistal placement), (b) Blunted papilla as a result, (c) Wax up fabrication.

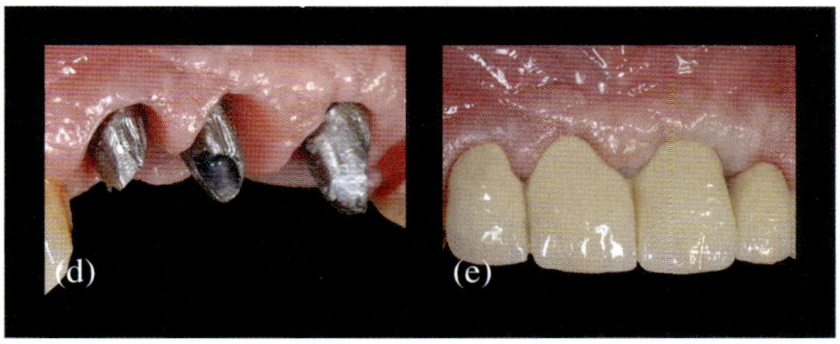

Figure 8.37 (d) Using angled abutments to solve the spacing resulted in regain papillary height, (e) Final case restored.

guidance for implant placement in the ideal position (see Figure 8.38a–j).

The ideal implant 3D position will improve the relationship between the proposed restoration and the implant and the final hard and soft tissue response (Buser et al. 2004). In other words, the faulty position of an implant fixture influences the gingival collar shape and color, if placed in a too distant an incisal position (Al-Sabbagh 2006; Buser et al. 2004) (see Figure 8.39a–o).

Implant angulation is determined by the trajectory of the drill while it proceeds into the bone (Greenstein,

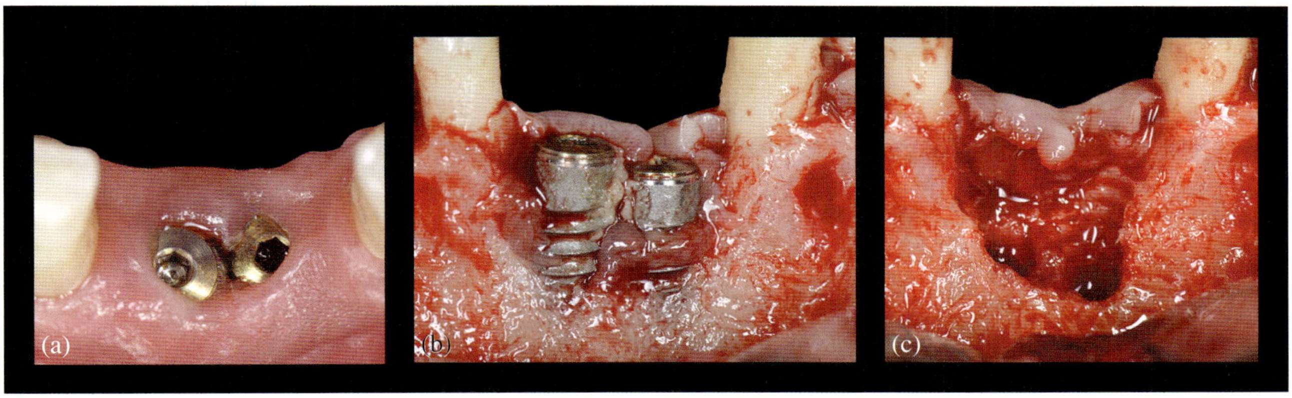

Figure 8.38 (a) Faulty mesiodistal implant positioning, (b) Mucoperiosteal flap reflected showing clinical signs of bone resorption as a result of faulty positioning, (c) Resultant defect after implant removal.

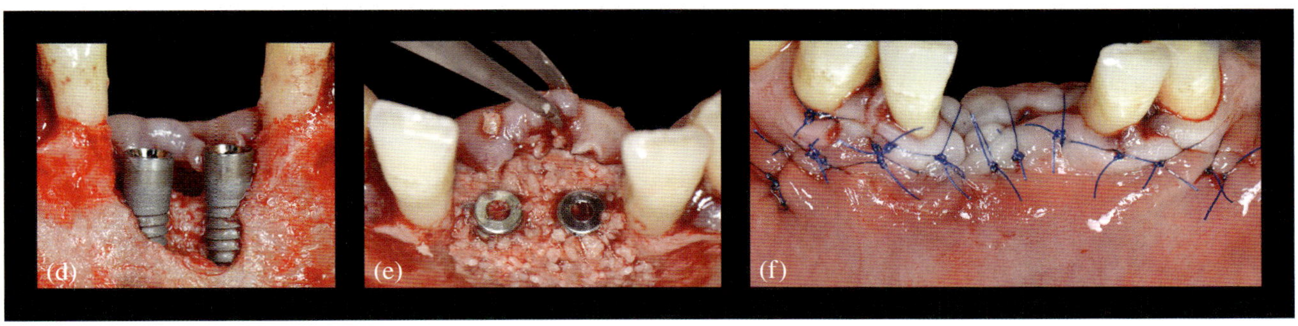

Figure 8.38 (d) New two narrow diameter implants positioned, (e) The defect is grafted with particulated bone graft, (f) Flap sutured.

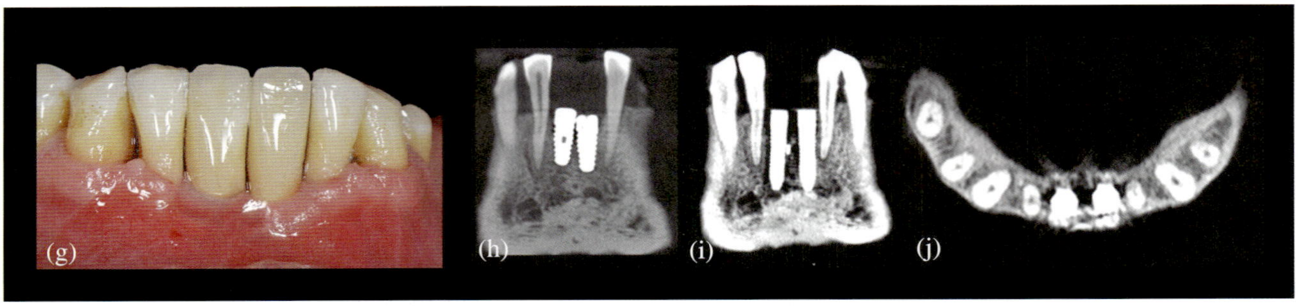

Figure 8.38 (g) Case finally restored, (h) Preoperative CBCt view, (i) and (j) Post-operative CBCT view.

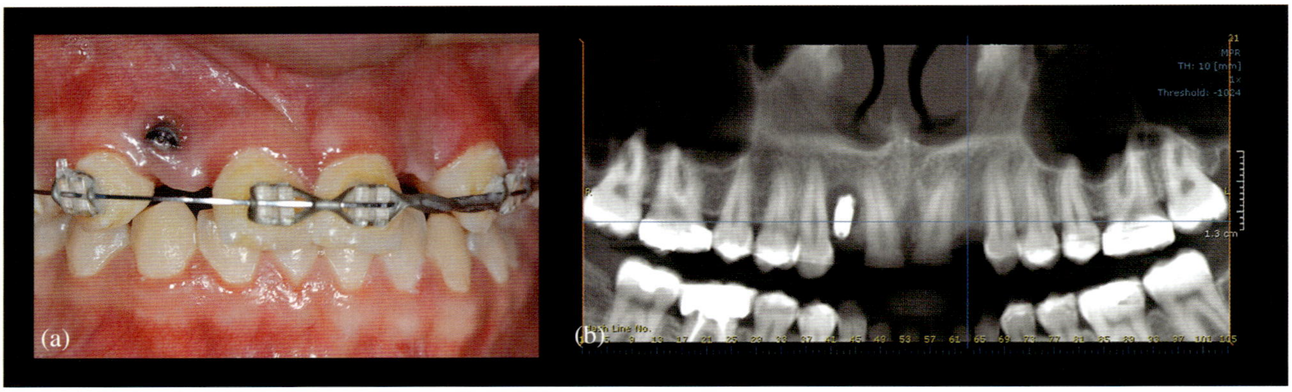

Figure 8.39 (a) Clinical view of poor implant angulation replacing missing lateral incisor, (b) Radiographic view CBCT showing poor implant positioning.

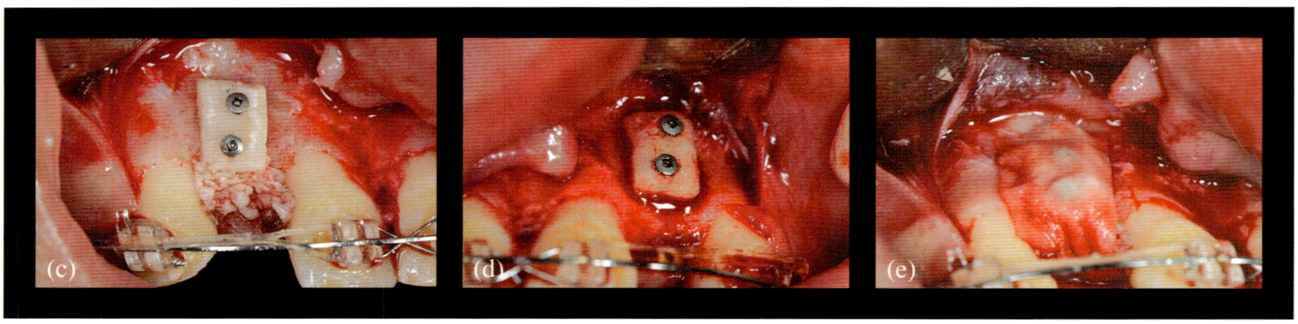

Figure 8.39 (c–e) Optimizing the ridge condition by addition of two onlay cortical cancellous bone graft and a collagen membrane.

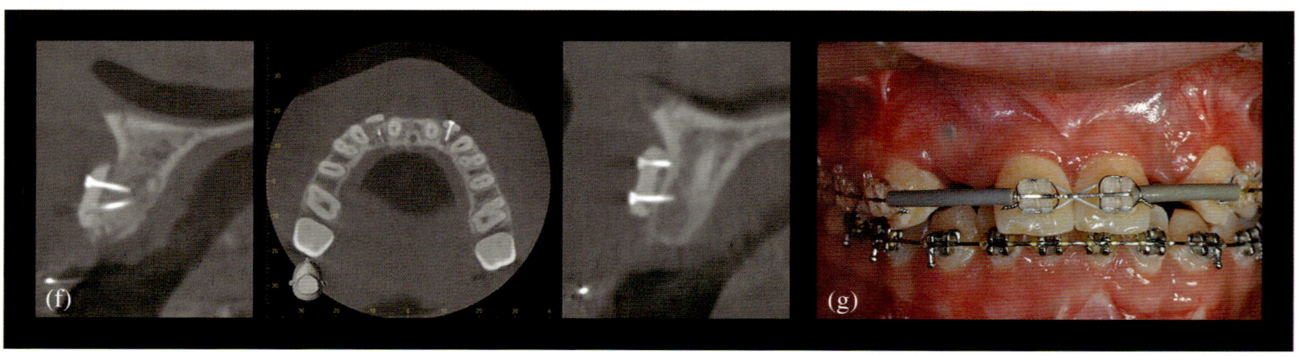

Figure 8.39 (f) Post-operative CBCT showing the graft in place, (g) Two months post grafting showing thinning of the related soft tissues.

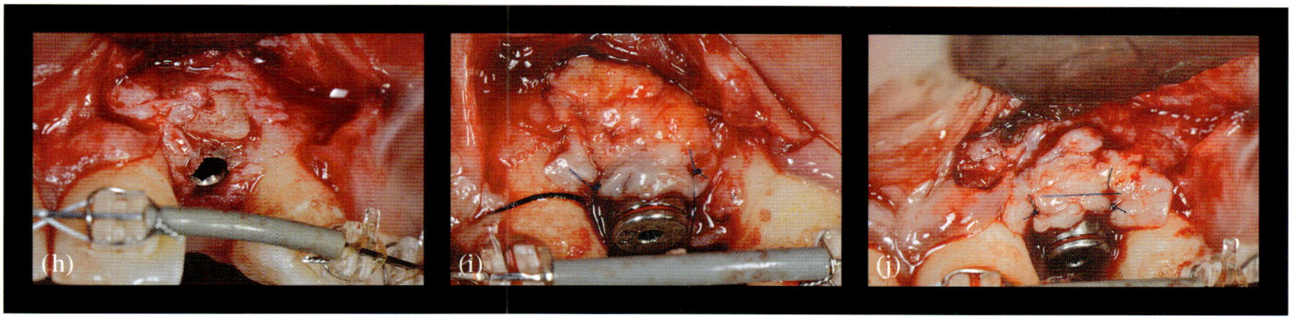

Figure 8.39 (h) Clinical view of the two incorporated grafts with the two implants placed, (i) and (j) Connective tissue graft stabilized to improve tissue keratinization.

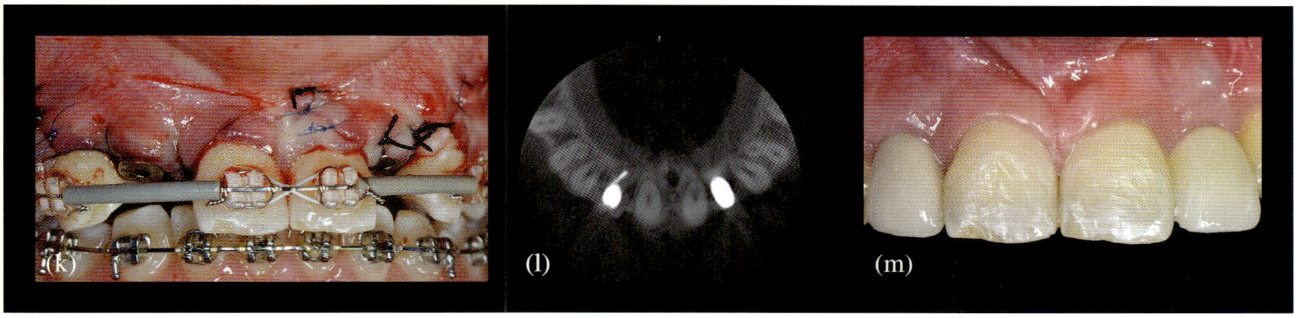

Figure 8.39 (k) Flap sutured, (l) CBCT scan showing implants in place, (m) Case finally restored.

Cavellaro and Tarnow 2008). It is easy to manage miss-angulation of the implant fixture up to 15°; (most of the available prefabricated angled abutments are in 0–15° configurations). To correct more severe implant angulation problems, custom-milled abutments can help to correct the situation (e.g. 25°, 35°). However, the off-axis load will be of great concern. When using an angled abutment, there must be a sufficient transmucosal space to allow the transition of the angulated abutment collar in to the oral environment to attach the implant-supported crown, which might lead to the possibility of a fracture of the coronal aspect of an implant, screw fracture, or abutment screw loosening as a result of high stresses and occlusal load placed on the implant–abutment interface (Buser et al. 2004; Froum et al. 2011). These complications will be exaggerated in the posterior area due to greater masticatory forces. From a functional perspective, if severe implant angulation cannot be avoided, additional implants can be placed to provide a supplementary surface area of support and avoid the previously mentioned complications if there is available restorative space (Lundgren and Laurell 1984; Greenstein et al. 2008; Pjetursson et al. 2004) (see Figure 8.40a–e).

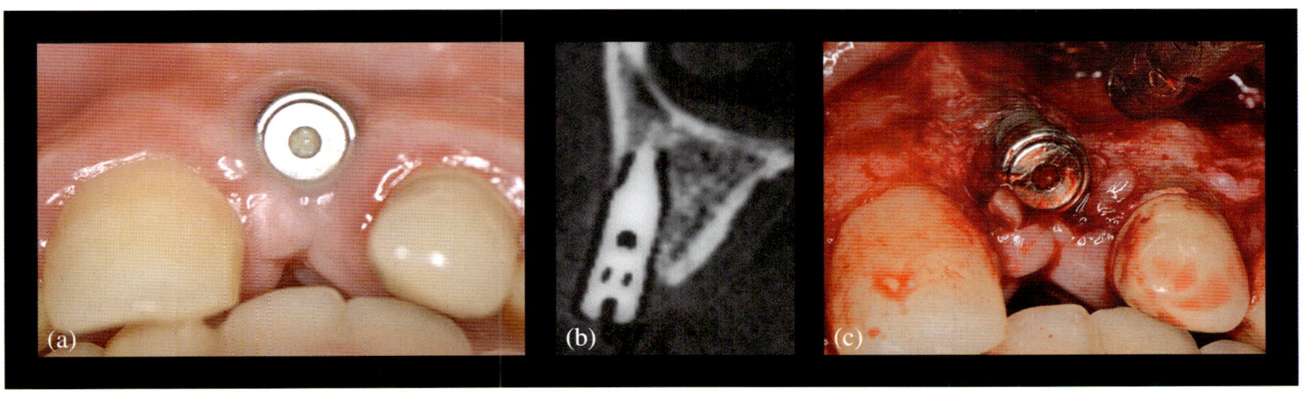

Figure 8.40 (a) Too far labially placed implant, (b) CBCT showing complete violation of the labial plate of bone, (c) Incisal views showing the violation of the labial plate of bone due to poor implant position.

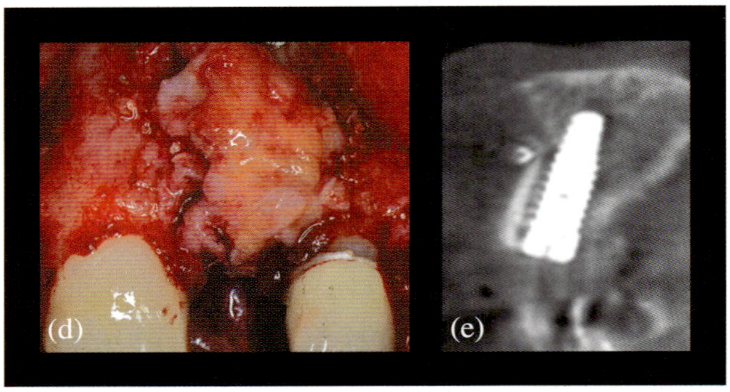

Figure 8.40 (d) Mono cortical block graft is stabilized to restore the labial plate of bone deficiency along with connective tissue graft, (e) CBCT scan showing implant in the correct position along with the grafted.

Attempts (Guerrero et al. 1999; Warden and Scuba 2000) have been made to correct implant misplacement by performing a segmental osteotomy around the osseous housing of the implant fixture, moving the segment to the required ideal position, and stabilizing it with microplates and screws. The possibility of using segmental maxillary or mandibular osteotomies to reposition an alveolar segment with its implants may be an effective method to treat misplacements (Jensen 2006). The procedure requires delicate surgical maneuver with minimal stripping of the periosteum to ensure an uninterrupted blood supply to the segment, promote faster healing, and avoid necrosis for the segment. The titanium microplate used for rigid fixation is micro-sized and placed strategically in a position that does not require postsurgical removal. A longer period of immobilization is indicated and the occlusion should be checked to eliminate any premature contacts. A surgical guide is made before the osteotomy is carried out accordingly to determine the ideal position of the segment. However, the limited space between the existing natural root and the implant fixture sometimes makes the osteotomy clinically inapplicable. Additional limitations may include insufficient keratinized tissues to cover the surgical site, any existing anatomical landmark, and risk of site morbidity (Hur et al. 2010) (see Figure 8.41a–e). A balance of benefits between using this technique and implant removal should be made.

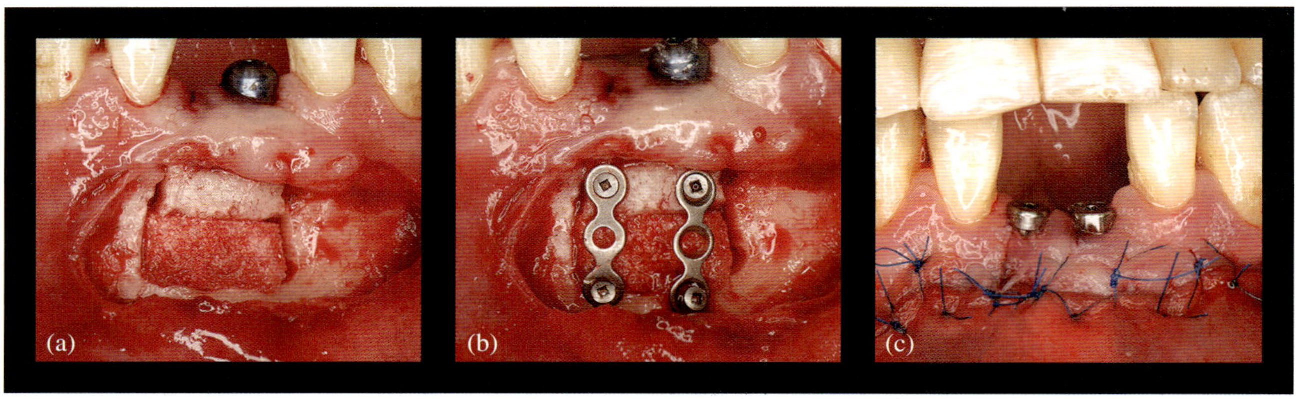

Figure 8.41 (a–c) Too deep implants positioning treated with sandwich osteotomy.

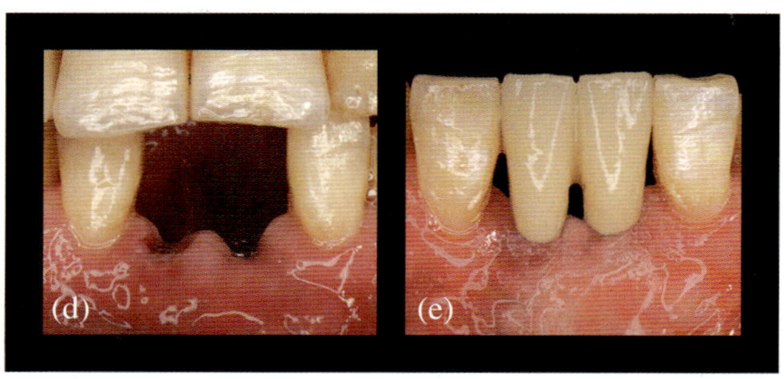

Figure 8.41 (d) and (e) Post-operative view showing implants with proper position.

Another clinical suggestion for restoring a partially edentulous area in patients with compromised oral hygiene or unfavorably positioned implants is the use of an implant-supported milled metal bar with an acrylic resin partial over denture (Asvanund and Morgano 2004). When dental implants were poorly positioned, ZAAG (Zest Anchors, Inc., Escondido, CA, USA) attachments were used with a milled bar to restore the partially edentulous area with a parallel-sided milled bar to prevent the prosthesis from rotating labiolingually. The method might improve the patient's speech, function, and esthetics.

Another implant positioning complication is the proximity of the implant fixture to the tooth apex, this occurs because of not using a surgical guide, the arbitrary placement of the dental implant fixtures and the lack of preoperative planning. The risk of a retrograde peri-implantitis increases when the distance between the tooth and implant apexes is shorter and when the time between the endodontic procedure and the implantation is also shorter (Tozum et al. 2006; Zhou et al. 2009).

Retrograde peri-implantitis is uncommon, I must say that it is rare; however, authors suggested that placement of an implant might trigger a latent periapical pathology (Quirynen et al. 2005) from the adjacent teeth. The process of implant placement could result in activation of this latent response either due to overheating or contamination or a combination of both. Recent evidence suggests the existence of an autoimmune response in the periapical area in relation to an antigen which may be microbial in origin (Wahlgren et al. 2002). This activation could have resulted in rapid bone loss in a short time. The importance of periodic clinical and radiographic examination of implants that are placed adjacent to endodontically treated teeth must be emphasized and a shorter recall program could be considered to identify and manage retrograde peri-implant bone loss in its early stages (Mohamed et al. 2010).

The involved risks of treating retrograde peri-implantitis was described by Levitt (2003), who recorded a dysesthesia produced during carrying out an apicectomy of the implant, pain and swelling.

Examples of implant misplacements that have led to serious consequences, such as placing implants in the proximity to the mental foramen (Kim 2011), the clinician must take into consideration the anterior looping of the interior alveolar nerve and the available bone above the mental foramen, because the inferior alveolar nerve often rises as it approaches the mental foramen (Kraut and Chahal 2002). The patient should be referred for microsurgery if total anesthesia persists or if, after 16 weeks, dysesthesia is ongoing (Misch and Wang 2008, as cited in Day 1994; Nazarian, Eliav and Nahlieli 2003).

Many studies have reported favorable patient responses to inferior alveolar nerve repairs. All have emphasized the need for repair before Wallerian degeneration of the distal portion of the inferior alveolar nerve has occurred; because this degeneration is a slow process, repair is possible four to six months after the injury has occurred (Kraut and Chahal 2002) (see Figure 8.42a–n).

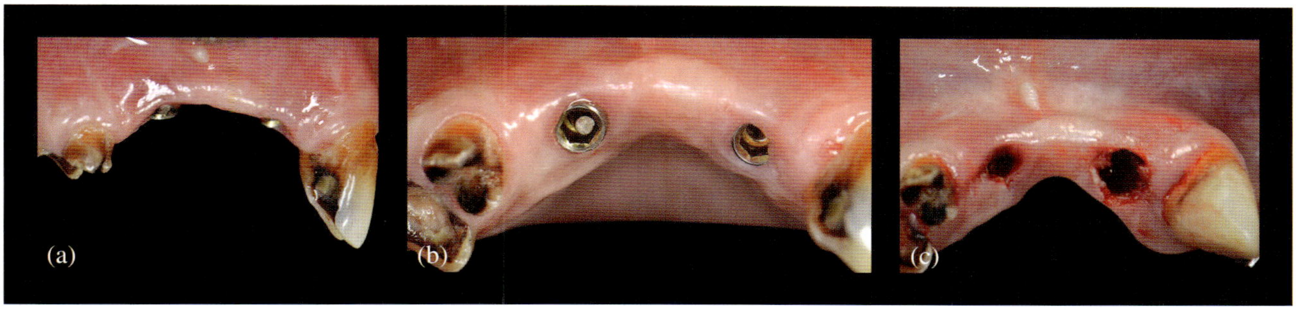

Figure 8.42 (a) and (b) Improper mesiodistal positioning of two implants placed in the pre-maxilla that is completely un restorable, (c) Implants removed.

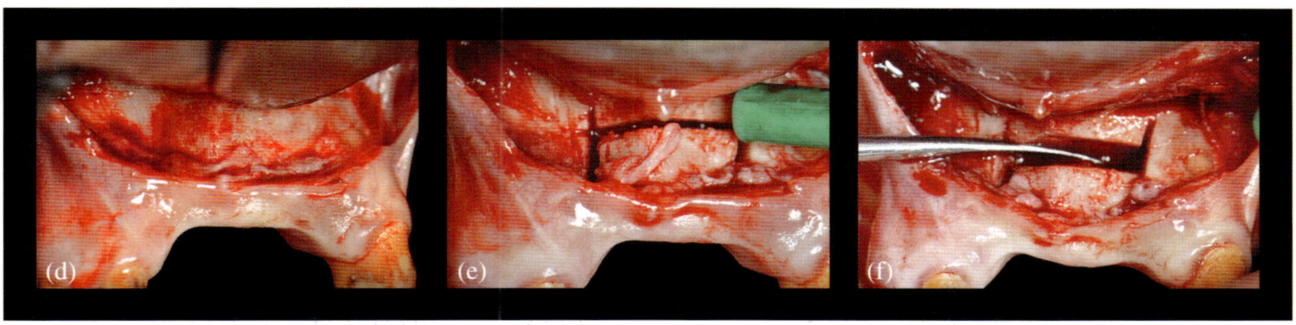

Figure 8.42 (d) Two months later sandwich osteotomy is planned for enhancing the vertical bone loss, (e) Sandwich osteotomy outlined with piezzotome bone cutting tip, (f) The bone block is mobilized.

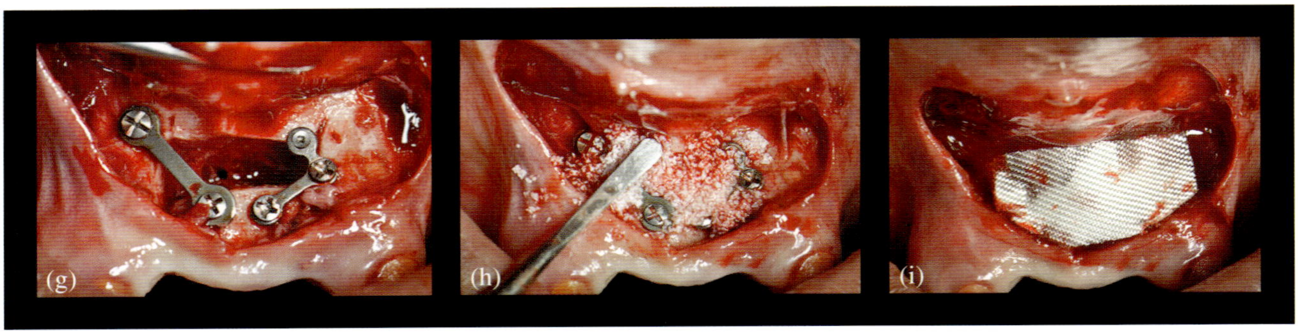

Figure 8.42 (g) The bone block is stabilized with titanium microplates to the basal bone, (h) Bone voids filled with particulated bone graft, (i) Collagen membrane placed on top.

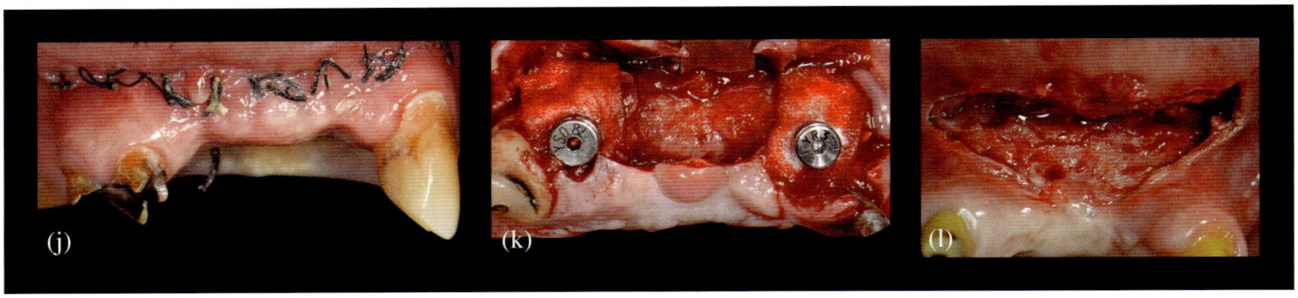

Figure 8.42 (j) One week post flap closure, (k) Four months later two implants are placed, (l) Enhancement of the vestibular depth, removal of the epithelium.

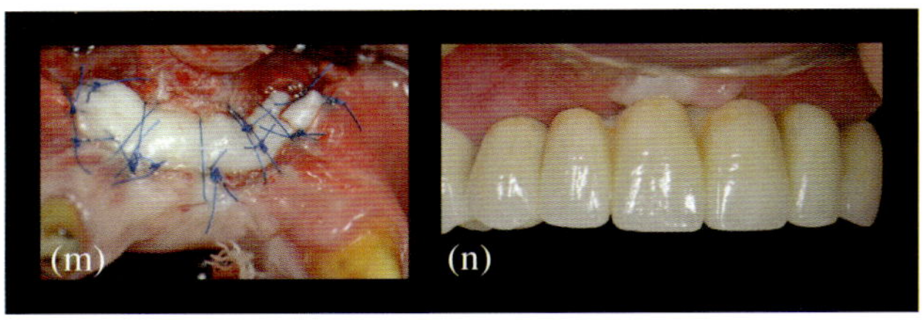

Figure 8.42 (m) Onlay keratinized tissue graft is placed to enhance keratinization, (n) New implants placed, final case restored.

Also, the risk of maxillary sinus membrane perforation exists as a result of a tear in the Schneiderian membrane occurring along the periphery of the osteotomy (Zijderveld et al. 2008). In general, small tears (<5–8 mm) are mitigated simply by folding the membrane up against itself as it is elevated (Chanavaz 1990). Larger tears might be repaired with collagen or a fibrin adhesive (Karabuda, Arisan and Ozyuvaci 2006). The displacement of implants into the maxillary sinus can result in a foreign-body reaction and may present a risk for the development of maxillary sinusitis (Galindo et al. 2005). The natural ciliary movement in the maxillary sinus will transport foreign material toward the ostium (Hunter et al. 2009). An implant can easily migrate into the sinus without apparent force in the posterior maxilla (Peleg, Garg and Mazor 2006). The implants must be immediately retrieved endoscopically via the transnasal route to avoid inflammatory complications (Ueda and Kaneda 1992). Patients who smoke have an added risk factor, which can significantly jeopardize results (Abt 2009; Cochran et al. 2009; Garg 2010; Lindfors et al. 2010) (see Figure 8.43a–r).

Possible therapeutic options for treating implant malposition usually depend on the degree of malpositioning:

1) In mild misalignments, angled abutments or screw-retained abutments can be used, which might help to solve a minor misalignment.
2) In moderate malposition, custom-milled abutments can be used to solve other space problems or malposition to a limited extent. These abutments should receive a screw-retained restoration later on. Surgical corrections, often described in the current literature as segmental osteotomies, appear possible from a medical perspective and are recommended in very few individual cases, keeping in mind that these procedures require a meticulous assessment of possible additional complications. Complete and comprehensive patient information is mandatory.

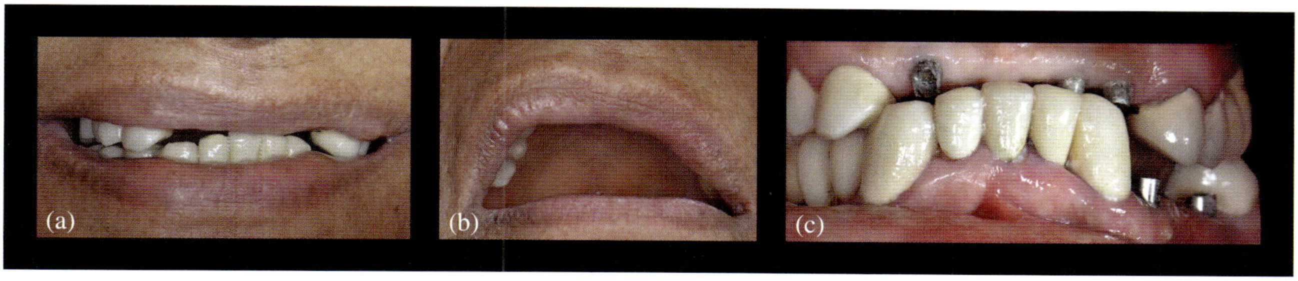

Figure 8.43 (a) Pre-operative view poor oral esthetics as a result of poor planning and poor implant positioning, (b) Loss of lip support as a result of anterior teeth loss, (c) Frontal view showing the over eruption of the mandibular anterior teeth.

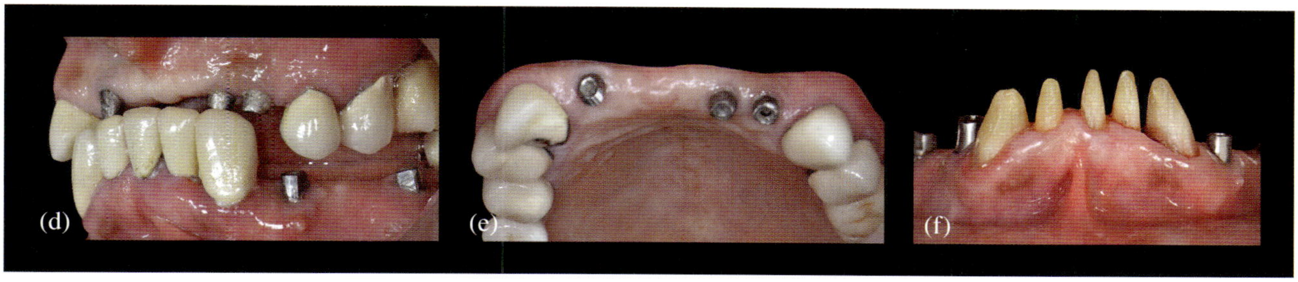

Figure 8.43 (d) Side view showing over eruption of the maxillary posterior teeth with over all bite collapse, (e) Loss of the pre maxilla contour as a result of long term teeth loss, (f) Intra operative view of the anterior mandible that warrants osseous recession.

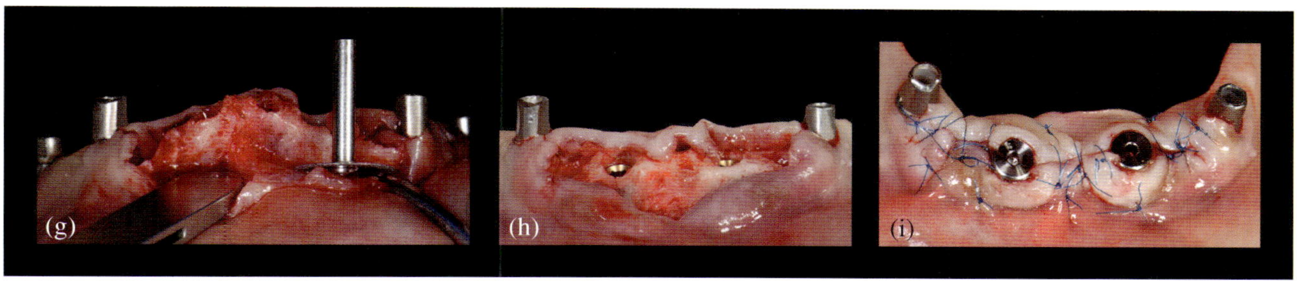

Figure 8.43 (g) Osteotomy of the anterior mandibular alveolar ridge, (h) After osseous trimming and flattening of the bone profile implant placed, (i) Flap closure showing an important periosteal tie suture that is important to tie the excess soft tissues together thus preserving the keratinized tissues.

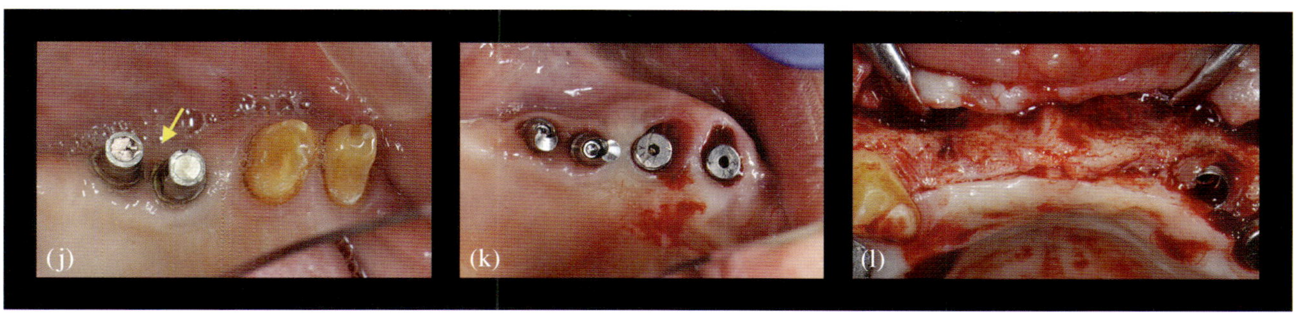

Figure 8.43 (j) and (k) Managing the posterior maxilla, angulated abutments placement to allow a better prosthetic space, and natural teeth removal both sides to allow better support, (l) Intra operative view of the anterior maxilla post old implants removal.

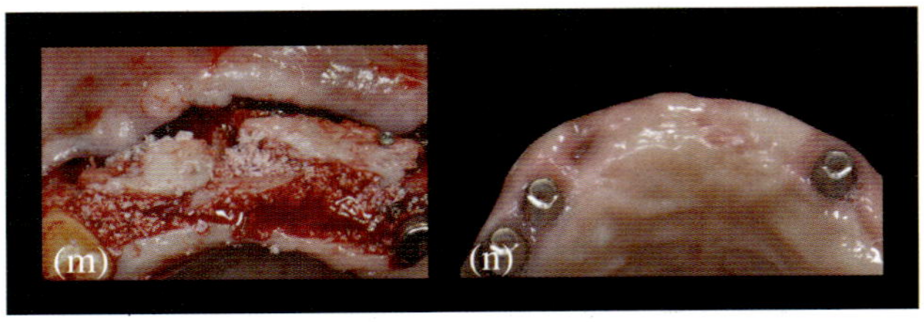

Figure 8.43 (m) Two composite autografts being stabilized to the pre maxilla to realign the list contour, (n) Final healing of the pre maxilla showing enhanced maxillary contour.

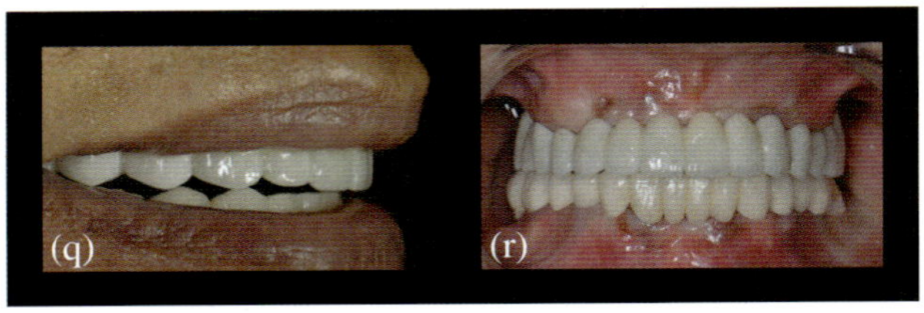

Figure 8.43 (q) The lost lip support is restored, (r) Both arches in occlusion.

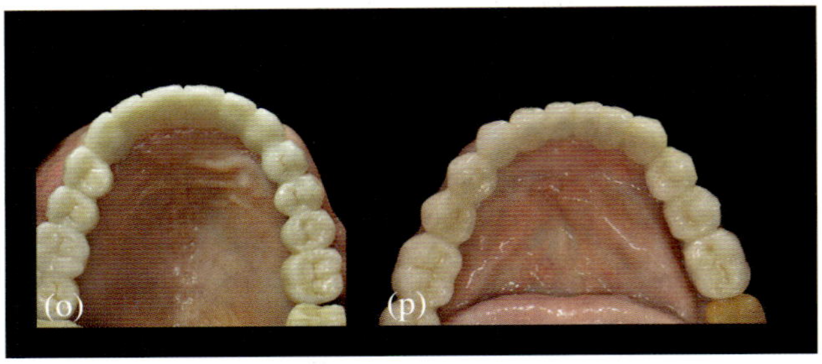

Figure 8.43 (o) and (p) Both arches finally restored.

3) In cases where the implant fixture is severely mispositioned there will be no choice but implant removal and reinserting a new implant simultaneously or at a later stage, which is the easiest solution to treat malposed implants.

References

Abt, E. (2009). Smoking increases dental implant failures and complications. *Evid. Based Dent.* 10 (3): 79–80.

Al-Sabbagh, M. (2006). Implants in the esthetic zone. *Dent. Clin. North. Am.* 50 (3): 391–407.

Asvanund, C. and Morgano, S.M. (2004). Restoration of unfavorably positioned implants for a partially endentulous patient by using an overdenture retained with a milled bar and attachments: a clinical report. *J. Prosthet. Dent.* 91 (1): 6–10.

Bach, N., Baylard, J.F., and Voyer, R. (2004). Orthodontic extrusion: periodontal considerations and applications. *J. Can. Dent. Assoc.* 70 (11): 775–780.

Berglundh, T. and Lindhe, J. (1996). Dimension of the periimplant mucosa. Biological width revisited. *J. Clin. Periodontol.* 23 (10): 971–973.

Blair, F.M., Wassell, R.W., and Steele, J.G. (2002). Crowns and other extra-coronal restorations: preparations for full veneer crowns. *Br. Dent. J.* 192 (10): 561–564. 567–571.

Block, M.S., Kent, J.N., and Guerra, L.R. (1997). *Implants in Dentistry*. Philadelphia, PA: W.B. Saunders Co.

Boyd, R.L. (2009). Periodontal and restorative considerations with clear aligner treatment to establish a more favourable restorative environment. *Compend. Contin. Educ. Dent.* 30 (5): 280–282. 284, 286–288.

Brunski, J.B., Puleo, D.A., and Nanci, A. (2000). Biomaterials and biomechanics of oral and maxillofacial implants: current status and future developments. *Int. J. Oral Maxillofac. Implants* 15: 15–46.

Burger, E.H. and Klein-Nulend, J. (1999). Responses of bone cells to biomechanical forces *in vitro*. *Adv. Dent. Res.* 13: 93–98.

Buser, D., Martin, W., Belser, U.C. et al. (2004). Optimizing esthetics for implant restorations in the anterior maxilla: anatomic and surgical considerations. *Int. J. Oral Maxillofac. Implants* 19 (Suppl): 43–61.

Buser, D., Mericske-Stern, R., Bernard, J.P. et al. (1997). Long-term evaluation of non-submerged ITI implants. Part 1: 8-year life table analysis of a prospective multi-center study with 2359 implants. *Clin. Oral Implants Res.* 8 (3): 161–172.

Buser, D., Mericske-Stern, R., Dula, K., and Lang, N.P. (1999). Clinical experience with one-stage, non-submerged dental implants. *Adv. Dent. Res.* 13: 153–161.

Buskin, R., Castellon, P., and Hochstedler, J.L. (2000). Orthodontic extrusion and orthodontic extraction in preprosthetic treatment using implant therapy. *Pract. Periodontics Aesthet. Dent.* 12 (2): 213–219. quiz 220.

Carlsson, L., Rostlund, T., Albrektsson, B. et al. (1988). Removal torques for polished and rough titanium implants. *Int. J. Oral Maxillofac. Implants* 3 (1): 21–24.

Carranza, F.A. Jr. and Jolkovsky, D.L. (1991). Current status of periodontal therapy for furcation involvements. *Dent. Clin. North. Am.* 35 (3): 555–570.

Casap, N., Tarazi, E., Wexeler, A. et al. (2005). Intraoperative computerized navigation for flapless implant surgery and immediate loading in the edentulous mandible. *Int. J. Oral Maxillofac. Implants* 20: 92–98.

Chanavaz, M. (1990). Maxillary sinus: anatomy, physiology, surgery, and bone grafting related to implantology – eleven years of surgical experience. *J. Oral Implantol.* 16 (3): 199–209.

Chari, H. and Shaik, K. (2016). Preprosthetic surgery: review of literature. *IJSS Case Rep. Rev.* 3 (4): 9–16.

Chen, C.M., Tseng, Y.C., Huang, I.Y. et al. (2004). Interdisciplinary management of dental implant patient: a case report. *Kaohsiung J. Med. Sci.* 20 (8): 415–418.

Chin, M. and Toth, B.A. (1996). Distraction osteogenesis in maxillofacial surgery using internal devices: review of five cases. *J. Oral Maxillofac. Surg.* 54 (1): 45–53.

Chun, Y.S., Row, J., Yang, S.J. et al. (2000). Management of extruded maxillary molars to accommodate a mandibular restoration: a clinical report. *J. Prosthet. Dent.* 83 (6): 604–606.

Cochran, D.L., Schou, S., Heitz-Mayfield, L.J. et al. (2009). Consensus statements and recommended clinical procedures regarding risk factors in implant therapy. *Int. J. Oral Maxillofac. Implants* 24 (Suppl): 86–89.

Consolo, U., Bertoldi, C., Urbani, G., and Zaffe, D. (2000). Clinical evaluation, radiologic and histologic analysis in mandibular alveolar distraction procedures. Preliminary study. *Minerva Stomatol.* 49 (10): 475–484.

Cuoghi, O.A., Bosco, A.F., de Mendonça, M.R. et al. (2010). Multidisciplinary treatment of a fractured root: a case report. *Aust. Orthod. J.* 26 (1): 90–94.

Daftary, F. (1995). Natural esthetics with implant prosthesis. *J. Esthet. Dent.* 7: 9–17.

Danza, M., Zollino, I., Avantaggiato, A. et al. (2011). Distance between implants has a potential impact of crestal bone resorption. *Saudi Dent. J.* 23 (3): 129–133.

Davidoff, D. (1996). Developing soft tissue contours for implant supported restorations: a simplified method for enhanced aesthetics. *Pract. Periodontics Aesthet. Dent.* (8): 507–513.

Day, R.H. (1994). Microneurosurgery of the injured trigeminal nerve. *Oral Maxillofac. Surg. Knowledge Updat.* 1: 91–116.

Elaskary, A.S. (2000). Multi-faceted aspects of implant esthetics: the anterior maxilla. *Implant Dent.* 10: 182–191.

Elaskary, A.S., Meffert, R.M., and Griffin, T. (1999a). Why do dental implants fail? Part I. *Implant Dent.* 8: 173–185.

Elaskary, A.S., Meffert, R.M., and Griffin, T. (1999b). Why do dental implants fail? Part II. *Implant Dent.* 8: 265–277.

Elaskary, A.S. (2008). *Fundamentals of Aesthetic Implant Dentistry*, 2e. U.S.A: Wiley-Blackwell Pub. Co.

English, C.E. (1993). Biomechanical concerns with fixed partial dentures involving implants. *Implant Dent.* 2: 221–242.

Erkut, S., Arman, A., Gulsahi, A. et al. (2007). Forced eruption and implant treatment in posterior maxilla: a clinical report. *J. Prosthet. Dent.* 97 (2): 70–74.

Evans, C.D. and Chen, S.T. (2008). Esthetic outcomes of immediate implant placements. *Clin. Oral Implants Res.* 19 (1): 73–80.

Friedman, N. (1955). Periodontal osseous surgery: osteoplasty and ostectomy. *J. Periodontol.* 26: 257–259.

Froum, S., Casanova, L., Byrne, S., and Cho, S.C. (2011). Risk assessment before extraction for immediate implant placement in the posterior mandible: a computerized tomographic scan study. *J. Periodontol.* 82 (3): 395–402. Epub 2010.

Gaggl, A., Schultes, G., and Kärcher, H. (2000). Vertical alveolar ridge distraction with prosthetic treatable distractors: a clinical investigation. *Int. J. Oral Maxillofac. Implants* 15 (5): 701–710.

Galindo, P., Sánchez-Fernández, E., Avila, G. et al. (2005). Migration of implants into the maxillary sinus: two clinical cases. *Int. J. Oral Maxillofac. Implants* 20 (2): 291–295.

Garcia, A.G., Martin, M.S., Vila, P.G., and Maceiras, J.L. (2002). Minor complications arising in alveolar distraction osteogenesis. *J. Oral Maxillofac. Surg.* 60: 496–501.

Garg, A. (2010). Pathophysiology of tobacco use and wound healing. *Dent. Implantol. Updat.* 21 (1): 1–4.

Geckili, O., Sakar, O., Yurdakuloglu, T. et al. (2011). Multidisciplinary management of limited interocclusal space: a clinical report. *J. Prosthodont.* 20 (4): 329–332.

Goodacre, C.J., Brown, D.T., Roberts, W.E., and Jeiroudi, M.T. (1997). Prosthodontic considerations when using implants for orthodontic anchorage. *J. Prosthet. Dent.* 77 (2): 162–167.

Gores, R.J., Hayes, C.K., and Unni, K.K. (1989). Post mortem examination of six maxillary core-vent implants. Report of a case. *J. Oral Maxillofac. Surg.* 47 (3): 302–306.

Greenstein, G., Cavallaro, J., and Tarnow, D. (2008). Practical application of anatomy for the dental implant surgeon. *J. Periodontol.* 79 (10): 1833–1846.

Grunder, U., Gracis, S., and Capelli, M. (2005). Influence of the 3-D bone-to-implant relationship on esthetics. *Int. J. Periodontics Restorative Dent.* 25: 113–119.

Guerrero, C.A., Laplana, R., Figueredo, N., and Rojas, A. (1999). Surgical implant repositioning: a clinical report. *Int. J. Oral Maxillofac. Implants* 14 (1): 48–54.

Hämmerle, C.H. and Jung, R.E. (2003). Bone augmentation by means of barrier membranes. *Periodontol.* 33: 36–53.

Heithersay, G.S. and Hirsch, R.S. (1993). Tooth discoloration and resolution following a luxation injury: significance of blood pigment in dentin to laser Doppler flowmetry readings. *Quintessence Int.* 24 (9): 669–676.

Hempton, T.J. and Dominici, J.T. (2010). Contemporary crown-lengthening therapy: a review. *J. Am. Dent. Assoc.* 141 (6): 647–655.

Hermann, G. (2000). Primary stability of oral implants. *Int. Mag. Oral Implantol.* (1): 22–24.

Holst, S., Hegenbarth, E.A., Schlegel, K.A., and Holst, A.I. (2007). Restoration of a nonrestorable central incisor using forced orthodontic eruption, immediate implant placement, and an all-ceramic restoration: a clinical report. *J. Prosthet. Dent.* 98 (4): 251–255.

Hunter, W.L. 4th, Bradrick, J.P., Houser, S.M. et al. (2009). 'Maxillary sinusitis resulting from ostium plugging by dislodged bone graft: case report. *J. Oral Maxillofac. Surg.* 67 (7): 1495–1498. doi: 10.1016/j.joms.2009.03.033.

Hur, Y., Tsukiyama, T., Yoon, T.H., and Griffin, T. (2010). Double flap incision design for guided bone regeneration: a novel technique and clinical considerations. *J. Periodontol.* 81 (6): 945–952.

Iglhaut, M. (2003). Implant surgical guide and positioning system – a case report. *Int. Mag. Oral Implantol.* (1): 389–391.

Ilizarov, G.A. and Deviatov, A.A. (1969). Surgical lengthening of the shin with simultaneous correction of deformities. *Ortop. Travmatol. Protez.* 30: 32–33.

Ingber, J.S. (1974). Forced eruption. I. A method of treating isolated one and two wall infrabony osseous defects-rationale and case report. *J. Periodontol.* 45 (4): 199–206.

Ingle, J. and Bakland, L. (2002). *Endodontics*, 5e. Hamilton: BC Decker.

Jaffin, R.A. and Berman, C.L. (1991). The excessive loss of Branemark fixtures in type IV bone: a 5-year analysis. *J. Periodontol.* 62 (1): 2–4.

Jansen, C.E. and Weisgold, A. (1995). Presurgical treatment planning for the anterior single-tooth implant restoration. *Compendium* 16: 746–763.

Jemt, T. (1991). Failures and complications in 391 consecutively inserted fixed prostheses supported by Brånemark implants in edentulous jaws: a study of treatment from the time of prosthesis placement to the first annual checkup. *Int. J. Oral Maxillofac. Implants* 6 (3): 270–276.

Jensen, O.T. (2006). Alveolar segmental "sandwich" osteotomies for posterior edentulous mandibular sites for dental implants. *J. Oral Maxillofac. Surg.* 64 (3): 471–475.

Jivraj, S. and Chee, W. (2006). Treatment planning of implants in posterior quadrants. *Br. Dent. J.* 201: 13–23.

Johansson, C. and Albrektsson, T. (1987). Integration of screw implants in the rabbit: a 1-yr follow-up of removal torque of titanium implants. *Int. J. Oral Maxillofac. Implants* 2 (2): 69–75.

Johnson, G.K. and Sivers, J.E. (1986). Forced eruption in crown-lengthening procedures. *J. Prosthet. Dent.* 56 (4): 424–427.

Jonsson, B. and Siemssen, S.J. (1998). Arced segmental mandibular regeneration by distraction osteogenesis. *Plast. Reconstr. Surg.* 101: 1925.

Kanomi, R. (1997). Mini-implant for orthodontic anchorage. *J. Clin. Orthod.* 31 (11): 763–767.

Karabuda, C., Arisan, V., and Ozyuvaci, H. (2006). Effects of sinus membrane perforations on the success of dental implants placed in the augmented sinus. *J. Periodontol.* 77 (12): 1991–1197.

Karthik, K., Sivakumar, S., and Thangaswamy, V. (2013). Evaluation of implant success: a review of past and present concepts. *J. Pharm. Bioallied Sci.* 5 (Suppl. 1): S117–S119.

Keller, E.E., Tolman, D., and Eckert, S. (1998). Endosseous implant and autogenous bone graft reconstruction of mandibular discontinuity: a 12-year longitudinal study of 31 patients. *Int. J. Oral Maxillofac. Implants* 13 (6): 767–780.

Kendrick, S. and Wong, D. (2009). Vertical and horizontal dimensions of implant dentistry: numbers every dentist should know. *Inside Dent.* (July-Aug): p2–p5.

Kennedy, B.D., Collins, T.A., and Kline, P.C. (1998). Simplified guide for precise implant placement: a technical note. *Int. J. Oral Maxillofac. Implants* 13: 684–688.

Kim, S.G. (2011). Clinical complications of dental implants. In: *Implant Dentistry – A Rapidly Evolving Practice*, vol. 2, chapter 20 (ed. I. Turkyilmaz), 467–490. Rijeka, Croatia: InTech.

Kline, R., Hoar, J.E., Beck, G.H. et al. (2002). A prospective multi-center clinical investigation of a bone quality-based dental implant system. *Implant Dent.* 11 (3): 224–234.

Korayem, M., Flores-Mir, C., Nassar, U., and Olfert, K. (2008). Implant site development by orthodontic extrusion. A systematic review. *Angle Orthod.* 78 (4): 752–760.

Koyanagi, K. (2002). Development and clinical application of a surgical guide for optimal implant placement. *J. Prosthet. Dent.* 88: 548–552.

Kraut, R.A. and Chahal, O. (2002). Management of patients with trigeminal nerve injuries after mandibular implant placement. *J. Am. Dent. Assoc.* 133 (10): 1351–1354.

Kravitz, N.D., Kusnoto, B., Tsay, T.P., and Hohlt, W.F. (2007a). Review the use of temporary anchorage devices for molar intrusion. *J. Am. Dent. Assoc.* 138 (1): 56–64.

Kravitz, N.D., Kusnoto, B., Tsay, P.T., and Hohlt, W.F. (2007b). Intrusion of over erupted upper first molar using two orthodontic miniscrews. A case report. *Angle Orthod.* 77 (5): 915–922.

Lee, E.A. (2004). Aesthetic crown lengthening: classification, biologic rationale, and treatment planning considerations. *Pract. Proced. Aesthet. Dent.* 16 (10): 769–778.

Lee, J.H., Frias, V., Lee, K.W., and Wright, R.F. (2005). Effect of implant size and shape on implant success rates: a literature review. *J. Prosthet. Dent.* 94 (4): 377–381.

Levitt, D.S. (2003). Apicoectomy of an endosseous implant to relieve paresthesia: a case report. *Implant Dent.* 12 (3): 202–205.

Lindfors, L.T., Tervonen, E.A., Sandor, G.K., and Ylikontiola, L.P. (2010). Guided bone regeneration using a titanium-reinforced ePTFE membrane and particulate autogenous bone: the effect of smoking and membrane exposure. *Oral Surg. Oral Med. Oral Pathol. Oral Radiol. Endod.* 109 (6): 825–830.

Livas, C., Jongsma, A.C., and Ren, Y. (2013). Enamel reduction techniques in orthodontics: a literature review. *Open Dent. J.* 7: 146–151.

Lundgren, D. and Laurell, L. (1984). Occlusal forces in prosthetically restored dentitions: a methodological study. *J. Oral Rehabil* 11 (1): 29–37.

Malathi, K., Anand, A., Karthikeyan, R., and Sagar, G. (2014). Coronoplasty. *J. Dent. & Med. Sci.* 13 (9): 64–67.

Malmgren, O., Malmgren, B., and Frykholm, A. (1991). Rapid orthodontic extrusion of crown root and cervical root fractured teeth. *Endod. Dent. Traumatol.* 7 (2): 49–54.

Mantzikos, T. and Shamus, I. (1997). Forced eruption and implant site development: soft tissue response. *Am. J. Orthod. Dentofac. Orthop.* 112 (6): 596–606.

Mantzikos, T. and Shamus, I. (1999). Forced eruption and implant site development: an osteophysiologic response. *Am. J. Orthod. Dentofac. Orthop.* 115 (5): 583–591.

Maynard, J.G. and Wilson, R.D. (1979). Physiologic dimensions of the periodontium significant to the restorative dentist. *J. Periodontol.* 50: 170–174.

Meffert, R.M. (1992). Treatment of failing dental implants. *Curr. Opin. Dent.* 2: 109–144.

Miller, T.E. (1995). Orthodontic and restorative procedures for retained deciduous teeth in the adult. *J. Prosthet. Dent.* 73 (6): 501–509.

Minsk, L. (2000). Tooth extrusion as an adjunct to periodontal therapy. *Compend. Contin. Educ. Dent.* 21 (9): 768–770. 772, 774 passim. No abstract available.

Misch, C.E. (1995). The maxillary anterior single tooth implant aesthetic health compromise. *Int. J. Dent. Symp.* 3 (1): 4–9.

Misch, C.E., Goodacre, C.J., Finley, J.M. et al. (2005). Consensus conference panel report: crown-height space guidelines for implant dentistry – part 1. *Implant Dent.* 14 (4): 312–318.

Misch, C.E. and Resnik, R. (2012). Mandibular nerve neurosensory impairment following dental implant surgery: management and protocol. *Implant Dent.* 19 (5): 378–386.

Misch, C.E., Wang, H.L., Misch, C.M. et al. (2004). Rationale for the application of immediate load in implant dentistry: part I. *Implant Dent.* 13 (3): 207–217.

Misch, K. and Wang, H.L. (2008). Implant surgery complications: etiology and treatment. *Implant Dent.* 17 (2): 159–168.

Mohamed, J., Shivakumar, B., Sudarsan, S. et al. (2010). Retrograde peri-implantitis. *J. Indian Soc. Periodontol.* 14 (1): 57–65.

Narayan, S., Narayan, T.V., and Jacob, P.C. (2011). Correction of gummy smile: a report of two cases. *J. Indian Soc. Periodontol.* 15 (4): 421–424.

Nazarian, Y., Eliav, E., and Nahlieli, O. (2003). Nerve injury following implant placement: prevention, diagnosis and treatment modalities. *Refuat Hapeh Vehashinayim* 20 (3): 44–50.

Nebot, V.X., Rodríguez-Ciurana, R.X., Rodado, A.C., and Maribel, S. (2006). Benefits of an implant platform modification technique to reduce crestal bone resorption. *Implant Dent.* 15: 313–320.

Nugala, B., Kumar, B.S., Sahitya, S., and Krishna, P.M. (2012). Biologic width and its importance in periodontal and restorative dentistry. *J. Conserv. Dent.* 15 (1): 12–17.

Obwegeser, H.O. (1966). *Conference on Comprehensive Oral Surgery*. Washington, DC: American Society of Oral Surgeons.

O'Neal, R.B. and Butler, B.L. (2002). Restoration or implant placement: a growing treatment planning quandary. *Periodontol. 2000* 30: 111–122.

Oesterle, L.J. and Wood, L.W. (1991). Raising the root. A look at orthodontic extrusion. *J. Am. Dent. Assoc.* 122 (7): 193–198.

Ohenell, L., Palmquist, J., and Brånemark, P.I. (1992). Single tooth replacement. In: *Advanced Osseointegration Surgery Applications in the Maxillofacial Region* (ed. P. Worthington and P.I. Brånemark), 211–132. Carol Stream, IL: Quintessence Publishing Co.

Parel, S.M. and Sullivan, D.Y. (1989). *Esthetics and Osseointegration*. Dallas, TX: Taylor Publishing.

Park, H.S., Bae, S.M., Kyung, H.M., and Sung, J.H. (2001). Micro-implant anchorage for treatment of skeletal class I bi-alveolar protrusion. *J. Clin. Orthod.* 35 (7): 417–422.

Park, H.S., Lee, S.K., and Kwon, O.W. (2005). Group distal movement of teeth using microscrew implant anchorage. *Angle Orthod.* 75 (4): 602–609.

Peleg, M., Garg, A.K., and Mazor, Z. (2006). Predictability of simultaneous implant placement in the severely atrophic posterior maxilla: a 9-year longitudinal experience study of 2132 implants placed into 731 human sinus grafts. *Int. J. Oral Maxillofac. Implants* 21 (1): 94–102.

Pjetursson, B.E., Tan, K., Lang, N.P. et al. (2004). A systematic review of the survival and complication rates of fixed partial dentures (FPDs) after an observation period of at least 5 years. *Clin. Oral Implants Res.* 15 (6): 667–676.

Potashnick, S.R. (1998). Soft tissue modeling for the esthetic single-tooth implant restoration. *J. Esthet. Dent.* 10: 121–131.

Potashnick, S.R. and Rosenberg, E.S. (1982). Forced eruption: principles in periodontics and restorative dentistry. *J. Prosthet. Dent.* 48 (2): 141–148.

Quirynen, M., Vogels, R., Alsaadi, G. et al. (2005). Predisposing conditions for retrograde peri-implantitis, and treatment suggestions. *Clin. Oral Implants Res.* 16 (5): 599–608.

Rose, T.P., Jivraj, S., and Chee, W. (2006). The role of orthodontics in implant dentistry. *Br. Dent. J.* 201 (12): 753–764.

Rosenstiel, S.F. (1998). *Contemporary Fixed Prosthodontics*. Harcourt Brace.

Sabri, R. (1989). Crown lengthening by orthodontic extrusion. Principles and technics. *J. Parodontol.* 8 (2): 197–204.

Salama, H. and Salama, M. (1993). The role of orthodontic extrusive remodeling in the enhancement of soft and hard tissue profiles prior to implant placement: a systematic approach to the management of extraction site defects. *Int. J. Periodontics Restorative Dent.* 13 (4): 312–333.

Schluger, S. (1949). Osseous resection: a basic principle in periodontal surgery. *Oral Surg. Oral Med. Oral Pathol.* 2 (3): 316–325.

Seibert, J.S. and Salama, H. (1996). Alveolar ridge preservation and reconstruction. *Periodontol. 2000* 11: 69–84.

Sennerby, L., Thomsen, P., and Ericson, L.E. (1992). A morphometric and biomechanic comparison of titanium implants inserted in rabbit corical and cancellous bone. *Int. J. Oral Maxillofac. Implants* 7: 62–71.

Sharma, A., Rahul, G., Poduval, S., and Shetty, K. (2012). Short clinical crowns (SCC) – treatment considerations and techniques. *J. Clin. Exp. Dent.* 4 (4): e230–e236.

Shenoy, V.K. (2012). Single tooth implants: pretreatment considerations and pretreatment evaluation. *J. Interdiscip. Dentistry* 2: 149–157.

Sivakumar, I. and Sivakumar, A. (2014). Intrusion of an overerupted molar using orthodontic miniscrew implant: a preprosthodontic therapy. *Contemp. Clin. Dent.* 5 (3): 422–424.

Sohn, D.S., Lee, J.K., and An, K.M. (2008). Minor tooth movements using microimplant anchorage: case reports. *Implant Dent.* 17 (1): 32–39.

Spalding, P.M. and Cohen, B.D. (1992). Orthodontic adjunctive treatment in fixed prosthodontics. *Dent. Clin. North Am.*, July 36 (3): 607–629.

Stewart, R.E. and Prescott, G.H. (1976). *Oral Facial Defects*, 1e, 151. St. Louis, MI: The CV Mosby Co.

Szmukler-Moncler, S., Salama, H., Reingewirtz, Y. et al. (1998). Timing of loading and effect of micromotion on bone-dental implant interface: review of experimental literature. *J. Biomed. Mater. Res.* 43: 192–203.

Tardieu, P., Vrielinck, L., and Escolano, E. (2003). Computer-assisted implant placement. A case report: treatment of the mandible. *Int. J. Oral Maxillofac. Implants* 18: 599–604.

Tondelli, P.M., Kay, F.A., and Kuabara, M.R. (2014). Orthodontic extrusion as an aid in oral rehabilitation. *Oral Health Dent. Manag.* 13 (2): 223–228.

Tozum, T.F., Sencimen, M., Ortakoglu, K. et al. (2006). Diagnosis and treatment of a large periapical implant lesion associated with adjacent natural tooth: a case report. *Oral Surg. Oral Med. Oral Pathol. Oral Radiol. Endod.* 101 (6): e132–e138.

Uckan, S., Dolanmaz, D., Kalayci, A., and Cilasun, U. (2002). Distraction osteogenesis of basal mandibular bone for reconstruction of the alveolar ridge. *Br. J. Oral Maxillofac. Surg.* 40 (5): 393–396.

Ueda, M. and Kaneda, T. (1992). Maxillary sinusitis caused by dental implants: report of two cases. *J. Oral Maxillofac. Surg.* 50 (3): 285–287. Update, 21 (1): 1–4.

Urbani, G. (2001). Alveolar distraction before implantation: a report of five cases and a review of the literature. *Int. J. Periodontics Restorative Dent.* 21 (6): 569–579.

van Steenberghe, D., Naert, I., Bossuyt, M. et al. (1997). The rehabilitation of the severely resorbed maxilla by simultaneous placement of autogenous bone grafts and implants: a 10-year evaluation. *Clin. Oral Investig.* 1 (3): 102–108.

Wahlgren, J., Salo, T., Teronen, O. et al. (2002). Matrix metalloproteinase-8 (MMP-8) in pulpal and periapical inflammation and periapical root-canal exudates. *Int. Endod. J.* 35: 897–904.

Warden, P.J. and Scuba, J.R. (2000). Surgical repositioning of a malposed, unserviceable implant: case report. *J. Oral Maxillofac. Surg.* 58: 433–435. Washington, DC: American Society of Oral Surgeons; 1966.

Wheeler, R.C. (1950). *A Text Book of Dental Anatomy and Physiology*, 2e. Philadelphia, PA: W.B. Saunders Co.

Wheeler, R.C. (1974). *Dental Anatomy, Physiology and Occlusion*, 5e. Philadelphia, PA: W.B Saunders Co.

Yao, C.C., Lee, J.J., Chen, H.Y. et al. (2005). Maxillary molar intrusion with fixed appliances and mini-implant anchorage studied in three dimensions. *Angle Orthod.* 75 (5): 754–760.

Yousef, H., Luke, A., Ricci, J. et al. (2005). Analysis of changes in implant screws subject to occlusal loading: a preliminary analysis. *Implant Dent.* 14: 378–385.

Zhou, W., Han, C., Li, D. et al. (2009). Endodontic treatment of teeth induces retrograde peri-implantitis. *Clin. Oral Implants Res.* 20 (12): 1326–1332.

Zijderveld, S.A., van den Bergh, J.P., Schulten, E.A., and ten Bruggenkate, C.M. (2008). Anatomical and surgical findings and complications in 100 consecutive maxillary sinus floor elevation procedures. *J. Oral Maxillofac. Surg.* 66 (7): 1426–1438.

9

Treatment Complications and Failures with Dental Implants

9.1 Introduction

The installation of osseointegrated oral implants in partially edentulous patients proved an efficacious therapy for restoring missing natural teeth (Gunne et al. 1992, 1994; Jemt 1986; Jemt et al. 1989, 1992; Jemt and Lekholm 1993; Nevins and Langer 1993; Zarb and Schmitt 1990). Although the success rate of dental implants is relatively higher than other treatment alternatives, some factors such as bone quality, surgical trauma, or bacterial contamination during implant surgery have been associated with early failures and reduced success rates (Esposito et al. 1998).

In spite of the gained popularity of dental implants among practitioners, a limited number of studies analyzed the impact of the clinician's experience or training on the outcome of dental implant therapy. A 1993 survey conducted by the American Dental Association reported that dental training varied widely among clinicians who placed implants (Kohavi et al. 2004). The report emphasized not only the wide availability of training modules in the USA and global implant education activities and hands-on courses, but also a lack of courses and educational modules that are specially focused on treating and managing implant-related complications. It was also recommended that surgical predicaments associated with implant dentistry should be well studied in the various educational programs.

A study (Lambert et al. 1997) reported that implants placed by inexperienced surgeons (less than 50 implants) failed twice as often as those placed by experienced surgeons who placed 50 implants or more. Inexperienced surgeons had more failures in the first nine cases (5.9%) than more experienced surgeons (2.4%). However, the number of implants placed by clinicians did not necessarily reflect their own clinical experience, and it was the author's recommendation that it is important for postgraduate educational modules that focus only on managing and avoiding implant related complications.

Implant surgical complications occur frequently in dental practice and knowledge in the management of these cases is essential. The aim of this chapter is to highlight the challenges of treatment for plan-related, anatomy-related, and procedure-related surgical complications as well as to discuss the etiology, management, and treatment options required to achieve a satisfactory treatment outcome, and to outline the relative risk factors involved.

The highest recorded failure rate with dental implants occurs with low bone density, as evidenced in a 10-year Brånemark study (Brånemark et al. 1977), which showed that fixture failures in maxillary type IV bone is 44%. A relationship between periodontal disease and peri-implantitis was established based on the findings of increased gram-negative, anaerobic flora with high levels of spirochetes associated with failing or failed implants (Esposito et al. 1998). English (1993) stated that implant-supported fixed partial dentures may fail for numerous reasons. He listed leverage, torsion, occlusal overload, and poor oral hygiene as primary causative factors, thus expanding the scope of factors that cause implant failure. Elaskary et al. (1999a, b) emphasized improper patient selection, accumulation of bacterial plaque because of poor oral hygiene practice, traumatic occlusion, poor prosthetic construction, and poor bone preparation as factors contributing to the breakdown of otherwise successful implants. Att and Stappert (2003), Chee and Jivraj (2007), and Montes et al. (2007) concluded that overall treatment planning and patient selection are among the influential factors for implant success and that unidentified host conditions might add higher risk. Moy et al. (2005) reported the influence of age to the success rate of dental implants, they stated that the older patients (more than 60 years old) are more liable and at higher risk of dental implant complications and failures. (see Figure 9.1a–c).

Advances in Esthetic Implant Dentistry, First Edition. Abdelsalam Elaskary.

Companion website: www.wiley.com/go/elaskary/esthetic

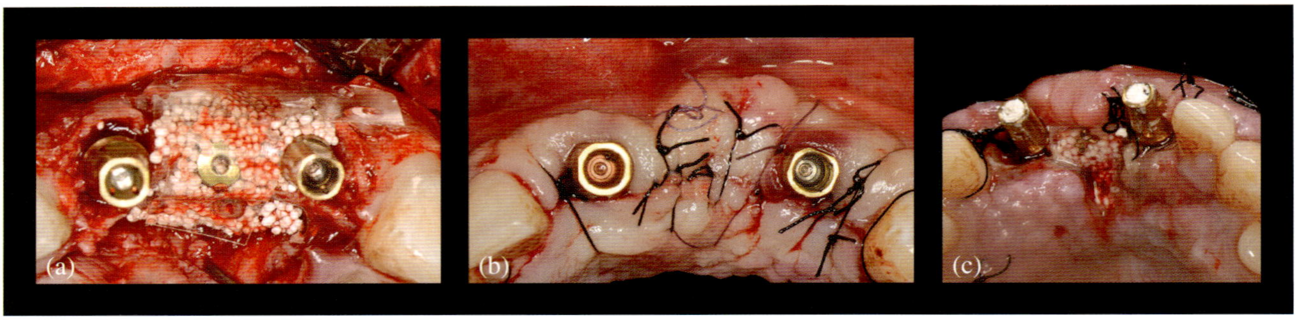

Figure 9.1 (a) Implant placement with simultaneous bone grafting procedure is made, (b) Optimal soft tissue closure, (c) Wound sloughing, bone grafting exposure as a result of smoking.

Goodacre et al. (2003) conducted a report that details the most common reasons for implant related treatment complications and failures. The following six categories of clinical complications are associated with an implant prosthesis: surgical, implant loss, bone loss, peri-implant soft tissue, esthetic/phonetic, and mechanical. They also listed the frequency of complications related to implant over dentures. Sanz et al. (2010) studied the influence of physiological modeling response of the labial plate of bone to the overall success of implant supported restorations placed in immediate sites. Ashley et al. (2003) described the different clinical pictures of implant deterioration conditions whether they are ailing, failing, or failed. Abt (2009) studied the effect of cigarette smoking on the success rate of dental implant-supported restorations. Keller et al. (2004) reported on the effect of systemic disorders such as osteoporosis and their impact on the overall dental implant therapy.

Berglundh et al. (2002), in a meta-analysis of various studies, indicated the biological and technical reasons for dental implants loss prior to functional loading is expected to occur in about 2.5% of all implants placed in implant therapy that includes more than one implant and when routine procedures are used. Implant loss during function occurred in about 2–3% of implants supporting fixed restorations, while in overdenture therapy >5% of the implants can be expected to be lost during a five-year period. A higher incidence of soft tissue complications was reported for patients treated with implants supporting overdentures. There is limited information regarding the occurrence of peri-implantitis and implants exhibiting bone loss ≥2.5 mm. Implant fracture is a rare complication and occurs in <1% of all implants during a five-year period. The incidence of technical complications related to implant components and suprastructures was higher in overdentures than in fixed reconstructions. It was concluded that implant loss was most frequently described (reported in about 100% of studies), while biological complications were considered in only 40–60% and technical complications in only 60–80% of the studies. This observation indicates that data on the incidence of biological and technical complications may be underestimated and should be interpreted with caution.

Some clinical pictures that can indicate or predict implant-related complications and failures, in most cases connecting screw loosening is the major warning sign for the early stage of failure when overload is the influential factor. It indicates increased load on the implant components or increased torque as in single tooth replacements. The screw loosening creates microgaps between the abutment and the implant interface (a favorable place for bacteria to populate) and subsequently irritates the gingiva, causing bleeding and edema, connecting screw fracture when overload exceeding the normal values, gingival bleeding, pocketing, fracture of the prosthetic components, and angular bone loss, pain is not common (Dewan et al. 2015).

9.1.1 Implant Failure Terms

Elaskary et al. (1999a, b) defined implant failure as the total failure of the implant to fulfill its purpose (either functional, esthetic, or phonetic) due to mechanical or biological reasons. Dental implants may fail for different reasons, with an array that differentiates between a failure and a complication. Esposito et al. (1998) stated that this definition includes biological failures (related to biological processes) and mechanical failure of the component (including fractures of implants, coatings, connecting screws, and prostheses), and included fractures of the implant connecting screws and prosthesis as failures.

Meffert (1992) proposed a classification of failure including ailing, failing, and failed implants. He described ailing implants as those showing radiographic bone loss without inflammatory signs or mobility. Such implants do not pose any indication of failure, but with the progression of bone loss, they could be at a higher risk of failure. Failing implants are characterized by progressive bone loss, signs of inflammation, and no mobility. These implants are usually in a reversible state (the condition can be treated). It is therefore necessary to determine and eliminate the etiological factor(s) causing such a condition. While failed implants are these are implants with progressive bone loss with clinical mobility and that are not functioning, implants are usually encapsulated (Dewan et al. 2015). Surviving implants applies to implants that are still in function but have not been tested against success criteria. For an implant is considered to be in an intermediate situation between successful and failing implants until proper evaluation is made Roos et al. (1997).

Tonetti and Schmid (1994) classified dental implant failures chronologically as early and late failures. (1) Early failure: failure to establish osseointegration. Causes of early failure include infection, inferior surgical technique, systemic disease, incompatible host site, and graft loss due to smoking or pressure on the surgical site. (2) Late failure: breakdown of an established osseointegration. Causes of late failure include overloading the implant, cantilevers, incorrectly fitting prosthesis, and parafunctional habits (Parithimarkalaignan and Padmanabhan 2013).

Peri-implant diseases (as a result of bacterial invasion) are categorized into two types: peri-implant mucositis and peri-implantitis. Peri-implant mucositis (as shown in Figure 9.2) is characterized by inflammation of the soft tissues surrounding the implant without any signs of bone loss. The clinical signs of peri-implant mucositis include bleeding, inflammation, with no evidence of radiographic bone loss. Mucositis is often reversible, however, it is considered as a precursor to peri-implantitis (Dewan et al. 2015). Mombelli et al. (1987) first described the term peri-implantitis (as shown in Figure 9.3a and b) as an infectious disease with many features common to periodontitis. Peri-implantitis is defined as an inflammatory process affecting the tissue around an implant in function that has resulted in loss of supporting bone (Derks et al. 2016) (see Figure 9.4a and b). Roos-Jansaker et al. (2007) described peri-implantitis as a condition in which implants with varying degrees of bone loss are accompanied by a probing depth of 4 mm, bleeding on probing, and purulent discharge on gentle probing. Berglundh, Zitzman and Donati (2011) defined peri-implantitis with a probing depth of 6 mm and in combination with bleeding on probing and clinical attachment loss of at least 2.5 mm (see Figure 9.5).

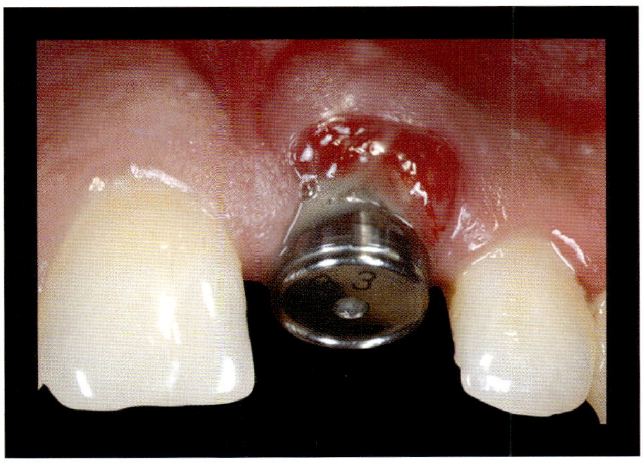

Figure 9.2 Classic clinical picture of peri-implant mucosities.

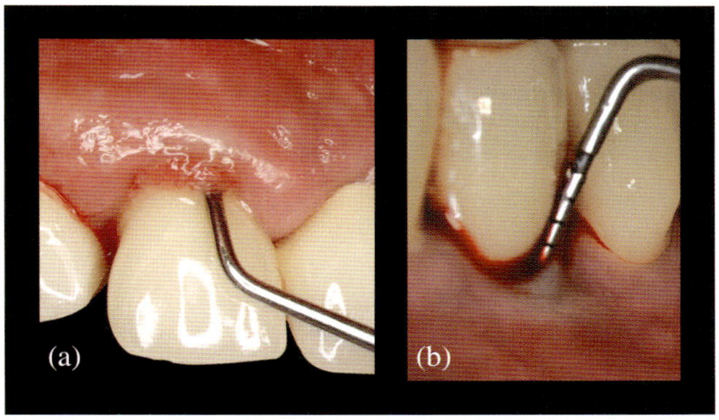

Figure 9.3 (a) Pocketing is a cardinal sign for peri-implantitis, (b) Bleeding upon probing is another cardinal sign for peri implantities.

Froum and Rosen (2012) proposed a classification that differentiated peri-implantitis according to the severity of inflammation and extent of bone loss around the implant (see Figure 9.6a and b). This classification is based on three different clinical stages of peri-implantitis; early, moderate, and advanced. A probing depth of at least 4 mm and radiographic bone loss of less than 25% of the total implant length defines early. In moderate peri-implantitis, 6 mm probing depth and radiographic bone loss of 25–50% of the total implant length, and at least 8 mm with more than 50% of radiographic bone loss, with reference to the implant length, is termed advanced peri-implantitis (see Figures 9.7a, b and 9.8a, b).

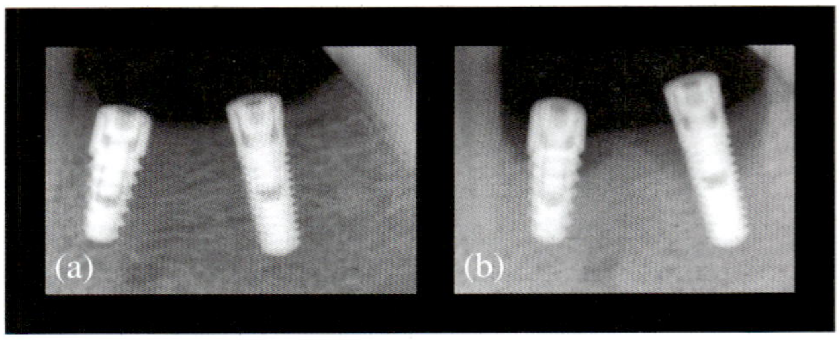

Figure 9.4 (a) Two implant placed in healed ridge, (b) Two years later developed peri-implant tissue breakdown.

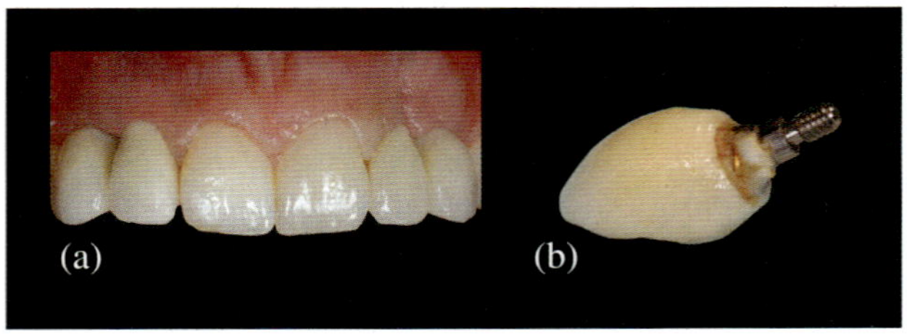

Figure 9.7 (a) Implant supported restoration treating missing two lateral incisors, (b) Note the cement treatment underneath the abutment.

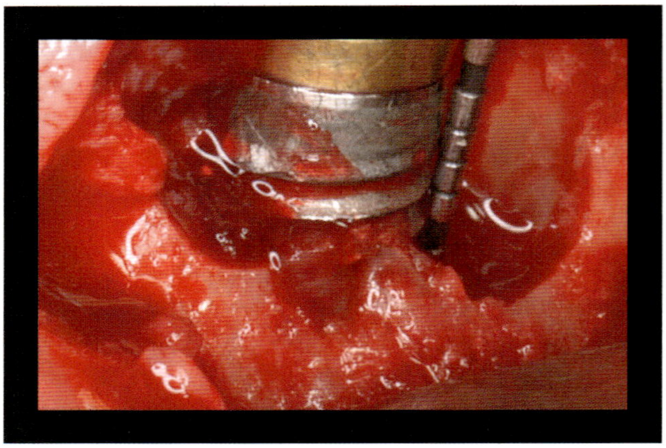

Figure 9.5 Bone destruction around dental implant as a result of peri implant tissue infection.

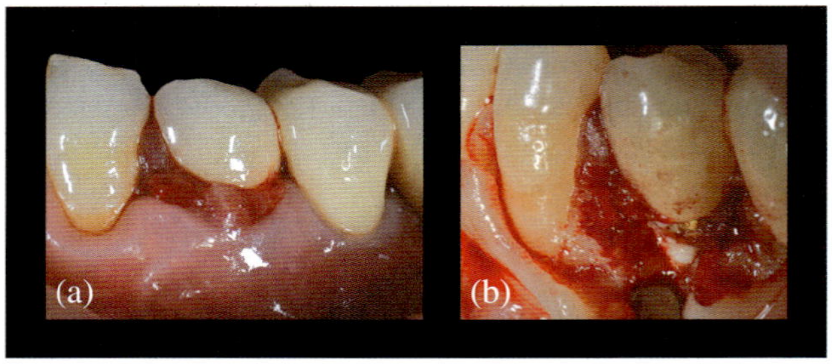

Figure 9.8 (a) and (b) Per implant tissue infection indicating residual cement irritation.

Another novel classification was introduced by Caton et al. (2018) who have published an introductory paper that presents an overview for the new classification of periodontal and peri-implant diseases and conditions;

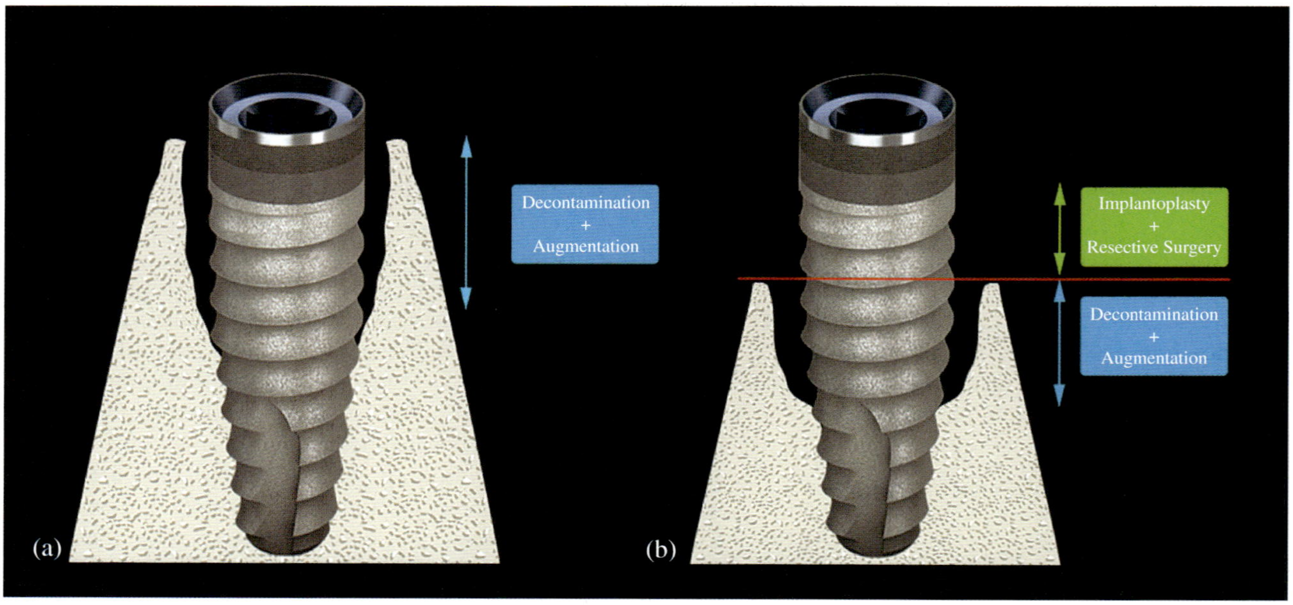

Figure 9.6 (a) and (b) Repair strategies for treating peri implantitis surgically.

they have classified peri-implant diseases into: Peri-implant health that was defined both clinically and histologically, was characterized by an absence of visual signs of inflammation and bleeding on probing. Peri-implant health can exist around implants with normal or reduced bone support. Peri-implant mucositis is characterized by bleeding on probing and visual signs of inflammation, while there is a strong evidence that peri-implant mucositis is caused by plaque, there is very little evidence for non-plaque induced peri-implant mucositis. Peri-implant mucositis can be reversed with measures aimed at eliminating the plaque. Peri-implantitis was defined as a plaque-associated pathologic condition occurring in the tissue around dental implants, characterized by inflammation in the peri-implant mucosa and subsequent progressive loss of supporting bone. Peri-implant mucositis is assumed to precede peri-implantitis. Peri-implantitis is associated with poor plaque control and with patients with a history of severe periodontitis. The onset of peri-implantitis may occur early following implant placement as indicated by radiographic data. Peri-implantitis, in the absence of treatment, seems to progress in a non-linear and accelerating pattern. Hard and soft tissue implant site deficiencies that are larger ridge deficiencies can occur at sites associated with severe loss of periodontal support, extraction trauma, endodontic infections, root fractures, thin buccal bone plates, poor tooth position, injury, and pneumatization of the maxillary sinuses. Other factors affecting the ridge can be associated with medications and systemic diseases reducing the amount of naturally forming bone, tooth agenesis, and pressure from prostheses.

9.2 Prevalence of Implant-related Treatment Complications

The prevalence of peri-implant diseases has been reported in the literature; however, considerable variations among these studies are noted. Albrektsson and Isidor (1994) reported peri-implantitis in 6.47% of the implants included in their review. Zitzmann and Berglundh (2008) showed that the frequency of peri-implantitis varied between 28 and 56% of the participants and 12 and 43% of individual implants. Papathanasiou et al. (2016) conducted a survey to investigate the perceived prevalence, etiology, and management of peri-implant mucositis and peri-implantitis by periodontists in the United States. A 20-question survey was developed. Periodontists currently practicing in the United States were contacted by e-mail that contained a link to access a survey. Two hundred and eighty periodontists (79.3% males: 62.9% with >10 years in practice and 75.7% in private practice) completed the survey. Most (96.1%) of the participants were placing implants (58.3% for >10 years and 32.4% >150 implants/year). The majority reported that the prevalence of peri-implant mucositis and peri-implantitis in their practices was up to 25% but was higher in the general US population and that up to 10% of implants must be removed due to peri-implantitis. There was agreement among contributing etiologic factors such as: (1) plaque; (2) smoking; (3) adverse loading; (4) oral hygiene. They concluded that most participants reported seeing peri-implant pathology in up to 25% of their patients. A significant heterogeneity was recorded in relation to the instruments used for debridement, use and type of surgical treatment (debridement/resective/regenerative), and the study indicated the absence of a standard therapeutic protocol results in significant empirical use of therapeutic modalities. Most of the participants believed peri-implantitis treatment to be moderately effective.

Numerous surgical complications have been identified in implant literature, including mild bleeding, neurosensory disturbance, adjacent tooth devitalization, mandibular fracture, life-threatening hemorrhage, air emboli, implant displacement into the mandibular spaces or to the maxillary sinus, screwdriver aspiration, etc. Although mandibular fractures, secondary to the placing of implants, are an infrequent complication, they have been widely described in the literature in the past. This complication occurs when implants are placed in the atrophic mandible, and usually occur in elderly patients seeking implant treatment in the anterior area to improve their chewing abilities. Raghoebar et al. (2000) described four cases of mandibular fractures related to the placing of implants in atrophic alveolar processes. During the period 1990–2000, 2734 implants were placed in the edentulous mandible with a maximum height of the symphysis of 15 mm; two patients suffered mandibular fractures during the insertion or explantation of the implants (Pelayo et al. 2008). On other occasions, the mandibular fractures are related to complex surgical techniques, such as the transposition or lateralization of the inferior alveolar nerve. The occurrence of mandibular fracture in conjunction with implant surgery placement was reported in three studies with four fractures recorded among 1523 patients treated. The mean incidence was 0.3% with a range from 0.2 to 0.8% (Goodacre et al. 2003).

Out of 379 patients, 92 were identified as being affected by factors like ecchymosis and hematomas, for a mean incidence of 24% and a range from 12 to 30% (Goodacre et al. 2003). Data related to the incidence of neurosensory disturbance after surgery occurred with a mean incidence of 7% with a range from 0.6 to 39%. Four studies provided data demonstrating that the incidence of disturbance is significantly lower after one year (Goodacre et al. 2003).

Data regarding implant loss with maxillary implant-fixed complete dentures were provided in nine studies with a mean loss of 10% (443 of 4559 implants). In the mandible a 3% mean loss was recorded (255 of 9991 implants) from the combined data of 14 studies. With implant overdentures, the mean maxillary implant loss was 19% (209 of 1103 implants) and the mean mandibular implant was 4% (242 of 5683 implants); with implant-fixed partial dentures, the maxillary and mandibular implant loss rates were the same. A mean loss of 6% was recorded for both arches in 16 out of the 20 studies evaluated for implant loss with single crowns. Implant length has an impact on the success of implant-supported restorations In the 10 mm long or less category, (10%). Implants failed with the implants greater than 10 mm long (3%) (Kotsovilis et al. 2009). Peri-implant soft tissue complications that have been reported include fenestration/dehiscence, gingival inflammation/proliferation, and fistulas. The most common postoperative complication is wound dehiscence, which sometimes occurs during the first 10 days after implant placement surgery (Greenstein et al. 2008), exposure of the graft material or barrier membrane may occur as a result of flap tension, continuous mechanical trauma, or continuous wound irritation from an existing prosthesis, incorrect incision design, and faulty flap handling as recorded by Park and Wang (2005).

The fenestration/dehiscence of soft tissue around dental implants ranged between 2 and 13% (Goodacre et al. 2003). A mean prosthesis screw loosening of 7% was calculated. Esthetic deficiencies were recorded in seven studies. A mean complication incidence of 10% was reported. The average loosening with implant single crowns that used early screw designs was 25% and 2% fracture of abutment screws (Goodacre et al. 2003).

Sussman (1998) has recorded the possible damage of an adjacent tooth by implant placement that may cause the tooth to become non-vital, and the tooth may require subsequent endodontic treatment. Ideally, 1.5–2 mm of bone should be present between an implant and the adjacent tooth (Greenstein et al. 2008). To prevent a latent infection of the implant from the potential endodontic lesion, endodontic treatment should be accurately performed (Sussman 1998). Discrepancies between the apical and crestal interdental spaces as a result of mesial or distal tipping of the roots can be corrected orthodontically (Annibali et al. 2009a).

9.3 Anatomical Related Treatment Complications

Anatomical related complications, such as rupture of the Schneiderian membrane, may occur during attempts to place dental implants in the posterior maxilla. The Schneiderian membrane, which is characterized by periosteum overlaid with a thin layer of pseudociliated stratified respiratory epithelium, constitutes an important barrier for the protection, lavage, and defense of the sinus cavity (Ardekian et al. 2006). When sinus membrane perforation occurs, it may represent a window for bacterial penetration and invasion into the grafted area (Zijderveld et al. 2008). Failure to a-traumatically elevate the Schneiderian membrane and isolate the grafted bone in the confined lifted area can lead to an alteration of the normal mucociliary flow patterns, causing retention of secretions and infections around the foreign body (Ward et al. 2008). However, the occurrence of iatrogenic sinus membrane perforations during surgery does not seem to be related to sinusitis in healthy individuals (Ardekian et al. 2006).

Schneiderian membrane perforation, which occurs in 10–60% of all procedures (Ardekian et al. 2006; Pikos 1999; Proussaefs 2004), increases when anatomical variations such as a maxillary sinus septum, spine, or sharp edge are present (Chanavaz 1990; van den Bergh et al. 2000). Sharper angles located at the inner walls of the maxillary sinus in the vicinity presents a higher risk of perforation (Zijderveld et al. 2008). Clinicians are urged to thoroughly study the CBCT scan of the patient prior to performing any maxillary sinus elevation technique with simultaneous bone grafting. The maxillary sinus anatomy and location of septa should be assessed; Graziani et al. (2005) suggested aborting the sinus grafting procedure once a major perforation has occurred.

Another complication described in the literature is the displacement of the implants into the maxillary sinus cavity. While in some cases implant migration causes sinusitis, in many patients it remains asymptomatic (Graziani et al. 2005).

Hemorrhage could occur in the anterior mandible, which has an arterial supply provided by three main arteries: the lingual, facial, and inferior alveolar (Flanagan 2003). Accidental perforation the mandibular lingual bone cortex may cause arterial bleeding at the lingual cortex caused by severing a terminal branch of the sublingual, submental arteries, and mylohyoid. Submental, sublingual, and mylohyoid arteries might be anastomosed. Many of these blood vessels penetrate the alveolar mucosa in the anterior tooth region, and many distal branches of the vessels also finally penetrate the bone. This seems to explain why many vascular injuries are encountered around the mandibular anterior tooth lingual region during implant surgery (Fujita et al. 2012). The high risk of damaging the arteries of the floor of the mouth (below the mylohyoid floor) is explained by the close proximity and insertion of the vessels into the lingual cortex and the sublingual fossa. A real potential threat when the arteries are injured causes a massive internal hemorrhage below the floor of the mouth, expanding swelling occurs and air way stenosis results from the displacement of the tongue. Hemorrhage is prevented from escaping into the oral cavity because it is guarded by the mylohyoid muscle. Sometimes hemorrhage and swelling occurs one hour after implant placement injury, which explains the need to retain the suspected patient in the waiting room for some time after operating in the anterior mandible. Using short implants would definitely reduce the likelihood of the occurrence of this complication, which would not cause any compromise to the overall function. Hemorrhage may be controlled by compression, or ligation. Bimanual compression should be attempted from the floor of the mouth from one end and underneath the lower mandible from the other side to control it. If these attempts failed, rushing the patient to an emergency room, to allow patent airway via intubation might be necessary. CBCT seems to be the best presurgical option for the prevention of such complications, as it shows the area of the vascular branch entries to the anterior mandibular region through the bone canals and generally provides a three-dimensional image of the bone structures (De Vera, Calleja and García 2008).

Haemorrhage may occur as a result of perforating the posterior palatine artery during implant placement in the retromolar trigone of the maxilla, or the pterygoid apophyses. To minimize the potential danger of vascular injury in this area, preparation of the implant bed using osteotomes can be used to avoid using drills, or opting for another implant location may also be considered. Keller et al. (1997) described the potential danger of placing dental implants in irradiated mandibles, in the mandible; the inferior alveolar nerve is midway between the buccal and lingual cortical plates in the first molar region (Tammisalo et al. 1992). In about 1% of patients, the mandibular canal bifurcates in the inferior superior or medial lateral planes. Thus, a bifurcated mandibular canal will manifest more than one mental foramen. This may not be seen on panoramic or periapical films. Accordingly, Dario suggested that clinicians should consider obtaining a preoperative tomogram (now a CBCT) to avoid nerve injuries prior to implant placement above the inferior alveolar canal (Greenstein and Tarnow 2006).

Other anatomical related complications in implant placement surgery are neurosensory alterations, which manifest during the immediate postoperative period in the form of anesthesia, hypoesthesia, paresthesia, or dysesthesia. The sensory disturbances produced following implant placement in the mandible are the result of injury to one or more of the branches of the mandibular nerve, which includes the inferior alveolar nerve, the mental nerve, or the lingual nerve. Damage to one of these nerves may produce inadvertent biting in the affected area, tongue, lip, or cheek, drooling, pain and changes in mastication. Complex surgical techniques, such as the transposition and lateralization of the inferior alveolar nerve, or the excessive intrusion of the drill or implant into the mandibular canal, can lead to nerve injury, so caution must be exercised when performing such procedures. The lingual nerve can be damaged by the accidental raising of lingual flaps, lingual anesthesia using the inferior alveolar nerve block, or even by excessive separation of the soft tissue from the lingual cortex during surgical removal of the third molar.

The inferior alveolar nerve may be affected by perforating the mandibular canal during drilling or by positioning the implant close to the canal and the subsequent formation of an adjacent hematoma that presses against the nerve, which may cause neuroma. For this reason, for the placement of dental implants in the mandible, an anesthetic technique by infiltration of the mandible has been proposed, with the aim of maintaining sufficient sensation to indicate the proximity of the roof or the inferior alveolar nerve during implant placement (Walton 2000). Preventative measures suggested are correct presurgical planning using the appropriate radiographic techniques, placing implants at least 5 mm from the mental foramen and 2 mm from the mandibular canal. CBCT scan should be used to identify the anatomical structures involved in the area for implantation and also to perform correct surgical planning. A mean incidence of neurosensory disturbance incidence after implant surgery was 6.1% (Goodacre et al. 1999) to 7% (Goodacre et al. 2003). Nerve damage can have results ranging from mild paresthesia to complete anesthesia or even disabling dysesthesia (Misch and Wang 2008). Nerve injuries may be caused indirectly by postsurgical intra-alveolar edema resulting in a neuroma or hematomas that produce a temporary or long-standing pressure increase, especially inside the mandibular canal. Direct traumas are the most frequent causes of nerve injury and may occur through five mechanisms: compression, stretch, cut, overheating, and accidental puncture (Annibali et al. 2009b). Finally, prolonged pressure from neuritis may lead to the permanent degeneration of the affected nerve (Park and Wang 2005). The mental nerve is at particular risk of iatrogenic injury (Bartling, Freeman and Kraut 1999). In long-term edentulous patients, it may be very close to the bone surface or the top of the crest. The nerve injury may cause one of the following conditions: Paresthesia: Any altered sensation including pain, numbness, tingling, aching, warmth, cold, and burning. Dysesthesia: Any altered sensation that is unpleasant. Hyperalgesia: Exaggerated response to mild painful stimuli (due to decrease in pain threshold). Allodynia: Pain caused by stimuli that is normally not painful. Anesthesia: Total loss of feeling or sensation (Misch and Resnik 2010).

For implants placed in the atrophic posterior mandible, the routine use of intraoperative periapical radiographs during the drilling sequence can help avoid the risk of injury to the inferior alveolar nerve. The clinician needs to determine safe distances between the implant and the inferior alveolar canal, thus avoiding the risk of injury to the nerve (Burstein, Mastin and Le 2008); tilting implant fixtures may help avoid anatomical structures (Dreiseidler et al. 2009).

There are limited reports available in the literature documenting the effect of surgical experience on the accuracy of implant placement. Surgical experience may have more impact in complex cases, especially if the anatomy at the implant recipient site varies significantly from the prosthetically planned position.

9.4 Predictability of Regenerative Materials and Techniques

Our bones have a marvelous natural design, continuously rejuvenating through a finely tuned equilibrium of bone resorption and new bone formation. To understand the worth of bone grafting, one has to be conjugated with bone tissue and its significance. The anatomical and functional components of human bone include: (1) organic matrix, which makes up 40% of the weight of bone and is composed of type I collagen, proteoglycans, cytokines, and growth factors; (2) mineralized matrix, making up 60% of the weight of bone and composed of hydroxyapatite crystals: Ca10 (PO4)(OH)2; (3) cells: osteoprogenitor cells (from mesenchymal cells), osteoblasts, osteoclasts, and osteocytes (mature bone cells in the bone matrix that it previously secreted as osteoblasts; (4) vascular and nutrition distribution: bone receives 5–10% of cardiac output, arterial supply, lymphatics, and venous return: (5) neurological: autonomic in function; (6) marrow; which serves both hematopoietic and osteogenic functions; (7) periosteum, which is the 'outer fibrous envelope,' a source of osteoprogenitor cells, neurovascular distribution, and blood supply; (8) endosteum, which is the 'inner osteogenic layer,' a thin layer of connective tissue that lines the surface of the bony tissue that forms the medullary cavity of long bones; and (9) communication system, which is a network including Haversian and Volksmann's canals, canaliculi, lacunae, and extracellular fluid (Amini, Laurencin and Nukavarapu 2012).

On the basis of the physical structural composition, bone may be classified as: (1) compact bone, is a dense, solid bone found at the outer cortical layer of maxilla or mandible or the cortical plate of the extraction socket; (2) trabecular bone is located between the cortical plates of the maxilla or mandible and may also be referred to as spongy or cancellous bone; (3) woven (embryonic) bone is a less-organized, poorly mineralized bone and is the first type of bone observed in a healing extraction site; and (4) lamellar bone is a secondary structure of bone arranged in a typical layered fashion (Amini et al. 2012).

On the osseous cellular level, osteoblasts and osteocytes are derived from osteoprogenitor cells, but osteoclasts are derived from the same cells that differentiate to form macrophages and monocytes (Bilezikian, Raisz and Marti 2008). Osteoprogenitor cells are the undifferentiated stem cells and differentiate into preosteoblastic and mature osteoblastic cells lining the endosteal surfaces of bone. They robustly produce alkaline phosphatase, an enzyme that has a role in the mineralization of bone, as well as many matrix proteins (Carlsson, Bergman and Hedegård 1967b).

An osteoblast is the "bone-forming" cell responsible for deposition and calcification of the extracellular bone matrix. The osteocyte is a mature, fully differentiated osteoblast that is surrounded by mineralized bone matrix. While it is no longer active in terms of forming bone matrix, it does play a role in cell-to-cell communication. The osteoclast cell is responsible for the resorptive aspect of bone modeling and remodeling. All of these cells are regulated via secreted enzymes such as collagenase and lysosomal enzymes (Tevlin et al. 2014).

As a result of the continuous demand to provide optimal implant osseous housing, numerous grafting materials and techniques have been proposed in the past four decades. Advances in biomaterials research and the development of new and improved surgical techniques and armamentarium have allowed the placement of dental implants in deficient alveolar ridge areas. The ultimate goal for these bone-grafting procedures is to amend osseous deficiencies of the jaws. In a cohort study by Petersson, Lindh and Carlsson (1992), 20% of the maxillary edentulous patients needed bone-grafting procedures before the placement of dental implants, which gives an insight into the vast demand for using regenerative materials and techniques.

Alveolar bone volume is often reduced after tooth extraction for many reasons, (Esposito et al. 2008; Khoury and Buchmann 2001; Rocchietta, Fontana and Simion 2008). After tooth extraction an average alveolar bone loss of 1.5–2 mm (vertical) and 40–50% (horizontal) occurs within six months (Liu and Kerns 2014; Van der Weijden, Dell'Acqua and Slot 2009). Most alveolar dimensional changes occur during the first three months (Schropp et al. 2003). If no treatment to restore the lost dentition is performed, then continued bone loss occurs with up to 40–60% of ridge volume lost in the first three years (Bernstein et al. 2006; Carlsson et al. 1967a; Tallgren 2003).

The loss of vertical bone height poses great challenges for dental implant placement due to surgical difficulties and anatomical limitations (Rocchietta et al. 2008). This lack of sufficient bone volume, if unresolved, is eventually detrimental to the final treatment outcome with respect to implant success, prosthetic rehabilitation, and long term survival (Rocchietta et al. 2008; Tolman 1993). Early on several bone grafting techniques and materials were developed to fulfill the high demand for treating a defective alveolar ridge. These include guided bone regeneration with or without particulate bone grafting, ridge splitting, distraction osteogenesis, orthodontic tooth movement through a deficient ridge, and grafting of bone blocks harvested intraorally, extraorally, or from cadaveric (allogeneic) sources (Chiapasco, Zaniboni and Rimondini 2007; Roccuzzo et al. 2007; Sacco and Chepeha 2007; Von Arx and Buser 2006; Von Arx, Hardt and Wallkamm 1996).

9.4.1 Etiology of Bone Grafting Complications

It is the author's personal opinion that the most frequent treatment complications are those related to regenerative therapy, because bone deficiency before implant placement can pose a challenge to many clinicians. These complications challenge the clinicians' ability to identify etiologies and provide proper and timely management of these problems. It is also the author's personal opinion that regenerative complications often occur because of the poor management of the overlying soft tissue, or the poor response of the soft tissue to surgical manipulations. The author strongly recommends that a superior level of basic surgical knowledge regarding the manipulation of soft tissue must be obtained and perfected prior to learning the art and science of bone regeneration therapy.

9.4.1.1 Soft Tissue Influence on the Regenerative Therapy Outcome

Adequate soft-tissue coverage of any grafted bone is mandatory to the overall success of regenerative therapy, as it protects the graft material and isolates it from the oral environment (Abrahamsson 2011). With increasing alveolar ridge size by bone grafting complements, the related soft tissue is manipulated so it is elongated to allow a tension-free coverage of the bone graft components. There is always an increased risk of graft exposure with these manipulations, for many reasons that include the patient's oral hygiene, the patient's habits, and the patient's systemic condition, and the operator's skills. Therefore, the assessment of soft tissue parameters should be encouraged to identify any possible long-term complications of grafting therapy (see Figure 9.9a & b).

Cordaro et al. (2011) and Chiapasco et al. (2007) studied several soft tissue related clinical parameters including: modified plaque index, modified bleeding index, and probing depth. Hiatt and Schallhorn (1973) found that the degree of regeneration directly correlates with the adequacy of soft tissue cover and the surface area of the vascularized defect bony walls, implying that primary wound coverage is fundamental for bone regeneration. Tolman (1995) and Brener (2006) indicated that wound dehiscence was directly related to implant failure.

The clinician should inspect the planned graft recipient site for soft tissue phenotype, including quality, amount of keratinized mucosa, tissue thickness, high muscle attachments, and pre-existing scarring. Any inflammation of the

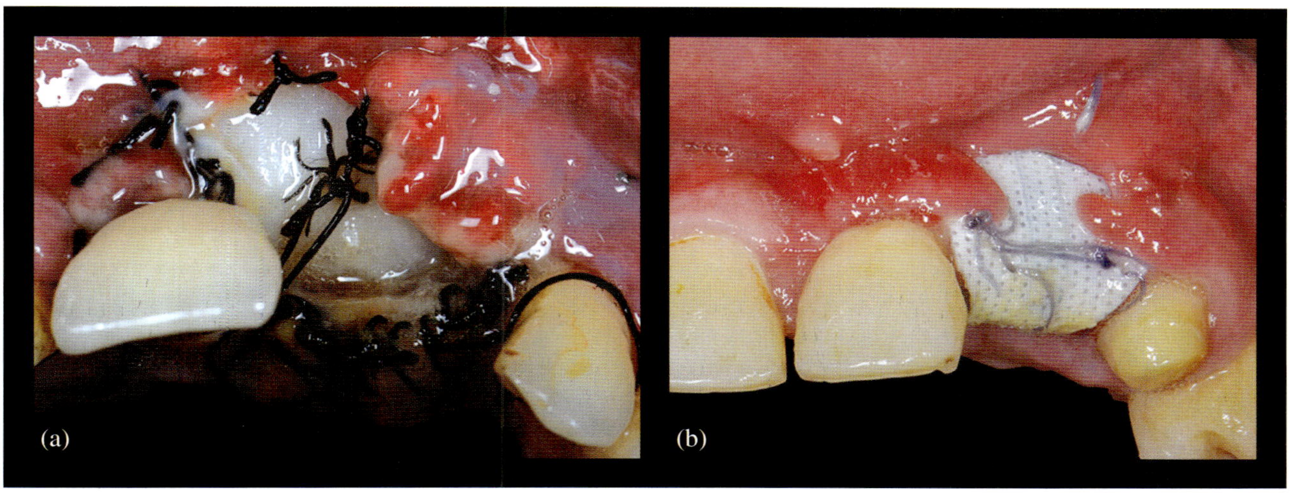

Figure 9.9 (a) Sever sloughing as a result of smoking. (b) Poor technical skills managing soft tissues that lead to sever wound sloughing.

overlying soft tissues should be resolved before surgery. Soft tissue-borne prostheses may require adjustment and presurgical tissue conditioning with liners. Poor oral hygiene must be corrected by both patients and hygienists, the decision on whether to correct defective soft tissue prior or along with graft placement remains a controversial issue (Ioannou et al. 2015).

Preregenerative soft tissue optimization provides better tissue quality and thicker tissue to maintain flap closure (see Figure 9.10a–c). Short vestibular depth or muscle attachments may also be managed during soft tissue corrective surgery to increase the zone of keratinized tissue by using autogenous free gingival grafts or allograft dermis, or a palatal pedicle connective tissue graft can be used when the overlying mucosa is thin in the recipient site. In this way, the soft tissue volume may be enhanced, which ensures a vascular supply to the graft (Froum 2013).

When staged soft tissue corrective surgery is planned, it should be performed at least eight weeks before bone graft surgery to allow incorporation of grafted tissue and re-establishment of vascularity to the area. Pre-existing scar tissue can also cause resistance to adaptation of the wound margins. In addition, scar tissue compromises the blood supply and healing of the flaps and reduces flap resiliency. For this reason, the retreatment of failed augmentation cases is more complicated and should be managed by experienced surgeons (see Figure 9.11a–c). However, it is the author's personal opinion that repeated oral corrective surgeries at the same site leads to soft tissue rigidity and scar tissue formation that can limit flap mobility and impede vascular supply to the flap. Therefore minimizing the number of surgeries (whenever possible) offers a better surgical outcome of the regenerative procedure.

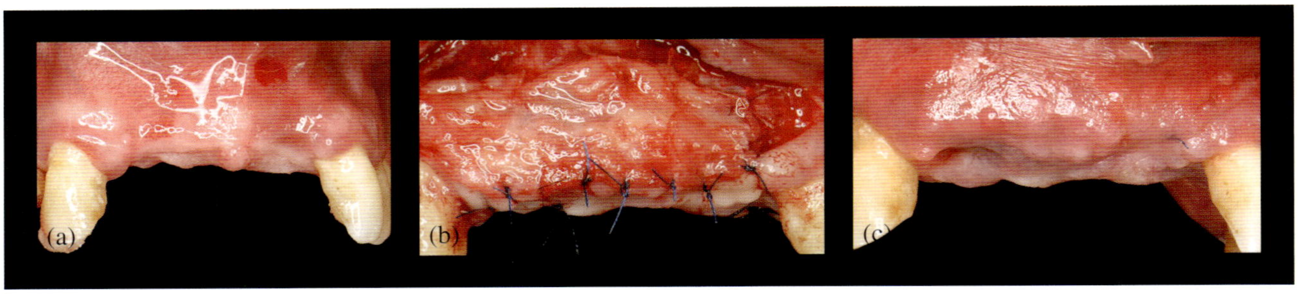

Figure 9.10 (a) Lack of keratinize tissue band related to missing anterior teeth that requires both bone grafting as well as enhancement of the soft tissue status, (b) Inlay connective tissue graft is placed and partially secured, (c) Four weeks post soft tissue grafting showing improvement in the keratinized tissue band.

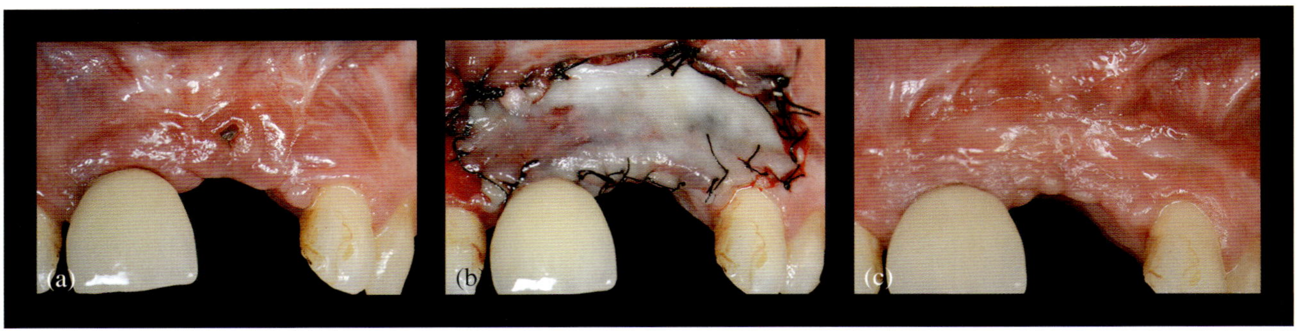

Figure 9.11 (a) Multiple scar tissue formation and narrowing of the vestibule due to multiple surgeries, (b) Onlay keratinized tissue graft stabilized, (c) Final healing showing improved keratinized tissue graft.

Basic surgical skills and knowledge in soft tissue management should be obtained prior to performing bone grafting surgeries; crestal incisions maintain vascular supply to the flap because blood vessels on the labial side don't anastomose with the palatal side (Talwar 2012). Incisions made significantly palatal to the ridge in the maxilla and buccal to the ridge in the posterior mandible can result in wound breakdown due to postoperative tissue necrosis. Divergent releasing incisions remote to the defect produce a broad-based flap that facilitates closure and also maintains a sufficient blood supply. It is pererable to make the primary crestal incision by bisecting the keratinized mucosa.

To provide more length and elasticity to the flap, several steps are taken to advance the soft tissue flap over any bone graft. The mucoperiosteal flap reflection should extend well beyond the localized area of bone repair. Secondary vertical or oblique releasing incisions also improve flap mobility. The greatest limitation to flap advancement over the bone graft is periosteum rigidity. A horizontal incision is made, through the thin periosteal layer along the deepest area of the facial flap. The periosteal incision should extend along the entire base of the flap and connect to the borders of the vertical releasing incisions. It is important that the periosteal incision remains superficial. After the periosteal releasing incision is made, the flap is tested and stretched to assess closure without tension. If resistance to adapting the wound margins is noted then further flap release can be obtained with blunt dissection through the periosteal release and beyond the vestibular depth (Misch 1999). In the maxilla, the palatal tissue is rigid and can't be mobilized, lingual flap advancement can be obtained in the posterior mandible by reflecting the mucoperiosteal flap to the mylohyoid muscle attachment and using a finger to stretch and release or brush the thin periosteum (see Figure 9.12a–g).

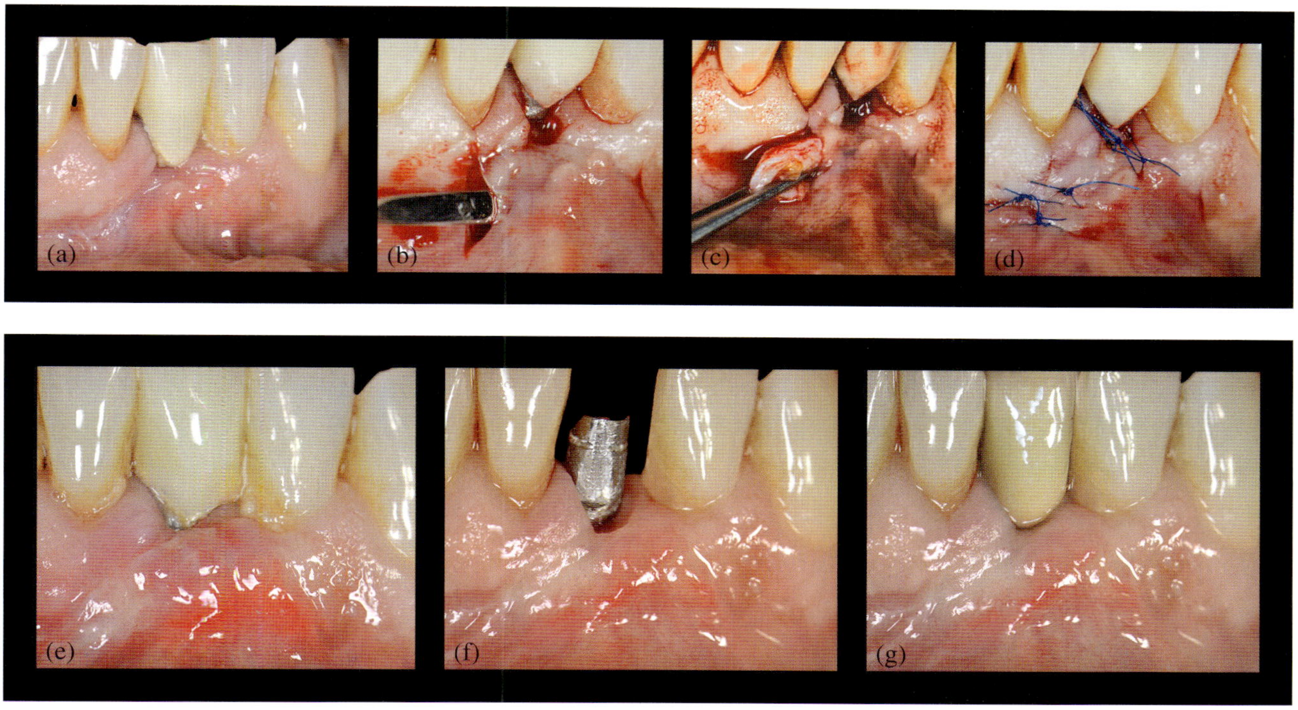

Figure 9.12 (a) Scar tissue formation, Soft tissue defect post implant placement, (b) Verticular sulcular incision (tunnel), (c) Connective tissue graft inserted, (d) Flap sutured, (e) One week post-surgery, (f) One month post-surgery, (g) Six months post-surgery.

It is common to end up with reduced vestibular depth after regenerative therapies due to advancement of the facial flap over the graft. Although it is important that the flap margins are well approximated, the sutures should not be pulled too tightly or ischemia will occur. The flaps should be closed over the bone graft with suture materials that maintain their tensile strength until the wound has completely healed (Misch and Moore 1989). The addition of supplemental growth factors has been reported to enhance and accelerate soft tissue wound healing (Marx, Carlson and Eichstaedt 1998). Platelet-rich plasma has been shown to improve the healing of skin graft donor sites (Monteleone, Marx and Ghurani 2000). Many clinicians have anecdotally observed the positive effect of autologous growth factors on soft-tissue healing. The various cytokines and mediators found in the alpha granules of the platelets promote angiogenesis and collagen synthesis (Cromack, Porras-Reyes and Mustoe 1990). This may enhance soft tissue healing and diminish the risk of wound dehiscence and bone graft exposure to the oral cavity. However the use of autologous growth factors should be only considered as a healing promoter not as regenerative material.

The development of recombinant human platelet-derived growth factor (rhPDGF) provides another strategy for improving wound healing and preventing complications (Kaigler, Cirelli and Giannobile 2006). This form of the growth factor is estimated to be 1000 times the strength of autologous platelet-rich plasma and avoids the need for procuring blood for centrifuging. The liquid rhPDGF may be soaked into a thin collagen sponge and placed over the graft site before closure. However, the capacity of these growth factors to promote bone formation is questioned and debatable.

The postoperative management of wound dehiscence (see Figure 9.13) when it occurs after bone grafting procedure is based on the biological principle that the graft is non-viable until revascularized. No attempt should be made to resuture or manipulate the surrounding flaps as the edematous soft tissue is inflamed and friable. Once bone graft material is exposed to the oral cavity the bone graft is contaminated with the oral bacteria. at this stage the bone graft would not offer any clinical benefit. Even if it is not removed and did not cause any tissue reactions, it loses its potential for bone formation. Minimal sharp protruding edges of any block bone graft should be smoothed and reduced with a coarse diamond bur or any trimming forceps, if any soft tissue defect appears, then it might be covered with a partial thickness soft tissue pedicle flap rotated from the adjacent tissues, If more than 2 mm of the bone graft becomes exposed the prognosis is poor and graft removal should be considered (Carlson and Monteleone 2004). Also, the duration of the graft exposure to the oral environment is crucial, the literature did not answer the question one how long could the bone graft be exposed to the oral environment and still be viable for regeneration (see Figure 9.14a–e).

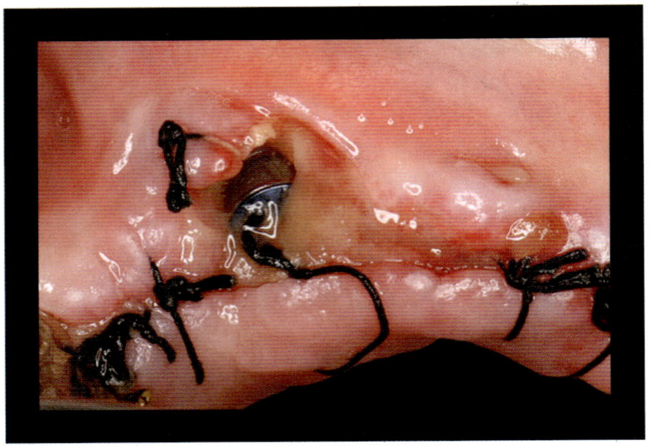

Figure 9.13 Bone graft is lost due to wound dehiscence.

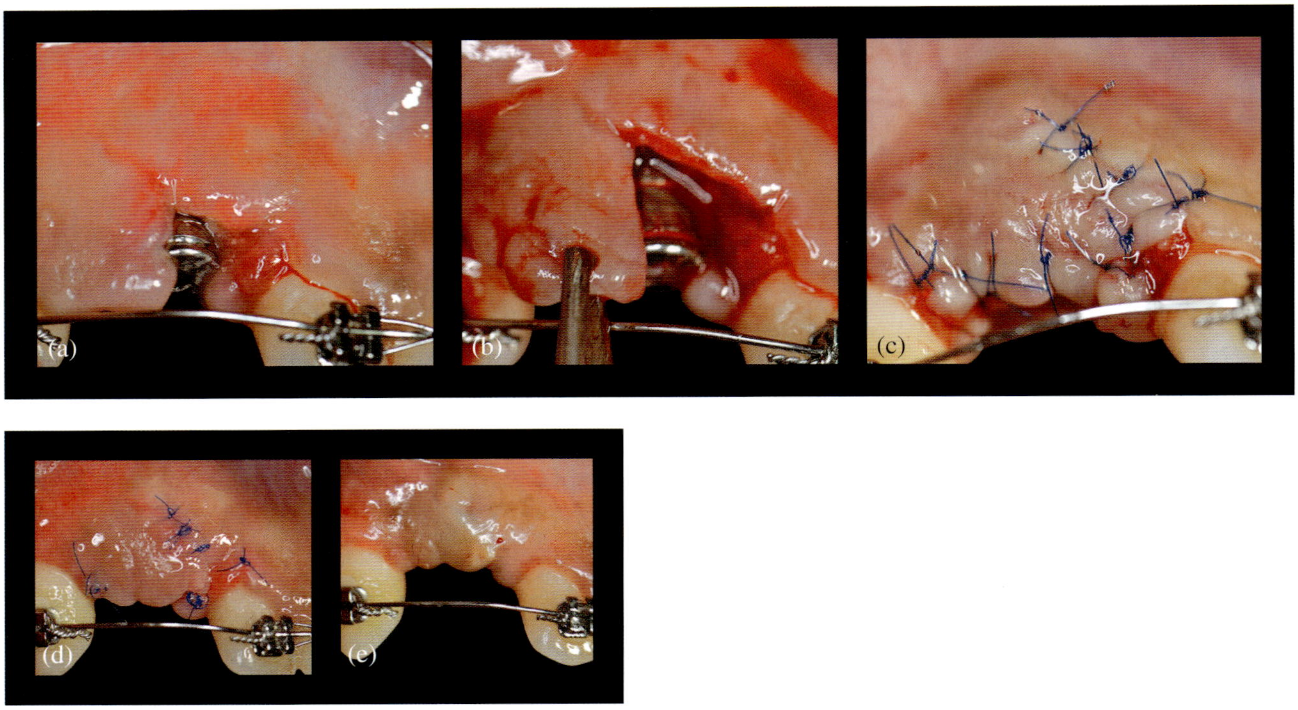

Figure 9.14 (a) Dehiscence around an implant from the labial side, (b) De-epithelializing wound edges and flap mobilization, (c) Medial mobilization of the flap and suturing, (d) One week post healing, (e) One month post healing with enhancement of the keratinized tissue quality and dehiscence coverage.

Oral wound Dehiscence at the incision probably is the most common postoperative complication of implant surgery (Cranin 1999; Dominici 1988) (see Figure 9.15a–d).

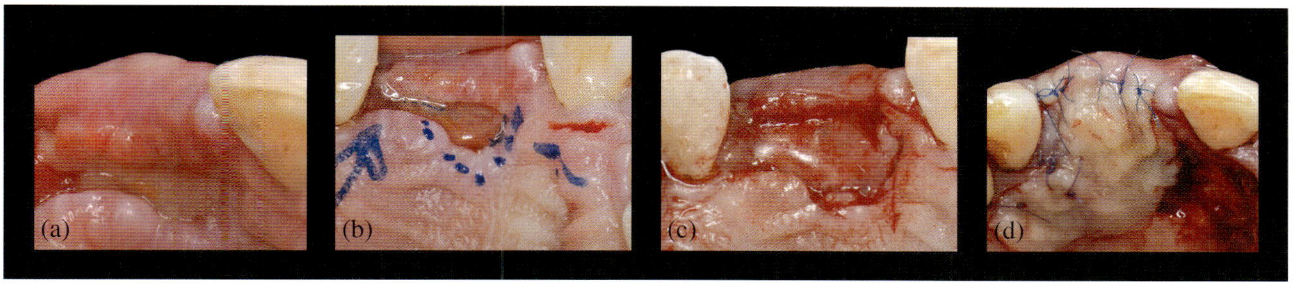

Figure 9.15 (a) Wound sloughing on top of grafted alveolar ridge defect, (b) Outlines of the flap, (c) Freshening wound edges, (d) Rotated palatal pedicle to the labial site to cover the defect.

Wound healing is influenced by a number of local and systemic factors. Superficial infections can occur along the suture line. Postoperative infection of soft tissue sometimes can be attributed to insufficient tightening of the cover screw, preoperative contamination, or retained sutures (Beirne and Worthington 1991; Jovanovic, Spiekermann and Richter 1992) (see Figures 9.16–9.18a, b, 9.19a–b, and 9.20a–c). Infection, if present, could prevent connective tissue repair and perpetuate the inflammatory response, causing neutrophils to release lysosomal enzymes, which results in proteolysis (tissue breakdown). Furthermore, local bacteria of the granulating surface occasionally inhibit epithelialization, especially certain streptococcus and pyogencus (Aligower 1981; Trowbridge and Emling 1997).

General factors interfering with wound healing include age, low serum protein, vitamins C, A, and K, reduced number of erythrocytes, histamine liberators,

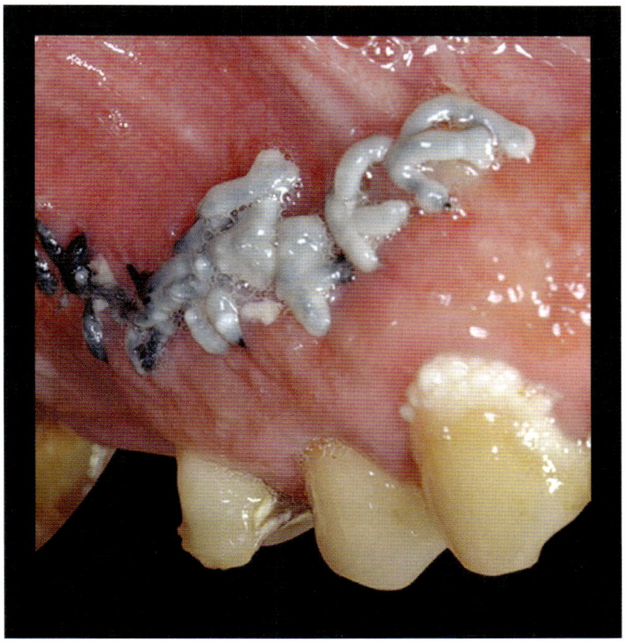

Figure 9.17 Plaque accumulation around suture that predicts poor healing.

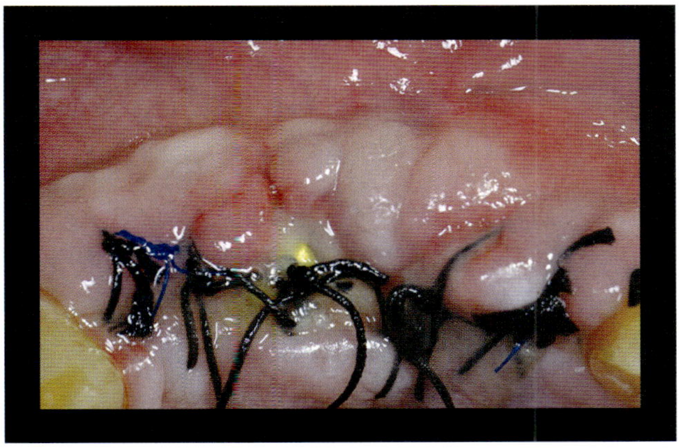

Figure 9.16 Classic clinica picture of wound sloughing as a result of flap closure under tension.

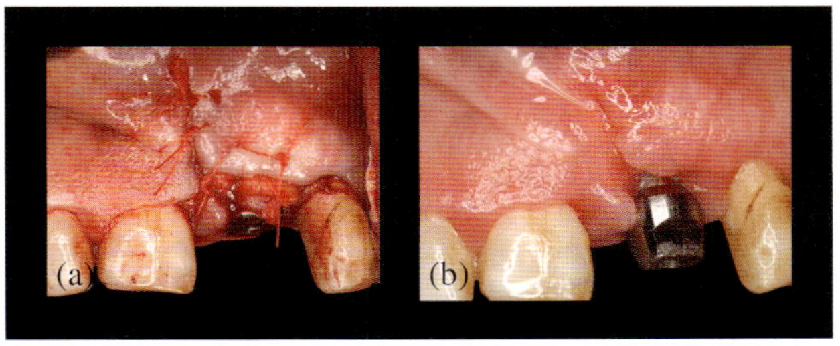

Figure 9.18 (a) Poor flap design, poor suturing technique, (b) Poor healing outcome.

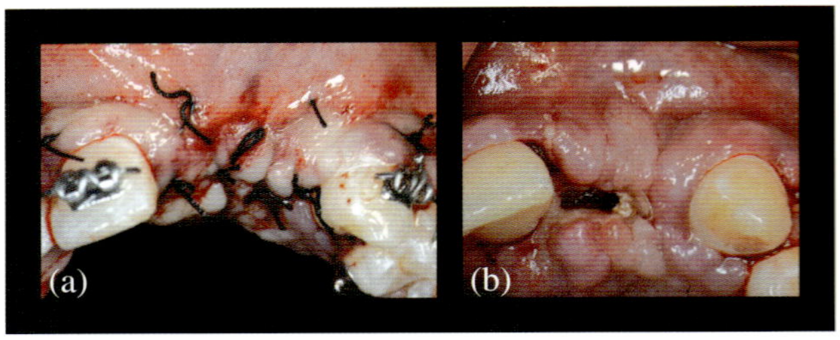

Figure 9.19 (a) Poor flap relaxation, poor suturing technique, (b) Incision line opening.

and hormone imbalance (Aligower 1981). Pathologic conditions that cause poor vascularity and decrease an inflammatory response, like uncontrolled diabetes mellitus, anemia, uremia, collagen disorders, and jaundice, have been reported to play a role in wound healing impairment (Shelton 1991). In general, the most important cause of delay in wound healing is interference with the microcirculation (Beirne and Worthington 1991). This can result either from local damage to the vessels by traumatic surgical maneuvers, or oral habits such as cigarette smoking (Klokkevold and Han 2007). The tobacco influence for promoting vasoconstriction might explain its effect on oral wounds, as it is a major contributor to wound dehiscence; a cessation protocol should be applied to patients who smoke to reduce the tendency of oral wound complications. A protocol was developed in which patients who smoked stopped smoking one week before dental implant placement, followed by eight more weeks without smoking to allow initial healing. The efficacy of a preoperative and postoperative smoking cessation protocol may benefit the patient. A prospective evaluation of this protocol in a pilot trial with 78 patients having over 200 implants showed an implant failure rate of 12% in the patients who followed the smoking cessation protocol compared with 38% in those who continued to smoke (Bain 1996).

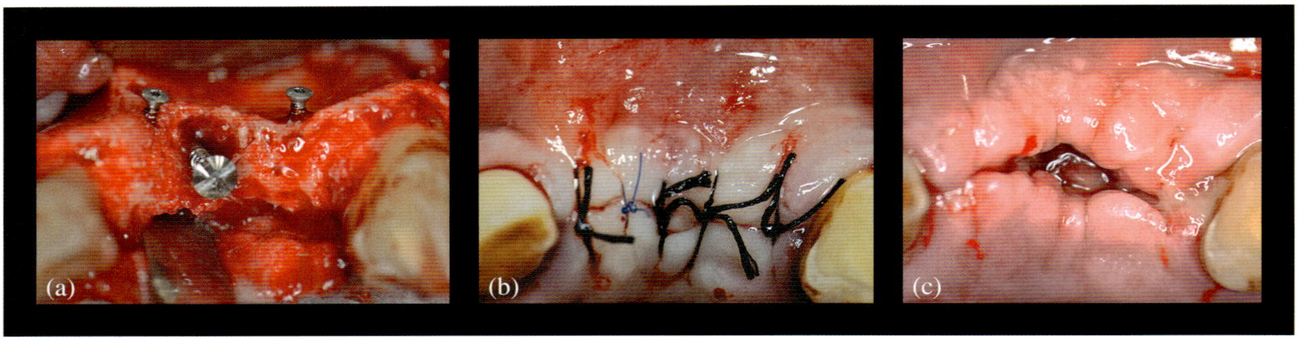

Figure 9.20 (a) Three screws were used to tent the grafting complex, (b) Wound closure is attempted (note the tension on the suture line), (c) Wound opened due to tension.

9.4.1.2 Influential Factors to Wound Healing

The primary objective of dental suturing is to adapt and retain surgical flaps to promote hemostasis and optimal healing. The failure of a suture to secure a wound closure is usually the result of undoing or tearing of a knot (Aligower 1981). The selection of correct suturing material and proper selection of the needle contributes to overall wound healing (Aligower 1981) (see Figures 9.21a–c).

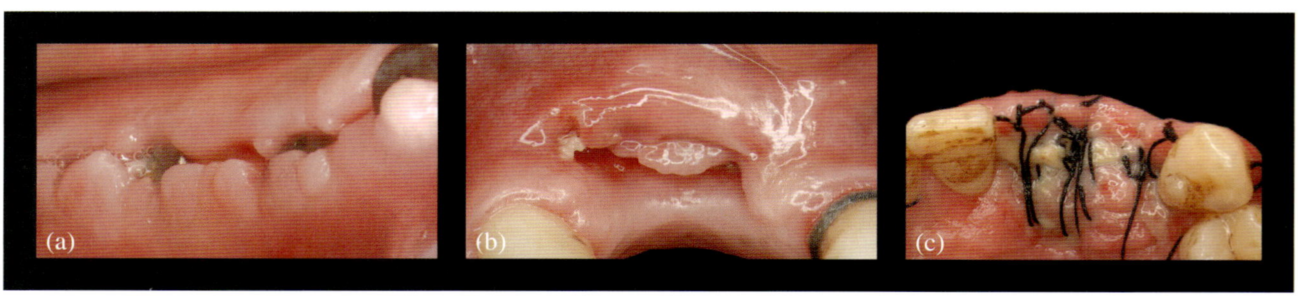

Figure 9.21 (a–c) Minor, moderate and critical flap dehiscence.

As a result of the inability to approximate tissue flaps, flaps closed under tension, the opened suture line could result in an exposed area of alveolar bone, contributing to necrosis, pain, significant bone loss, and delayed healing (Giglio and Laskin 1998). Suturing that is too tight can inhibit blood flow to the flap or lead to oral tissue laceration and lead to wound margin necrosis with dehiscence formation (Politis et al. 2016). When an extensive grafting procedure is performed with an increased operative time, multiple mucoperiosteal stripping often occurs in an attempt at primary wound closure, and a compromised blood supply is expected (Collins and Collins 1998). Wound breakdown would occur if the muccoperiosteal flap is lacerated as a result. Tissue phenotype pays an important role in oral wound healing.

When keratinized tissue band is insufficient, soft tissue closure will be performed on non-attached or vestibular tissues, the fragile edges become inflamed and lose the major part of their tensile strength 24–48 hours after surgery (George and Krishnamurthy 2013).

Suturing is yet another critical treatment step in soft tissue management. The optimal suture material has the following characteristics:

1) A minimal size that holds the wound edges together to minimize tissue trauma and piercing. The tensile strength of the suture need never exceed the tensile strength of the tissue.
2) Facilitates easy passage through tissue with minimal drag.
3) Allows precise knot placement.
4) Allows smooth tie-down and a decreased tendency to incarcerate tissue (Van Winkle and Hastings 1972).

The main requirements for any optimal suture material are (1) sterility, (2) non-electrolytic, (3) non-capillary, (4) non-allergenic, (5) non-carcinogenic, (6) non-ferromagnetic, (7) minimally reactive to the tissues, (8) high tensile strength to secure wound edges with no cutting or tearing, (9) shrinkage resistance, (10) pliability for ease of handling, and (11) consistent uniform diameter.

Sutures need to be either resorbable or non-resorbable or monofilament or multifilament. The monofilament sutures pass through tissue easier than multifilament sutures and do not attract microorganisms that may cause suture line infection (Lysimachos et al. 2010). They are also tied down easily. On the other hand, multifilament sutures attain greater tensile strength and flexibility, but are liable to attract bacteria (see Figure 9.22a–f).

Resorbable sutures might be naturally or synthetically absorbed by hydrolysis, which offers minimal tissue reaction. During the first stage of the absorption process, tensile strength diminishes in a gradual, almost

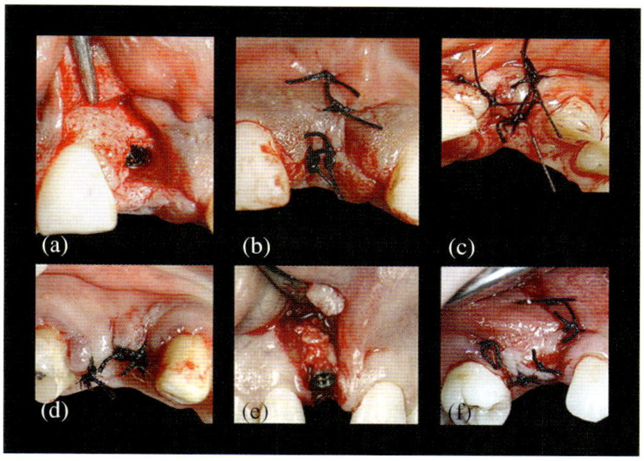

Figure 9.22 (a–f) Examples of faulty soft tissue management and suturing.

linear fashion. The second stage often follows with considerable overlap, characterized by loss of suture body mass. Both stages exhibit leukocytic cellular responses that serve to remove cellular debris and suture material from the line of tissue approximation. Drawbacks of resorbable sutures are infection and premature absorption due to exposure to tissue fluids in the oral cavity; non-resorbable sutures offer more tensile strength and less tissue reaction. Good examples of non-resorbable sutures are black silk and nylon. Nylon is a very inert suturing material because it causes minimum tissue reaction and provides the least inflammatory response around it. Even if it is left for a longer time in the oral wounds, it does not seem to cause any bacterial aggregation around it. However, its sharp edges can cause oral ulcers when it is located at the site of a moving organ such as the tongue or the lips. Needles should cause the least trauma to the tissues and should be as small as possible to minimize tissue piercing. They should be sharp, rigid, and corrosion resistant. Sutures should be removed using aseptic and sterile techniques. The steps for suture removal are:

1) Clean with antiseptic solution or swabbing material.
2) Pick up one end of the suture with thumb forceps and cut as close to the skin as possible where the suture enters the skin.
3) Gently pull the suture strand out though the side opposite the knot with the forceps.

Incision design is yet another factor to oral wound healing; the two most popular incisions for placement of implants are crestal and vestibular incisions. Although not well documented, disadvantages of crestal flap designs include a higher incidence of wound dehiscence and increased difficulty in managing knife-edge ridges and the possibility of flap perforation (Moy, Weiniaender and Kennedy 1989). Vestibular incisions can offer advantages of not having the implant or bone grafts located directly under the incision. Therefore, there is less chance that dehiscence will result in implant exposure; however, there is generally more edema and greater patient discomfort with this type of incision. Also, suture placement and removal are more difficult, and the flange of any transitional prosthesis might impinge on the incision (Hunt et al. 1996; Moy et al. 1989) (see Figures 9.23a and b).

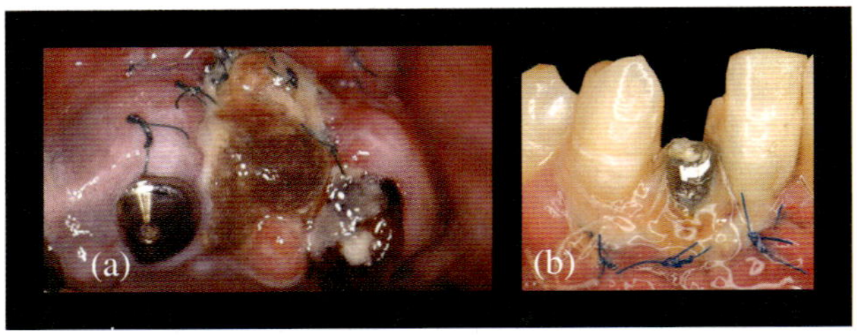

Figure 9.23 (a) and (b) Soft tissue necrosis due to improper flap design.

An incision that is too small results in excessive retraction on the flap and increases the risk of tearing the mucosa. Torn mucosal flaps will likely undergo necrosis, delay healing, and possibly contribute to implant failure (Giglio and Laskin 1998).

Generally speaking, the standard protocol for delayed submerged implant installation in the esthetic zone first entails administering a local anesthetic solution. Next, a crestal incision is made slightly on the palatal aspect or in the mid-crestal position. The incision ends at the distal surface of the teeth adjacent to the buccal and palatal aspect of the alveolar crest. Buccal-relieving incisions are only made when necessary, that is, excluding the interproximal papilla. Subsequently, the buccal and palatal mucoperiosteal flaps are then reflected carefully to ensure minimal atraumatic soft tissue handling. However, conservative flap design is becoming a routine treatment discipline in modern esthetic dental implantology. Although it is becoming an integral part of any esthetic treatment plan, it avoids unnecessary tissue reflection while providing sufficient access to the underlying structures during implant surgery. A number of incision designs are used during implant placement at first-stage surgery. Many clinical benefits have evolved from these designs, which that have contributed to today's routine clinical practice (Becker and Becker 1996; Palacci 2004). Most of the currently available techniques aim to preserve natural esthetics and fulfill the standard operative standards for mucoperiosteal flap management (see Figure 9.24a and b).

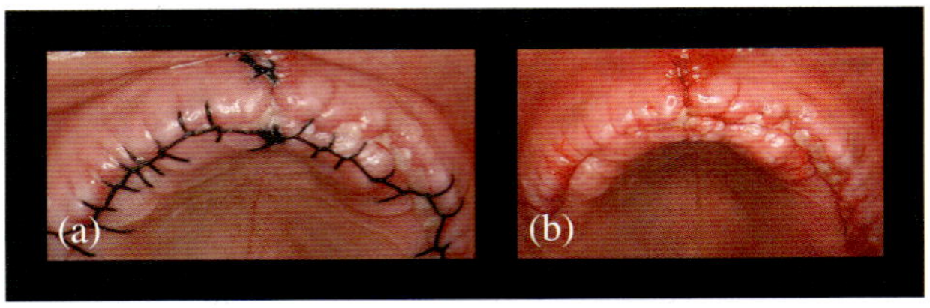

Figure 9.24 (a) Optimal tissue healing on the right side of the patient while tissue sloughing due to the mechanical trauma from eating on the left side, (b) Case after suture removal showing the poor wound healing on the left side.

The periostium is an important factor influencing the healing of oral wounds. Periosteal integrity and vascularity are considered important elements in wound healing post-surgery, and angiogenesis may be important for designing a flap and a suturing method that gives a stable postoperative result. Nobuto and others (2005) have monitored the role of the periosteum in tissue healing and postoperative angiogenesis. They investigated the role of the periosteal vascular plexus in the healing process and used 3D and ultrastructural monitoring of the angiogenic process after elevation of the mucoperiosteal flap. Mucoperiosteal flap surgery was performed on nine adult beagle dogs. The periosteal vascular plexus was observed at three, five, and seven days after surgery in histological specimens in which blood vessels were injected with India ink under a light microscope, in ultrathin sections under a transmission electron microscope and in acryl plastic vascular cast specimens under a scanning electron microscope. On day three after surgery, new blood vessels, formed through sprouting, bridging. In addition, island-like structures consisting of clustered immature endothelial cells were noted in the repaired tissue. On days five to seven after surgery, 3D observation of vascular casts clarified that these new blood vessels had a sinus-like morphology in the interstitium of the periosteal vascular plexus. These new sinusoidal vessels exhibited a stereoscopic structure with increased continuity as the blood vessels matured and the ultrastructural vascular endothelium was thinned (see Figures 9.25a and b).

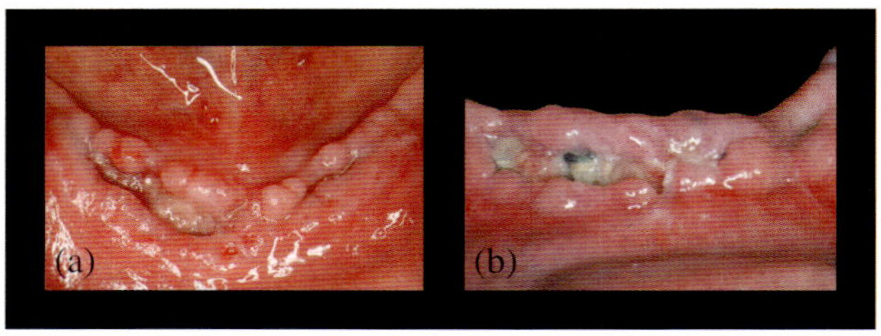

Figure 9.25 (a) and (b) Flap dehiscence due to the poor flap design and the continuous muscle pull along the wound edges.

The study concluded that after mucoperiosteal flap elevation, the periosteal vascularity exhibited potent blood vessel-forming activity through various angiogenic mechanisms and through repair activity. Therefore, clinicians should minimize periosteal manipulation as much as possible during the surgery to maintain the maximum tissue reparative capacity. Surgical entries to install an implant fixture within the bone have several modalities, and each one offers a clinical benefit and has a clinical indication. The modalities can vary greatly and include a delayed submerged implant placement protocol (crestal and vestibular approaches), flapless non-submerged implant placement protocol, delayed non-submerged protocol, immediate implant placement protocol with complete soft tissue closure that is currently rarely used, and immediate implant placement protocol without complete soft tissue closure (Block and Kent 1991; Brånemark 1972).

9.4.1.3 Management of Mucoperiosteal Flap Dehiscence

Tissue healing requires only a daily debridement and wound toilet using antibacterial mouthwash until the tissue closes by secondary intention (Cranin 1999). When dehiscence occurred, any attempt to resuture the dehiscent wound will not attain any additional benefit. It was also recommended that the wound should be immediately re-sutured after the margins have been freshened with a scalpel. This redemption might be accompanied by bone reduction maneuvers to prevent bone necrosis (Collins and Collins 1998).

The following factors are worth recognizing before considering the successful management of dehiscent wounds (Sadig and Almas 2004): (1) the cause of the dehiscence should be determined; (2) site of the dehiscence; (3) the length of the dehiscence and flap design; (4) the condition of the wound margins and amount of remaining attached gingiva; (5) the anatomic shape of the ridge crest ridge, thick, broad, thin, or knife edged; (6) the presence or absence and type of bone graft and regenerative membrane; (7) the underlying and adjacent living tissue, and whether it consists of vessels, muscles, or nerves; (8) the time elapsed since the wound breakdown took place; (9) the presence or absence of soft tissue infection, edema, or hematoma; (10) the presence or absence of denuded or necrotic bone; (11) the age and the underlying systemic condition of the patient; and (12) compliance to postoperative instructions and availability of the patient for frequent follow-up appointments.

In a protocol for management of a dehiscent wound in implant therapy, Sadig and Almas (2004) proposed a treatment plan according to the wound condition and patient considerations. For protocol P-1, a small dehiscent wound around 1–2 cm presented within 24–48 hours post-surgery at any site in the mouth, the clinician may immediately resuture the dehiscence followed by regular monitoring. For protocol P-2, when P-1 was unsuccessful and the time elapsed is more than two to three days, with a large dehiscence of 2–3 cm, exposed bone but not necrotic, wound margins not abused or fragile, or even in the presence of a bone graft or membrane, the clinician may consider excision of wound margins before resuturing (see Figure 9.26). As for protocol P-3, when wound margins are traumatized in the anterior region of the mouth the bone is left exposed but not necrotic with the presence of lacerated non-attached gingival. In such a situation, wound debridement with antibiotic added to the isotonic solution adjuncts the treatment along with thorough irrigation and mouth washings with chlorhexidine or iodine solution every other day. The clinician needs to cover the denuded bone with dressing iodine followed by gradual reduction in dressing size and wound monitoring for three to six weeks until healing by secondary intention. For protocol P-4, if there is denuded necrotic bone in the posterior mandibular region of the mouth with an extremely knife-edged residual ridge and the patient is elderly and debilitated, it is recommended that the bone graft be removed and any necrosed bone be trimmed until fresh bone is reached with resultant fresh bleeding. Implant removal could also be carried out if the implant is infected, becomes mobile or interferes with tissue closure; a large mobilization of the mucoperiosteal flap buccally and lingually should be performed to cover the denuded bone, followed by suturing, and an antibiotic regimen should be started for a minimum of 10 days.

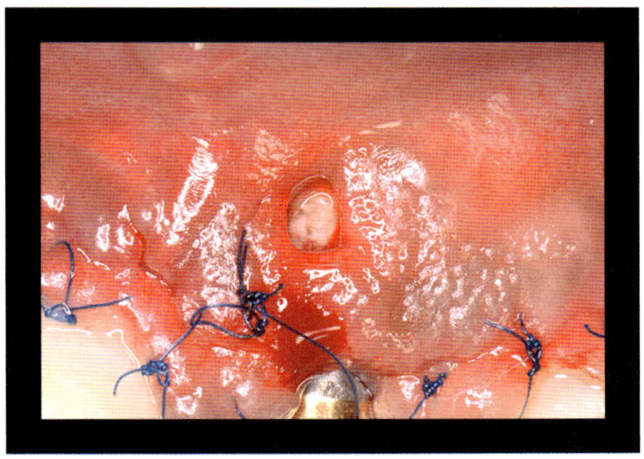

Figure 9.26 Wound dehiscence on top of grafted bone as a result of poor tissue handling and poor soft tissue quality.

It is the author's experience that, depending upon the extent of flap dehiscence, the complication may be described as *minor*, *moderate*, or *critical*. (1) For a *minor flap* margins dehiscence the clinician may leave the wound clean and maintain the site with chlorohexidine application and vigorous saline irrigation; (2) *Moderate flap* margins dehiscence, it depend on the duration of the graft exposure: when the graft is recently exposed (few days), a buccal or palatal pedicle rotated flap is elevated, rotated to the lacerated site and sutured to the freshened edges. If the patient presents with an exposed bone graft that occurred more than (few days) previously, the graft should be removed completely, the site curetted well, irrigated with normal saline, and any regrafting attempts abandoned till complete healing occurs.

A rotated palatal subepithelial connective tissue graft (RPSCTG) may be used to cover the graft materials. After administration of local anesthesia on the palatal donor site, two parallel palatal incisions are made from the right first molar area and run anteriorly to the crestal incision line to obtain pedicled connective tissue. The superficial epithelial tissue is dissected with a sharp blade (No. 15 c) and retracted posteriorly; subsequently, the deep subepithelial connective tissue flap is dissected, elevated, and rotated anteriorly to cover the exposed graft site and sutured. In the donor site, the superficial epithelial flap was placed in its original position and sutured. Postoperatively, antibiotic coverage continued for a week along with saline water mouth gargle. (3) In *critical flap marginal dehiscences*, when the implant or bone augmentation site is lacking keratinized tissue and the graft exposure area is fresh (only a few days), a coronally repositioned flap is performed along with a connective tissue graft underneath it to enhance the keratinized tissue band; acellular dermal matrix (ADM) (AlloDerm BioHorizons, Birmingham, AL, USA) can be used after wound healing under the flap to enhance soft tissue quality. ADM is an acellular dermal matrix designed to serve as a biologic scaffold for normal tissue remodeling. ADM contains both the structure and the biochemical information to direct normal revascularization and cell repopulation, preserved proteoglycans and proteins direct the patient's own cells to initiate revascularization and cell repopulation. Grafted ADMs maintain their ultrastructural acellular matrix integrity and do not provoke a rejection or inflammatory response in host tissues (Eppley 2000; Wainwright et al. 1996) (see Figure 9.27a–c).

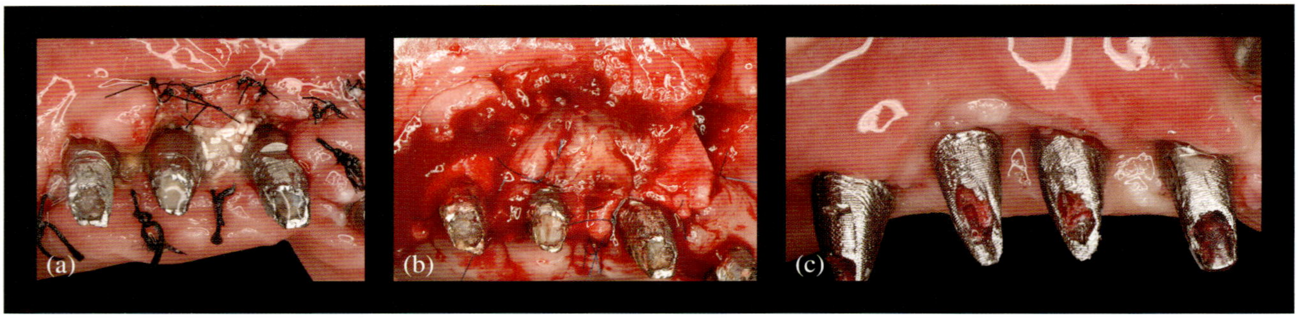

Figure 9.27 (a) Critical flap dehiscence with bone graft exposure to the oral cavity, (b) Connective tissue graft is placed on top to bulk the labial profile, (c) The final tissue healing four weeks post-surgery.

Batista and Batista (2001) showed in a case report that soft tissue fenestration in bone graft surgery could be managed by using ADM, which promoted completed soft tissue healing without exposing the grafted material. In addition, they reported a six months, follow-up for the use of this material to correct ridge deformities. Recently, AlGhamdi and Buhite (2008) recommended the routine use of ADM prior to any block grafting procedure in order to minimize the risk of soft tissue fenestration. The histologic appearance of ADMs and CTGs is similar (Cummings, Kaldah; and Allen 2005; Harris 2003). ADMs have been successfully used in the treatment of gingival recession (Aichelmann-Reidy et al. 2001; Henderson et al. 2001; Mahn 2001; Tal et al. 2002), bone regeneration (Fowler et al. 2000; Griffin et al. 2004), and soft tissue ridge augmentation (Harris 2003; Mahn 2003). However, the use of the ADM requires intensive clinical training.

9.4.2 Treatment Complications with the Use of Autografts

Despite various alternatives, the autologous bone graft still remains the graft of choice for bone volume restoration procedures (Nkenke et al. 2007), with optimal quality, quantity, and a high clinical predictability being the main reasons that make this type of graft a favorite. The autologous graft is still generally considered as most effective, and with success rates as high as 95%, it is considered 'the gold standard' (Rabelo et al. 2010; Roccuzzo et al. 2004) due to the absence of immunological reactions, its osteoinductive and osteoconductive properties, and the presence of osteoprogenitor cells along with growth factors (Rabelo 2010). Autologous grafts can be classified as extraoral or intraoral (Rabelo 2010). Schwartz-Arad, Levin and Sigal (2005) concluded that intraoral bone graft surgery is a predictable surgical procedure with a high success rate (see Figure 9.28a–c). Intraoral grafts offer the advantages of eliminating the need for hospitalization, and lower morbidity and discomfort for the patient (da Silva and Camilli 2006; Misch 1997; Rabelo et al. 2010). The main disadvantages of using autogenous bone grafts are postoperative complications such as dental-related complications, mucosal-related complications, skin sensory disturbances, temporary limitation of the mouth opening, and sometimes an altered facial contour (Cordaro et al. 2011; Misch 1997; Rabelo et al. 2010).

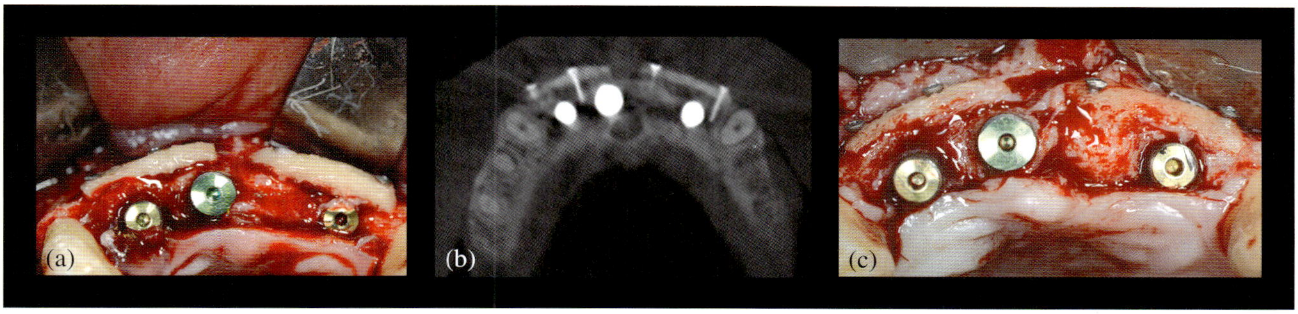

Figure 9.28 (a) Two onlay moncortical graft stabilized with titanium screws, (b) CBCT scan showing the complete restoration of the labial contour, (c) Three months post healing showing excellent incorporation of the graft.

The mandibular body, ramus, the symphysis, the coronoid processes, the anterior maxillary sinus wall, the tuberosity, the zygomatic bone, tori, and the anterior nasal spine can be potential donor sites for autogenous grafts. The most commonly used of these donor sites are the mandibular body, ramus, and symphysis. Ramus bone grafts (Acocella et al. 2010; Fakhry 2011) are dense, with a small amount of marrow bone, providing enough bone quantity for treating the defects of one to three teeth and requiring four to six months for integration. The symphysis area is described as an easily accessible area, with a suitable cortical and cancellous bone volume and higher cancellous bone mass, and may provide enough bone to treat the defects of one to six teeth, although it presents an increased rate of resorption (see Figure 9.29a–c) (Cranin 2001; Gapski et al. 2001; Raghoebar et al. 2007).

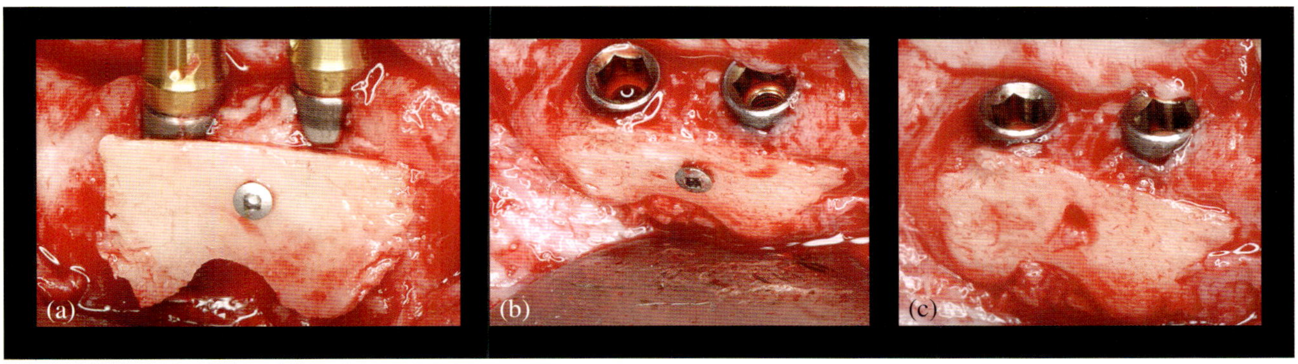

Figure 9.29 (a) Monocortical autograft is being used to restore an osseous defect related to dental implants placed in the premolar area, (b) and (c) Four months post grafting showing an excellent graft incorporation.

The block graft is structurally stable and gives immediate stability for dental implants. Fixation of an onlay graft to the recipient site can influence the fate of a graft (Phillips and Rahn 1990). A poor stabilized graft may become separated from the host site and encapsulated. Fixation screws for the onlay graft should be tightened to ensure close adaptation to host bed.

Autogenous block grafts (cortico-cancellous) are usually composed of an outer cortical layer surrounding the inner trabecular bone. During the first week, the graft becomes the center of an inflammatory reaction, then the inflammatory reaction subsides, and osteoclastic activity starts. The block also acts as a scaffold or a barrier to allow ingrowth of vessels and the accumulation of osteoblasts. A new bone structure is formed by creeping substitution and a lamellar bone develops. During the following months, this bone gradually calcifies but it takes about a year for it to reach its normal physical strength. Stable levels of biological properties will not be reached until about two years after grafting when a mixture of viable and necrotic bone will be clearly visible under the microscope (Sheikh et al. 2015a).

9.4.2.1 Donor Site Complications

Barone and Covani (2007) suggested that one of the major disadvantages of an autologous graft is morbidity of the donor site. This may cause serious related compilations including poor acceptance by many patients. Among the frequently occurring complications is that of postoperative bleeding, which can be controlled by continuous pressure, hematoma formation, wound sloughing, when iliac crest is chosen as a donor site, it can result in severe pain; other complications include gait disturbance, infection, fracture of the iliac crest, hematoma (Myeroff and Archdeacon 2011), scars, and sensory disturbance (Joshi and Kostakis 2004). Iliac grafts possess a rich source of pluripotent or osteogenic precursor cells (Joshi and Kostakis 2004) but they also possess a large amount of graft resorption postoperatively (Antoun et al. 2001).

Sensory disturbances in the lower lip and mental area as a result of chin graft harvesting was noted in 16% of harvesting procedures involving symphysis, while 8.3% involving the mandibular ramus area reported some sensory disturbances (Cordaro et al. 2002), also teeth sensory alterations could occur as a result of injury to the teeth roots adjacent to the graft harvesting area (Raghoebar et al. 2000).

9.4.2.2 Recipient Site Complications

9.4.2.2.1 Infection

The incidence of post-operative infection following onlay autogenous bone graft surgery is usually low (Lindeboom, Tjiook and Kroon 2006). Although an aseptic technique has been found acceptable for dental implant surgery (Günther, Scharf and Puhl 1993), clinicians should consider using an aseptic technique during more extensive and prolonged reconstructive procedures to avoid graft contamination with subsequent infection (Carlson and Monteleone 2004) (see Figure 9.30a–c).

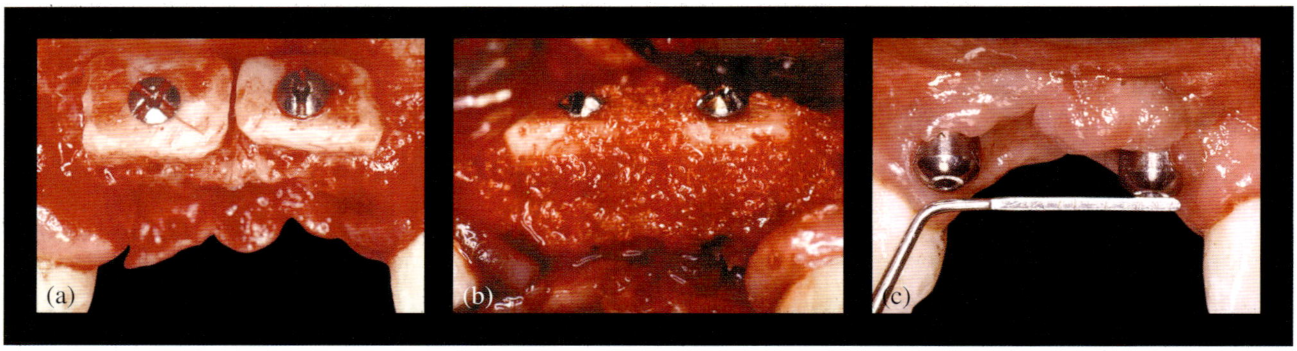

Figure 9.30 (a) Two chin cortico-cancellous block grafts secured with two titanium screws to restore a horizontal bone defect, (b) Particulated bone graft to fill the voids, (c) Graft failure due to poor soft tissue management.

The graft should be handled with caution, bone graft should be stored in sterile normal saline after harvesting rather than a moist sponge or towel to maintain cellular viability (Steiner and Ramp 1988), and the time elapsed between graft harvest and placement should be minimized. Aseptic surgical conditions and working over sterile drapes are advised. The bone graft should always be held with a bone clamp, or Allis forceps during transfer and manipulation rather than using gloved fingers. The risk of graft contamination by glove powder is documented (Field 1997), however an accidental contact from the glove to the graft can occur without causing any problems, because usually the graft makes contact with the exterior side of the glove, not the interior side that has the powder. Soaking the graft in 10% povidone–iodine solution for 10 minutes has been found to eliminate surface bacteria without altering the histologic integrity of the graft (Hooe and Steinberg 1996), however, it is unknown if it later the osteogenic and osteoinductive properties of the graft. Saliva contamination may be another factor for graft contamination. Antisialagogue agents, where suggested, such as glycopyrrolate, may be administered preoperatively to decrease salivary flow, which may carry bacteria into the grafted site.

When extraoral donor sites are be used (tibia, ilium), a strict complete aseptic sterile technique must be followed. The skin is prepped with antiseptic solution and the surgical field is isolated with sterile drapes, the patient should be placed on prophylactic antibiotics starting with a loading dose one hour prior to surgery and continuing for one week (Lindeboom et al. 2006; Misch 1992). Preoperative chlorhexidine rinsing can reduce the bacterial contamination of intraorally harvested bone grafts (Young et al. 2002a) wound dehiscence is associated with a higher incidence of postoperative infection of the graft recipient site (Albrektsson and Johansson 2001).

Signs of graft-related infection include edema, swelling, redness, induration, purulence exudate, wound sloughing, and graft piercing through the soft tissue. If these signs are recent, then the use of a wide spectrum combination antibiotic therapy is advised (i.e. amoxicillin + metronidizole), with follow-up two weeks after antibiotic therapy. If the adverse signs have subsided two weeks after antibiotic therapy, then the infection is resolved; however, if the symptoms recur, then graft removal should be considered immediately.

For late infections, i.e. the patient presented with signs of infection that lasted for longer than one week, graft removal is the only choice.

For frank infections that invaded the bone graft block, the bone graft should be removed immediately and soft tissue closure attempted with antibiotics coverage and saline irrigation to the site. Signs of frank infections are well known to clinicians; therefore, when any of the signs are observed a thorough examination to confirm the presence of the infection should be made.

9.4.2.2.2 Bone Graft Remodeling and Resorption

The embryologic origin of an autologous bone graft has been suggested as a predictor of graft resorption. More recent studies emphasized the importance of the microarchitecture of the bone used for grafting over embryologic origin (Manson 1994; Ozaki and Buchman 1998). The bone graft is remodeled and replaced with new bone over time (creeping substitution) (Manson 1994). Bone cells, in higher concentration in the cancellous marrow, survive the transplantation and produce osteoid matrix (Manson 1994). Autogenous bone grafts must become revascularized to incorporate the host bed. The cancellous portion of the graft revascularizes more rapidly than the cortex (Burchardt 1983). Membranous bone grafts, from the mandible or calvarium, have been found to reveal a lower resorption rate than grafts from endochondral sites, such as the iliac crest. Denser cortical bone grafts resorb less than more porous cancellous bone grafts when used for onlay bone augmentation (Ozaki and Buchman 1998). Monocortical bone grafts from the mandible exhibit minimal resorption and maintain their dense quality, making them ideal for onlay augmentation before implant placement. Upon incorporation the volume loss of cortical bone grafts used for onlay augmentation is less than 20%. Corticocancellous bone grafts from the ilium are associated with greater resorption, owing to the thinner outer cortex and more porous cancellous component, which may lead to a 40% loss of graft size. Whereas the greatest change in the width of a corticocancellous graft occurs in the first 3 months, the volume loss in height stabilizes after one year (Nyström et al. 1996). It is prudent to overbuild the reconstructed ridge in anticipation of some volume loss upon healing (see Figure 9.31a–c).

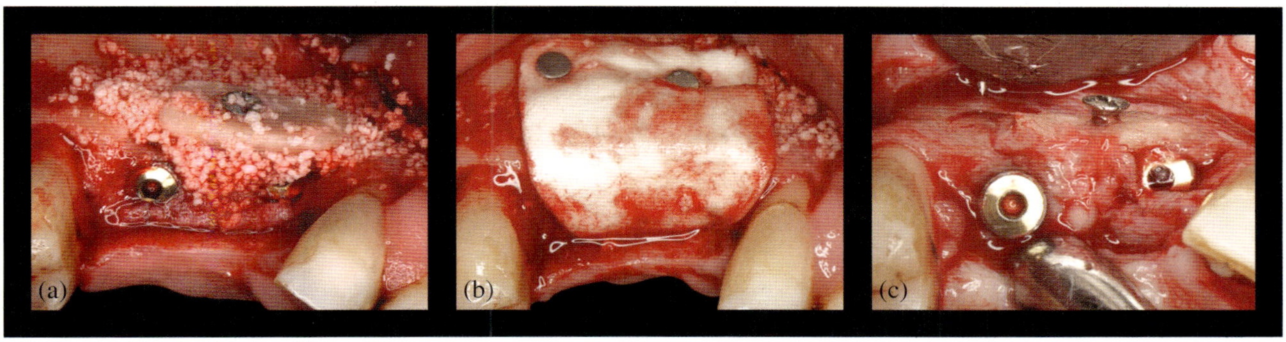

Figure 9.31 (a) Showing implants placed, (Tapered Internal, BioHorizons, Birmingham, AL, USA) along with mono-cortical mandibular block stabilized with titanium fixation screw (KLS Martin, GmbH, Tuttilngen, Germany), (b) Collagen resorbable membrane (Mem-Lock, BioHorizons, Birmingham, AL, USA) is taced by (Auto Tac, BioHorizons, Birmingham, AL, USA) in order to minimize the amount of post grafting bone resorption, (c) Four months post grafting at the implant uncovery, excellent graft incorporation (take) however, the graft showing 10–20% of size reduction (showing under the flat head of the screw).

9.4.2.2.3 Soft Tissue Thinning and Dehiscence

Wound dehiscence occurs after a grafting procedure is the most common recipient site complication with onlay autogenous bone augmentation. The early exposure of the bone graft, within the first two to three weeks post-surgery, often leads to graft failure due to the vulnerability of the graft at this particular time. The clinician should take all possible precautions to avoid post-operative wound sloughing. Wound dehiscence has a direct impact on the rapid graft failure. The most common cause for incision line opening is a lack of tension-free flap adaptation (see Figures 9.32 and 9.33a–c). The periodontal health and endodontic status of teeth adjacent to the graft recipient site should be evaluated prior to grafting. It may be prudent to extract compromised or hopeless teeth prior to grafting, especially if infection is present (Misch 2007). The marginal bone height on the teeth bordering the bone defect determines the level that may be achieved with vertical bone augmentation (see Figure 9.34a–c).

The clinician should inspect the planned graft recipient site, including quality, amount of keratinized mucosa, tissue thickness, high muscle attachments, frenum, and scarring. Poor hygiene under pontics should be recognized and managed prior to surgery. Any teeth requiring extraction directly within the bone graft site should be planned for removal several weeks prior to surgery.

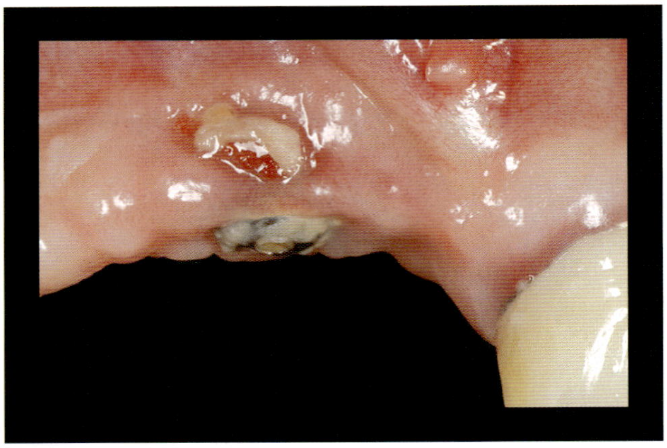

Figure 9.32 Graft exfoliation with soft tissue thinning.

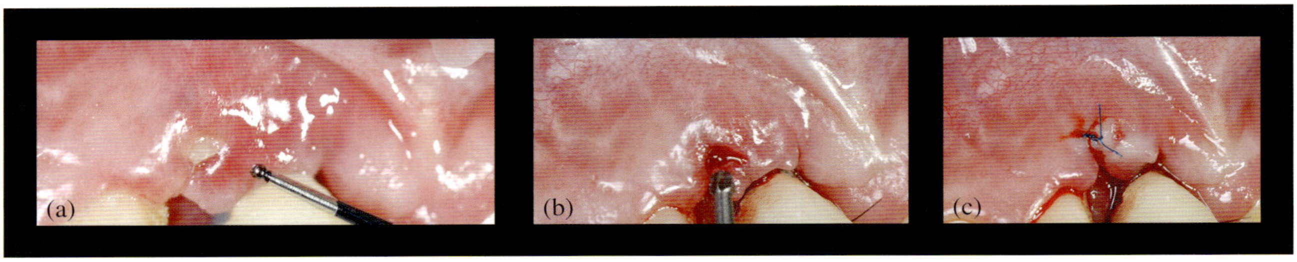

Figure 9.33 (a) Autograft piercing the soft tissue as a result of poor graft preparation, (b) Using a carbide round pair to remove the sharp edges of the graft, (c) Wound edges approximated.

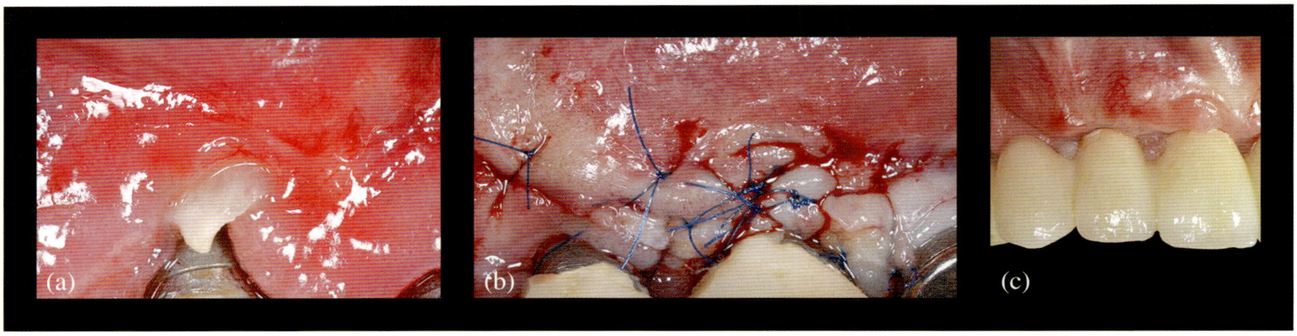

Figure 9.34 (a) Monocortical autograft piercing a thin mucosa, (b) Graft was trimmed down, wound edges approximated after flap relaxation has been made, (c) Three months post healing.

With the use of autogenous block grafts, and after a few months of healing, a frequent clinical picture that always arises is thinning of the soft tissue around fixation screws or membrane fixation pins. This results from several factors that include improper positioning of the fixation screw (not flush to the level of the bone graft), incomplete tightening of the positioning screw to the end, the inability to prepare the screw holes, and use of faulty type screws. These screws could be left for a long time without removal, unless the patient is esthetically concerned, or it pierced through the soft tissues (see Figures 9.35a–c, 9.36a, b, and 9.37a, b).

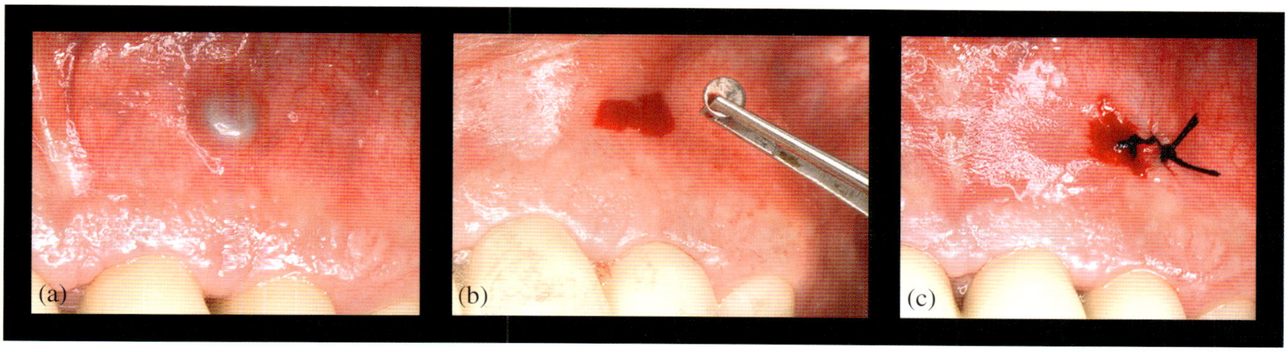

Figure 9.35 (a) Three months post using membrane tac (Auto Tac, BioHorizons, Birmingham, AL, USA), (b) Very conservative many incision to expose the tac, (c) Suturing of the incision.

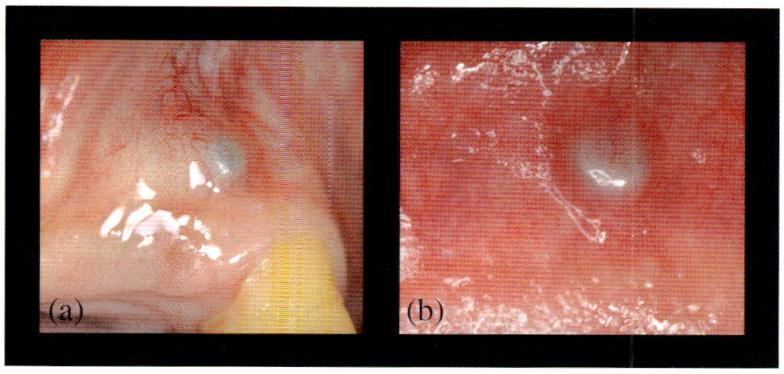

Figure 9.36 (a) and (b) Examples of soft tissue thinning over screws.

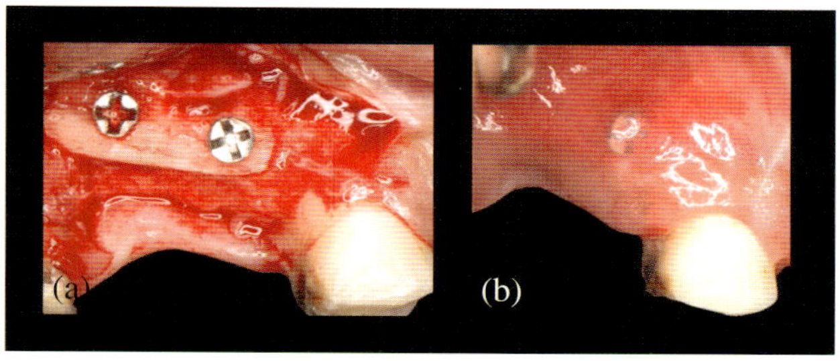

Figure 9.37 (a) Clinical view of a monocortical block after three months of placement, (b) Thinning of the soft tissue on top of the titanium fixation screw.

9.4.2.2.4 Fracture of the Graft

The use of monocortical grafts involves a greater risk for graft fracture than using corticocancellous grafts (Nyström et al. 1996) due to its minimized thickness, which can be liable to fracture while handling. Accurate preparation of the autogenous block grafts should be made with extreme caution (Jensen 1994; Matsumoto et al. 2002) (see Figure 9.38). The trimming of the block and the size of the block harvested make additional factors that contribute to the fracture of the graft (Buser et al. 2002). The placement of the block graft to its donor bed requires meticulous handling and advanced clinical skills. Tightening of the fixation screws should be considered to avoid over-tightening, which may lead to a block graft fracture when pressed against the recipient bed. Any removable prosthetics should be totally relieved at the graft location to avoid pressure on the graft structure. When an implant is to be placed at the same time as the grating procedure, there is a greater risk of force transferring to the graft that may lead to fracture via a wedging effect. If the graft is broken, then the graft disposal becomes mandatory and the whole procedure may need to be aborted. Graft fracture may also occur as a result of poor preparation of the host site bed (Wang, Waite and Steinhauser 1976).

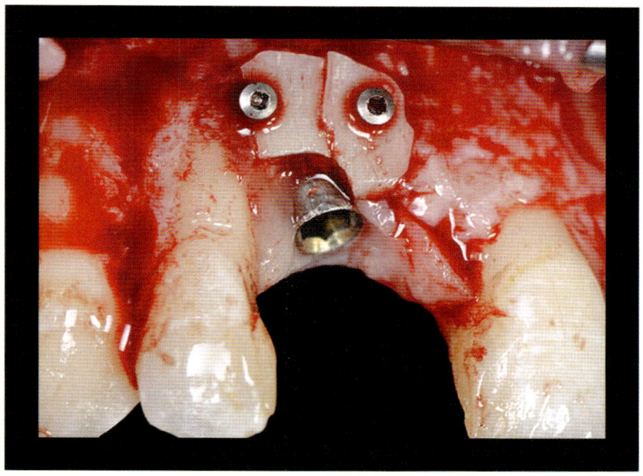

Figure 9.38 Bone graft fracture.

The presence of any sharp protruding edges on the bone graft may be smoothed and reduced with a coarse diamond bur. If more than half the bone graft becomes exposed, the prognosis is poor and graft removal should be considered (see Figures 9.39, 9.40, 9.41 and 9.42a–c).

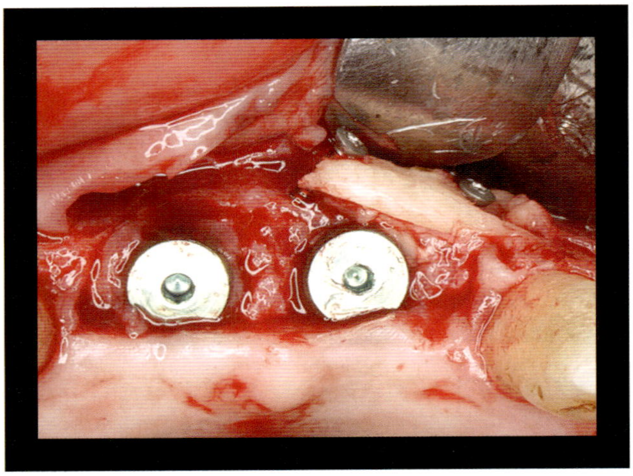

Figure 9.39 Graft failure, note the soft tissue intervening between the graft and the host bed.

Cancellous bone grafts have been reported to be more resilient and revascularize faster, which gives the additional benefit of overcoming graft fracture (Carlson and Monteleone 2004). It may be concluded that sequestration of a bone graft may occur as a consequence of poor clinical experience. The optimal host bed preparation expedites revascularization of the graft, and improves the graft incorporation (De Carvalho, Vasconcellos and Pi 2000) provided that the graft was positioned correctly so that nourishment can reach the graft itself. Decortication of the recipient site improved graft fit and significantly improved the outcome (De Carvalho et al. 2000). Corticocancellous block grafts require less adjustment as the portion of cancellous bone will often mold to the ridge. An understanding of vascular patterns within the oral cavity is important to prevent poor healing. Incisions to expose

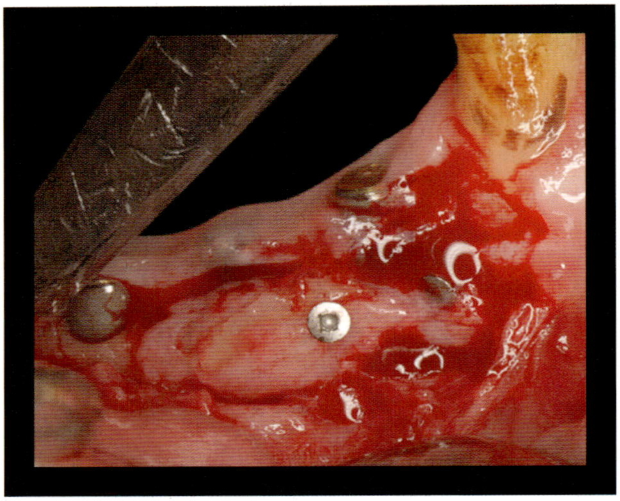

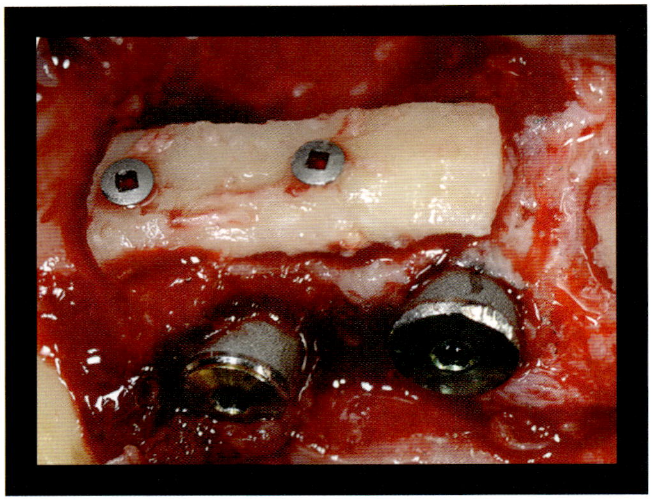

Figures 9.40 and 9.41 Two clinical examples of Improper graft position that is not fixed on the defect site.

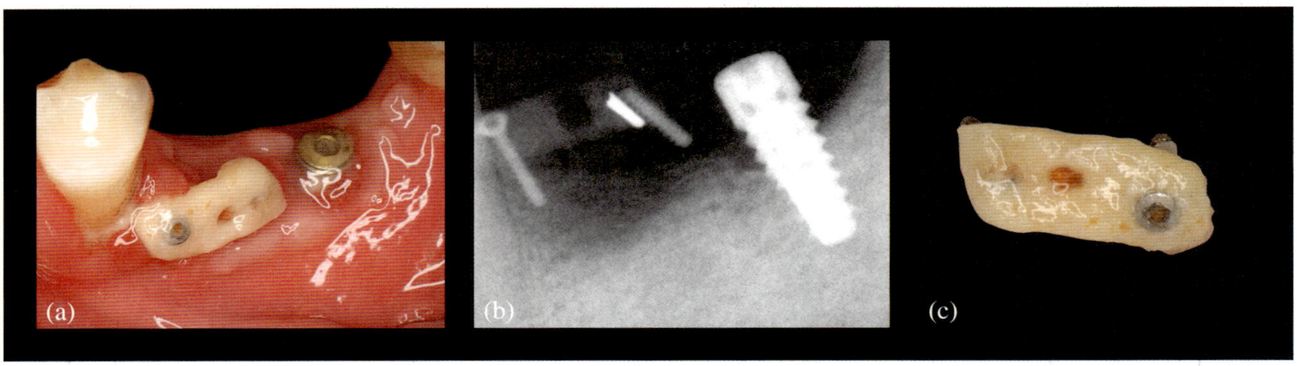

Figure 9.42 (a) Graft exfoliation (necrosis), note the soft tissue creeping underneath the graft leaving it exposed to the oral cavity environment, faulty graft position, (b) Radiographic view showing osseous defect related to the graft as well as the adjacent implant, (c) The necrotic graft removed.

the recipient site are typically made along the ridge crest. As blood vessels facial to the ridge do not cross over to the palatal or lingual regions, a crestal incision maintains vascular supply to the flaps (Whetzel and Sanders 1997) (see Figure 9.43a–z1).

The bone defect and graft recipient site are usually exposed and prepared prior to a bone graft harvest. This allows a better evaluation of the requirements of the bone repair and minimizes the time from bone harvest to graft placement. Harvesting the block from the donor site first may risk obtaining a bone graft that is too small. An accurate graft size should be ascertained by CBCT preoperatively (see Figures 9.44a, b and 9.45a, b).

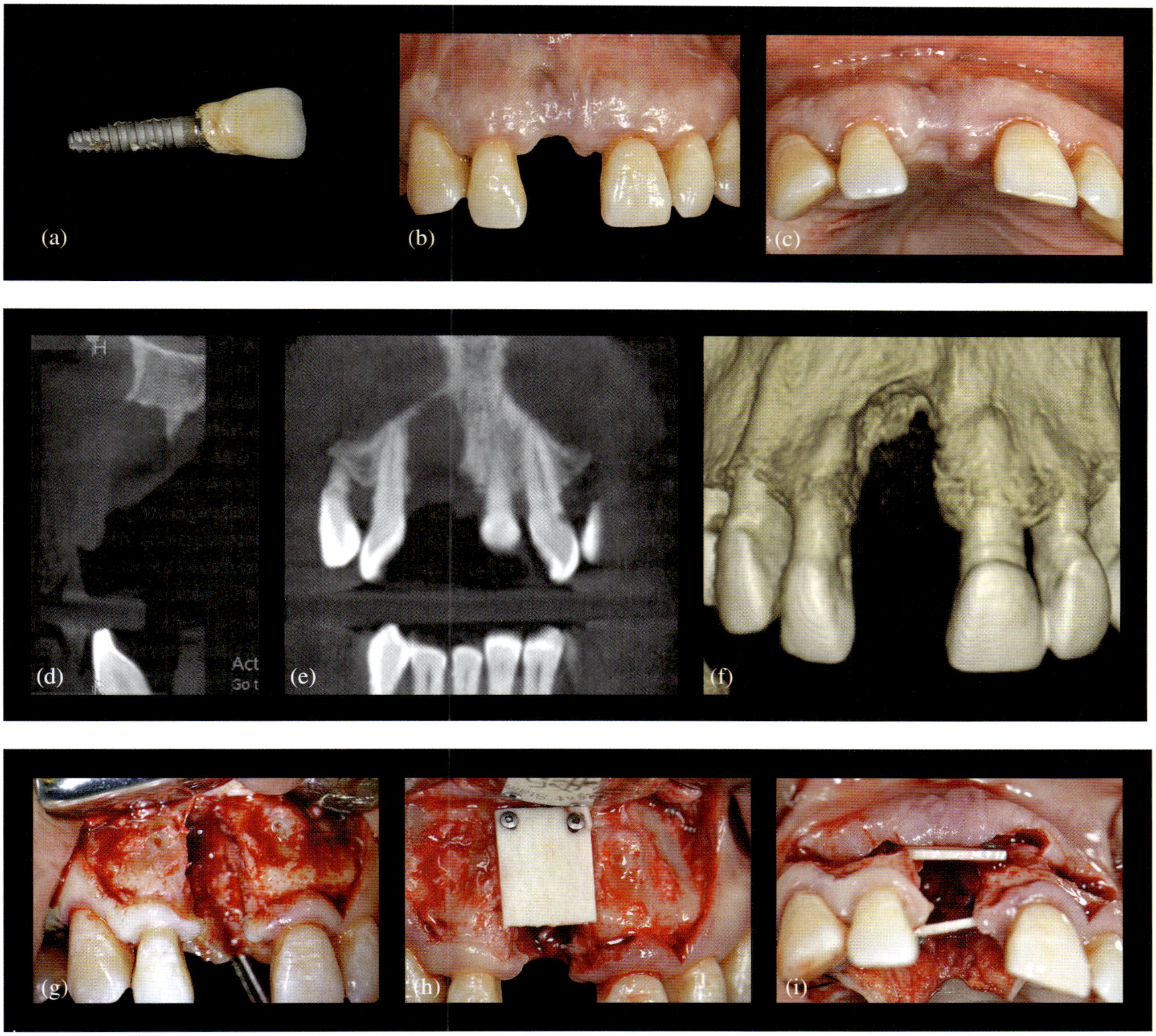

Figure 9.43 (a) Six months post restorative implant failure along with the grafted bone, (b) and (c) Clinical view showing the resultant osseous defect both facially and incisally, (d–f) CBCT scan images showing lost both labial and palatal plates of bone, (g) Intraoperative view showing the defect with the flap reflected, (h) Monocortical allograft is stabilized both labially and palatally, (i) Incisal view of the grafted plates.

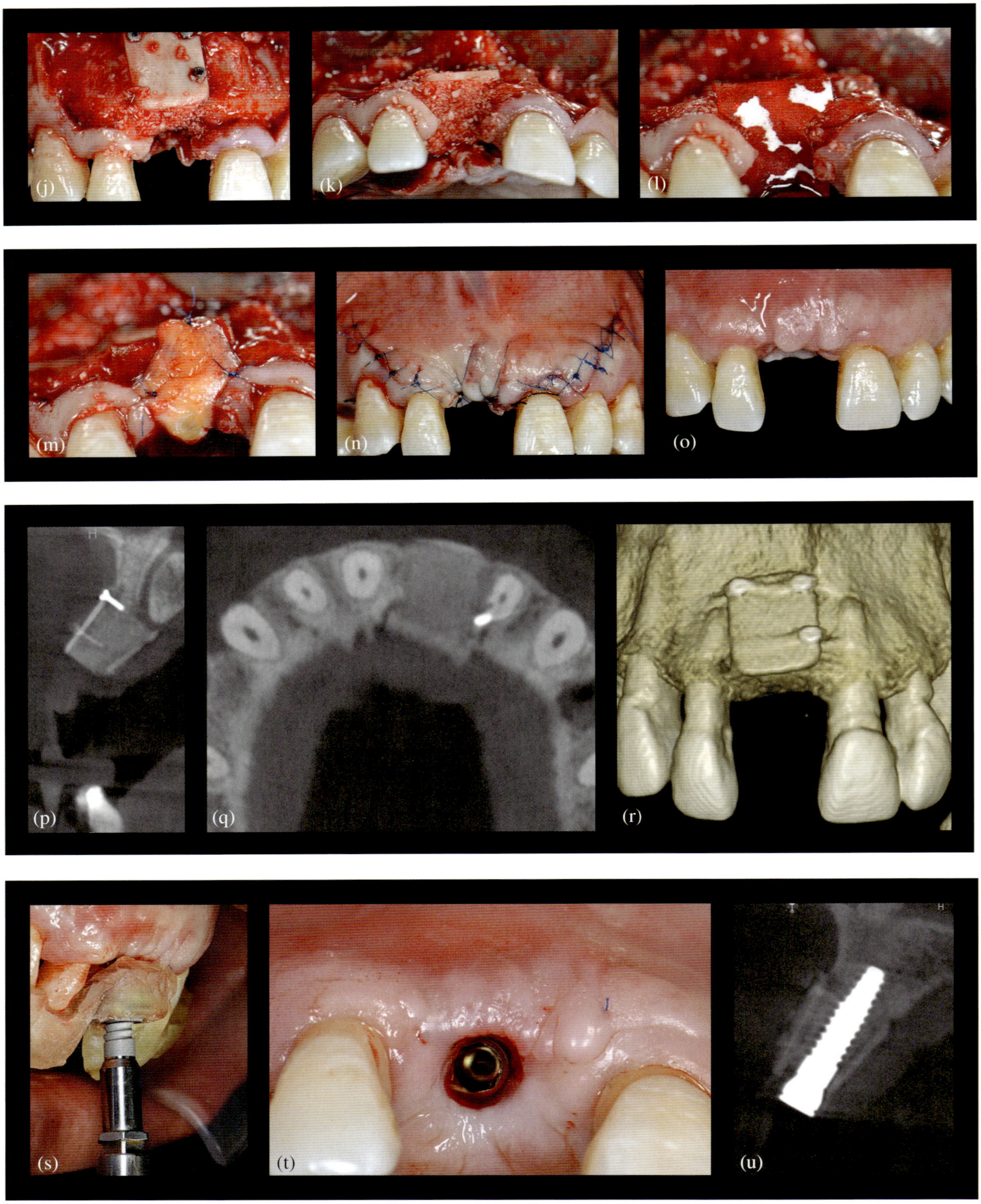

Figure 9.43 (j) and (k) Voids filled with particulated graft, (l) Collagen membrane is placed and stabilized to cover the grafted bone, (m) Connective tissue graft is sutured on top, (n) Flap sutured, (o) One week post healing, (p–r) CBCT views showing grafts in position, (s) CAD/CAM surgical guide in place for implant insertion, (t) Intraoperative view showing the implant in place, (u) CBCT view showing implant position within the two plates of bone.

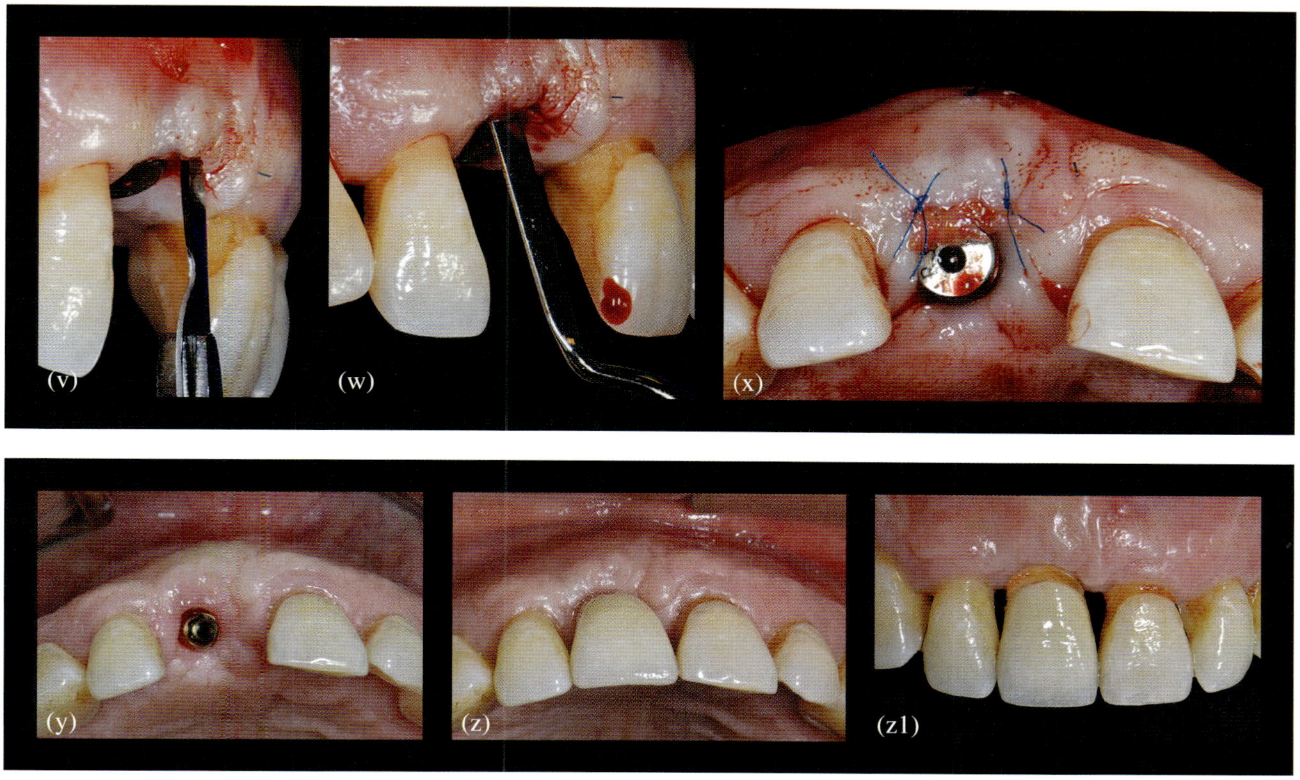

Figure 9.43 (v–x) Attempting to place a connective tissue graft to enhance the labial contour from the cervical area, (y) Final tissue healing and maturation, contour regain. (z) Incisal view with the final restoration in place showing the completed treatment. (z1) Facial view of the case finalized.

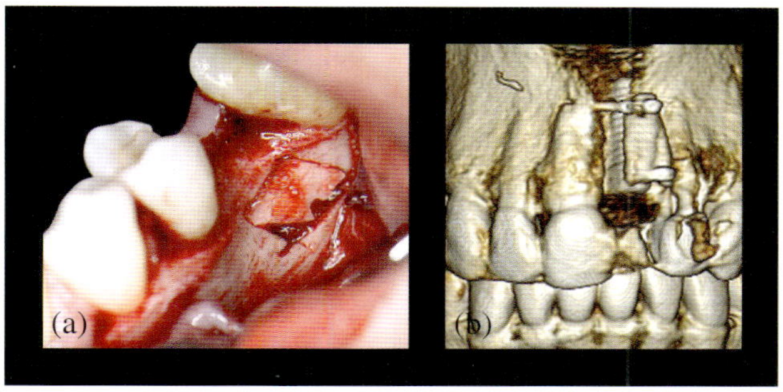

Figure 9.44 (a) and (b) Examples of insufficient graft size.

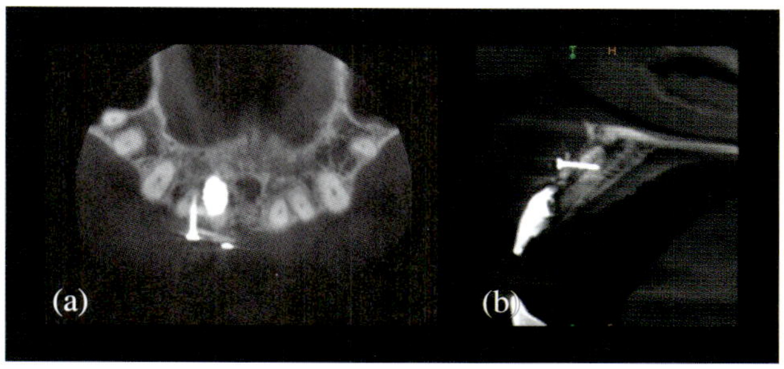

Figure 9.45 (a) and (b) CBCT views showing the faulty position (inside the natural tooth root) of the titanium screw.

9.4.3 Complications with Allographs

Bone allograft transplants are now being widely used by dental practitioners more than any other bone augmentation material. This is probably due to the ease of use and preparation, and the availability of allografts from many networks of tissue banks (Tomford et al. 1983; Kozak, Heilman and O'Brien 1994). Regretfully, the source of these grafts and the means of their preparation are not always consistent (Lavernia et al. 2004). Cadaver bone has been transplanted with considerable success since the beginning of the twentieth century and in large numbers for the past few decades. To obtain optimal results with grafting procedures and to safeguard recipients, the clinician must possess full knowledge of the biologic properties of allograft bone (see Figure 9.46a–c).

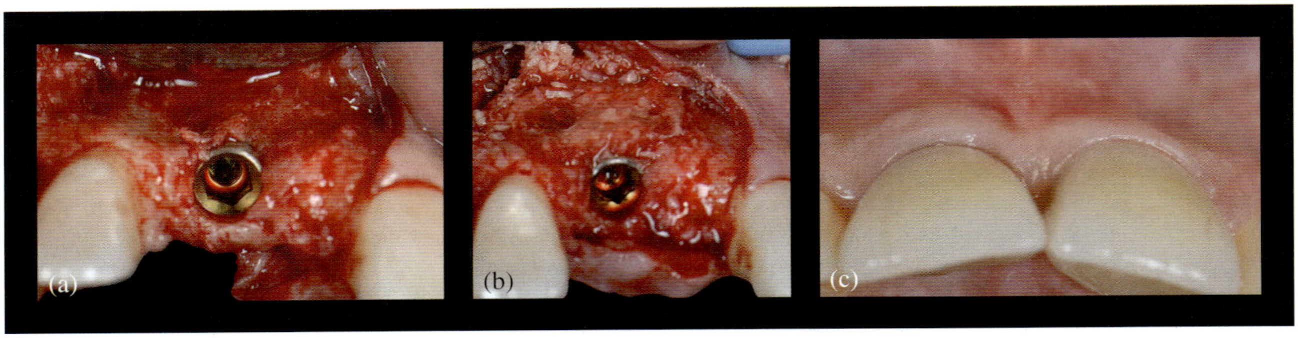

Figure 9.46 (a) An Implant is placed showing labial bone dehiscence, (b) The bone defect was grafted with particulated autogenous bone mix and covered with PDLLA membrane and stabilized with resorbable screws (KLS Martin, GmbH, Tuttilngen, Germany, SonicWeld), (c) Final case restored showing enhanced soft tissue contours with the complete restoration of labial profile.

The biologic properties and safety of allograft bone was demonstrated by Hyatt and Butler (1957) and Kreuz et al. (1951); the demand for allogeneic bone increased precipitously. This resulted in an increase in the number of tissue banks, which had substantial variations in techniques for allograft excision and preparation. The accurate and strict control of tissue banks for monitoring the processing of allografts worldwide is not consistent with the prevention of disease transmission.

Bone allografts can be obtained and prepared in several ways. There is comprehensive donor screening and rigorous disease surveillance using donor medical history, advanced laboratory methods, blood and marrow culture testing, and post-mortem examination. Using these measures minimizes the risk of transmitting disease to the recipient (see Figure 9.47a–h).

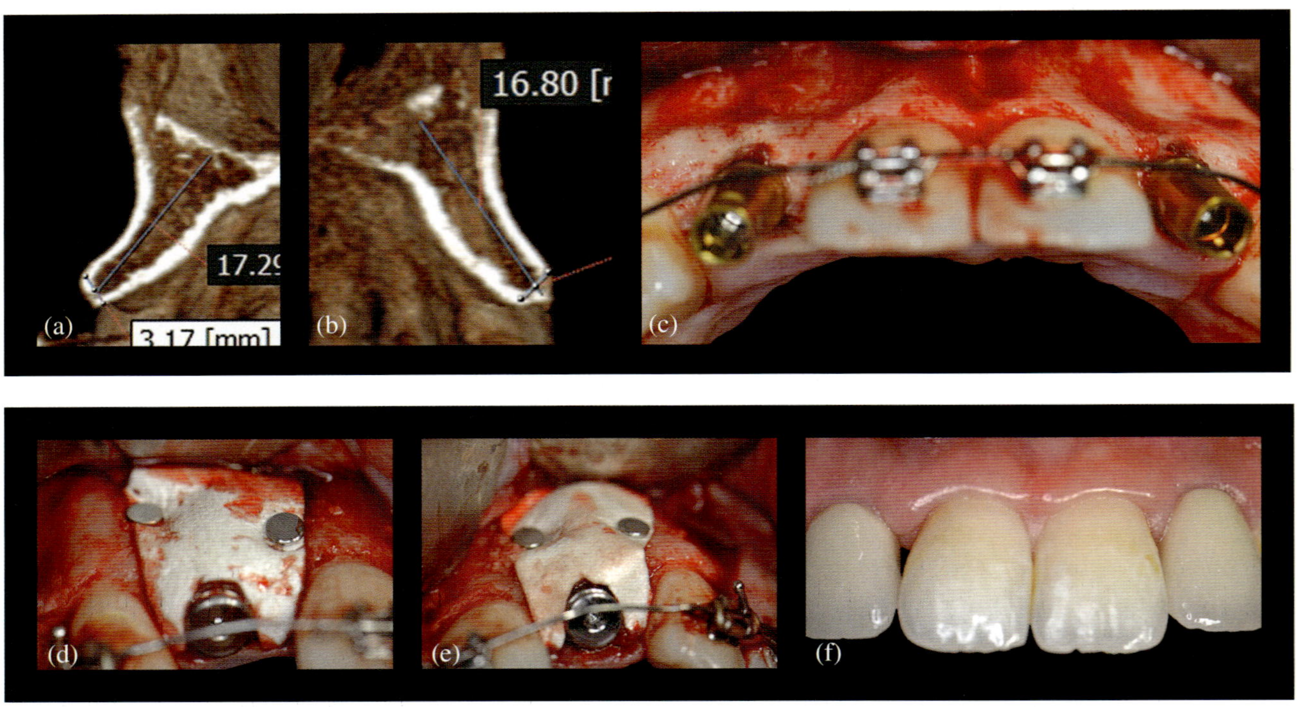

Figure 9.47 (a) and (b) CBCT scan showing deficient buccolingual width of the alveolar ridge, (c) Two implants placed leaving labial dehiscence, (d) and (e) Allograft particles were placed, stabilized and covered with collagen membrane and two membrane tacs (Auto Tac, BioHorizons, Birmingham, AL, USA), (f) Case restored.

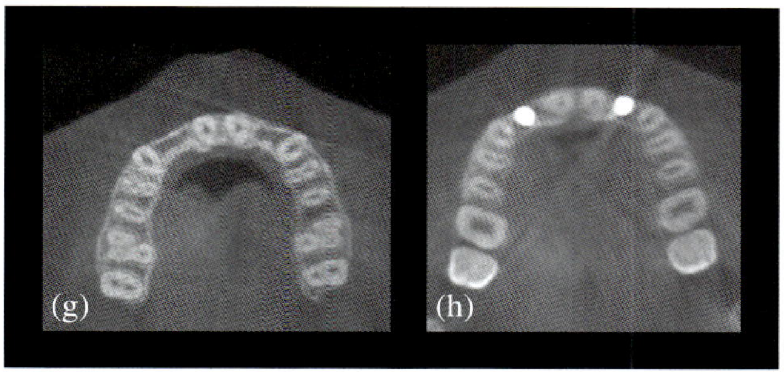

Figure 9.47 (g) and (h) Pre and post grafting picture with one year follow-up showing no bone formed labial to the implant surface in spite the fact that the grafting procedure were optimal which indicates the lack of the predictability of using allografts alone.

9.4.3.1 Inconsistent Regenerative Outcome and Questionable Osteoinduction

The effectiveness of demineralized bone grafts may differ depending on the age and gender of the donor, the residual mineral, the particle size, or the preparation method. According to Salyer et al. (1992), the success and safety of demineralized bone implants as well as different characteristics of the product, including its osteoinductive potential, depend on the technological process used to produce them. Studies have examined the ability of commercial demineralized freeze-dried bone allografts (DFDBA) to induce new bone formation to assess whether the broad variation in clinical response was due to differences in the preparations or due to variations in the host response. It was found that wide variations in commercial bone bank preparations of DFDBA do exist, including the ability to induce new bone formation, even within the same bank (Committee on Research, Science and Therapy of the American Academy of Periodontology 2001); however, the committee did not offer a solid statement on the osteogenic capacity of DFDBA. Commercial bone banks do not verify the specific amount of BMPs or any level of inductive capacity in any graft material they sell. Therefore, graft quality cannot be considered standard. Delaying the procurement of donor bone after death, improper storage conditions, or other processing factors may play a significant role in the bioactivity of an allograft that makes its way to the clinician's office (Holtzclaw et al. 2008).

If DFDBA particles remain in the site for longer than a year acting as a bone matrix, they may weaken the host bone and delay normal bone formation, possibly by interfering with the osteoclast's ability to resorb the DFDBA particles (Grover et al. 2011). When DFDBA is used in particulate form, particle size also appears to be an important variable in its success as a bone inductive material. Particles in the range 125–1000 μm possess a higher osteogenic potential than particles smaller than 125 μm. Optimal particle size appears to be between 100 and 300 μm. This may be due to a combined effect of surface area and packing density (Schwartz et al. 1996). Very small DFDBA particles elicit a macrophage response and are rapidly resorbed with little or no new bone formation. Tissue banks providing DFDBA usually have the graft material in various particle sizes, and they offer a range with variable particle size. Particle size from 250 to 750 μm is the most frequently available. Glowacki and Mulliken (1985) developed the technology of preparing demineralized bone implants in powder form. Powder provides the maximum surface area necessary for interaction with recipient target cells, which stimulates endochondral proliferation. Glowacki et al. (1981) demonstrated that the extent of bone induction is a function of the surface area of the implanted bone.

Gendler (1986) introduced micro perforations in the demineralized bone, which, according to his long-term experience, are centers of new bone formation. He assumed that the mechanism of osteoinduction of demineralized perforated bone is similar to that described for other forms of demineralized bone matrix although the micro perforations, in his opinion, enhance osteoinduction. Thus, the presence of micro perforations in demineralized bone allograft also affects the osteogenic potential of the graft. It is the author's opinion that the use of the allograft particles alone does not give the required osteogenic response because the bone particles go through a series of processes that probably lose their osteogenicity. As there is no proof of the presence of bone morphogenic proteins inside the graft particles is questionable and requires further research to confirm it. The clinician must understand the capacity and the clinical outcome of all the grafting materials used and be able to make the right choice for a long-term successful outcome. Usually after the placement of the allogeneic grafts, there is no second re-entry to check bone formation. In other words, clinicians do not perform another surgical re-entry to check graft viability, they only check with the radiographs. The presence of radio opacity in the radiographic view does not confirm the viability of the grafted bone. Some researchers suggest that irradiation interferes with osteoinduction (Singh, Singh and Singh 2016), others suggest that a dose of radiation (2.5 Mrad) used by most tissue banks for the sterilization of bone tissue does not destroy the bone induction properties of allografts (Tallentire and IAEA 1990). Therefore, sterilization processing may be an important contributor to variability in the osteoinductive properties of DFDBAs. There are two major concerns regarding the use of bone allografts: antigenicity, and the risk of disease transmission (see Figures 9.48a–e and 9.49a–f).

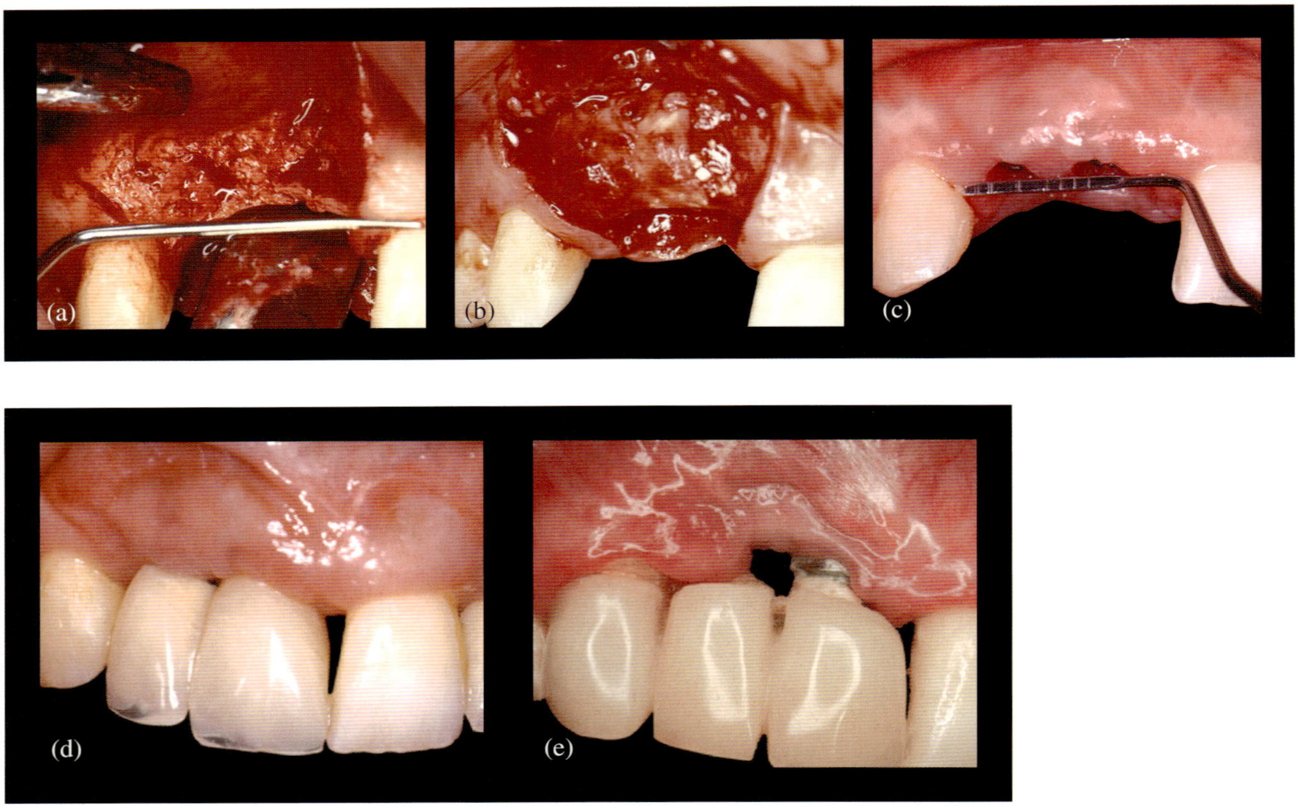

Figure 9.48 (a) Deficient vertical bone height, (b) Successful bone grafting procedure, (c) The regain of natural tissue architecture, (d) Final restoration in place, (e) Graft resorption and disintegration two years post restorative due to the poor systemic condition of the patient (uncontrolled diabetes).

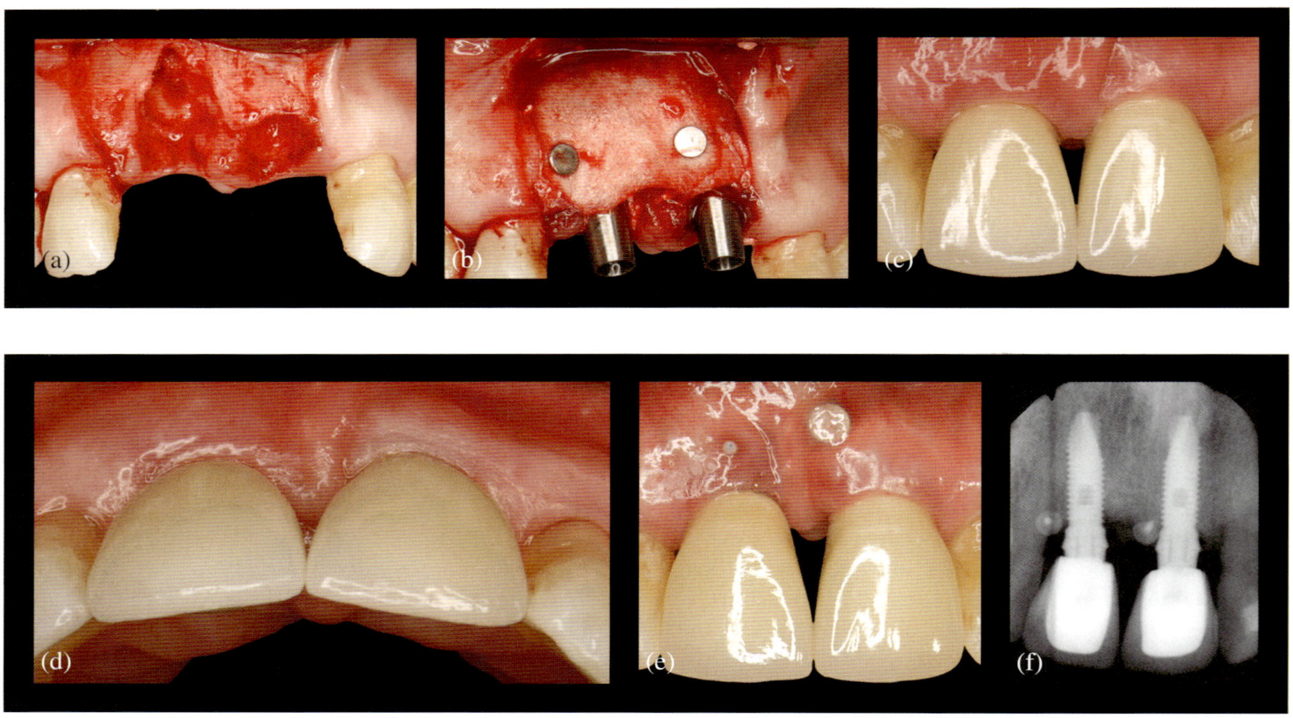

Figure 9.49 (a) Mucopreosetal flap reflected and teeth were extracted revealing bone deficiencies, (b) Two implants (Spline, Sulzer Medica, Carlesbad, CA, USA) bone allograft (Mineross, BioHorizons, Birmingham, AL, USA) was placed and a collagen membrane (Biomend, Sulzer Medica, Carlesbad, CA, USA) and tacked with membrane tacs (Auto Tac, BioHorizons, Birmingham, AL, USA), (c) and (d) Frontal and incisor view for the case finally restored with two PFM crowns at the year 2002, (e) Post insertion view at 2002 and three years later 2005 showing gingival recession, (f) Radiographic view at the time of implant placement 2002 and three years later showing advanced bone loss.

Because of the increased risk of disease transmission, gamma irradiation or ethylene oxide is used to secondarily sterilize the allografts. Residuals due to inadequate evacuation following ethylene oxide or radiation sterilization may also contribute to the variability in the graft response. Residual levels of ethylene oxide in the graft have been shown to be toxic to fibroblasts and appear to cause morphologic changes in fibroblasts that may or may not be reversible (Buck et al. 1989). Ethylene oxide may produce inflammation and impair healing, unless it or its byproducts are removed from the graft. More infections were found with the use of non-resorbable membrane for the GBR procedure compared with a bioabsorbable membrane over a bovine bone in a xenograft study (Friedmann et al. 2011). Selection of a suitable membrane and proper timing of membrane removal may reduce the risk of infection. Contamination with oral saliva is probably a major factor leading to bone graft infection (Glaser et al. 2004) (see Figure 9.50a–c).

With the use of allografts, antigenicity poses particular health risks that involve an exaggerated host response to implanted materials from other human donors. However, the possible immune reaction is considerably diminished with allografts but still remains a factor to consider, as does the risk of disease transmission such as HIV. Smith, Young and Kearney (1996) showed that, even at doses at which tissue quality begins to be compromised (1.5–2.5 Mrads), irradiation failed to be virucidal for HIV type 1 (see Figures 9.51a–c and 9.52a–f).

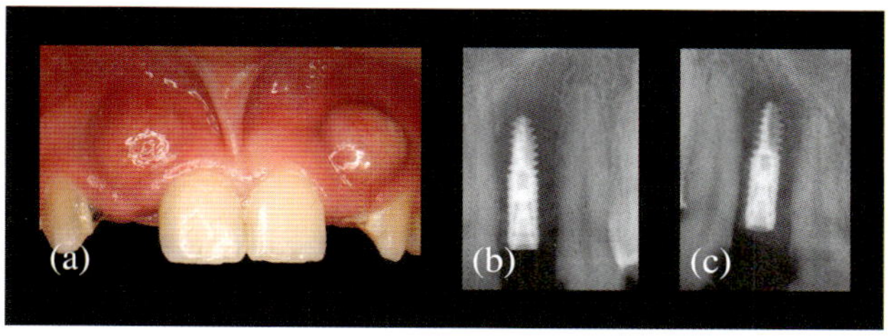

Figure 9.50 (a) Clinical view showing soft tissue swelling three weeks post implant placement as a result of infection, (b) and (c) Radiographic views showing sever bone resorption related to both implants.

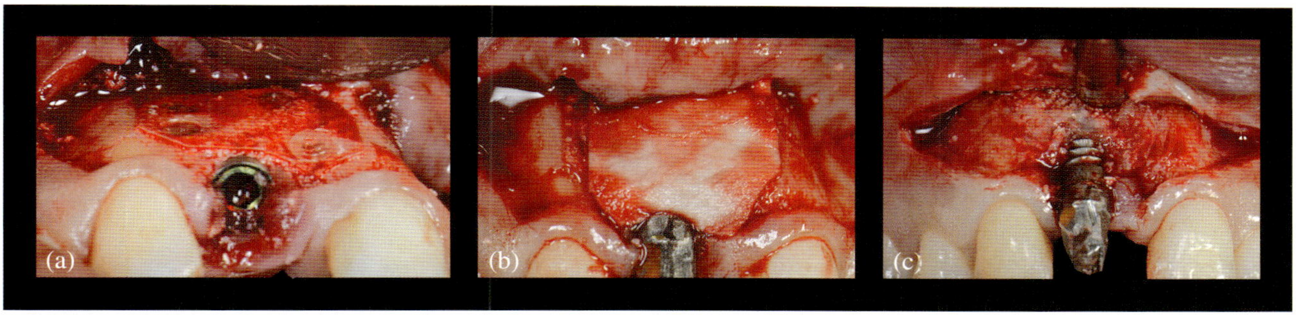

Figure 9.51 (a) The resultant osseous defect is grafted with allograft, (b) The graft is covered with collagen membrane, (c) Bone allograft failure as a result of immunologic reaction.

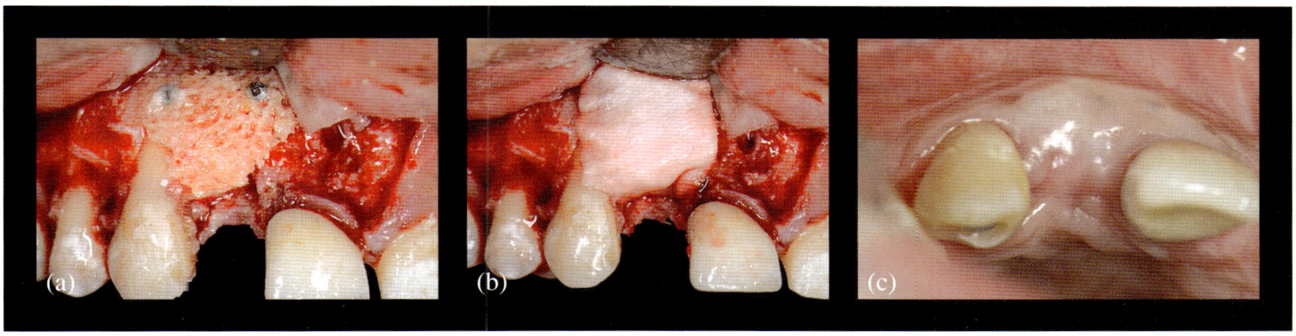

Figure 9.52 (a) Cancellous allograft is trimmed and stabilized to treat 3D osseous defect, (b) Collagen membrane covering the graft, (c) Two weeks postoperative healing.

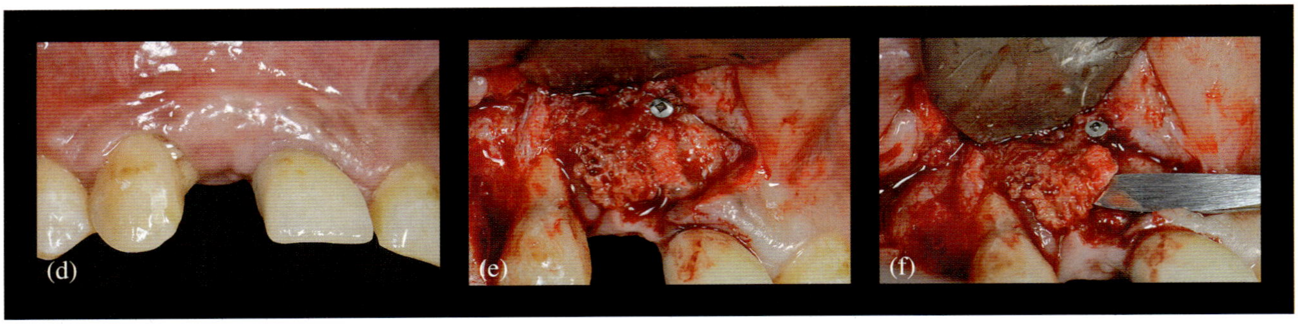

Figure 9.52 (d) Pus oozing from the side indicating infection, (e) Flap reflection showing resorption of the graft, (f) Graft removal.

Another form of allograft is the block form, which are available as monocortical blocks, corticocancellous blocks, also known as the J blocks, and the cancellous blocks. Due to the large size of the graft, the sterilization process is probably questioned more than the particle size. In a study by Chaushu et al. (2010) a total of 101 consecutive patients (62 females and 39 males; mean age 44 ± 17 years) with implant-supported restoration of 137 severe atrophic alveolar ridges augmented with cancellous bone-block allografts were treated. Recipient site complications associated with block grafting (infection, membrane exposure, incision line opening, and perforation of mucosa over the grafted bone, partial graft failure, total graft failure, and implant failure) were recorded. Partial and total bone-block graft failure occurred in 10 (7%) and 11 (8%) of 137 augmented sites, respectively (see Figure 9.53a–d).

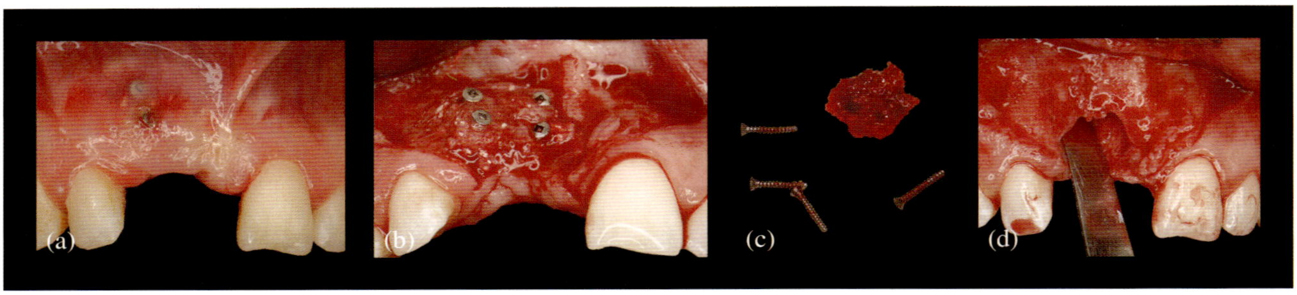

Figure 9.53 (a) Fourmonths post grafting showing marked redness and screw exfoliation, (b) Mucopreosteal flap reflected, (c) Bone graft removed due to morbidity, (d) Resultant osseous defect.

The implant failure rate was 12 (4.4%) of 271. Soft tissue complications included membrane exposure (42 (30.7%) of 137), incision line opening (41 (30%) of 137), and perforation of the mucosa over the grafted bone (19 (14%) of 137). Infection of the grafted site occurred in 18 (13%) of 137 bone blocks. Therefore it was concluded that the alveolar ridge deficiency location had a statistically significant effect on the outcome of recipient site complications. More complications were noted in the mandible compared to the maxilla. Failures caused by complications were rarely noted in association with cancellous block grafting.

In another histologic and histomorphometric study, Dellavia et al. (2016) treated 20 partially edentulous patients either with iliac crest fresh-frozen allograft blocks (14 patients) and with autografts (6 patients). The results revealed a decreasing proportion of blood vessels from the apical to the coronal portions, with a more lacunae in the apical portion and fewer vessels in the coronal portion than in the autograft group. Thus it was concluded that fresh-frozen allografts cannot be considered as successful and safe in alveolar bone reconstruction as autogenous bone grafting.

In yet another recent study, Deluiz et al. (2016) analyzed adverse events associated with placement of fresh-frozen bone allografts (FFBAs) during alveolar ridge augmentation and to assess one-year survival of dental implants placed in reconstructed sites. They enrolled 58 consecutive patients (15 males and 43 females, aged 38–76 years; mean age: 58 ± 9.2 years) requiring maxillary bone reconstruction prior to implant placement. A total of 268 implants was subsequently placed in sites reconstructed with fresh-frozen bone allografts. Infection occurred in six (10.34%) individuals, dehiscence in five (8.62%), and mucosal perforation in seven (12.07%). Adverse outcomes categorized as partial and total graft loss occurred in four (6.90%) and three (5.17%) patients, respectively. The implant failure rate was 16 (5.97%) of the 268 fixtures placed in 12 (20.70%) of 58 patients. The study concluded that infection and suture dehiscence are significantly correlated with graft loss in a maxillary FFBA augmentation (see Figure 9.54a–r).

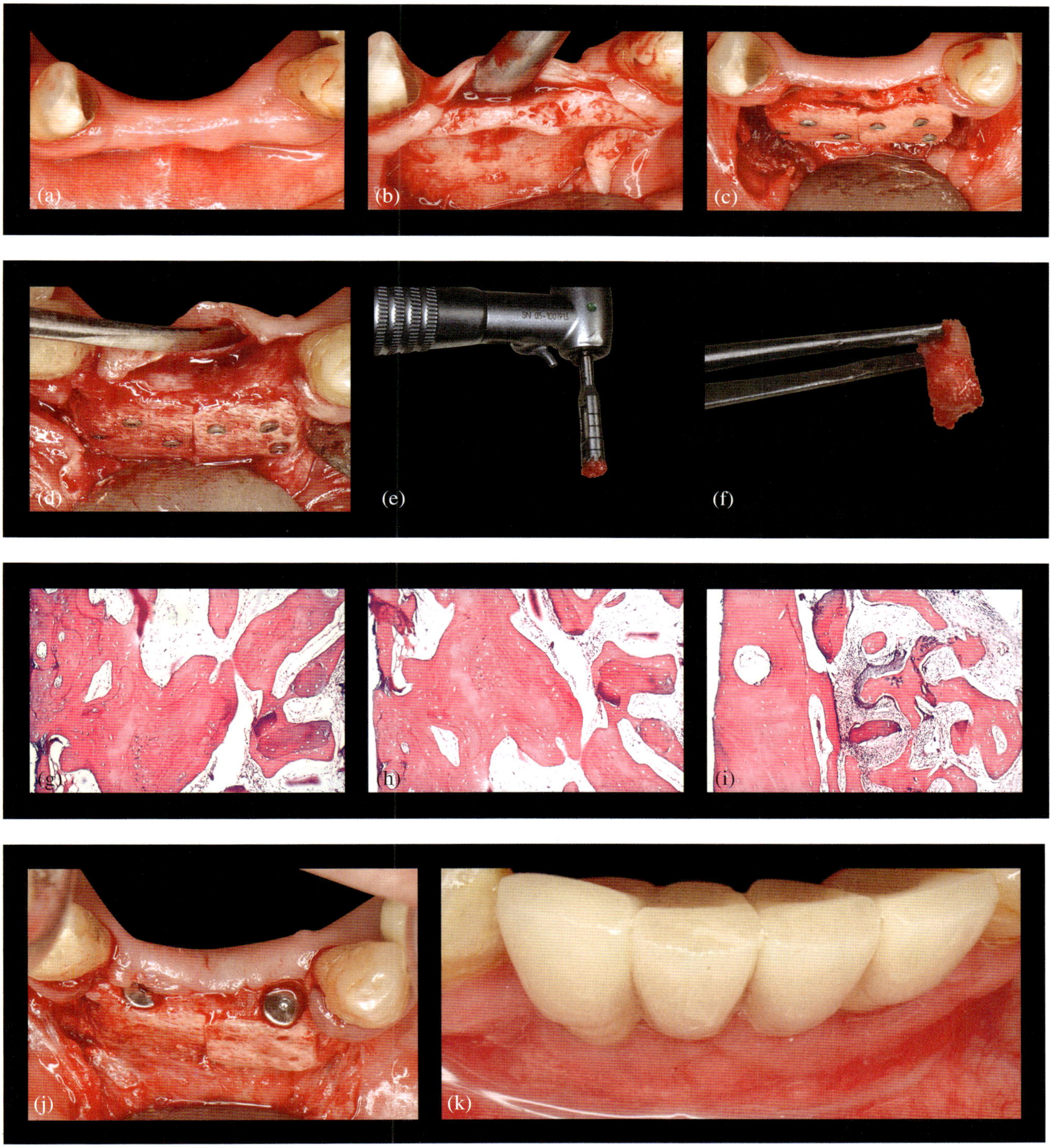

Figure 9.54 (a) Preoperative view of horizontally deficient anterior lower mandible, (b) Meuco periosteal flap is reflected revealing severe horizontal osseous deficiency, (c) Two allograft cortico-cancellus blocks (Puros Allograft, Zimmer dental, Carlesbad, CA, USA) stabilized by titanium microscrews (KLS Martin,GmbH, Tuttilngen, Germany), (d) Four month post-surgery revealing the integration of the bone blocks to recipient bed, (e) and (f) Trephine core is being harvested to confirm the nature of regenerated bone, (g–i) A histological decalcified H & E stained section showing multiple bone trabeculea (Woven bone). Rhythmic pattern of bone formation (resting lines) highly cellular, (j) Two implants are placed, (k) Final prostheses in place.

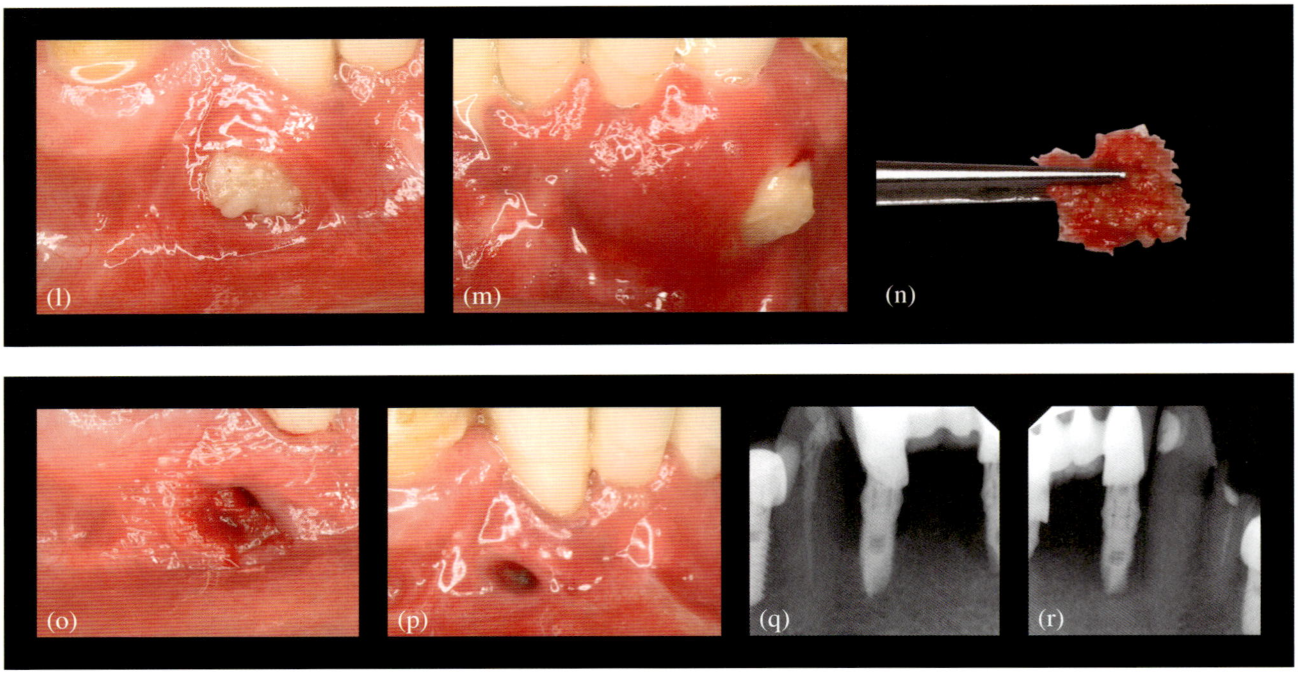

Figure 9.54 (l) and (m) One year post grafting showing graft morbidity and exfoliation, (n) The exfoliated graft, (o) The resultant defect at the time of graft removal, (p) One week post graft removal, (q) and (r) Radiographic view showing the resultant osseous defect.

9.4.4 Complications with Alloplasts

Alloplastic bone graft materials are synthetic materials developed to overcome the inherent problems associated with allografts (Hench 1998). The major advantages of alloplastic materials include their high abundance relative to natural materials, no risk of disease transmission and very low antigenicity (Shetty and Han 1991). Alloplastic materials have an osteoconductive character without any potential for osteoinduction, and are mainly used as a filler in osseous defects and as a matrix for new bone formation. Numerous alloplastic materials and forms are available such as tri-calcium phosphate which is a porous form of calcium phosphate. TCP has two crystallographic forms, α-TCP and β-TCP (Hashimoto-Uoshima et al. 1995); another form of TCP is dicalcium phosphate dihydrate (DCPD) called Brushite that claimed to offer (partial osteogenesis) generation of varying amounts of woven bone and fibrovascular tissue (Bauer and Muschler 2000) (see Figure 9.55). Another new form called biphasic calcium phosphate (BCP) is a mixture of HA and $Ca_3(PO_4)$.

Another alloplastic material, synthetic HA, has been used for a long time in bone regeneration for use in a variety of forms: porous non-resorbable, solid non-resorbable, and resorbable (non-ceramic, porous) (Sheikh et al. 2015b; Tevlin et al. 2014). However, HA have limited *in vivo* resorption and remodeling capacity and although unsuitable for bone augmentation, it is a rather good for space making and defect filling (Petrovic et al. 2012) (see Figure 9.56a–d).

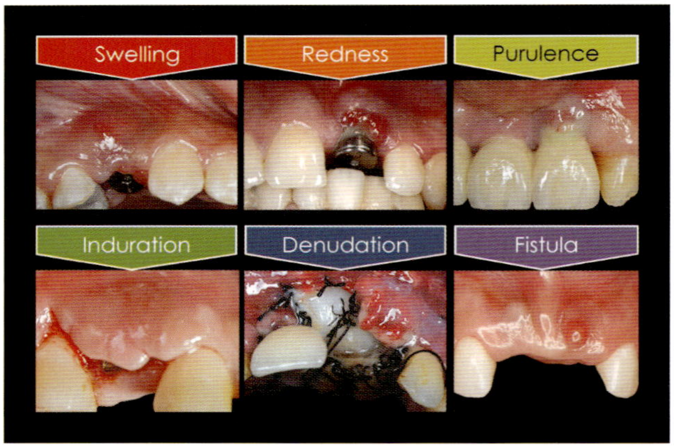

Figure 9.55 Signs and symptoms of bone graft infection.

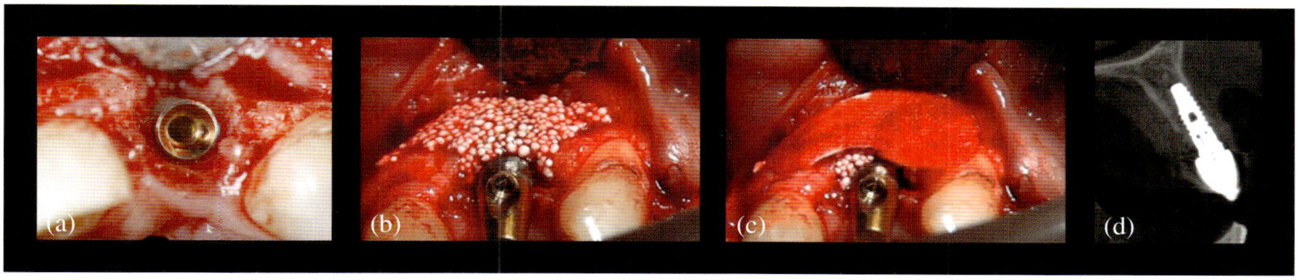

Figure 9.56 (a) Loss of the labial plate of bone that mandates grafting, (b) Alloplast material was used to graft the defect, (c) Collagen membrane was used to cover the graft material, (d) Two years CBCT scan showing the total absence of the grafted material which indicates the lack of predictability of the alloplasts.

Bioactive glass is also another form that gained popularity in the past decade; it is available in several particle sizes and is composed of silicon dioxide (45%), calcium oxide (24.5%), sodium oxide (24.5%), and phosphorus pentoxide (6%) (Schepers et al. 1991). Studies claimed that bioactive glass has several clinical benefits that include retarding epithelial down-growth to the site (Hallman and Thor 2008; Stanley et al. 1997; Wilson 1993). Another form of osteoconductive material, Bioceramics, has been claimed to possess degradation and progressive replacement by lamellar true bone (Barinov et al. 2006) (see Figures 9.57a–c and 9.58a–c).

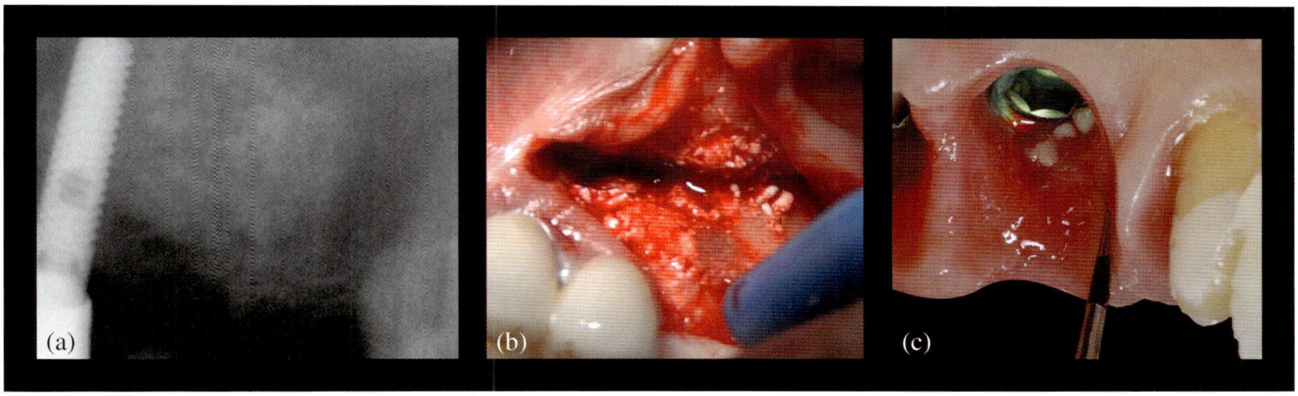

Figure 9.57 (a) and (b) Five years post maxillary sinus grafting with alloplastic showing adhesion of the particles to the periosteum, (c) Retained alloplastic bone graft particles in the gingival crevices for over two years.

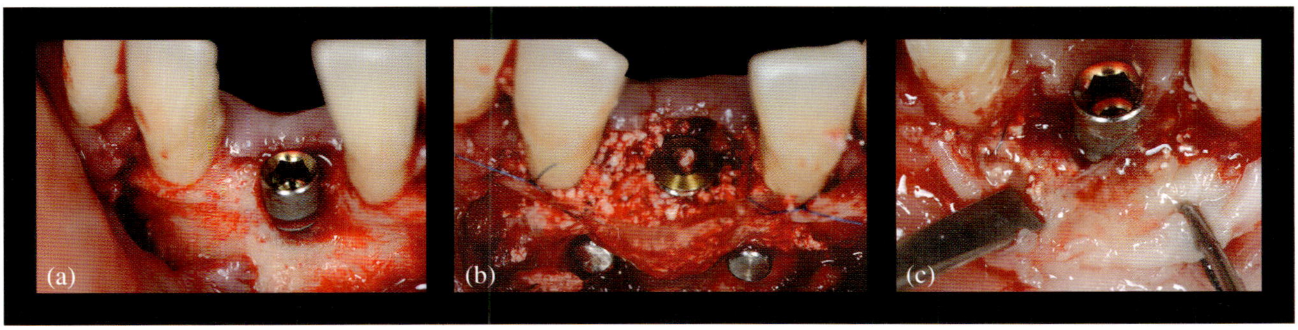

Figure 9.58 (a) Bone dehiscence around an implant, (b) Alloplast material is placed to treat the defect, (c) Three months post-operative showing complete resorption of the alloplast material.

The best clinical outcome of the osteoconductive variants is the better understanding of its function and merit of use, most of the osteoconductive materials (alloplasts) is used only as a filler to fresh extraction site or limited to filling cup shaped osseous defects or offering a scaffold. The efficacies of grafting materials are variable. Most of the conducted studies have many variables, such as the type of defects, the host, the systemic condition impact, the operator's skills, and soft tissue condition at closure. Many other commercially driven studies question the reality behind the use of alloplasts and most studies have evaluation periods of one or two years, which is considered limited for the overall assessment of the material (see Figure 9.59a–d).

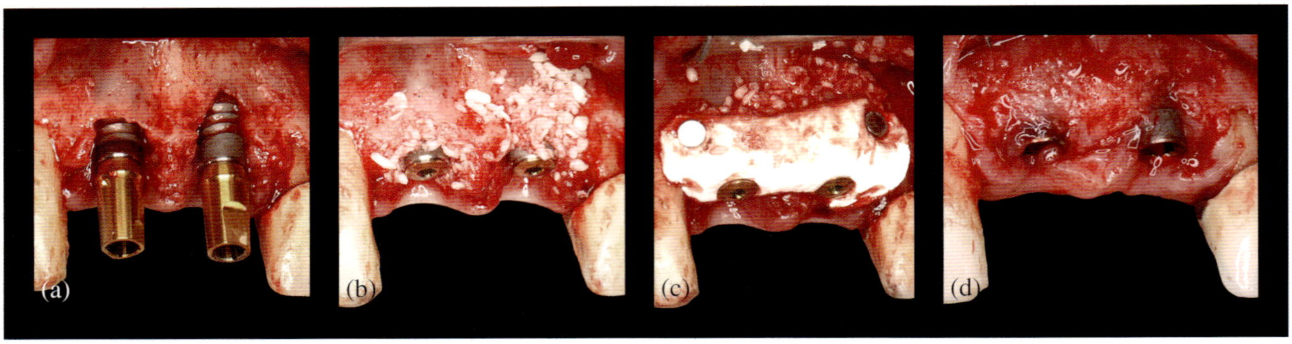

Figure 9.59 (a) Two implants placed (Tapered Internal, BioHorizons, Birmingham, AL, USA), (b) The labial bone defect is grafted with osteoplast material, (c) Collagen membrane is placed and secured with the cover screw, (d) Four months post grafting showing the poor regenerative outcome of the osteoplast.

There have been many attempts to enhance the clinical outcome of alloplasts, like adding platelet-rich plasma (PRP) to tri-calcium phosphate ß-TCP, the osseous regenerating capacity was increased to 38%. Nevertheless, a resorption rate of 32–43% was reported, where the type and quality of the crystal content of the graft material was a dominant factor controlling the rate of resorption (Cabezas-Mojón et al. 2012; Reinhardt and Kreusser 2000).

It is the author's long-term clinical assessment of the use of alloplasts that they have a questionable efficacy for bone regeneration; it is the author's opinion that alloplastic materials may only be used as adjuncts to more osteogenic autogenous grafting materials. They cannot be depended on purely and entirely as having bone-forming potential. Alloplasts should be approached with caution and should not be overestimated as an osteogenic material. The short-term assessment of the alloplast materials has mislead many practitioners to use it for regenerative purpose, but most of the studies did not offer a long term assessment of the material, and most practitioners assessed the efficacy of the materials radiographically, which in reality does not reflect the osteogenic potential of the material.

9.4.5 Complications with Titanium Mesh

Boyne et al. (1985) introduced the concept of a titanium mesh scaffold to be used as an alternative to traditional barrier membranes. The advantage purported at the time was the ability to offer significantly increased and continued space maintenance during the healing phase to allow bone regeneration to occur with fewer concerns about failure if the mesh became exposed. Titanium has been used extensively in numerous surgical applications because of its many inherent physical benefits: its low density and corresponding low weight, its ability to withstand high temperatures and its resistance to corrosion. The low density of titanium provides both high-strength and lightweight dental materials (Artzi et al. 2003; Von Arx and Kurt 1999). It has been used in guided tissue regeneration methods. Titanium-reinforced non-resorbable membranes retain their three-dimensional shape with a specific height and width overcoming the main inherent problem with regular occlusive or non-occlusive barriers (Lekholm et al. 1993), space making, with titanium mesh; the regenerative space is completely preserved by the physical geometry of the mesh. Since that time, numerous studies have reported the success of this technique in achieving a significant amount of osseous regeneration in implant site development procedures (Longoni et al. 2007; Proussaefs and Lozada 2006) (see Figure 9.60a–d and 9.61a–b).

Proussaefs and Lozada (2006) in a histomorphometric study used titanium mesh for localized alveolar ridge augmentation. An equal mixture of autogenous bone graft and inorganic bovine mineral was used. Titanium mesh was submerged for 8.47 months. Out of 17 patients, early mesh exposure (two weeks) was observed in two patients and late exposure (>3 months) was observed in four patients. The histomorphometric evaluation concluded that the average area of all 17 core sections occupied by new bone was 36.47%, which makes the amount of bone regenerated look complete to the clinician's eye, but under the microscope, the

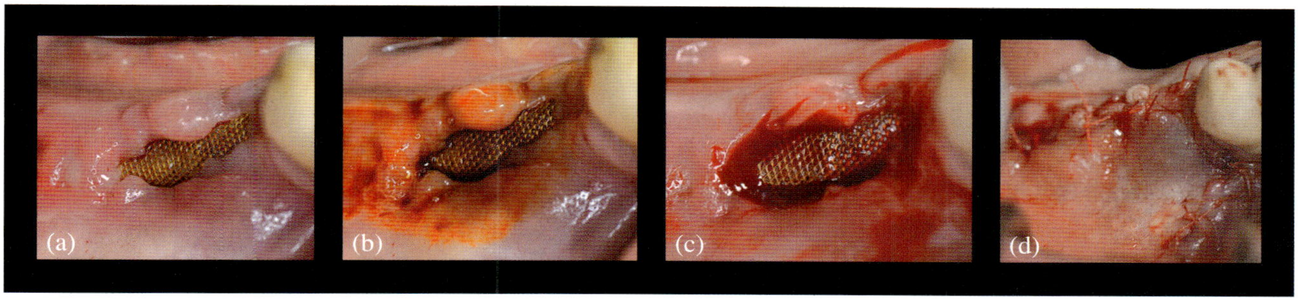

Figure 9.60 (a) Dendunudation of soft tissue on top of previously placed titanium mesh, (b) Disinfecting the site with iodine solution, (c) Freshening the wound edges (removing the epithelial margins), (d) Flap closure.

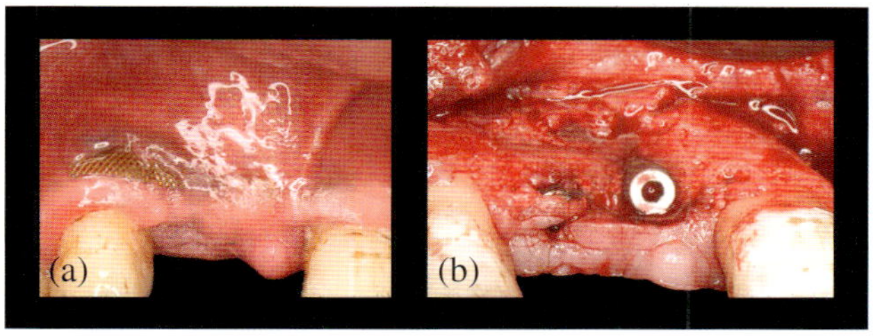

Figure 9.61 (a) Late mesh exposure (Three months), (b) Note the very poor regenerative outcome due to the mesh exposure.

bone formed constitutes almost one third of the formed mass under the mesh. In order to overcome such limitations, the use of deproteinized inorganic bovine bone has been developed as a xenogeneic graft material that can be mixed with autogenous bone graft. The rationale of mixing autogenous bone with the graft is to combine the scaffold properties of the xenograft with the osteogenic and osteoinductive properties of the autograft (Misch and Dietsh 1993) (see Figures 9.62a, b, 9.63a, b, and 9.64a, b).

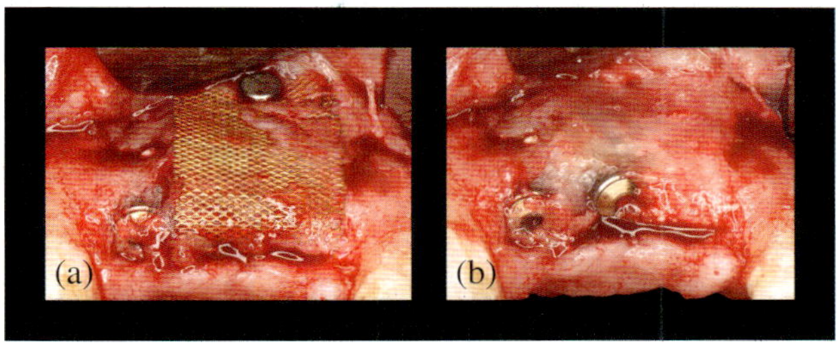

Figure 9.62 (a) Three months post healing showing the titanium mesh in place, (b) Frontal view showing poor regenerated bone underneath the mesh.

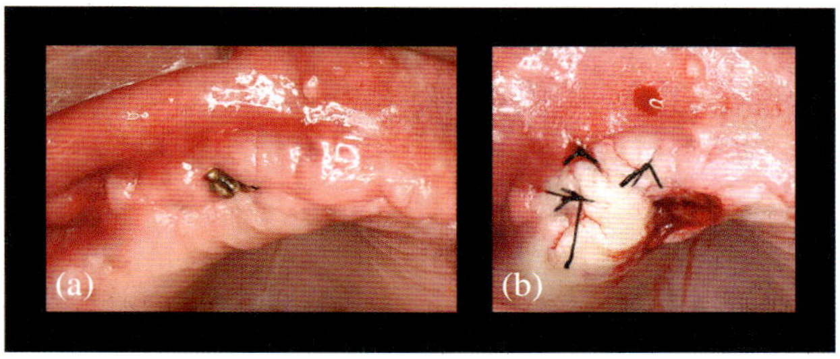

Figure 9.64 (a) One week post-surgery picture showing early soft tissue dehiscence, (b) Rotated palatal flap is used to correct the dehiscence.

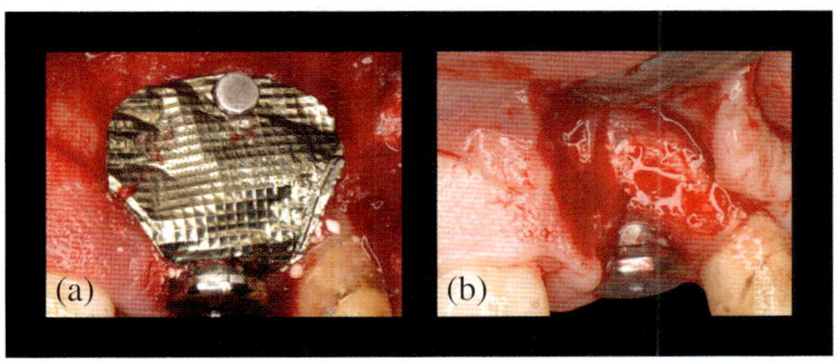

Figure 9.63 (a) Titanium membrane (Frios Bone Shields, Dentsply Friadent, Mannheim, Germany) was tacked apically with (Auto Tac, BioHorizons, Birmingham AL, USA) and inciosally with the cover screw, note that the edges of the membrane is close to the flap edges which indicates the improper flap design as well as the faulty application of the titanium mesh around the neck of a non-submerged implant fixture, (b) The Clinical outcome that indicates the failure of the bone grafting procedure with no bone regeneration due to the exposure of the titanium mesh.

The majority of mesh exposure cases occurred in patients with thin tissue phenotypes; this was related to the increased thickness of the pseudo-periosteum layer observed under the mesh and the lower bone quality in the area of exposure (Poli et al. 2014). Buser et al. (1990) stated that the predictability of guided bone regeneration is significantly compromised by infection of membrane sites, and the retention of the shape cannot be anticipated (see Figure 9.65a and b).

In fact, the use of titanium mesh involved numerous complications, that included soft tissue dehiscence on top of the mesh; blockage of the periosteal blood supply by ingrowth of the angiogenic cells, resulting in slow healing; and poor quality bone regenerated underneath the mesh. Rominger and Triplett (1994) documented 14% of infections in (nine membranes) and

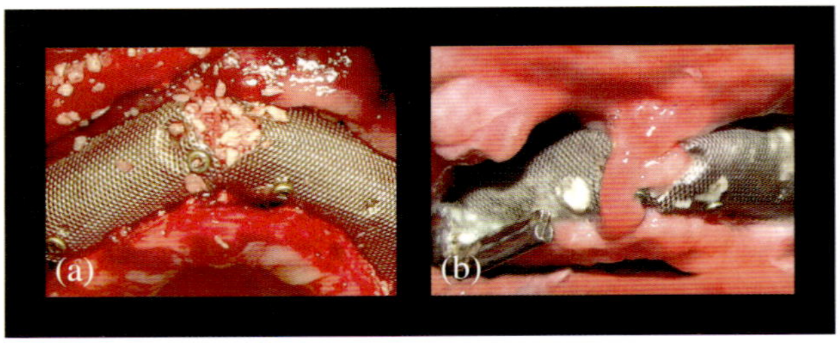

Figure 9.65 (a) A titanium mesh is being placed exceeding the biological original ridge size, (b) Severe soft tissue sloughing due to suture rupture.

14% of dehiscence with exposure of the mesh. These findings were also confirmed by a study by Maiorana et al. (2001), in which exposure of titanium mesh led to early graft resorption in the exposed area of about 15–25%. Clinical management of titanium mesh exposure includes the complete removal of the exposed mesh when the soft tissue is thin, and the exposure area is large, decontamination of the implant surface, and re-grafting along with soft tissue modification for complete coverage of the area (see Figures 9.66a–c and 9.67a, b).

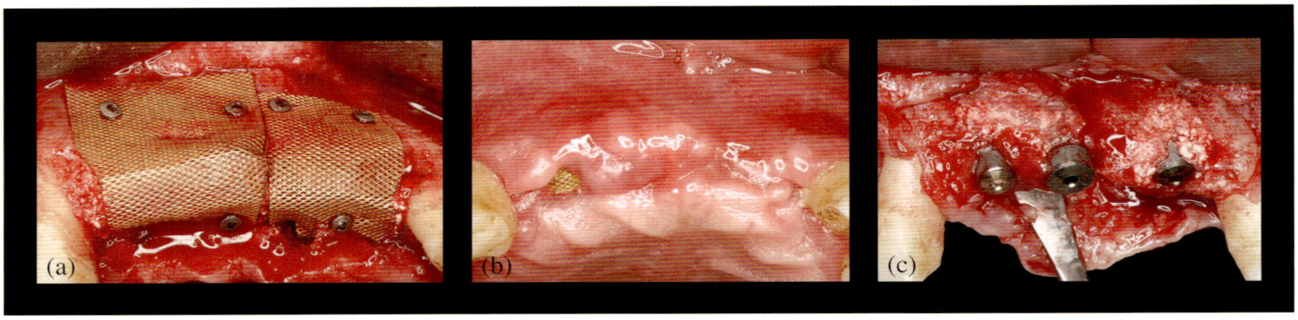

Figure 9.66 (a) Titanium mesh is stabilized with two micro screws (KLS Martin, GmbH, Tuttilngen, Germany), (b) One month post healing showing soft tissue dehiscence exposing the titanium mesh to the oral environment, the soft tissue opening was maintained with clorohexdine daily, (c) Four months post grafting showing reduced amount of regenerated bone due to the exposure of the titanium mesh to the oral environment.

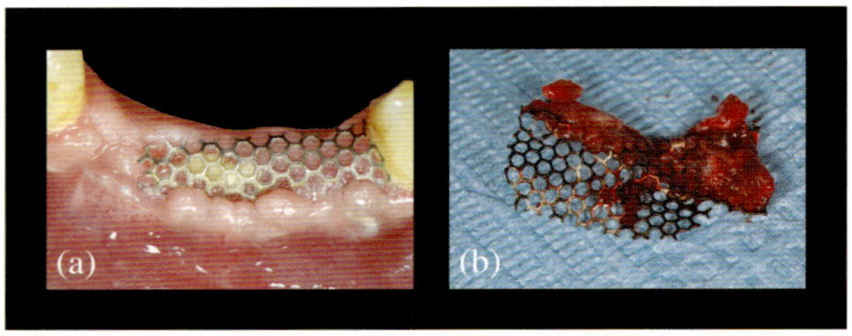

Figure 9.67 (a) and (b) Late titanium mesh exposure and underlying soft tissue adhesions.

Levine et al. (2014) presented part of a large, consecutive series study on the use of a titanium mesh scaffold for GBR. They concluded that complications related to early exposure and early removal of the barrier membrane make this technique less predictable when significant regeneration is required, while soft tissue adhesion makes titanium mesh more difficult to remove.

9.4.6 Predictable Guidelines for Regenerative Procedure

In the following section, some clinical guidelines are detailed to offer a reliable regenerative outcome and to maximize the treatment outcome.

9.4.6.1 Identify the Nature of the Defect

The accurate identification and understanding of the nature of the osseous defect to be grafted is of great importance, once the nature of the defect is identified, whether a cup-shaped defect or a two-dimensional defect, or a three-dimensional defect. Methods to amend the ridge are now proposed according to the known limitations and success rate of each method, grafting materials are chosen accordingly, the selection according to the speed of resorption of the material or the particle size etc. The identification of the local bone type (the bone density) standpoint will also predict the treatment outcome and mandates special materials and techniques to be elected. The ability of the clinician to identify the tissue phenotype involved in the surgical approach is highly important and will definitely contribute to the fate of the regenerative procedures immensely.

Therefore, acquaintance with the currently available classifications related to alveolar ridge defect has become mandatory. Lekholm and Zarb (1985) have classified a five-degree scale for alveolar bone resorption status (A to E) and jaw bone quality on a four-degree scale (1–4). Cawood and Howell (1988) offered a classification system of the edentulous jaws based on the assumption that gradual atrophy follows the loss of teeth. The edentulous maxilla is classified as class 1–6. The key factors in achieving implant stability are bone quantity and bone quality. Friberg, Jemt and Lekholm (1991) showed an overall implant failure rate of 38% in edentulous maxillary type 4 bone and a 7% failure rate of 7 mm long implants compared to less than 1% in implants longer than 10 mm. The impact of bone structure on implant stability was also shown by Jaffin and Berman (1991) with a failure rate of 44% in type 4 bone compared to 3.6% in types 1–3 (see Figures 9.68a–d and 9.69a–i). The ability of the clinician to detect the nature and type of the bone defect present is of high value as each individual osseous defect requires its own predictable approach and treatment alternatives, which allows the clinician to anticipate the fate of the procedure prior to starting and convey it to the patient.

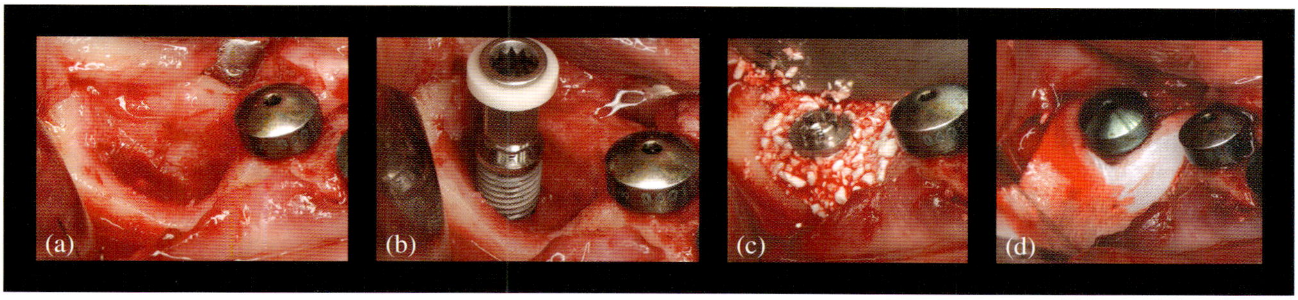

Figure 9.68 (a–d) Cup shape osseous defect that gives high predictability to bone grafting procedures outcome.

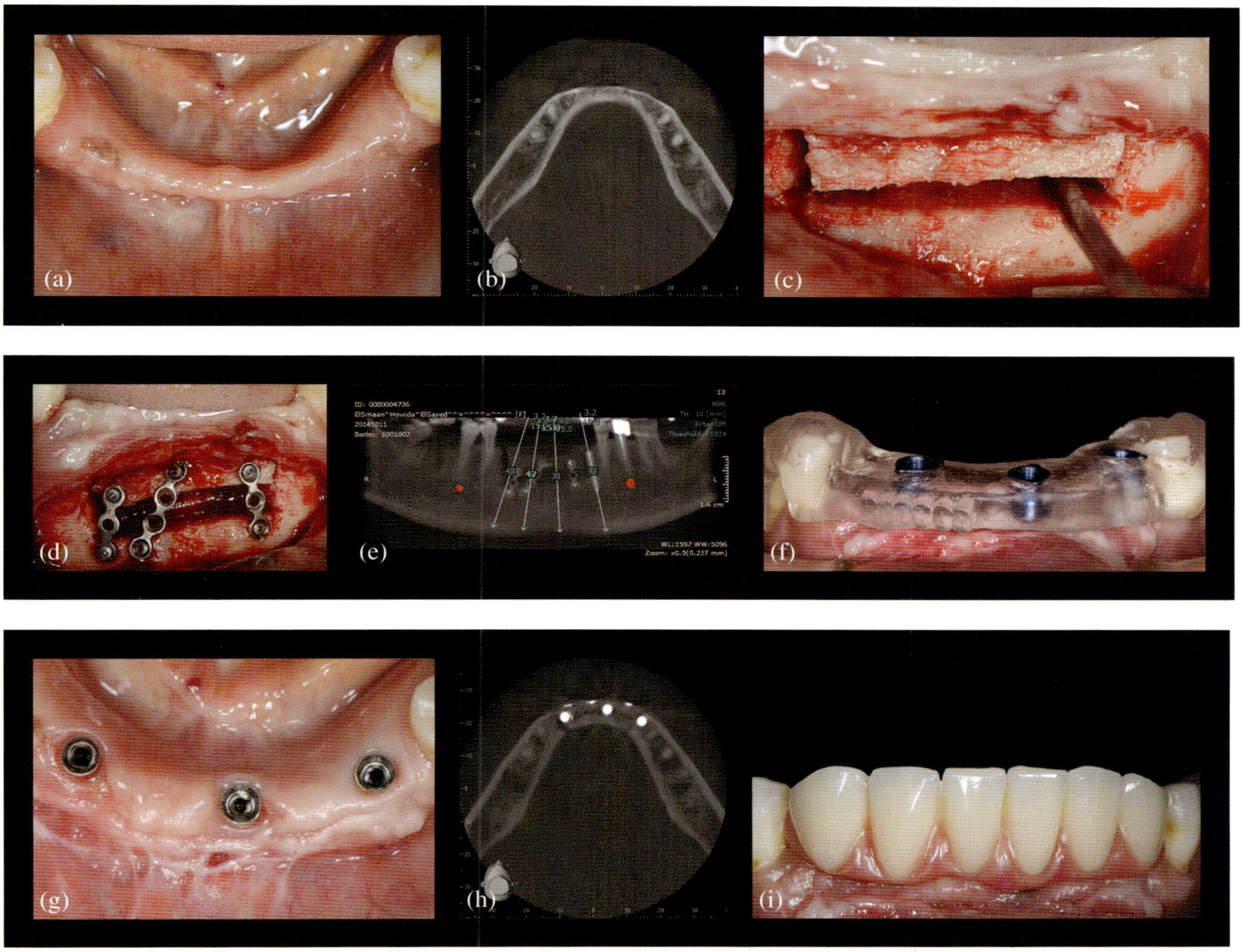

Figure 9.69 (a) and (b) Clinical and radiological views showing severe vertical ridge deficiency which indicates a different unusual treatment approach. (c) Mobilized osteotomy performed, (d) Titanium microplates are used to stabilize the mobilized block, (e) CBCT four months post-surgery for planning the future implants position, (f) CAD-CAM surgical guide in place, (g) Two months post implant placement healing, (h) CBCT showing Implants in place, (i) Final screw-retained prosthesis in place.

On the other hand, cells within cancellous bone are responsible for at least 60% of the patient's bone healing capacity. The periosteum in a young, healthy patient contributes an additional 30%. Cells in the cortical bone are responsible for only 10% of bone healing (Sandberg and Aspenberg 2016). As the cancellous compartment decreases, the reservoir for osteoblasts does as well. Computerized tomography can reveal the ratio of cancellous bone to cortical bone at the recipient site prior to surgery (see Figure 9.70).

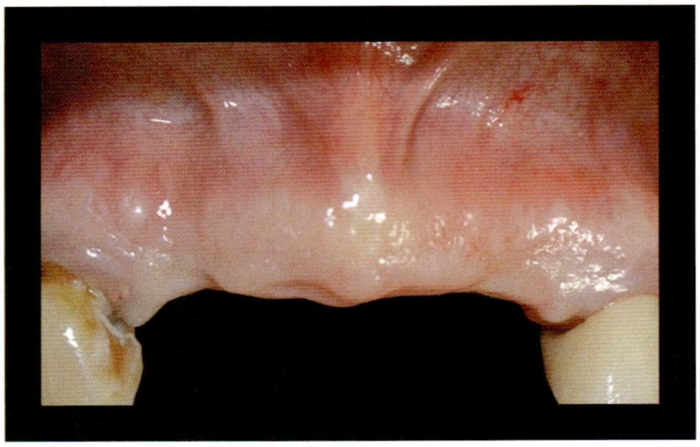

Figure 9.70 The phenotype (the quality of the soft and hard tissues) dictates the decision making and the operative approach to a great extent.

9.4.6.2 Predict the Host Response

Many systemic inflictions to the patient's health could directly impact the overall success of surgery, for example, diabetes, blood pressure, depression, osteoporosis etc. A reduction in mandible bone mass has been weakly correlated to cortical bone reduction in other parts of the skeleton, but no relationship to maxillary bone mass has been shown (see Figure 9.71a–o).

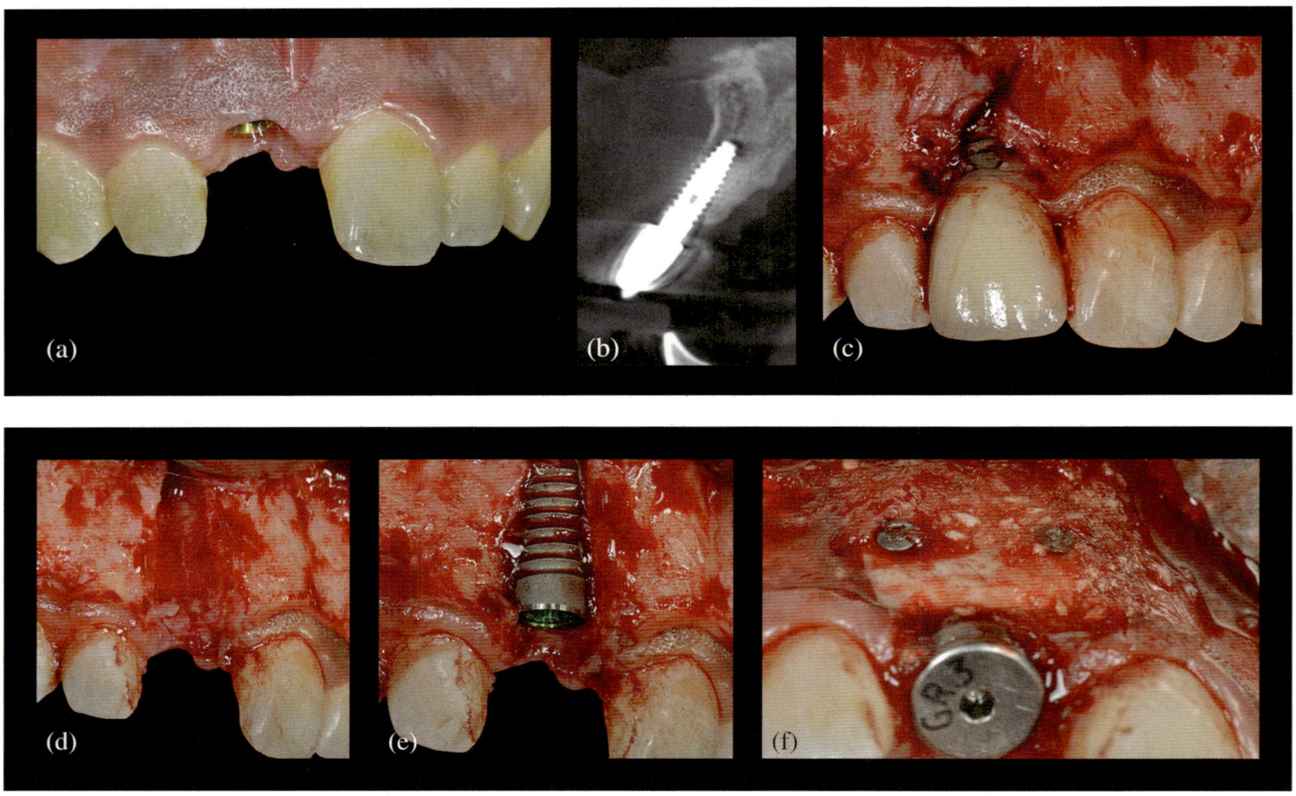

Figure 9.71 (a) Two month post-surgery showing after the peri-implant tissue profiling. (b) CBCT scan showing loss of the labial plate of bone and failed bone graft as a result of smoking. (c) Intra operative view showing the failed implant supported restoration, (d) Implant removed and bone is cleaned, degranulated, (e) A new implant fixture is placed, (f) Mono-cortical allograft is placed and stabilized with micro titanium screws.

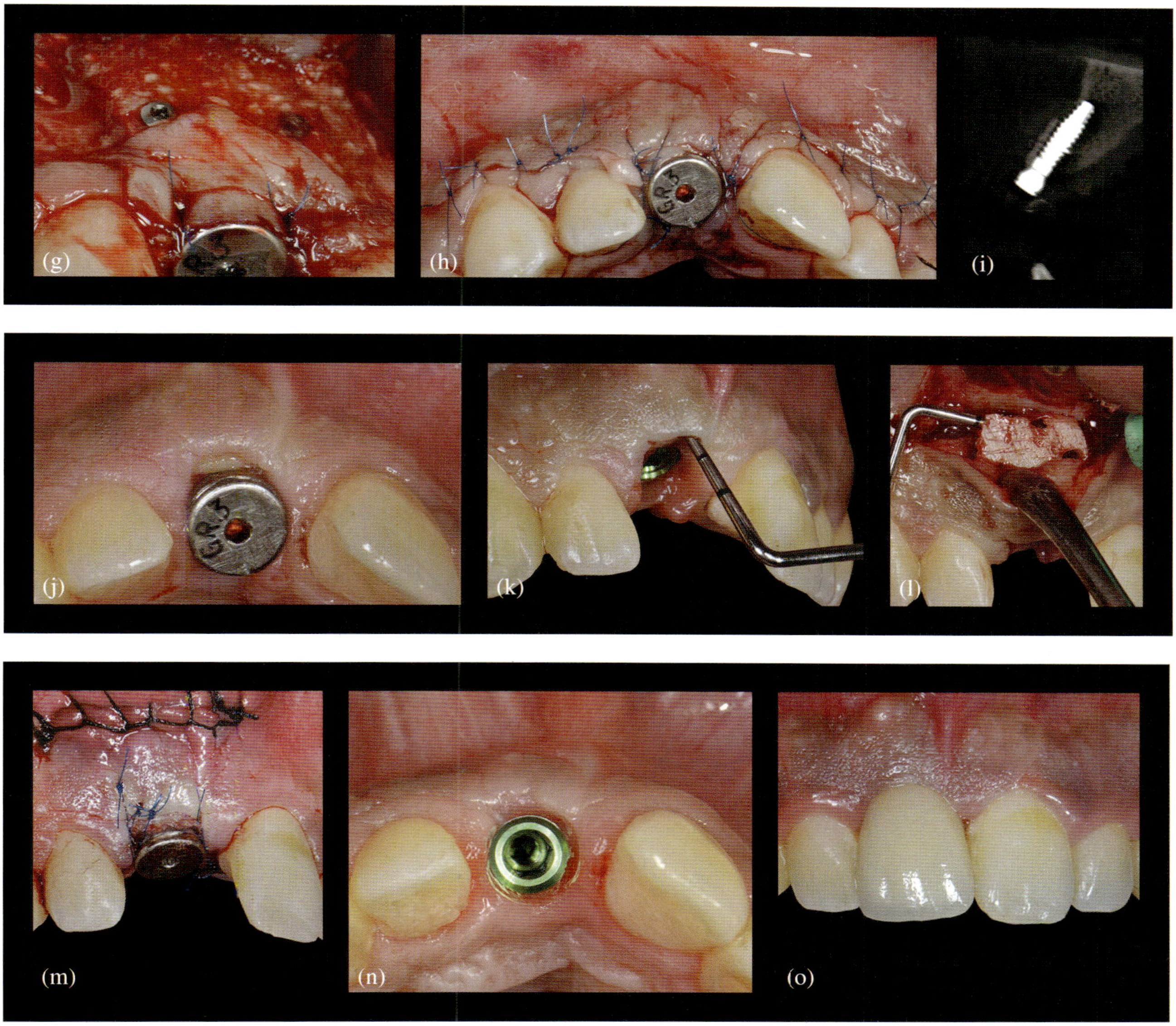

Figure 9.71 (g) Connective tissue graft is stabilized, (h) Flap closure attempted around the healing collar, (i) Immediate post op CBCT showing the graft is in place, (j) Two month post grafting, a clinical picture shows exposure of the bone graft, indicates its failure, (k) Pocketing along the graft surface and lack of epithelial attachment, (l) Vestibular incision is made to void crestal incision that might induce recession, the allograft cortical sheet is removed easily, (m) Connective tissue graft is positioned and flap closed, (n) Final healing one week post-operative, (o) Final case restored.

Patients are urged to reveal any ongoing medical treatment and/or any medications they are taking as well as any influencing habits. It highlights contraindications or important areas of concern for dental implant therapy (Sabes et al. 1970), it can also provide useful information on the potential prognosis of implant treatment (Halstead 1982; Misch 1982). The following areas of medical risks (Wakley and Baylink 1988) associated with dental implant placement can be evaluated through a detailed medical history or physical and laboratory examination, as dealing with medically compromised patients should be approached with caution. Some of the patients seen daily could be already contraindicated to implant therapy, some of them should be well controlled before the treatment, and others should be postponed for some time. Therefore, the complete understanding of the medical background of the patients prior to surgery becomes mandatory. The clinician should have an idea of the health profile of the patient just by gathering data from the patient him/herself, and should any suspicious symptoms exists, then the patient should be referred to his/her physician to investigate the condition and deliver a clear report. Following this protocol could save patients from many of the potential complications during the course of the treatment.

Renal disease is a major concern to dental implant therapy, which should be carefully evaluated initially through the medical history, because epinephrine and norepinephrine are naturally produced in the medulla of the kidney and are responsible for the regulation of blood pressure, myocardial contraction, and excitability. Glucocorticoids from the cortex is responsible for regulation of carbohydrates, fat, and protein metabolism. Hypo-function of the adrenal gland may lead to Addison's disease, which is manifested by weight loss, hypotension, and nausea with or without vomiting. Oral manifestation is hyper-pigmentation of lips and gingiva. The hyperfunction causes Cushing's syndrome, manifested by a moon face, hypertension, and decreased collagen production. Patients suffer from poor wound healing, osteoporosis and an increased risk of infection. Normal creatinine levels are 0.7–1.5 mg 100 ml^{-1} and any disturbance may indicate kidney dysfunction and warrants further investigation; if ignored it may lead to osteoporosis and decreased bone healing. Patients that have any chronic renal problems should receive additional steroids prescribed by an experienced physician. Blood dyscrasias such as anemia, leukemia, bleeding/clotting disorders, etc., also have an impact on dental implants. Mild anemia has many intra-oral symptoms; fatigue, anxiety, and sleeplessness, while chronic anemia is characterized by shortening of breath, abdominal pain, bone pain, tingling of the extremities, muscular weakness, headache, fainting, change in heart rhythm, and nausea. Oral symptoms of anemia include a sore, painful, smooth reddish tongue, loss of taste sensation, and paresthesia of oral tissues. Anemia might have some further complications including impaired bone maturation and development, while a faint large trabecular pattern of bone may appear radiographically, which indicates a 25–40% loss of trabecular pattern (Elaskary 2008).

Decreased bone density affects the initial implant placement and may influence the initial amount of mature lamellar bone forming at the interface of osseointegrated implants. Preoperative and postoperative antibiotics should be administered and hygiene appointments should be scheduled more frequently. The anemic condition should be corrected. On the other hand, the blood leukocytic disorders entails leukocytosis, which is either due leukemia, neoplasm, acute hemorrhage and/or diseases associated with acute inflammation, necrosis or leukopenia, which may accompany certain infections (e.g. hepatitis), or bone marrow damage (from irradiation therapy). Both conditions may cause complications that compromise the success of dental implant therapy, as infection, edema, and bleeding can be a common event due to thrombocytopenia. The treatment plan should shift towards a more conservative approach when dealing with leukocytic disorders. Vitamin D is yet another factor considered to be influential to implant therapy; it is synthesized in the liver, skin, kidney, intestine, and parathyroid gland. It helps to increase absorption of calcium and phosphate from the intestine and kidney. Deficiency of vitamin D is called 'osteomalacia.' Oral findings of osteomalacia are a decrease in trabecular bone, indistinct lamina dura, and an increase in the tendency to chronic periodontal disease. Hyperparathyroidism also has distinctive oral findings including loss of lamina dura, loosening of the teeth, and altered trabecular bone pattern (ground glass appearance). Central and peripheral giant cell tumors may develop. Implants are relatively contraindicated in cases of hyperparathyroidism. Patients with severely compromised immune systems, and severe gastrointestinal diseases (e.g. hepatitis, malabsorption, etc.) should also be excluded from any surgical intervention for dental implant installation. Patients with musculoskeletal diseases (e.g. osteoporosis, osteopetrosis, and osteitis deformas (Paget's disease)) that show a slowly progressive bone disease due to increased osteoblastic activity, are usually marked by increased serum alkaline phosphates and calcium levels. Bony enlargement could be palpated and appears radiographically as cotton wool shape. The patient is therefore predisposed to osteosarcoma. In such conditions, dental implants are totally contraindicated. Osteoporosis is a common oral bone disease that influences implant placement; the problem arises from an imbalance between the rates of bone resorption and formation. The resorption process dominates, the cortical plates become thinner, the trabecular bone pattern more discrete, and advanced demineralization occurs. Osteoporosis affects females twice as much as males, especially after the menopausal period (Elaskary 2008). It does not constitute an absolute contraindication for dental implants, but it influences the treatment path. Precautions should include: estrogen therapy intake, dietary calcium intake, progressive bone loading, and implant designs should be greater in width and coated with hydroxyapatite to increase bone contact (Wakley and Baylink 1988).

Some situations or predicaments preclude the success of implant therapy because they compromise the body's health either generally or locally. Pregnancy, persistent oral infections, AIDS, neurologic disorders (e.g. stroke, palsy, mental retardation, etc.) which may render a patient incapable of maintaining adequate oral hygiene on a daily basis, and malignancies are examples of such contraindicating situations for dental implant therapy (Smiler 1987).

Smoking is increasingly cited in the literature as a risk factor in soft tissue healing (Rees et al. 1984), periodontal health, and implant therapy (Bergström and Preber 1994). There are several controversial points of views concerning smoking in relation to dental implant failure; modern science has proven that there is a potential increased risk of smoking on the long- and short-term success of dental implants (Gorman et al. 1994). A study by Persson, Bergström and Gustafsson (2003) evaluated the soft tissue response towards smoking and they stated that tobacco smoking has considerable negative effects on the outcome of periodontal treatment. The reason might be related to altered neutrophil activity in terms of elastase and/or matrix metalloproteinase-8 (MMP-8), as well as in the protease inhibitor alpha-1-antitrypsin (a-1-AT) and alpha-2- macroglobulin (a-2-MG) activities. The study included 15 smoking and 15 non-smoking patients with moderate to severe periodontitis receiving surgical treatment. Clinical examinations and collection of GCF were carried out prior to surgery and one and five weeks following treatment. The elastase activity was measured with a chromogenic low-molecular substrate and the levels of a-1-AT, a-2-MG, and MMP-8 with enzyme-linked immunosorbent assay. Results showed unaltered levels of a-1-AT, a-2-MG, and MMP-8 in smokers following surgery. In non-smokers, the levels of a-1-AT and a-2-MG increased, whereas MMP-8 levels decreased. The levels of elastase remained in both smokers and non-smokers. The results indicated that in the presence of smoking, the levels of a-1-AT, a-2-MG, and MMP-8 remained unaltered during the recovery period following surgical treatment. This is interpreted as a possible interference of smoking with the treatment response and may, in part, explain the clinical evidence of poor treatment outcome in patients who smoke. That probably explains the statement that excludes smokers from periodontal and implantology treatment till they follow a strict cessation protocol. Another study (Henemyre et al. 2003) determined the effect of physiologically relevant nicotine levels on porcine osteoclast function as measured by resorption of calcium phosphate. The study used pure nicotine that was diluted in medium to the following concentrations: 0.03, 0.15, 0.30, 0.60, and 1.50 μM. Porcine osteoclasts were seeded onto calcium phosphate multi-test slides and incubated at 37 °C with half media changes every 24 hours. Cells received 0, 0.15, 0.30, 0.60, and 1.50 μM nicotine, or 25 nM parathyroid hormone (PTH). Osteoclast resorption was quantified by measuring the resorbed surface area of the calcium phosphate substrate. The study showed an increased number of osteoclasts was directly related to an increasing nicotine concentrations; however, no correlation was found between osteoclast number and the amount of resorption. It was concluded that nicotine appears to stimulate osteoclast differentiation and the resorption of calcium phosphate, which is the major component of bone. Nicotine-modulated osteoclast stimulation may, in part, explain the increased rapidity of periodontal bone loss and refractory disease incidence in patients who smoke (Elaskary 2008).

Allergies are yet another source of concern. A thorough medical and dental history is important in identifying allergies that could dictate the use or avoidance of certain drugs of other substances in dental implant therapy. Due to its high passivity and biocompatibility, no allergies to titanium or titanium alloy have been reported in the dental literature (Bezzon 1993; Latta, McDougal and Bowles 1993). However, allergies to denture was reported (Hansen and West 1997) and restorative base metals such as chromium cobalt, nickel, and palladium-copper-gold alloys have appeared in research abstracts (Fieding and Hild 1993).

Patients with artificial joints may develop bacteremia due to implant surgery that can cause hematogenous seeding at the joint implants. It was hypothesized that bacteria may seed the prosthesis and cause infection due to dental procedures. Antibiotic coverage is preoperatively being highly indicated. The salivary glands and ducts must be inspected for any obstruction that may hinder normal salivary flow and intra-oral lubrication to any oral prosthesis and may mandate a change in the proposed prosthodontic plan. Liver function should be assessed because liver cirrhosis causes reduction in the synthesis of clotting factors, abnormal synthesis of fibrinogen and clotting proteins, vitamin K deficiency, enhanced fibrinolytic activity, and quantitative and qualitative platelet deficiency. Two of the more important functions of the liver that are influential to implantology procedures are the synthesis of clotting factors and the ability to detoxify drugs. Bilirubin altered range (total: 0.7 mg 100 ml^{-1}) indicates liver disease that affects tissue healing, drug pharmacokinetics, and long-term overall health of the patient. In minor procedures, postoperative control of bleeding should be applied by using bovine collagen and additional sutures (Elaskary 2008). Advanced surgical procedures require hospitalization to control hemorrhage. Any history of osteomyelitis or irradiation therapy in the region of the proposed implant receptor site should be well investigated; the relationship between dental implant failure and irradiation therapy is not quite clear. Irradiation for the treatment of oral cancer does not seem to reduce the survival rate of implants as compared to those placed in the non-irradiated jaws; the main problem with irradiated patients is decreased salivary flow (xerostomia) (Jisaander et al. 1997), the liability for infection due to the decrease in blood supply, and the possibility of osteoradionecrosis (Marx and Johnson 1987).

The complication of radiation starts when the dose exceeds 64 Gy (Murray et al. 1980). Some authors stated that the maxilla is more liable to failure with dental implants after irradiation therapy. The waiting period between the end of radiation therapy and implant placement is not definite. Some authors suggest three to six months (King, Casarett and Weber 1979). Others suggest six months, because after six months fibrosis is expected to begin in the irradiated tissues as a result of reduced cell reproducibility and progressive ischemia. Others recommend a 12 month waiting period (Albrektsson 1988). It seems that the failure rate of dental implants after oral radiotherapy is minimal; but it is recommended to wait for a longer healing period and to use hyperbaric oxygen therapy especially in the maxilla, to improve the healing capacity and avoid soft tissue ulceration as well as reducing fibrous tissue formation (Keller 1997).

Physical conditions and symptoms are not the only aspects an oral surgeon should evaluate and assess. A patient's psychological ability to commit to long-term treatment and maintenance programs must be an integral part of the examination and selection process. During the consultation, the clinician should determine whether the patient is psychologically capable of making the necessary long-term commitment. For example, phobic or highly anxious individuals may have low pain thresholds and refuse to present for treatment follow-ups. On the other hand, patients whose dental complaints stem from somatization disorders will probably not be satisfied with the results of implant therapy (Melamed 1989).

It is unfortunate that not every person may be considered mentally, psychologically, physically, and emotionally sound. As a result, some cases may contraindicate for dental implant therapy. Persons afflicted with acute psychiatric or psychological disorder are one such example. These disorders may be subdivided into (1) inability to understand information, follow instructions, or make reasonable decision (e.g. psychotic syndromes, severe neurotic conditions, or character disorders, etc.); (2) impaired memory or motor coordination necessary for routine oral hygiene (e.g. cerebral lesion syndromes, presenile dementia, etc.); and (3) chronic, severe drug addiction, because of a high propensity for poor motivation, inadequate nutrition, and lack of compliance with oral hygiene regimen (Smith, Silverman, Auclert 1989). As always, it is best to select candidates whose level of understanding and cooperation is superior, for that guarantees a successful end result (Elaskary 2008). Endocrine systemic diseases (e.g. uncontrolled diabetes, hyperthyroidism, pituitary/adrenal disorders, etc.), should be approached with caution, as 75% of patients with diabetes mellitus exhibit increased alveolar bone loss and inflammatory gingival changes that might affect osseointegration negatively. 'Hypoglycemia' is the most serious complication for diabetic patients during any dental procedure; it occurs as a result of excessive insulin levels, excessive hypoglycemic drugs, or inadequate food intake. Its symptoms include: weakness, nervousness, tremor, palpitations, and/or sweating, and in worse cases, confusion and agitation to seizure; coma is the final fate. Diabetes mellitus does not directly affect the failure of dental implants. A consensus expressed that the placement of implants in patients with metabolically controlled diabetes mellitus does not result in a greater risk of failure than in the general population; but a group study stated that patients with diabetes experience more infection in clean wounds than patients without diabetes (Goodson and Hunt 1979). The liability of infection is probably due to the thinning and fragility of the blood vessels, which alters the blood supply. In conclusion, current surgical opinion is that patients with well-controlled diabetes (below $250\,\mathrm{mg\,dl^{-1}}$) probably do not encounter inordinate operative risks, while patients with poorly controlled diabetes or high-risk patients (more than $250\,\mathrm{mg\,dl^{-1}}$) may frequently experience wound failure; therefore, patients with poorly controlled diabetes present more difficult management problems and postponement of the surgery is recommended until better control is achieved (Smith et al. 1992).

Alcohol consumption is detrimental to the success of dental implantology procedures (Sampson et al. 1996) because it contributes negatively to osteoporosis, osteopenia. This statement is supported by the studies which suggested that alcohol intake leads to a negative bone balance effect and progressive bone loss (Lindholm et al. 1991). This in turn may lead to insufficient bone volume for the application of dental implants. A study by Bombonato et al. (2004) evaluated the possible effect of alcoholic beverage administration on reparative bone formation around hydroxyapatite tri-calcium phosphate implants inside the alveolar socket in rats. The study confirmed that a significant delay in reparative bone formation was detected in the alveolus of alcoholic rats by using a histometric differential point counting method. A thorough physical examination prior to implant placement is imperative to assess the patient's present health status and to detect early signs of any undiagnosed disease. Bi-digital palpation of the lips, buccal mucosa, hard and soft palates, the oral pharynx and the submental, submandibular, and cervical lymph nodes should be made to assess the presence of any masses (Smith, Silverman, Auclert 1989). By gently grasping and lifting the tongue forward, upward and laterally, the floor of the mouth and the tongue can also be examined. Registering information and taking notes on past history are only one aspect of the presurgical stage of implant therapy. Recording the patient's vital signs (pulse, blood pressure, respiratory rate, and temperature) can be important in assessing the patient's present overall health. Other medical tests and/or consultations with the patient's physician may be necessary when compromised medical conditions exist or are suspected. It is important to note that the literature suggests evaluating medically compromised implant candidates on a patient-by-patient basis, as compromised medical status alone is not necessarily indicative of implant failure (Elaskary 2008; Elaskary et al. 1999a, b) (see Figure 9.72a–r).

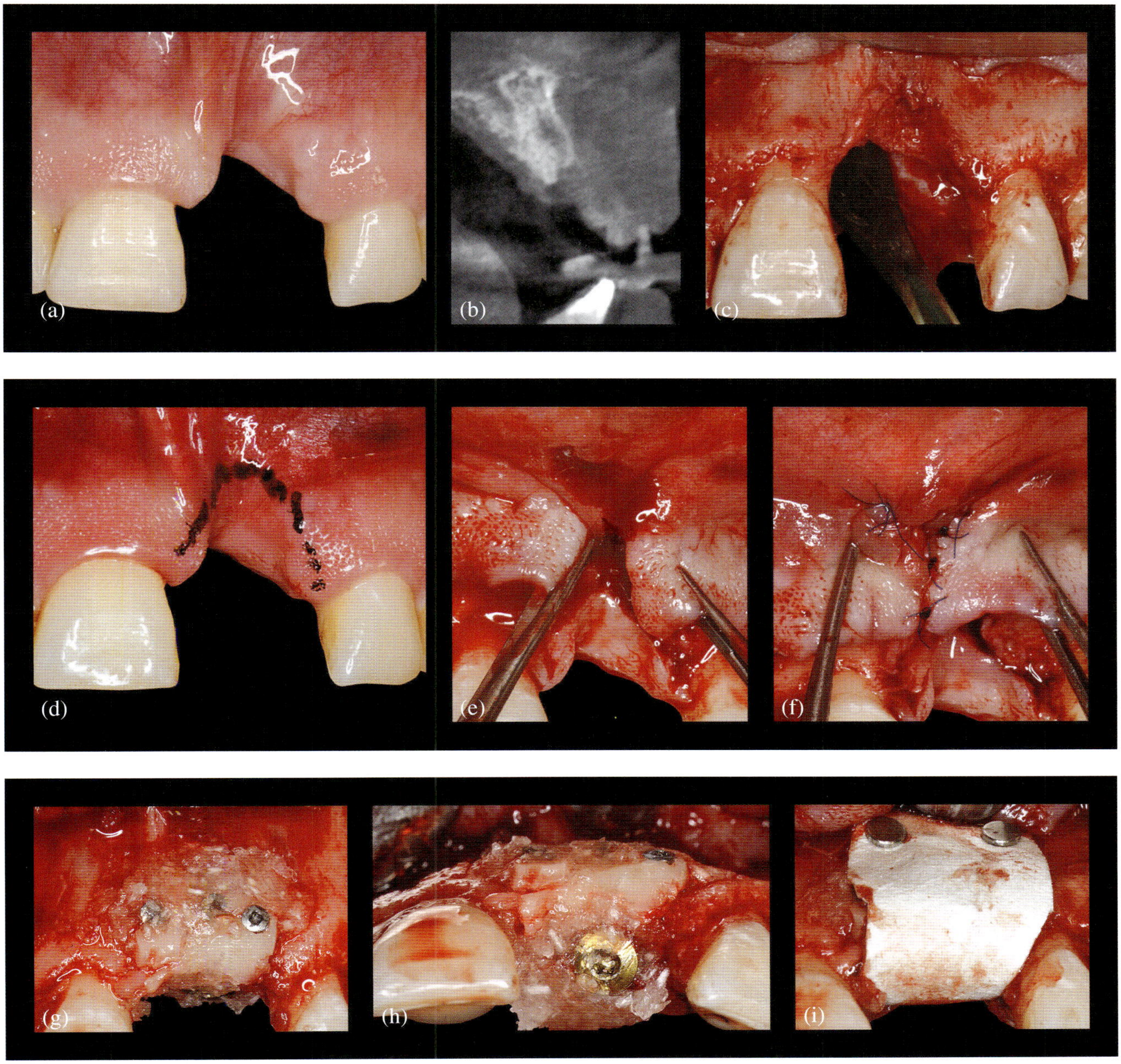

Figure 9.72 (a) Vertical bone loss related to maxillary left central incisor that requires a highly osteogenic grafting material, (b) CBCT scan showing complete loss of both labial and lingual plates of bone, (c) Inter-operative view showing the severity of the bone loss, (d) The black markings showing the incision line (inverted V letter), (e) Approximation of the wound edges, (f) Suturing of wound edges of the double papillary approximation flap, (g) Autogenous bone block harvested from the chin is stabilized with titanium screws (KLS Martin,GmbH, Tuttilngen, Germany), (h) 3.8 × 15 mm laser lock implant being inserted (Laser-lock, BioHorizons, Birmingham, AL, USA), (i) Collagen membrane (Mem-Lock, BioHorizons, Birmingham, AL,USA) is being stabilized by two membrane tacs (Auto Tac, BioHorizons, Birmingham, AL, USA).

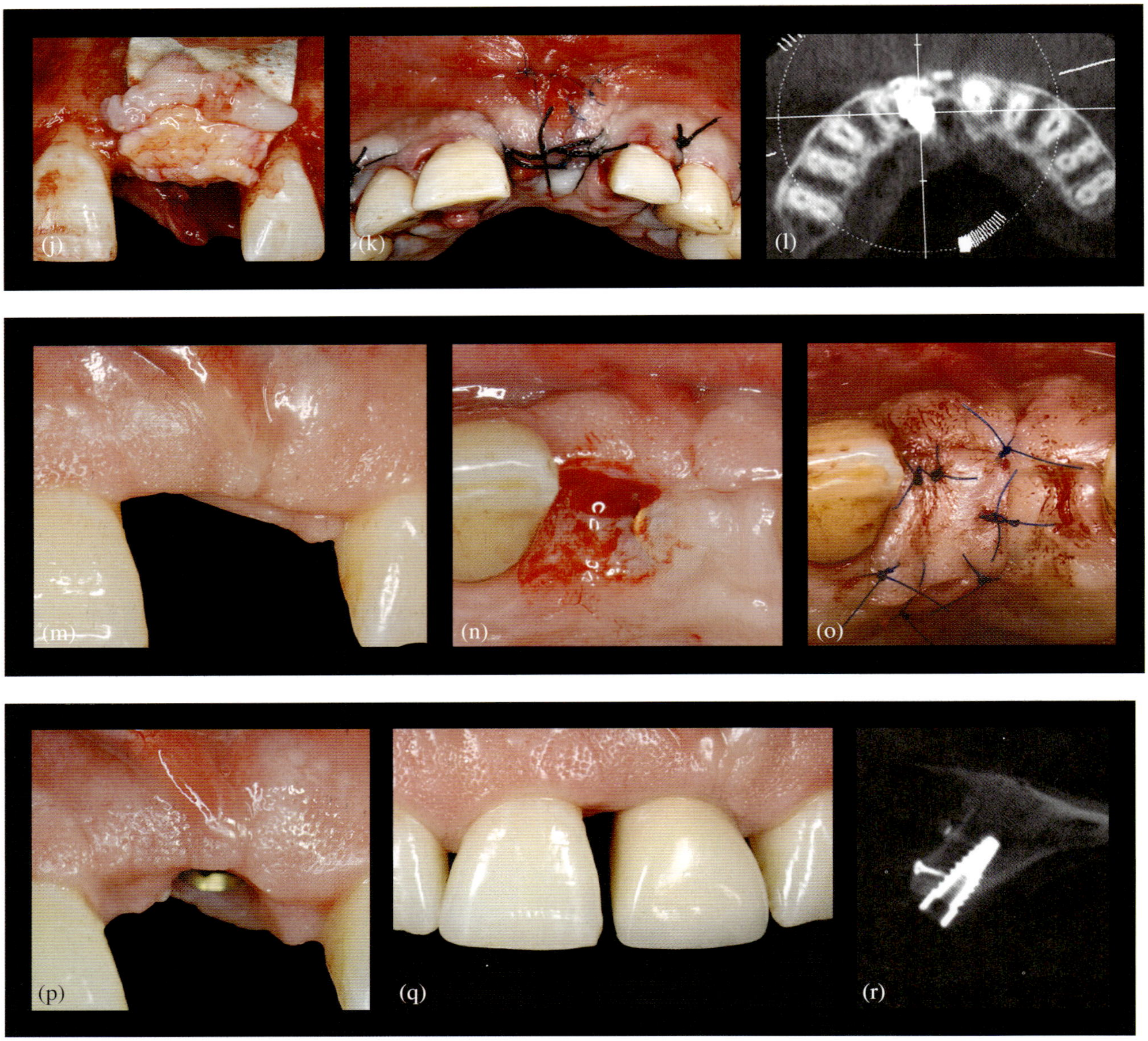

Figure 9.72 (j) Rotated pedicle connective tissue graft from the palate is positioned along the crest of the ridge to ensure maximum tissue volume and better quality of keratinize tissue, (k) Intraoperative view of flap sutured, (l) CBCT postoperative view showing regain of both lingual and buccal contour, (m) Post healing result, (n) De-epithelization the defective ridge, (o) Onlay keratinized graft is used to enhance the soft tissue condition, (p) One month post healing, (q) Final restoration inserted.

9.4.6.3 Optimal Soft Tissue Management and Closure

It is the author's personal opinion that optimizing soft tissue management is more important than the bone graft procedure itself, in the understanding that the bone graft fails easily when the overlying soft tissue fails; therefore, the success of the bone graft is strictly linked to the status of the soft tissue. The movement of the flap during the healing phase will cause fibrous tissues and epithelial cells to fill the defect and invade the graft, leaving much scar and fibrous tissue in place. All of the previous guidelines that have been listed to manage oral soft tissues should be carefully taken into consideration. The author's personal opinion is that when performing regenerative therapy, the clinician should start with soft tissue management and then commence with bone therapy, because in cases where the soft tissue is inadequate, or failed, then the regenerative procedure should be aborted. Start the regenerative procedure by managing the soft tissue first, thus ensuring that this soft tissue will protect and cover the regenerative material with no or few potential complications (see Figure 9.73).

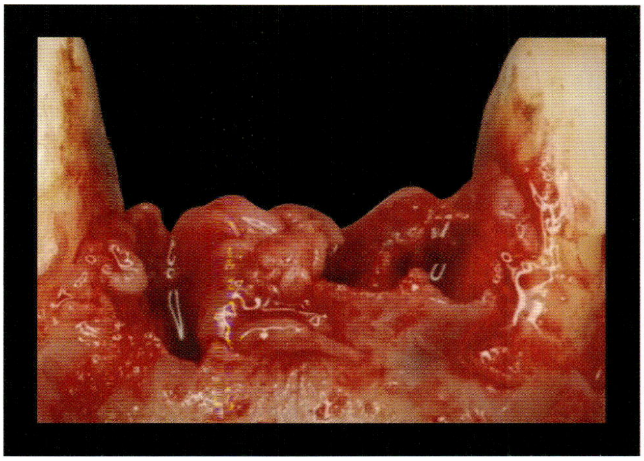

Figure 9.73 Removal of the inflammatory tissue is important prior to any grafting procedure, it controls to a great extent the success of the grafting procedure.

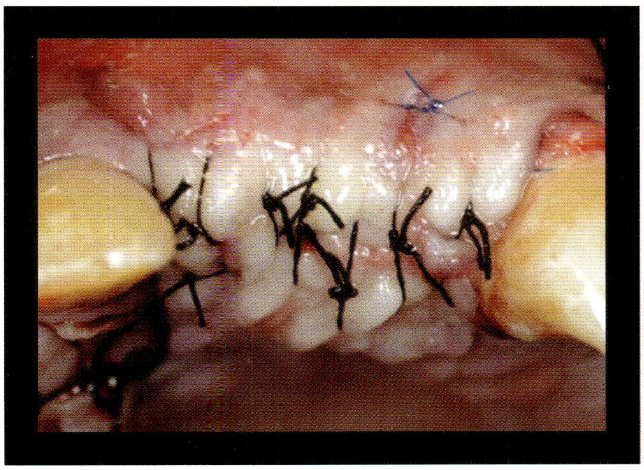

Figure 9.74 Delicate periosteal reflection, minimal tissue trauma, tension free sutures, and avoiding tissue laceration are all important factors to the success of any grafting procedure.

9.4.6.4 Stability and Space Making for Graft Material

One of the most important steps in regenerative therapy is to stabilize all the graft components, whether it is autogenous grafts, alloplasts or allografts. Placing the bone graft then covering it with a collagen membrane without stabilization is no longer an acceptable treatment modality; the graft must be stabilized to protect the coagulum underneath and to counteract against the healing pressure from the periosteum and minimize fibroblast invasion to the graft. When the graft particles are not stable following soft tissue closure, the particles become dispersed throughout the site via muscular movement or chewing. Fixation devices like bone screws, membrane tacs, wires, etc., must be used all the time with no exception. The fact that guided bone regeneration is based on isolating the grafted site from the surrounding soft tissue shows the value of stabilization. The GBR membrane keeps the faster growing tissues like epithelium, fibrous tissue, or gingival connective tissue out of the defect, allowing controlled regeneration to occur with vital bone formation. The application of bone graft material into the defect prevents the collapse of the collagen membrane and acts as a place holder for new regenerating bone and an osteoconductive scaffold for the growth of blood vessels and osteoblasts.

The stability of the grafting complex is one of the most important factors currently being overlooked by many clinicians. Stability of the grafting complex becomes a prior value to any regenerative procedure (see Figure 9.74).

By stabilizing the graft, sufficient space is preserved, and an adequate vascular supply ensured (see Figure 9.75a–c). Once you enable a space that is protected for the bone graft components, the regenerative procedure starts normally. Space making is an old topic that has been detailed by many authors over the years. Since the induction of the osteopromotion theory, it remains one of the most implant prerequisites in the field of regenerative dentistry.

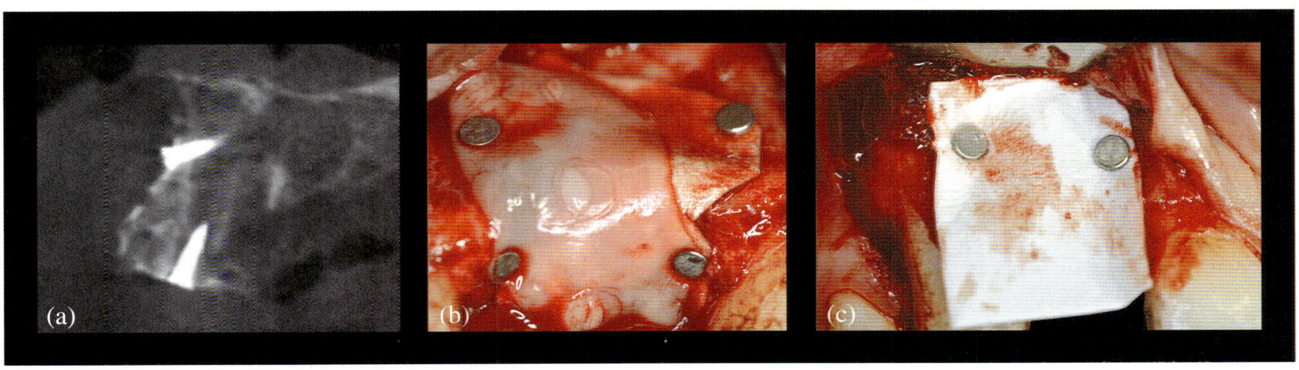

Figure 9.75 (a–c) Achieve stability of the grafted complex via using either membrane tacs or fixating screws is an absolute necessity for stabilizing the coagulum underneath the membrane.

9.4.6.5 Selection of Suitable Regenerative Approach & Material

The correct selection of the grating materials and technique used, depends on several factors that should be accounted for; the osteogenic potential of the graft components; the graft should attain certain osteogenic capacity; the graft matrix must contain or encourage population by osteoblasts; the economic condition of the patient; the ability of the clinician to use the materials selected; and the readiness of the materials in the office. A vast array of choices are now available to clinicians for a graft to be successful. Bone grafting is regeneration not repair, the term 'repair' implies the regaining of lost tissue; regeneration is a biologic process where not only is the tissue regained but also its form and function. The blood clot serves as the initial matrix where cells migrate and then serves as anchorage for the osteoblasts, therefore the need to stabilize the blood clot is also important. Numerous grafting materials and techniques are available in the marketplace. It is the clinician's responsibilty to select the best material and technique that will provide the optimal treatment outcome. The materials used for vertical bone augmentation is definitely different than those used for socket preservation, which explains the value of the selection of the best grafting material.

The author suggests a grafting recipe that may ensure a high predictability outcome of the regenerative procedure, the optimal particulated mix (OPM) is composed of a combination of two thirds of autograft bone chips and one third of deproteinized inorganic bovine bone (DBBM), preferably of equine origin. The bone graft mix is formed of autogenous bone chips harvested from the operating site using any commercially available bone scrapers and DBBM grafting material of an average particle size of 300 M (see Figure 9.76a–c). The reason for using autogenous bone is to ensure a high osteogenic potential of the graft and the rest is used as a filler to maintain a good body bulk of the graft, to ensure minimal graft remodeling postoperatively, and to minimize the postoperative graft reapportion with minimal or no antigenicity or possible tissue reaction. The primary data from the use of the OPM indicates a minimal remodeling rate, high regeneration capacity, ease of use, and less discomfort to the patient.

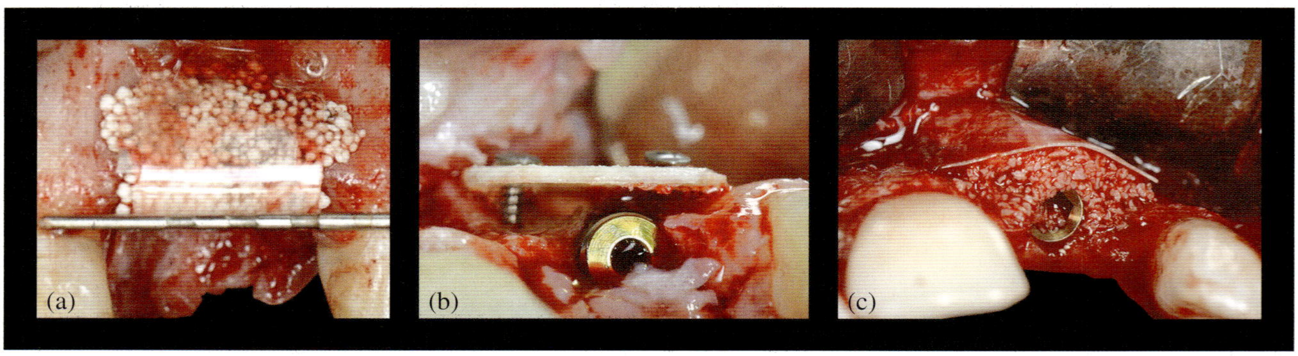

Figure 9.76 (a–c) Examples of space making.

Harvesting autogenous chips from donor sites can be accomplished using drills, piezoelectric curettes, bone scrapers, and manual curettes. Autogenous bone chips can also be harvested from an intra-oral donor site, such as the maxillary tuberosity, mandibular retromolar area, and the symphysis (Kainulainen et al. 2002, 2003) (see Figure 9.77).

The reasons behind selecting the bone chips as the preferred method of autogenous bone use is supported by the work conducted by Miron et al. (2011), who evaluated the ability of the graft to promote an osteogenic response in osteoblast cultures, with cell proliferation measured at one, two, three, and five days, in an *in vitro* study (pigs). They compared four types of autograft forms: (1) milled block grafts, (2) bone chips harvested via a bone scraper, (3) bone

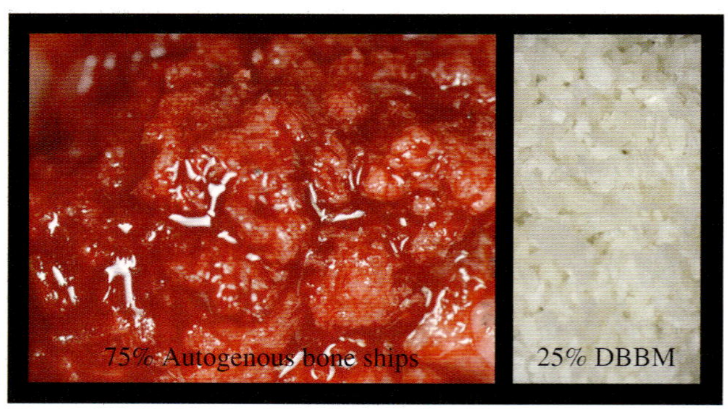

Figure 9.77 An optimal grafting mixture is proposed by the author that consists of 75% of autogenous bone chips and 25% of deprotinized inorganic xenograft for less resorption and providing bulk to the body of the graft.

slurry harvested using a bone trap, and (4) bone harvested via piezosurgery. The study concluded that osteoblasts seeded on bone mill and bone scraper samples exhibited significantly higher levels of collagen, osteocalcin, and osterix and produced more mineralized tissue, which explains the value of using the chips (see Figure 9.78a–c).

Bone collectors should not be used for this purpose, as it has a high potential for contaminating the bone (Young et al. 2002b) (see Figure 9.79a–c).

In conclusion, there is no specific recipe that can be implemented in all clinical situations, because this is not applicable in the oral cavity due to the many variables that exist. The clinician should learn the benefits and side effects of each method along with its clinical predictability, using the previously mentioned guidelines as a reference for any regenerative procedure that has been found to be highly advantageous and leads to a highly predicable regenerative outcome (see Figure 9.80 a–c).

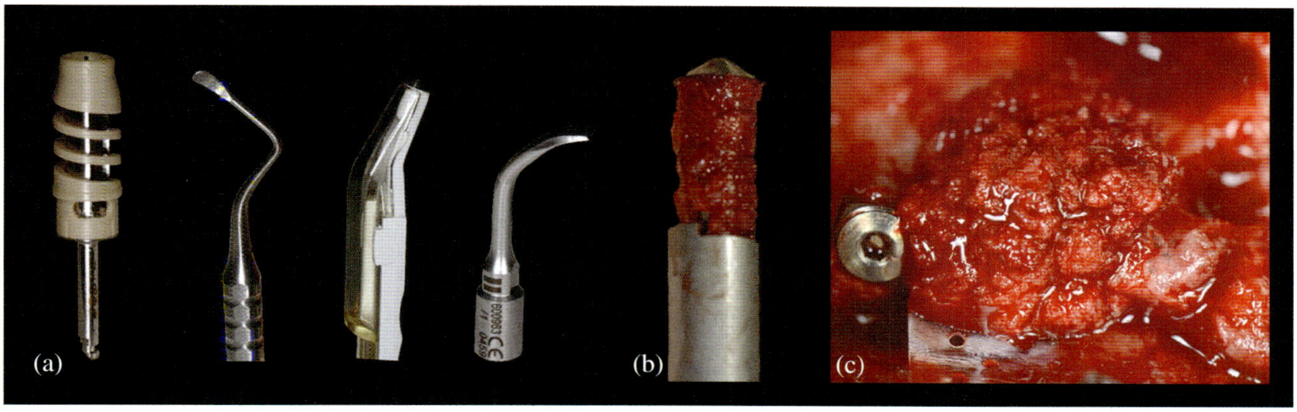

Figure 9.73 (a) Tools for autogenous bone chips harvesting Drills, Curettes, Scrapers, Peizzo surgery respectively, (b) and (c) an example of the right particulated bone grafting mixture that includes 75% of autogenous bone chips harvested with bone scrapper.

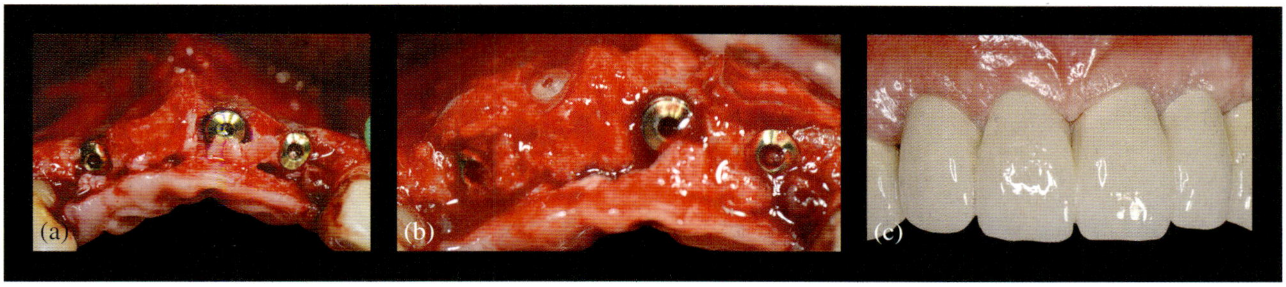

Figure 9.79 (a) Horizontal osseous defect in the anterior region, simultaneous Dental implants placement attempted along with non-staged grafting approach, (b) The defect was grafted with a particulate bone graft produced from harvested bone chips and mixed with one third alloplastic material, all covered with PDLLA membrane, (c) and (d) Incisal and frontal clinical views of the case finally restored.

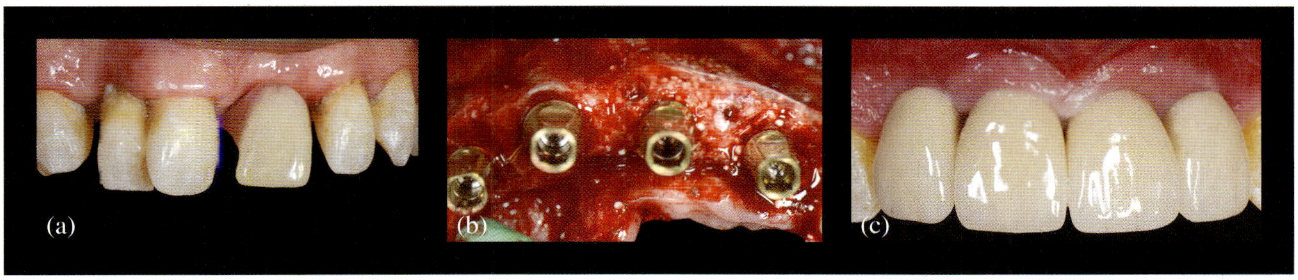

Figure 9.80 (a) Preoperative view missing osseous contours and missing central and lateral incisors, (b) The local defect is rafted with a particulate bone graft produced from harvested bone chips and mixed with one third alloplastic material, all covered with PDLLA membrane, (c) Final case restored.

References

Abrahamsson, P. (2011). Intra-oral soft tissue expansion and volume stability of onlay bone grafts. *Swed. Dent. J. Suppl.* (211): 11–66.

Abt, E. (2009). Smoking increases dental implant failures and complications. *Evid. Based Dent.* 10 (3): 79–80.

Acocella, A., Bertolai, R., Colafranceschi, M., and Sacco, R. (2010). Clinical, histological and histomorphometric evaluation of the healing of mandibular ramus bone block grafts for alveolar ridge augmentation before implant placement. *J. Craniomaxillofac. Surg.*, Apr 38 (3): 222–230.

Aichelmann-Reidy, M.E., Yukna, R.A., Evans, G.H. et al. (2001). Clinical evaluation of acellular allograft dermis for the treatment of human gingival recession. *J. Periodontol.* 72 (8): 998–1005.

Albrektsson, T. (1988). A multicenter report on osseointegrated oral implants. *J. Prosthet. Dent.* 60: 75–84.

Albrektsson, T. and Isidor, F. (1994). Consensus report of session IV. In: *Proceedings of the 1st European Workshop on Periodontology* (ed. N.P. Land and T. Karring), 365. Chicago, IL: Quintessence.

Albrektsson, T. and Johansson, C. (2001). Osteoinduction, osteoconduction and osseointegration. *Eur. Spine J.* 10 (Suppl. 2): S96–S101.

AlGhamdi, A.S. and Buhite, R.J. (2008). A new tunnel technique with acellular dermal matrix for soft tissue preparation prior to symphyseal block graft – a description of technique and case report. *J. Oral Implantol.* 34 (5): 274–281.

Aligower, M. (1981). Wound healing. In: *Wound Closure in the Operating Theater*, 1e, 20, 26, 28, 66. Germany: B. Braun and A.G. Melsungen.

Amini, A.R., Laurencin, C.T., and Nukavarapu, S.P. (2012). Bone tissue engineering: recent advances and challenges. *Crit. Rev. Biomed. Eng.* 40 (5): 363–340.

Annibali, S., La Monaca, G., Tantardini, M., and Cristalli, M.P. (2009a). The role of the template in prosthetically guided implantology. *J. Prosthodont.* 18 (2): 177–183.

Annibali, S., Ripari, M., La Monaca, G. et al. (2009b). Local accidents in dental implant surgery: prevention and treatment. *Int. J. Periodontics Restorative Dent.* 29 (3): 325–331.

Antoun, H., Sitbon, J.M., Martinez, H., and Missika, P. (2001). A prospective randomized study comparing two techniques of bone augmentation: onlay graft alone or associated with a membrane. *Clin. Oral Implants Res.* 12 (6): 632–639.

Ardekian, L., Oved-Peleg, E., Mactei, E.E., and Peled, M. (2006). The clinical significance of sinus membrane perforation during augmentation of the maxillary sinus. *J. Oral Maxillofac. Surg.* 64 (2): 277–282.

Artzi, Z., Givol, N., Rohrer, M.D. et al. (2003). Qualitative and quantitative expression of bovine bone mineral in experimental bone defects. Part 1: description of a dog model and histological observations. *J. Periodontol.* 74 (8): 1143–1152.

Ashley, E.T., Covington, L.L., Bishop, B.G., and Breault, L.G. (2003). Ailing and failing endosseous dental implants: a literature review. *J. Contemp. Dent. Pract.* 4 (2): 35–50.

Att, W. and Stappert, C. (2003). Implant therapy to improve quality of life. *Quintessence Int.* 34 (8): 573–581.

Bain, C.A. (1996). Smoking and implant failure. Benefits of a smoking cessation protocol. *Int. J. Oral Maxillofac. Implants* 11: 756–759.

Barinov, S.M., Rau, J.V., Cesaro, S.N. et al. (2006). Carbonate release from carbonated hydroxyapatite in the wide temperature rage. *J. Mater. Sci. Mater. Med.* 17 (7): 597–604.

Barone, A. and Covani, U. (2007). Maxillary alveolar ridge reconstruction with nonvascularized autogenous block bone: clinical results. *J. Oral Maxillofac. Surg.* 65 (10): 2039–2046.

Bartling, R., Freeman, K., and Kraut, R.A. (1999). The incidence of altered sensation of the mental nerve after mandibular implant placement. *J. Oral Maxillofac. Surg.* 57: 1408–1410.

Batista, E.L. Jr. and Batista, F.C. (2001). Managing soft tissue fenestrations in bone grafting surgery with an acellular dermal matrix: a case report. *Int. J. Oral Maxillofac. Implants* 16 (6): 875–879.

Bauer, T.W. and Muschler, G.F. (2000). Bone graft materials. An overview of the basic science. *Clin. Orthop. Relat. Res.* (371): 10–27. Review.

Becker, W. and Becker, B.E. (1996). Flap designs for minimization of recession adjacent to maxillary anterior implant sites: a clinical study. *Int. J. Oral Maxillofac. Implants* 11 (1): 46–55.

Beirne, O.R. and Worthington, P. (1991). Problems and complications in implant surgery: the surgeon's perspective. *Oral Maxillofac. Surg. Clin. North Am.* 3: 993–1000.

Berglundh, T., Persson, L., and Klinge, B. (2002). A systematic review of the incidence of biological and technical complications in implant dentistry reported in prospective longitudinal studies of at least 5 years. *J. Clin. Periodontol.* 29: 197–212.

Berglundh, T., Zitzmann, N.U., and Donati, M. (2011). Are peri-implantitis lesions different from periodontitis lesions?'. *J. Clin. Periodontol.* 38 (Suppl. 11): 188–202.

Bergström, J. and Preber, H. (1994). Tobacco as a risk factor. *J. Periodontol.* 65 (May suppl): 545–550.

Bernstein, S., Cooke, J., Fotek, P., and Wang, H.L. (2006). Vertical bone augmentation: where are we now? *Implant. Dent.* 15: 219–228.

Bezzon, O.L. (1993). Allergic sensitivity to several base metals: a clinical report. *J. Prosthet. Dent.* (70): 109–110.

Bilezikian, J.P., Raisz, L.G., and Marti, T.J. (2008). *Principles of Bone Biology*, 3e. Elsevier Publishing.

Block, M.S. and Kent, J.N. (1991). Placement of endosseous implants into tooth extraction sites. *J. Oral Maxillofac. Surg.* 49 (12): 1269–1276.

Bombonato, K., Brentegani, G., Thomazini, A. et al. (2004). Alcohol intake and osseointegration around implants: a histometric and scanning electron microscopy study. *Implant. Dent.* 13: 238–244.

Boyne, P.J., Cole, M.D., Stringer, D., and Shafqat, J.P. (1985). A technique for osseous restoration of deficient edentulous maxillary ridges. *J. Oral Maxillofac. Surg.* 43 (2): 87–91.

Brånemark, P.I. (1972). Rehabilitation with intra-osseous anchorage of dental prosthesis. *Tandlakartidningen* 844 (20): 662–663.

Brånemark, P.I., Hansson, B.O., Adell, R. et al. (1977). Osseointegrated implants in the treatment of the edentulous jaw. Experience from a 10-year period. *Scand. J. Plast. Reconstr. Surg. Suppl.* 16: 1–132.

Brener, D. (2006). The mandibular ramus donor site. *Aust. Dent. J.* 51: 187–190.

Buck, B., Malinin, T., and Brown, M. (1989). Bone transplantation and human immunodeficiency virus: an estimated risk of acquired immunodeficiency syndrome (AIDS). *Clin. Orthop.* (240): 129–136.

Burchardt, H. (1983). The biology of bone graft repair. *Clin. Orthop. Relat. Res.* (174): 28–42.

Burstein, J., Mastin, C., and Le, B. (2008). Avoiding injury to the inferior alveolar nerve by routine use of intraoperative radiographs during implant placement. *J. Oral Implantol.* 34 (1): 34–38.

Buser, D., Bragger, U., Lang, N.P., and Nyman, S. (1990). Regeneration and enlargement of jaw bone using guided tissue regeneration. *Clin. Oral Implants Res.* 1: 22–32.

Buser, D., Ingimarsson, S., Dula, K. et al. (2002). Long-term stability of osseointegrated implants in augmented bone: a 5-year prospective study in partially edentulous patients. *Int. J. Periodontics Restorative Dent.* 22 (2): 109–117.

Cabezas-Mojón, J., Barona-Dorado, C., Gómez-Moreno, G. et al. (2012). Meta-analytic study of implant survival following sinus augmentation. *Med. Oral Patol. Oral Cir. Bucal* 17 (1): e135–e139.

Carlson, E.R. and Monteleone, K. (2004). An analysis of inadvertent perforations of mucosa and skin concurrent with mandibular reconstruction. *J. Oral Maxillofac. Surg.* 62: 1103–1107.

Carlsson, G.E., Thilander, H., and Hedegard, B. (1967a). Histologic changes in the upper alveolar process after extractions with or without insertion of an immediate full denture. *Acta Odontol. Scand.* 25: 21–43.

Carlsson, G.E., Bergman, B., and Hedegård, B. (1967b). Changes in contour of the maxillary alveolar process under immediate dentures. A longitudinal clinical and X-ray cephalometric study covering 5 years. *Acta Odontol. Scand.* 25 (1): 45–75.

Caton, J. G., Armitage, G., Berglundh, T. et al. (2018). A new classification scheme for periodontal and peri-implant diseases and conditions – Introduction and key changes from the 1999 classification. *J. Clin. Periodontol.* 45 (Suppl 20): S1–S8. doi: 10.1111/jcpe.12935.

Cawood, J.I. and Howell, R.A. (1988). A classification of the edentulous jaws. *Int. J. Oral Maxillofac. Surg.* 17 (4): 232–236.

Chanavaz, M. (1990). Maxillary sinus: anatomy, physiology, surgery, and bone grafting related to implantology – eleven years of surgical experience (1979–1990). *J. Oral Implantol.* 16 (3): 199–209.

Chaushu, G., Mardinger, O., Peleg, M. et al. (2010). Analysis of complications following augmentation with cancellous block allografts. *J. Periodontol.* 81 (12): 1759–1764.

Chee, W. and Jivraj, S. (2007). Failures in implant dentistry. *Br. Dent. J.* 202 (3): 123–129.

Chiapasco, M., Zaniboni, M., and Rimondini, L. (2007). Autogenous onlay bone grafts vs. alveolar distraction osteogenesis for the correction of vertically deficient edentulous ridges: a 2–4-year prospective study on humans. *Clin. Oral Implants Res.* 18: 432–440.

Collins, T. and Collins, T. Jr. (1998). Surgical misadventures in implant placement. *Oral Maxillofac. Surg. Clin. North Am.* 2: 203–219.

Committee on Research, Science and Therapy of the American Academy of Periodontology (2001). Tissue banking of bone allografts used in periodontal regeneration. *J. Periodontol.* 72 (6): 834–838.

Cordaro, L., Amade, D.S., and Cordaro, M. (2002). Clinical results of alveolar ridge augmentation with mandibular block bone grafts in partially edentulous patients prior to implant placement. *Clin. Oral Implants Res.* 13: 103–111.

Cordaro, L., Torsello, F., Morcavallo, S., and di Torresanto, V.M. (2011). Effect of bovine bone and collagen membranes on healing of mandibular bone blocks: a prospective randomized controlled study. *Clin. Oral Implants Res.* 22: 1145–1150.

Cranin, A.N. (1999). Diagnosis and treatment of complications. In: *Atlas of Oral Implantology*, 2e (ed. A.N. Cranin), 418–419. St. Louis: Mosby.

Cranin, A.N. (2001). The implant Marshall plan. *J. Oral Implantol.* 27 (4): 163.

Cromack, D.T., Porras-Reyes, B., and Mustoe, T.A. (1990). Current concepts in wound healing: growth factor and macrophage interaction. *J. Trauma* 30: 129–133.

Cummings, L.C., Kaldahl, W.B., and Allen, E.P. (2005). Histologic evaluation of autogenous connective tissue and acellular dermal matrix grafts in humans. *J. Periodontol.* 76: 178–186.

Da Silva, R.V. and Camilli, J.A. (2006). Repair of bone defects treated with autogenous bone graft and low-power laser. *J. Craniofac. Surg.* 17 (2): 297–301.

Dario, L.J. (2002). Implant placement above a bifurcated mandibular canal: a case report. *Implant Dent.* 11 (3): 258–261.

De Carvalho, P.S., Vasconcellos, L.W., and Pi, J. (2000). Influence of bed preparation on the incorporation of autogenous bone grafts: a study in dogs. *Int. J. Oral Maxillofac. Implants* 15 (4): 565–570.

De Vera, J.L., Calleja, J.M., and García, M. (2008). Hematoma of the floor of the mouth and airway obstruction during mandibular dental implant placement: a case report. *Oral Maxillofac. Surg.* 12 (4): 223–226.

Dellavia, C., Giammattei, M., Carmagnola, D. et al. (2016). Iliac crest fresh-frozen allografts versus autografts in oral pre-prosthetic bone reconstructive surgery: histologic and histomorphometric study. *Implant. Dent.* 25 (6): 731–738.

Deluiz, D., Oliveira, L.S., Fletcher, P. et al. (2016). Histologic and tomographic findings of bone block allografts in a 4 year follow-up: a case series. *Braz. Dent. J.* 27 (6): 775–780.

Derks, J., Schaller, D., Håkansson, J. et al. (2016). Peri-implantitis – onset and pattern of progression. *J. Clin. Periodontol.* 43 (4): 383–388.

Dewan, S.K., Arora, A., Sehgal, M., and Khullar, A. (2015). Microstomia – a treatment challenge to a prosthodontist. *J. Clin. Diagn. Res.* 9 (4): ZD12–ZD13.

Dominici, J.T. (1988). Prosthodontic considerations in first stage implant failures. *Oral Maxillofac. Surg. Clin. North Am.* 10: 235–274.

Dreiseidler, T., Neugebauer, J., Ritter, L. et al. (2009). Accuracy of a newly developed integrated system for dental implant planning. *Clin. Oral Implants Res.* 20 (11): 1191–1199.

Elaskary, A.S. (2008). *Fundamentals of Aesthetic Implant Dentistry*, 2e. U.S.A: Wiley-Blackwell Pub. Co.

Elaskary, A.S., Meffert, R.M., and Griffin, T. (1999a). Why do dental implants fail? Part I. *Implant. Dent.* 8 (2): 173–185.

Elaskary, A.S., Meffert, R.M., and Griffin, T. (1999b). Why do dental implants fail? Part I. *Implant. Dent.* 8 (2): 265–277.

English, C.E. (1993). Implant-supported versus implant-natural-tooth-supported fixed partial dentures. *J. Dent. Symp.*, August 1: 10–15.

Eppley, B.L. (2000). Revascularization of acellular human dermis (alloderm) in subcutaneous implantation. *Aesthet. Surg. J.* 20: 291–295.

Esposito, M., Hirsch, J.M., Lekholm, U., and Thomsen, P. (1998). Biological factors contributing to failures of osseointegrated oral implants. (I). Success criteria and epidemiology. *Eur. J. Oral Sci.* 106 (1): 527–551.

Esposito, M., Grusovin, M.G., Kwan, S. et al. (2008). Interventions for replacing missing teeth: bone augmentation techniques for dental implant treatment. *Cochrane Database Syst. Rev.* 3: doi: 10.1002/14651858.CD003607.pub3.

Fakhry, A. (2011). The mandibular retromolar area as a donor site in maxillofacial bone grafting: surgical notes. *Int. J. Periodontics Restorative Dent.* 31: 275–283.

Fieding, A.F. and Hild, E.R. 1993 Maintaining the quality of life in the HIV patient through osseointegrated implants. Abstract. Second International Workshop on the Oral Manifestations of HIV Infection. San Francisco, Jan. 31 Feb. 3,.

Field, E.A. (1997). The use of powdered gloves in dental practice: a cause for concern? *J. Dent.* 25 (3–4): 209–214.

Flanagan, D. (2003). Important arterial supply of the mandible, control of an arterial hemorrhage, and report of a hemorrhagic incident. *J. Oral Implantol.* 29 (4): 165–173.

Fowler, E.B., Breault, L.G., and Rebitski, G. (2000). Ridge preservation utilizing an acellular dermal allograft and demineralized freeze-dried bone allograft: Part I. A report of 2 cases. *J. Periodontol.* 71: 1353–1359.

Friberg, B., Jemt, T., and Lekholm, U. (1991). Early failure in 4641 consecutively placed Branemark dental implants: a study from stage 1 to the connection of completed prostheses. *Int. J. Oral Maxillofac. Implants* 6: 142–146.

Friedmann, A., Gissel, K., Soudan, M. et al. (2011). Randomized controlled trial on lateral augmentation using two collagen membranes: morphometric results on mineralized tissue compound. *J. Clin. Periodontol.* 38: 677–685.

Froum, S.J. (2013). The team approach to managing dental implant complications: the periodontist's point of view. *Compend. Contin. Educ. Dent.* 34 (7): 4–9.

Froum, S.J. and Rosen, P.S. (2012). A proposed classification for peri-implantitis. *Int. J. Periodontics Restorative Dent.* 32 (5): 533–540.

Fujita, S., Ide, Y., and Abe, S. (2012). Variations of vascular distribution in the mandibular anterior lingual region: a high risk of vascular injury during implant surgery. *Implant. Dent.* 21 (4): 259–264.

Gapski, R., Wang, H.L., and Misch, C.E. (2001). Management of incision design in symphysis graft procedures: a review of the literature. *J. Oral Implantol.* 27: 134–142.

Gendler, E. (1986). Perforated demineralized bone matrix: a new form of osteoinductive biomaterial. *J. Biomed. Mater. Res.* 20 (6): 687–689.

George, R K. and Krishnamurthy, A. (2013). Microsurgical free flaps: controversies in maxillofacial reconstruction. *Ann. Maxillofac. Surg.* 3 (1): 72–79.

Giglio, J. and Laskin, D. (1998). Perioperative errors contributing to implant failure. *Oral Maxillofac. Surg. Clin. North Am.* 2: 197–202.

Glaser, B., Hodel, Y., Meyer, J., and Lambrecht, J.T. (2004). Bacterial contamination of bony particles from the bone collection trap. *Schweiz. Monatsschr. Zahnmed.* 114 (4): 337–341.

Glowacki, J., Altobelli, D., and Mulliken, J.B. (1981). Fate of mineralized and demineralized osseous implants in cranial defects. *Calcif. Tissue Int.* 33 (1): 71–76.

Glowacki, J. and Mulliken, J.B. (1985). Demineralized bone implants. *Clin. Plast. Surg.* 12 (2): 233–241. Review.

Goodacre, C.J., Kan, J.Y., and Rungcharassaeng, K. (1999). Clinical complications of osseointegrated implants. *J. Prosthet. Dent.* 81 (5): 537–552. Review.

Goodacre, C.J., Bernal, G., Rungcharassaeng, K., and Kan, J.Y. (2003). Clinical complications with implants and implant prostheses. *J. Prosthet. Dent.* 90 (2): 121–132.

Goodson, W.H. and Hunt, T.K. (1979). Wound healing and the diabetic patient. *Surg. Gynecol. Obstet.* 149: 600–608.

Gorman, L.M., Lambert, P.M., Morris, H.F. et al. (1994). The effect of smoking on implant survival at second stage surgery: DICRG interim report. *Implant. Dent.* 3: 165–168.

Graziani, F., Ducci, F., Tonelli, M. et al. (2005). Maxillary sinus augmentation with platelet-rich plasma and fibrinogen cryoprecipitate: a tomographic pilot study. *Implant. Dent.* 14: 63–69.

Greenstein, G. and Tarnow, D. (2006). The mental foramen and nerve: clinical and anatomical factors related to dental implant placement: a literature review. *J. Periodontol.* 77 (12): 1933–1943.

Greenstein, G., Cavallaro, J., Romanos, G., and Tarnow, D. (2008). Clinical recommendations for avoiding and managing surgical complications associated with implant dentistry: a review. *J. Periodontol.* 79 (8): 1317–1329.

Griffin, T.J., Cheung, W.S., and Hirayama, H. (2004). Hard and soft tissue augmentation in implant therapy using acellular dermal matrix. *Int. J. Periodontics Restorative Dent.* 24: 352–361.

Grover, V., Kapoor, A., Malhotra, R., and Sachdeva, S. (2011). Bone allografts: a review of safety and efficacy. *Indian J. Dent. Res.* 22 (3): 496.

Gunne, J., Astrand, P., Ahlén, K. et al. (1992). Implants in partially edentulous patients. A longitudinal study of bridges supported by both implants and natural teeth. *Clin. Oral Implants Res.* 3 (2): 49–56.

Gunne, J., Jemt, T., and Lindén, B. (1994). Implant treatment in partially edentulous patients: a report on prostheses after 3 years. *Int. J. Prosthodont.* 7 (2): 143–148.

Günther, K., Scharf, H.P., and Puhl, W. (1993). In vitro toxicity tests of bioceramics and bone transplants in fibroblast culture. *Biomed. Tech. (Berl)* 38 (10): 249–254.

Hallman, M. and Thor, A. (2008). Bone substitutes and growth factors as an alternative/complement to autogenous bone for grafting in implant dentistry. *Periodontol 2000* 47: 172–192.

Halstead, C. (ed.) (1982). *Physical Evaluation of the Dental Patient*, 74–81. St. Louis: Mosby.

Hansen, P.A. and West, L.A. (1997). Allergic reaction following insertion of a Pd-Cu-Au fixed partial denture: a clinical report. *J. Prosthodont.* 6: 144–148.

Harris, R.J. (2003). Soft tissue ridge augmentation with an acellular dermal matrix. *Int. J. Periodontics Restorative Dent.* 23: 87–92.

Hashimoto-Uoshima, M., Ishikawa, I., Kinoshita, A. et al. (1995). Clinical and histologic observation of replacement of biphasic calcium phosphate by bone tissue in monkeys. *Int. J. Periodontics Restorative Dent.* 15 (2): 205–211.

Hench, L.L. (1998). Bioactive materials: the potential for tissue regeneration. *J. Biomed. Mater. Res.* 41 (4): 511–518.

Henderson, R.D., Greenwell, H., Drisko, C. et al. (2001). Predictable multiple site root coverage using an acellular dermal matrix allograft. *J. Periodontol.* 72: 571–582.

Henemyre, C., Scales, D., Hokett, D. et al. (2003). Nicotine stimulates osteoclast resorption in a porcine marrow cell model. *J. Periodontol.* 74: 1440–1446.

Hiatt, W.H. and Schallhorn, R.G. (1973). Intraoral transplants of cancellous bone and marrow in periodontal lesions. *J. Periodontol.* 44: 194–208.

Holtzclaw, D., Toscano, N., Eisenlohr, L., and Callan, D. (2008). The safety of bone allografts used in dentistry: a review. *J. Am. Dent. Assoc.* 139: 1192–1199.

Hooe, W. and Steinberg, B. (1996). Management of contaminated bone grafts: an experimental in vitro study. *Oral Surg. Oral Med. Oral Pathol. Oral Radiol. Endod.* 82 (1): 34–37.

Hunt, B.W., Sandifer, J.B., Assad, D.A. et al. (1996). Effect of flap design on healing and osseointegration of dental implants. *Int. J. Periodontics Restorative Dent.* 16: 583–593.

Hyatt, G.W. and Butler, M.C. (1957). The procurement, storage, and clinical use of bone homografts. *Instr. Course Lect.* 14: 343–373.

Ioannou, A.L., Kotsakis, G.A., McHale, M.G. et al. (2015). Soft tissue surgical procedures for optimizing anterior implant esthetics. *Int. J. Dent.* 2015: 740–764.

Jaffin, R.A. and Berman, C.L. (1991). The excessive loss of Branemark fixtures in type IV bone: a 5-year analysis. *J. Periodontol.* 62 (1): 2–4.

Jemt, T. (1986). Changes in masticatory movement parameters within the chewing period in young dentate persons and patients rehabilitated with bridges supported by implants in the mandible. *J. Oral Rehabil.* 13 (5): 487–495.

Jemt, T. and Lekholm, U. (1993). Oral implant treatment in posterior partially edentulous jaws: a 5-year follow-up report. *Int. J. Oral Maxillofac. Implants* 8 (6): 635–640.

Jemt, T., Lekholm, U., and Adell, R. (1989). Osseointegrated implants in the treatment of partially edentulous patients: a preliminary study on 876 consecutively placed fixtures. *Int. J. Oral Maxillofac. Implants* 4 (3): 211–217.

Jemt, T., Book, K., Lindén, B., and Urde, G. (1992). Failures and complications in 92 consecutively inserted overdentures supported by Brånemark implants in severely resorbed edentulous maxillae: a study from prosthetic treatment to first annual check-up. *Int. J. Oral Maxillofac. Implants* 7 (2): 162–167.

Jensen, O.T. (1994). When is it really osseointegration? *J. Oral Maxillofac. Surg.* 52 (10): 1098.

Jisaander, S., Grenthe, B., and Alberius, P. (1997). Dental implant survival in the irradiate jaw: a preliminary report. *Int. J. Oral Maxillofac. Implants* 12: 643–648.

Joshi, A. and Kostakis, G.C. (2004). An investigation of post-operative morbidity following iliac crest graft harvesting. *Br. Dent. J.* 196 (3): 167–171. discussion 155.

Jovanovic, S.A., Spiekermann, H., and Richter, E.J. (1992). Bone regeneration around Ti dental implants in dehiscenced defect sites: a clinical study. *Int. J. Oral Maxillofac. Implants* 7: 233–245.

Kaigler, D., Cirelli, J., and Giannobile, W. (2006). Growth factor delivery for oral and periodontal tissue engineering. *Expert Opin. Drug Deliv.* 3 (5): 647–662.

Kainulainen, V.T., Sandor, G.K.B., Oikarinen, K.S., and Clokie, C.M.L. (2002). Zygomatic bone: an additional donor site for alveolar bone reconstruction. Technical note. *Int. J. Oral Maxillofac. Implants* 17: 723–728.

Kainulainen, V.T., Sandor, G.K.B., Oikarinen, K.S., and Clokie, C.M.L. (2003). The intraoral bone harvesting sites for osseous reconstruction in oral and maxillofacial surgery. *Oral Health* 93: 10–24.

Keller, E.E. (1997). Placement of dental implants in the irradiated mandible: a protocol without adjunctive hyperbaric oxygen. *J. Oral Maxillofac. Surg.* 55: 972–980.

Keller, J.C., Stewart, M., Roehm, M., and Schneider, G.B. (2004). Osteoporosis-like bone conditions affect osseointegration of implants. *Int. J. Oral Maxillofac. Implants* 19 (5): 687–694.

Khoury, F. and Buchmann, R. (2001). Surgical therapy of peri-implant disease: a 3-year follow-up study of cases treated with 3 different techniques of bone regeneration. *J. Periodontol.* 72: 1498–1508.

King, M.A., Casarett, G.W., and Weber, D.A. (1979). A study of irradiated bone: histologic and physiologic changes. *J. Nucl. Med.* 20: 1142–1149.

Klokkevold, P.R. and Han, T.J. (2007). How do smoking, diabetes and periodontitis affect outcomes of implant? *Int. J. Oral Maxillofac. Implants* 22: 173–198.

Kohavi, D., Azran, G., Shapira, L., and Casap, N. (2004). Retrospective clinical review of dental implants placed in a university training program. *J. Oral Implantol.* 30 (1): 23–29.

Kotsovilis, S., Fourmousis, I., Karoussis, I.K., and Bamia, C. (2009). A systematic review and meta-analysis on the effect of implant length on the survival of rough-surface dental implants. *Periodontol.* 80 (11): 1700–1718.

Kozak, J.A., Heilman, A.E., and O'Brien, J.P. (1994). Anterior lumbar fusion options. Technique and graft materials. *Clin. Orthop. Relat. Res.* (300): 45–51. Review of 1983 bone bank procedures.

Kreuz, F.P., Hyatt, G.W., Turner, T.C., and Bassett, A.L. (1951). The preservation and clinical use of freeze-dried bone. *J. Bone Joint Surg. Am.* 33-A (4): 863–872.

Laboda, G. (1990). Life-threatening hemorrhage after placement of an endosseous implant: report of case. *J. Am. Dent. Assoc.* 121: 201–204.

Lambert, P.M., Morris, H.F., and Ochi, S. (1997). Positive effect of surgical experience with implants on second-stage implant survival. *J. Oral Maxillofac. Surg.* 55 (Suppl. 5): 12–18.

Latta, G.H. Jr., McDougal, S., and Bowles, W.F. (1993). Response of known nickel-sensitive patient to a removable partial denture with a titanium alloy framework: a clinical report. *J. Prosthet. Dent.* 70: 109–110.

Lavernia, C.J., Malinin, T.I., Temple, H.T., and Moreyra, C.E. (2004). Bone and tissue allograft use by orthopaedic surgeons. *J. Arthroplast.* 19 (4): 430–435.

Lekholm, U., Becker, W., Dahlin, C. et al. (1993). The role of early versus late removal of GTAM membranes on bone formation at oral implants placed into immediate extraction sockets. An experimental study in dogs. *Clin. Oral Implants Res.* 4 (3): 121–129.

Lekholm, U. and Zarb, G.A. (1985). In patient selection and preparation. In: *Tissue Integrated Prostheses: Osseointegration in Clinical Dentistry* (ed. P.I. Branemark, G.A. Zarb and T. Albrektsson), 199–209. Chicago, IL: Quintessence Publishing Company.

Levine, R.A., Manji, A., Faucher, J., and Present, S. (2014). Use of titanium mesh in implant site development for restorative-driven implant placement: case report. Part 1: restorative protocol for single-tooth esthetic zone sites. *Compend. Contin. Educ. Dent.* 35 (4): 264): 267–277.

Lindeboom, J.A., Tjiook, Y., and Kroon, F.H. (2006). Immediate placement of implants in periapical infected sites: a prospective randomized study in 50 patients.

Oral Surg. Oral Med. Oral Pathol. Oral Radiol. Endod., June 101 (6): 705–710.

Lindholm, J., Steiniche, T., Rasmussen, E. et al. Bone disorder in men with chronic alcoholism: a reversible disease? *J. Clin. Endocrinol. Metab* 73: 118–124.

Liu, J. and Kerns, D.G. (2014). Mechanisms of guided bone regeneration: a review. *Open Dent. J.* 8: 56–65.

Longoni, S., Sartori, M., Apruzzese, D., and Baldoni, M. (2007). Preliminary clinical and histologic evaluation of a bilateral 3-dimensional reconstruction in an atrophic mandible: a case report. *Int. J. Oral Maxillofac. Implants* 22 (3): 478–483.

Lysimachos, G., Tsioli, P.V., Papaioannou, N. et al. (2010). Comparison of absorbable and nonabsorbable sutures for intradermal skin closure in cats. *Can. Vet. J.* 51 (7): 770–772.

Mahn, D.H. (2001). Treatment of gingival recession with a modified "tunnel" technique and an acellular dermal connective tissue allograft. *Pract. Proced. Aesthet. Dent.* 13: 69–74.

Mahn, D.H. (2003). Esthetic soft tissue ridge augmentation using an acellular dermal connective tissue allograft. *J. Esthet. Restor. Dent.* 15: 72–79.

Maiorana, C., Santoro, F., Rabagliati, M., and Salina, S. (2001). Evaluation of the use of iliac cancellous bone and anorganic bovine bone in the reconstruction of the atrophic maxilla with titanium mesh: a clinical and histologic investigation. *Int. J. Oral Maxillofac. Implants* 16 (3): 427–432.

Manson, P.N. (1994). Facial bone healing and bone grafts. A review of clinical physiology. *Clin. Plast. Surg.*, July 21 (3): 331–348. Review.

Marx, R.E. and Johnson, R.P. (1987). Studies in the radiobiology of osteoradionecrosis and their clinical significance. *Oral Surg. Oral Med. Oral Pathol.* 64: 379–390.

Marx, R.E., Carlson, E.R., and Eichstaedt, R.M. (1998). Platelet-rich plasma: growth factor enhancement for bone grafts. *Oral Surg. Oral Med. Oral Pathol.* 85: 638–646.

Matsumoto, M.A., Filho, H.N., Francischone, A.E., and Consolaro, A. (2002). Microscopic analysis of reconstructed maxillary alveolar ridges using autogenous bone grafts from the chin and iliac crest. *Int. J. Oral Maxillofac. Implants* 17 (4): 507–516.

Meffert, R.M. (1992). How to treat ailing and failing implants. *Implant. Dent.* 1 (1): 25–33.

Melamed, B.G. (1989). Psychological considerations for implant patients. *J. Oral Implantol.* 15 (4): 249–254.

Miron, R.J., Hedbom, E., Saulacic, N. et al. (2011). Osteogenic potential of autogenous bone grafts harvested with four different surgical techniques. *J. Dent. Res.* 90 (12): 1428–1433.

Misch, C.E. (1982). Medical evaluation of the implant candidate. Part II. *Int. J. Oral Implantol.* 10 (3): 11–18.

Misch, C.M. (1992). The pharmacologic management of maxillary sinus elevation surgery. *J. Oral Implantol.* 18: 15–23.

Misch, C.M. (1997). Comparison of intraoral donor sites for onlay grafting prior to implant placement. *Int. J. Oral Max. Fac. Implants.* 12: 767–776.

Misch, C.E. (1999). Implant design considerations for the posterior regions of the mouth. *Implant. Dent.* 8 (4): 376–386. Review.

Misch, C.E. (2007). Implants and the general practitioner. *Dent. Today* 26 (8): 48, 50, 52.

Misch, C.E. and Dietsh, F. (1993). Bone-grafting materials in implant dentistry. *Implant. Dent.* 2 (3): 158–167.

Misch, C.E. and Moore, P.A. (1989). Steroids and the reduction of pain, edema and dysfunction in implant dentistry. *J. Oral Implantol.* 6: 27–31.

Misch, C.E. and Resnik, R. (2010). Mandibular nerve neurosensory impairment after dental implant surgery: management and protocol. *Implant. Dent.* 19 (5): 378–386.

Misch, K. and Wang, H.L. (2008). Implant surgery complications: etiology and treatment. *Implant. Dent.* 17 (2): 159–168.

Mombelli, A., van Oosten, M.A., Schurch, E. Jr., and Land, N.P. (1987). The microbiota associated with successful or failing osseointegrated titanium implants. *Oral Microbiol. Immunol.* 2 (4): 145–151.

Monteleone, K., Marx, R.E., and Ghurani, R. 2000. Healing enhancement of skin graft donor sites with platelet rich plasma. Presented at the *82nd American Association of Oral and Maxilliofacial Surgeons Meeting*, San Francisco, CA, 22 September 2000.

Montes, C.C., Pereira, F.A., Thomé, G. et al. (2007). Failing factors associated with osseointegrated dental implant loss. *Implant. Dent.* 16 (4): 404–412.

Moy, K., Weiniaender, M., and Kenney, E.B. (1989). Soft tissue modifications of surgical techniques for placement and uncovering of osseointegrated implants. *Dent. Clin. North. Am.* 33: 665–679.

Moy, P.K., Medina, D., Shetty, V., and Aghaloo, T.L. (2005). Dental implant failure rates and associated risk factors. *Int. J. Oral Maxillofac. Implants* 20 (4): 569–577.

Murray, C.G., Harson, J., Daly, T.E., and Zimmerman, S. (1980). Radiation necrosis of the mandible: a 10 year study. Part II. Dental factors; onset, duration and management of necrosis. *Int. J. Radiat. Oncol. Biol. Phys.* 6: 549–553.

Myeroff, C. and Archdeacon, M. (2011). Autogenous bone graft: donor sites and techniques. *J Bone Joint Surg Am.* 93 (23): 2227–2236.

Nevins, M. and Langer, B. (1993). The successful application of osseointegrated implants to the posterior jaw: a long-term retrospective study. *Int. J. Oral Maxillofac. Implants* 8 (4): 428–432.

Nkenke, E., Eitner, S., Radespiel-Tröger, M. et al. (2007). Patient-centred outcomes comparing transmucosal implant placement with an open approach in the maxilla: a prospective, non-randomized pilot study. *Clin. Oral Implants Res.* 18: 197–203.

Nobuto, T., Suwa, F., Kono, T. et al. (2005). Microvascular response in the periosteum following mucoperiosteal flap surgery in dogs: 3-dimensional observation of an angiogenic process. *J. Periodontol.* 76 (8): 1339–1345.

Nyström, E., Ahlqvist, J., Kahnberg, K.E., and Rosenquist, J.B. (1996). Autogenous onlay bone grafts fixed with screw implants for the treatment of severely resorbed maxillae. Radiographic evaluation of preoperative bone dimensions, postoperative bone loss, and changes in soft-tissue profile. *Int. J. Oral Max. Fac. Surg.* 25 (5): 351–359.

Ozaki, W. and Buchman, S.R. (1998). Volume maintenance of onlay bone grafts in the craniofacial skeleton: micro-architecture versus embryologic origin. *Plast. Reconstr. Surg.* 102 (2): 291–299.

Palacci, P. (2004). Aesthetic treatment of the anterior maxilla: soft and hard tissue considerations. *Oral Maxillofac. Surg. Clin. North Am.* 16 (1): 127–137. vii.

Papathanasiou, E., Finkelman, M., Hanley, J., and Parashis, A.O. (2016). Prevalence, etiology and treatment of peri-implant mucositis and peri-implantitis: a survey of periodontists in the United States. *J. Periodontol.* 87 (5): 493–501.

Parithimarkalaignan, S. and Padmanabhan, T.V. (2013). Osseointegration: an update. *J. Indian Prosthodont. Soc.* 13 (1): 2–6.

Park, S.H. and Wang, H.L. (2005). Implant reversible complications: classification and treatments. *Implant. Dent.* 14 (3): 211–220.

Pelayo, L.J., Peñarrocha Diago, M., Martí Bowen, E., and Peñarrocha Diago, M. (2008). Intraoperative complications during oral implantology. *Med. Oral Patol. Oral Cir. Bucal* 13 (4): E239–E243.

Persson, L., Bergström, J., and Gustafsson, A. (2003). Effect of tobacco smoking on neutrophil activity following periodontal surgery. *J. Periodontol.* 74: 1475–1482.

Petersson, A., Lindh, C., and Carlsson, L.E. (1992). Estimation of the possibility to treat the edentulous maxilla with osseointegrated implants. *Swed. Dent. J.* 16: 1–6.

Petrovic, V., Zivkovic, P., Petrovic, D., and Stefanovic, V. (2012). Craniofacial bone tissue engineering. *Oral Surg. Oral Med. Oral Pathol. Oral Radiol.* 114: e1–e9.

Phillips, J.H. and Rahn, B.A. (1990). Fixation effects on membranous and endochondral onlay bone graft revascularization and bone deposition. *Plast. Reconstr. Surg.* 85: 891–897.

Pikos, M.A. (1999). Maxillary sinus membrane repair: report of a technique for large perforations. *Implant. Dent.* 8 (1): 29–34.

Poli, P., Beretta, M., Cicciù, M., and Maiorana, C. (2014). Alveolar ridge augmentation with titanium mesh. A retrospective clinical study. *Open Dent. J.* 8: 148–158.

Politis, C., Schoenaers, J., Jacobs, R., and Jimoh, O. (2016). Wound healing problems in the mouth. *Front. Physiol.* 7: 507.

Proussaefs, P. (2004). Use of the frontal process of the maxillary bone for implant placement to retain a nasal prosthesis: a clinical report. *Int. J. Oral Maxillofac. Implants* 19 (6): 901–905.

Proussaefs, P. and Lozada, J. (2006). Use of titanium mesh for staged localized alveolar ridge augmentation: clinical and histologic–histomorphometric valuation. *J. Oral Implantol.* 32 (5): 237–247.

Rabelo, G.D., de Paula, P.M., Rocha, F.S. et al. (2010). Retrospective study of bone grafting procedures before implant placement. *Implant. Dent.* 19 (4): 342–350.

Raghoebar, G.M., Stellingsma, K., Batenburg, R.H., and Vissink, A. (2000). Etiology and management of mandibular fractures associated with endosteal implants in the atrophic mandible. *Oral Surg. Oral Med. Oral Pathol. Oral Radiol. Endod.* 89 (5): 553–559.

Raghoebar, G.M., Meijndert, L., Kalk, W.W.I., and Vissink, A. (2007). Morbidity of mandibular bone harvesting: a comparative study. *Int. J. Oral Maxillofac. Implants* 22 (3): 359–365.

Rees, T.D., Liverett, D.M., and Guy, C.L. (1984). The effect of cigarette smoking on skin-flap survival in the face lift patient. *Plast. Reconstr. Surg.* 73: 911–915.

Reinhardt, C. and Kreusser, B. (2000). Retrospective study dental implantation with sinus lift and Cerasorb augmentation. *Dental Implantol.* 14: 18–26.

Rocchietta, I., Fontana, F., and Simion, M. (2008). Clinical outcomes of vertical bone augmentation to enable dental implant placement: a systematic review. *J. Clin. Periodontol.* 35: 203–215.

Roccuzzo, M., Ramieri, G., Spada, M.C. et al. (2004). Vertical alveolar ridge augmentation by means of a titanium mesh and autogenous bone grafts. *Clin. Oral Implants Res.* 15: 73–81.

Roccuzzo, M., Ramieri, G., Bunino, M., and Berrone, S. (2007). Autogenous bone graft alone or associated with titanium mesh for vertical alveolar ridge augmentation: a controlled clinical trial. *Clin. Oral Implants Res.* 18: 286–294.

Rominger, J.W. and Triplett, R.G. (1994). The use of guided tissue regeneration to improve implant osseointegration. *J. Oral Maxillofac. Surg.* 52: 106–112.

Roos, J., Sennerby, L., Lekholm, U. et al. (1997). A qualitative and quantitative method for evaluating implant success: a 5-year retrospective analysis of the Brånemark implant. *Int. J. Oral Maxillofac. Implants* 12 (4): 504–514.

Roos-Jansaker, A.M., Renvert, H., Lindahl, C., and Renvert, S. (2007). Surgical treatment of peri-implantitis using a bone substitute with or without a resorbable membrane: a prospective cohort study. *J. Clin. Periodontol.* 34 (7): 625–632.

Sabes, W.R., Green, S., and Craine, C. (1970). Value of medical diagnostic screening tests for dental patients. *J. Am. Dent. Assoc.* 80: 133–136.

Sacco, A.G. and Chepeha, D.B. (2007). Current status of transport-disc-distraction osteogenesis for mandibular reconstruction. *Lancet Oncol.* 8: 323–330.

Sadig, W. and Almas, K. (2004). Risk factors and management of dehiscent wounds in implant dentistry. *Implant. Dent.* 13: 140–147.

Salyer, K.E., Gendler, E., Menendez, J.L. et al. (1992). Demineralized perforated bone implants in craniofacial surgery. *J. Craniofac Surg.* 3: 55–62.

Sampson, H.W., Perks, N., Champney, T.H. et al. (1996). Alcohol consumption inhibits bone growth and development in young actively growing rats. *Alcohol. Clin. Exp. Res.* 20: 1375–1384.

Sandberg, O. and Aspenberg, P. (2016). Inter-trabecular bone formation: a specific mechanism for healing of cancellous bone. *Acta Orthop.* 87 (5): 459–465.

Sanz, M., Cecchinato, D., Ferrus, J. et al. (2010). A prospective, randomized-controlled clinical trial to evaluate bone preservation using implants with different geometry placed into extraction sockets in the maxilla. *Clin. Oral Implants Res.* 21 (1): 13–21.

Schepers, E., De Clercq, M., and Ducheyn, P. (1991). Bioactive glass particulate material as a filler for bone lesions. *J. Oral Rehabil.* 18: 439–452.

Schropp, L., Wenzel, A., Kostopoulos, L. et al. (2003). Bone healing and soft tissue contour changes following single-tooth extraction: a clinical and radiographic 12-month prospective study. *Int. J. Periodontics Restorative Dent.* 23: 313–323.

Schwartz, Z., Mellonig, J.T., Carnes, D.L. Jr. et al. (1996). Ability of commercial demineralized freeze-dried bone allograft to induce new bone formation. *J. Periodontol.* 67: 918–926.

Sheikh, Z., Sima, C., and Glogauer, M. (2015a). Bone replacement materials and techniques used for achieving vertical alveolar bone augmentation. *Materials (Basel)* 8 (6): 2953–2993.

Sheikh, Z., Najeeb, S., Khurshid, Z. et al. (2015b). Biodegradable materials for bone repair and tissue engineering applications. *Materials (Basel)* 8: 5744–5794.

Shelton, D.W. (1991). Basic surgical principles for implantology. In: *Endosteal Dental Implants* (ed. R.V. McKinney Jr.), 75–87. St. Louis: Mosby-Yearbook.

Shetty, V. and Han, T.J. (1991). Alloplastic materials in reconstructive periodontal surgery. *Dent Clin North Am.* 35 (3): 521–530.

Singh, R., Singh, D., and Singh, A. (2016). Radiation sterilization of tissue allografts: a review. *World J. Radiol.* 8 (4): 355–369.

Smiler, D.G. (1987). Evaluation and treatment planning. *J. Calif. Dent. Assoc.* 15 (10): 35–41.

Smith, R.A., Silverman, S. Jr., and Auclert, O. (1989). Recognition of malignancy and dysplasia in the dental implant patient. *J. Oral Implantol.* 15 (4): 255–258.

Smith, R.A., Berger, R., and Dodson, T.B. (1992). Risk factors associated with dental implants in healthy and medically compromised patients. *Int. J. Oral Maxillofac. Implants.* 7: 367–372.

Smith, C., Young, I., and Kearney, J. (1996). Mechanical properties of tendons: changes with sterilization and preservation. *J. Biomech. Eng.* 118: 56–61. doi: 10.1115/1.2795946.

Stanley, H.R., Hall, M.B., Clark, A.E. et al. (1997). Using 45S5 bioglass cones as endosseous ridge maintenance implants to prevent alveolar ridge resorption: a 5-year evaluation. *Int. J. Oral Maxillofac. Implants* 12 (1): 95–105.

Steiner, M. and Ramp, W.K. (1988). Short-term storage of freshly harvested bone. *J. Oral Maxillofac. Surg.* 46 (10): 868–871.

Sussman, H.I. (1998). Tooth devitalization via implant placement: a case report. *Periodontal Clin. Investig.* 20 (1): 22–24.

Schwartz-Arad, D., Levin, L., and Sigal, L. (2005). Surgical success of intraoral autogenous block onlay bone grafting for alveolar ridge augmentation. *Implant Dent.* 14 (2): 131–138.

Tal, H., Moses, O., Zohar, R. et al. (2002). Root coverage of advanced gingival recession: a comparative study between acellular dermal matrix allograft and subepithelial connective tissue grafts. *J. Periodontol.* 73: 1405–1411.

Tallentire, A. IAEA. 1990. Guidelines for industrial radiation sterilization of disposable medical products. IAEA-TECDOC-539. International Atomic Energy Agency, Vienna, Austria 1990

Tallgren, A. (2003). The continuing reduction of the residual alveolar ridges in complete denture wearers: a mixed-longitudinal study covering 25 years. 1972. *J. Prosthet. Dent.* 89: 427–435.

Talwar, B.S. (2012). A focus on soft tissue in dental implantology. *J. Indian Prosthodont. Soc.* 12 (3): 137–142.

Tammisalo, T., Happonen, R.P., and Tammisalo, E.H. (1992). Stereographic assessment of mandibular canal in relation to the roots of impacted lower third molar using multiprojection narrow beam radiography. *Int. J. Oral Maxillofac. Surg.* 21 (2): 85–89.

Tevlin, R., McArdle, A., Atashroo, D. et al. (2014). Biomaterials for craniofacial bone engineering. *J. Dent. Res.* 93: 1187–1195.

Tolman, D.E. (1993). Advanced residual ridge resorption: surgical management. *Int. J. Prosthodont.* 6: 118–125.

Tolman, D.E. (1995). Reconstructive procedures with endosseous implants in grafted bone: a review of the literature. *Int. J. Oral Maxillofac. Implants* 10: 275–294.

Tomford, W.W., Doppelt, S.H., Mankin, H.J., and Friedlaender, G.E. (1983). Bone bank procedures. Bone and tissue allograft use by orthopaedic surgeons. *Clin. Orthop. Relat. Res.* (174): 15–21.

Tonetti, M.S. and Schmid, J. (1994). Pathogenesis of implant failures. *Periodontol. 2000* 4: 127–138.

Trowbridge, H.D. and Emling, R.C. (1997). *Inflammation: A Review of the Process*, 5e, 149–167. Quintessence Publishing Co., Inc.

van den Bergh, J.P., ten Bruggenkate, C.M., Krekeler, G., and Tuinzing, D.B. (2000). Maxillary sinusfloor elevation and grafting with human demineralized freeze dried bone. *Clin. Oral Implants Res.* 11 (5): 487–493.

Van der Weijden, F., Dell'Acqua, F., and Slot, D.E. (2009). Alveolar bone dimensional changes of post-extraction sockets in humans: a systematic review. *J. Clin. Periodontol.* 36: 1048–1058.

Van Winkle, W. Jr. and Hastings, J.C. (1972). Considerations in the choice of suture material for various tissues. *Surg. Gynecol. Obstet.* 135 (1): 113–126.

Von Arx, T. and Buser, D. (2006). Horizontal ridge augmentation using autogenous block grafts and the guided bone regeneration technique with collagen membranes: a clinical study with 42 patients. *Clin. Oral Implants Res.* 17: 359–366.

Von Arx, T., Hardt, N., and Wallkamm, B. (1996). The time technique: a new method for localized alveolar ridge augmentation prior to placement of dental implants. *Int. J. Oral Maxillofac. Implants* 11: 387–394.

Von Arx, T. and Kurt, B. (1999). Implant placement and simultaneous ridge augmentation using autogenous bone and a micro titanium mesh: a prospective clinical study with 20 implants. *Clin. Oral Implants Res.* 10 (1): 24–33.

Wainwright, D., Madden, M., Luterman, A. et al. (1996). Clinical evaluation of an acellular allograft dermal matrix in full-thickness burns. *J. Burn Care Rehabil.* 17: 124–136.

Wakley, G.K. and Baylink, D.J. (1988). Systemic influences on the bone response to dental & orthopedic implant. *J. Oral Implantol.* 14: 285–311.

Walton, J.N. (2000). Altered sensation associated with implants in the anterior mandible: a prospective study. *J. Prosthet. Dent.* 83 (4): 443–449.

Wang, J.H., Waite, D.E., and Steinhauser, E. (1976). Ridge augmentation: an evaluation and follow-up report. *J. Oral Surg.* 34 (7): 600–602.

Ward, B.B., Terrell, J.E., and Collins, J.K. (2008). Methicillin-resistant *Staphylococcus aureus* sinusitis associated with sinus lift bone grafting and dental implants: a case report. *J. Oral Maxillofac. Surg.* 66 (2): 231–234.

Whetzel, T.P. and Sanders, C.J. (1997). Arterial anatomy of the oral cavity: an analysis of vascular territories. *Plast. Reconstr. Surg.* 100: 582–587.

Wilson, T.G. Jr. (1993). The current status of determining periodontal prognosis. *Curr. Opin. Periodontol.* 1993: 67–70. Review.

Young, M.P., Korachi, M., Carter, D.H. et al. (2002a). The effects of an immediately pre-surgical chlorhexidine oral rinse on the bacterial contaminants of bone debris collected during dental implant surgery. *Clin. Oral Implants Res.* 13: 20–29.

Young, M.P., Worthington, H.V., Lloyd, R.E. et al. (2002b). Bone collected during dental implant surgery: a clinical and histological study. *Clin. Oral Implants Res.* 13: 298–303.

Zarb, G.A. and Schmitt, A. (1990). The longitudinal clinical effectiveness of osseointegrated dental implants: the Toronto Study. Part II: The prosthetic results. *J. Prosthet. Dent.* 64 (1): 53–61.

Zijderveld, S.A., van den Bergh, J.P., Schulten, E.A., and ten Bruggenkate, C.M. (2008). Anatomical and surgical findings and complications in 100 consecutive maxillary sinus floor elevation procedures. *J. Oral Maxillofac. Surg.* 66 (7): 1426–1438.

Zitzmann, N.U. and Berglundh, T. (2008). Definition and prevalence of peri-implant diseases. *J. Clin. Periodontol.* 35 (8 Suppl): 286–291.

Index

Page locators in **bold** indicate tables. Page locators in *italics* indicate figures. The index uses letter-by-letter alphabetization.

Advances in Esthetic Implant Dentistry, First Edition. Abdelsalam Elaskary.

Companion website: www.wiley.com/go/elaskary/esthetic

e

f

g

s

t